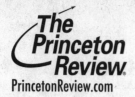

The Princeton Review®
PrincetonReview.com

THE BEST 167
MEDICAL
SCHOOLS

Malaika Stoll
and the Staff of The Princeton Review
2015 EDITION

PENGUIN RANDOM HOUSE

TPR Education IP Holdings, LLC
111 Speen Street, Suite 550
Framingham, MA 01701
E-mail: editorialsupport@review.com

A Penguin Random House Company

ISBN: 978-0-8041-2545-1
ISSN: 1943-1058

Printed in the United States of America on partially recycled paper.

Senior VP, Publisher: Robert Franek
Production: Best Content Solutions, LLC
Production Editor: Melissa Duclos-Yourdon
Editor: Kristen O'Toole
Account Manager: David Soto

9 8 7 6 5 4 3 2 1

Editorial
Robert Franek, Senior VP
Casey Cornelius, VP Content Development
Mary Beth Garrick, Director of Production
Selena Coppock, Managing Editor
Calvin Cato, Editor
Meave Shelton, Editor
Kristen O'Toole, Editorial Director
David Soto, Director of Content Development
Colleen Day, Editor
Aaron Riccio, Editor

Random House Publishing Team
Tom Russell, Publisher
Alison Stoltzfus, Publishing Manager
Ellen L. Reed, Production Manager
Dawn Ryan, Managing Editor
Kristin Lindner, Production Supervisor
Andrea Lau, Designer

Acknowledgments

Special thanks must go to the hundreds of med students and scores of admissions officers who have supplied information for this book over the years. This year's edition owes a great debt to the efforts of many: to Kristen O'Toole and Scott Harris for their editorial and design talents; to David Soto for heading the data collection efforts to Stephen Koch for managing communications with medical schools; and to Robert Franek, Publisher, for his enthusiasm and support.

Contents

Preface

For more than 25 years The Princeton Review has offered preparatory courses and tutoring for standardized tests such as the SAT, MCAT, LSAT, GRE, GMAT, and USMLE. More than 100,000 students took our courses last year, and hundreds of thousands have bought our *Cracking* series test-prep books. At the center of our approach is the desire to help students conquer the anxiety and sense of helplessness that have surrounded these entrance exams for so many years. The Princeton Review has long been an advocate of students' right to be informed consumers, and it works to make sure that information on these tests is readily accessible to all.

In addition to being consumers of entrance exams, students are also consumers of education. Before investing in a graduate degree, they have the right and the need to gather as much information as possible. We hope that this publication will provide students with a viable means of achieving this goal. The *Best 167 Medical Schools* contains the essentials students will need to answer basic and advanced questions regarding their lists of prospective medical schools. The 2015 edition contains 127 accredited allopathic schools in the United States, including Puerto Rico, 14 accredited allopathic schools in Canada, 1 school in the Caribbean which has the equivalent of allopathic accreditation, 20 accredited osteopathic schools, and a section profiling 5 accredited naturopathic schools in the United States and Canada.

When viewing individual schools listed in this year's guide, you will find the union of painstakingly researched school profiles coupled with school-specific statistical data. Each profile has been sent to the medical school for review prior to publication so that we may provide our readers with the most accurate and current information about the programs. The data presented was the most up-to-date available at the time of publication; students should consult the schools' websites for further information.

We hope this book will serve as an important guide as you research, gather, and consider information before embarking on your medical career, and we wish you the best of luck as you pursue your career in medicine. If you have questions, comments, or suggestions, we welcome them. Please give us your insights:

The Princeton Review
Best 167 Medical Schools
editorialsupport@review.com

We appreciate your input and want to make our books as useful to you as they can be.

Sincerely,
Kristen O'Toole
Editor
The Princeton Review Books

1 How to Use This Book

Although some people describe medical school education as somewhat canned— downplaying the differences between schools—differences do exist. Some differences, like the fact that a family medicine clerkship lasts two weeks at one school and eight at another, might not seem like a big deal, but such details may help convey a school's priorities. The school profile section of this guide will help you to discern such differences, and in doing so, match your interests with the school that can best fulfill them. But don't just use this book to decide where to apply; use it also as a resource to help you decide when to apply—or if you really want to apply at all. The detailed information about course offerings and facilities will help you prepare for interviews. Examine the profiles for descriptions of each program's fundamental academic approach and resources, the student body, and the school's emphasis as evidenced by the path its graduates take. These are all good points to bring up in an interview and will aid your decision of where to attend.

As you review the school profiles, keep the following in mind:

- Just as admissions offices rely too heavily on quantitative measures to evaluate candidates (MCAT and GPAs), applicants probably rely too much on school ranking in deciding where to apply and where to go to school. Often, the criteria for determining a school's ranking have little to do with how well a school will train you or how enjoyable your experience will be. Thus, you will find no quantitative rankings in this book.

- Our goal is to present accurate and complete descriptions of medical schools. Note that the admissions offices of each medical school had the opportunity to read and edit our write-ups. The data presented in this book was the most up-to-date at the time of publication. In deciding where to apply or where to go, you should consult the schools' websites in addition to using this book as part of your research. Take every opportunity to meet with medical students at the schools in which you are interested. Speak with more than just one student—and with students in different years—at each school.

- In response to managed care and other trends, many medical schools that traditionally focused on research or specialty medicine now claim to focus on primary care. Whether a school really has changed its focus may be partially gleaned from the percentage of graduates entering primary care fields. Note, however, that definitions of primary care vary (some include ob/gyn for example).

- In the Graduates section (under Students), a statistic on what percent of students match within their top one, two, or three residency preferences may appear. Less prestigious schools often have impressive rates. This is due in part because students only rank schools that they have a good chance of getting into (and at which they obtained an invitation to interview). In addition, students at less prestigious schools are less likely to enter highly specialized residency positions that are typically the most competitive. Please note that this stat is often misleading.

- For most schools, we list website addresses—they are often helpful and some include candid student opinions. Try to visit these websites before you make a commitment to apply, to interview, or to attend.

HOW THIS BOOK IS ORGANIZED

The 2015 edition of this book includes 141 U.S. and Canadian accredited allopathic medical schools. You may notice that we no longer list Puerto Rican schools separately from U.S. schools. The AAMC lists them under one umbrella, and so do we. The profile of each school is broken down into five text sections—Overview, Academics, Students, and Admissions. Three categories of hard stats supplement the general data in the allopathic profiles—Student Body, Admissions, and Cost and Aid—listed in the shaded sidebar column. We also created supplementary chapters of lists—including a general overview and admissions requirements—of the 20 accredited osteopathic schools, and of the 5 accredited naturopathic schools.

Here's what you will find in the various text and statistic sections for each school profile.

PROFILE

ACADEMICS

First, we give you a basic look at the academic program—quarter system or semester, pass/fail or honor, and USMLE requirements. Then we break it down in accordance with how your own studies will be broken down—Basic Sciences and Clinical Training—outlining the academic requirements and path of each. Here you will find out how much time you have to spend hunched over a book versus the fun part—hunched over, say, a cadaver. We will often use the term *selective* to describe certain clinical requirements. It means that students have some choice within a specified area: Selective courses are less "free" than an *elective* (which might also have some restrictions).

STUDENTS/CAMPUS LIFE

Discover where your potential classmates call home and who they are—percentage-wise. In the Student Life section, we describe what kind of recreation facilities are available, where you might live, where you might go out. We also include information about the graduates. Who are the grads of this school—primary care physicians, surgeons, public health administrators—and in what type of community do they choose to practice?

ADMISSIONS

The Requirements section details what the school is looking for in its prospective students. Pay special attention to the Suggestions section for some hints about how to impress the school. Then whip out your calendar—the Process section will tell you the dates you need to know and key stats about who gets interviews (and then who the lucky recipients of the fat envelopes are).

SIDEBAR

The shaded column next to each school listing contains the following information:

STUDENT BODY

Type: Is the school private or public? This is important information that is closely tied to the cost of tuition. In addition, public schools are often open only to state residents.

Enrollment: Total number of students enrolled in the medical school.

% male/female: Gender breakdown based on total enrollment.

% underrepresented minorities: Percentage of African Americans, Native Americans, Mexican Americans, and mainland Puerto Ricans in the total enrollment.

 # applied: The number of people who applied to the school in the most recently reported year, presented as the total number, and the number of out-of-state/province residents who applied.

 # accepted: The number of applicants who were accepted at the school in the most recently reported year. Also broken down in terms of total and out-of-state/province.

 # enrolled (out-of-state): The number of out-of-state applicants who were accepted who actually entered the school as first-year medical students in the most recently reported entering class.

Average age: The average age of the entering class.

FACULTY

Total faculty: The number of faculty employed by the medical school.

% female: Percentage of female faculty members.

% minority: Percentage of underrepresented minorities present on the faculty.

% part-time: Percentage of part-time faculty members.

Student-faculty ratio: The ratio of faculty members to enrolled students.

ADMISSIONS
Overall GPA
Average undergraduate grade point average of the students who matriculated in the most recently reported entering class.

MCAT
Average MCAT scores of the students who matriculated in the most recently reported entering class, broken down into the following areas: Biology, Physics, Verbal, and Essay.

Application Information
Outlines all the dates and facts you need to know:

Regular application: The latest date the school will accept all application materials for regular admission.

Regular notification: The latest date the school will notify prospective students of its decisions concerning regular admission.

Early application: The latest date the school will accept all application materials for the early decision plan.

Early notification: The latest date the school will notify prospective students of its decisions concerning admission to the early decision plan.

Are transfers accepted? Yes or No.

Admissions may be deferred? Yes or No.

Interview required? Yes or No.

Application fee: How much does it cost to apply?

Admissions requirements (required): Required qualifications in order for an applicant to be considered for admission into the school's program.

Admissions requirements (optional): Additional suggested qualifications for applicants—not required for admission.

Overlap schools: The other schools to which applicants are most likely to apply.

COSTS AND AID
Tuition & Fees
Most recent yearly tuition figures available for state residents and nonresidents. The amount of money students can expect to spend on books and fees is listed here as well.

Financial Aid
% students receiving aid: Percentage of medical students at the school receiving some sort of financial aid.

Average grant: The amount of money in grants students receive on average.

Average loan: The amount of money students borrow on average.

Average debt: How much do students owe when they get out?

2 So You Want to Be a Doctor . . .

A GLIMPSE AT MEDICINE IN THE TWENTY-FIRST CENTURY

Do you want to be a doctor? If your answer is yes, use this chapter to prepare yourself for what lies ahead. (This chapter can also prepare you for medical school interviews— you can impress interviewers with your knowledge of current trends in health care!) If you're not yet sure whether medicine is the career for you, this chapter will help you decide. Learn about current issues as well as potential future trends in health care, medicine, and physician practice. The purpose of this chapter is to provide a glimpse of what life will be like for you as a doctor. Although it is impossible to predict the future, research and analysis have allowed us to identify some of the issues that will shape medicine in the coming years.

DECISIONS, DECISIONS . . .

Becoming a doctor requires a real commitment, so your decision to pursue this career path should be an informed one. You should consider information from discussions with medical professionals as well as from books such as this one. Talk to as many doctors as you can. Find out how they spend their days and what they love and don't love about their professions. Think about whether you could fill their shoes and whether you would thrive in doing so. Always consider your source when gathering information. For example, television shows with exciting plots and attractive actors glamorize medicine, whereas newspapers sometimes do the opposite by highlighting negative trends and emphasizing scandals.

While you are fortunate to have hundreds of career options to choose from, having so many choices can be confusing and overwhelming. Don't let indecision paralyze you. Consider taking time off after college to work in medical or nonmedical fields, to travel, or to volunteer before applying to medical school. This type of experience serves the dual purpose of allowing you to assess your interest in medicine and giving you something to write about in your medical school application essays (not to mention that it can be fun and meaningful, depending on what you do). The chapter in this book on nontraditional medical school applicants discusses several alternative paths to medical school. In deciding whether medicine is the career for you, you should also reflect on the paths that you won't be taking. Are you deciding between being a teacher or a doctor? Why not teach for a year or two and then reconsider medical school? The skills you learn teaching will help you explain medical issues to patients if you decide to become a physician.

Perhaps you feel that there are too few rather than too many career possibilities from which to choose. Some people consider medicine, law, and other obvious professions because they just don't know what else is out there. In this situation, there is nothing like spending a couple of years in the real world. This will expose you to various professions and career options. Even working for a temp agency can be beneficial; it can provide exposure to a number of fields and organizations. Learning about other options might confirm your interest in medicine or could lead you in another direction. Either way, it will be a valuable use of your time.

WHAT IT TAKES TO BE A DOCTOR

In some ways, being a doctor in the United States in the twenty-first century is similar to being a doctor in any number of cultures during just about any time period. There are a few traits that are essential, no matter where you are or what century you're in. Consider the following questions:

Do you want to spend your life helping others?
Doctors heal people, save lives, and help others—often through direct, face-to-face interactions. If this is your motivation, you're in good company. However, there are other altruistic careers out there, all of which involve less schooling and less debt than medical school. The desire to help others should be one, but not your only, reason for becoming a doctor.

Do you enjoy working hard?
Medicine is an incredibly challenging field. This was the case a hundred years ago when doctors worked to fight yellow fever, polio, and influenza, and it is the case today as health professionals try to prevent and treat heart disease, cancer, AIDS/HIV, and influenza, while dealing with the constraints of managed care. Consider medicine only if you love challenges and you know you want tremendous challenge in your professional life. As you read through this chapter, think about whether the challenges involved in practicing medicine are the ones that appeal to you. For example, a physician who is 20 years out of medical school is still expected to be familiar with the latest medical developments. One of the challenges of practicing medicine is a commitment to lifelong learning.

Are you interested in science and health issues?
If you enjoyed some aspects of your science courses (few people enjoy all aspects of pre-medical course work) and you find yourself drawn to health issues, there is a good

chance that you will enjoy studying and practicing medicine. Although medicine has changed significantly over the years, its roots remain in basic science.

Do you like working with different people?

With the exception of a few fields, medicine involves working with people, many of whom may be very different from you. If science interests you but working with people does not, you may wish to consider a PhD rather than an MD (this choice also involves less debt). You might also look into an MD that allows you to do only research.

WHAT IT'S LIKE TO BE A DOCTOR

What is life like as a doctor in the twenty-first century? Although it varies a great deal depending on specialty, geographic region, employment situation, and so on, we can get a general idea by examining recent data.

PATIENT CARE

Most doctors—90 percent—spend their time seeing patients; in fact, they see 20 to 25 patients per day on average. Doctors generally work in one of three situations: solo, as part of a group practice, or as an employee of a hospital or organization. The most common reason people go to the doctor is for some sort of checkup or test. Other common reasons for doctor visits are respiratory (allergies, the flu), gastrointestinal (heart burn, nausea), and psychological (e.g., depression) complaints. An important responsibility of the primary care physician is to identify potentially serious issues during routine examinations. On the other side of the spectrum, a major challenge for doctors with highly specialized training (e.g., oncologists, cardiologists, and surgeons) is to work intensely to save and improve lives. The most common causes of mortality (death) in the United States are listed below.

Top 10 Causes of Mortality in the United States[1]

1. Heart disease

2. Cancer

3. Chronic lower respiratory diseases (e.g., emphysema, asthma, bronchitis).

3. Stroke

5. Accidents

6. Alzheimer's disease

---

[1] National Center for Health Statistics. Leading Causes of Death. www.cdc.gov/nchs/lcod.htm. Accessed June 24, 2013.

7. Diabetes mellitus (diabetes type 2)

8. Influenza and pneumonia

9. Nephritis, nephrotic syndrome, and nephrosis (kidney disease)

10. Intentional self-harm (suicide)

Note that all of the above except Alzheimer's and accidents are preventable. Preventive medicine and the interdisciplinary approach are important elements of practicing medicine.

WORKLOAD AND COMPENSATION

On average, doctors work 60 hours per week. Obstetricians work longer hours, 62 per week, while the typical psychiatrist works shorter hours, 49 per week. Although their annual incomes have decreased over the past few years, physicians are still among the highest paid professionals in the country. The following table presents median annual income for nine areas of practice. Incomes listed are after expenses (such as staff and malpractice insurance) but before taxes.[2]

Medical Field	Annual Income
Anesthesiology	$337,000
General/Family Practice	$175,000
Internal Medecine	$185,000
Ob/Gyn	$242,000
Pathology	$247,000
Pediatrics	$173,000
Psychiatry	$186,000
Radiation Therapy	$349,000
Surgery	$279,000

The figures listed above do not account for residents, who are notoriously underpaid. The national median salary for a resident is about $35,000. In the interest of patient safety, there have been some efforts—at the state and hospital level, and among residents themselves—to limit the number of hours that residents work each week. These efforts have been somewhat successful. However, despite the rules limiting the workweek to 80 hours, many residents continue to work more than 100 hours per week. Why are residents required to work so hard? In part, it's because hospitals depend on residents as a cheap source of labor, since they are paid much less than other physicians and somewhat less than nurses and other health professionals.

[2] Source: Medscape Physician Compensation Report 2013. www.medscape.com/features/slideshow/compensation/2013/public. Accessed June 24, 2013.

PRESTIGE

Almost universally, being a doctor carries prestige. Doctors are generally thought to be smart, well educated, hardworking, caring, and dedicated. Even in this era of managed care and malpractice lawsuits, doctors are well respected. In a recent Harris poll, Americans ranked "doctor" as one at the most prestigious professions/occupations.[3] You should consider the degree to which having a prestigious career is important to you. Other health professions, although perhaps less glamorous, also involve healing and helping others.

TRENDS IN MEDICINE IN THE TWENTY-FIRST CENTURY

Several trends in medicine that began during the past few decades are likely to continue well into the twenty-first century. These trends have implications for you, the aspiring doctor. They will impact the nature of your work, the structure of the organization in which you work, your salary, the relationship you have with patients, and above all, the quality of the health care you deliver.

In the sections that follow, we consider some important trends affecting medicine in the twenty-first century.

Trends in Medicine in the Twenty-First Century

1. Development of new technology.

2. Increased health care costs.

3. Evolution of health care delivery and payment systems.

4. Greater reliance on primary and preventive care.

5. More guidelines for patient care.

6. A possible surplus of physicians, at least in certain specialty areas.

7. Improved gender and ethnic diversity among physicians.

8. An aging patient population.

9. The emergence of new ethical issues.

10. Changes in academic medicine and medical education.

Note that the above list is by no means complete. Also, the trends listed are inter-related and are not necessarily in order of importance.

[3] The Harris Poll #86. "Firefighters, Scientists and Doctors Top List as 'Most Prestigious Occupations.'" August 4, 2009. www.harrisinteractive.com/vault/Harris-Interactive-Poll-Research-Pres-Occupations-2009-08.pdf. Accessed June 24, 2013.

NEW TECHNOLOGY

Medicine and health care has improved during the past few decades largely because of technological advancement; there are probably even more exciting developments on the horizon. The term *technology* is often used broadly. In the health care arena, it means the development of new drugs, procedures, techniques, and means of communication that, if used correctly, have the potential to improve diagnosis, care, and patient outcomes.

- **Medications and Procedures.** The increase in life expectancy over the past few decades is partially due to improvements in medications and procedures. For example, the death rate due to heart disease is declining because of better drugs (hypertension, heart, and cholesterol medications) and surgical techniques.

- **Laboratory Techniques.** Often, improvements in laboratory tools or techniques lead to important discoveries. For example, better tools allowed the human genome to be mapped.

- **The Internet.** Patients who are Internet users arrive at their doctor's office well informed about their illnesses. On the other hand, the Internet houses a great deal of misinformation. The physician who is Web savvy can guide patients to informative websites and web-based support groups. The Internet is an invaluable tool for research.

- **Telemedicine.** Telemedicine is defined by the American Telemedicine Association as *"the use of medical information exchanged from one site to another via electronic communication for the health and education of the patient or health care provider and for the purpose of improving care."* Sharing of radiographic images and patient information (X rays, MRIs) via computer between physicians is an important current application. In the future, we may see telemedicine bring the expertise of specialists to rural or other remote areas.

- **Other Computer Applications.** Computerized database systems are used for billing and patient records. Some physicians take advantage of software programs made for handheld devices. These can be used for note-taking, reference, or even patient management. Not surprisingly, it is often the younger doctors (and medical students) who are the most comfortable with computer technology. Interest in and understanding of relevant computer applications can give you an advantage when it comes to working with older, more experienced doctors; instead of just learning from them, you will have something to contribute. The key is being able to explain, teach, and pass on your knowledge effectively.

HEALTH CARE COSTS

The United States spends more money per capita on health care than any other country in the world. Some believe that the United States offers the best medical care in the world, thereby justifying the high cost. Others note that, according to indicators such as life expectancy and infant mortality, the United States lags behind other industrialized countries. In 1960, 6 percent of the United States Gross Domestic Product (the sum total of all expenditures, by all people, in a given country) went to health care. In 2011, that figure climbed to 17.9 percent, meaning that nearly a fifth of the GDP went to health-related goods and services.[4] There are many theories as to what has caused this escalation, two of which are discussed below.

Technology

As discussed above, technological advances usually serve to improve health care and health outcomes. However, technology is often cited as a major cause of rising health care costs. When new tools are developed and advertised, hospitals and physicians may feel pressure to purchase and use them, even if the benefit of the new device is still questionable. Someone ultimately pays for such purchases, and thus we see rising health care costs. The MRI—an imaging device that, for about $2,000, provides pictures of a patient's organs—is often thought to be overused in this country. For example, there are more MRI machines in Orange County, California, than in all of Canada.[5] It is important to remember, however, that technological advances can also serve to reduce costs. By preventing illness and reducing the spread of disease, new vaccines (anti-influenza, for example) lower the cost of treatment for society overall. New surgical instruments and the development of medication in pill form facilitate the use of out-patient procedures instead of expensive hospital stays.

Incentives

Patients are generally far removed from the cost of their care and, therefore, have little incentive to keep costs down. Employers and the government—not patients themselves—foot most of the bill for health care, creating a system of "third-party payers."[6] Some believe that since patients don't pay much for their own health care, they overuse it, thereby driving government and employer health care expenditures up.

As a physician, you will undoubtedly feel pressure to keep health care costs down. In many practice settings, doctors are scrutinized on the basis of the cost of the tests and treatments they prescribe. For example, primary care doctors are sometimes encouraged to limit referrals to specialists. All doctors may be monitored for overuse of expensive tests and equipment. Physicians face difficult decisions as they attempt to provide excellent care at a lower cost: if a patient has a slim chance of benefiting from

[4] World Bank. data.worldbank.org/indicator/SH.XPD.TOTL.ZS. Accessed June 24, 2013.

[5] "By the Numbers: Health Care Costs." *Scientific American*. April 1999.

[6] The United States relies largely upon an employer-based health care financing system, which means that most people (60 percent) receive health benefits through their work. In other words, employers pay for employees' health care—typically by taking responsibility for paying monthly premiums. Twenty percent of the population receives government health care benefits in the form of Medicare (everyone over 65 is eligible) or Medicaid (eligibility based on financial need).

an expensive treatment, should that treatment be employed? The physician must balance the cost of treating with the risk of not treating.

HEALTH CARE DELIVERY SYSTEMS

The push for management of health care costs has led to the growth of managed care. One of the most important trends of the past few decades has been the replacement of simple fee-for-service plans by the growth of the managed care industry.

Fee-for-Service

Before managed care, health care was delivered on a *fee-for-service* basis. Medicare (federally funded health insurance for those over 65 years of age) remains a fee-for-service program. Under a fee-for-service system, doctors and hospitals perform a service (a check-up, an operation, etc.) and charge a fee for the service. Typically, the patient's health insurance company pays the fee for whatever medical service the patient wants or needs. The patient pays the health insurance company a monthly premium or, if the patient has health benefits from his employer, the employer pays the monthly premiums. The insurance company calculates monthly premiums based on how much it pays out to hospitals and doctors each year for all people enrolled in the insurance plan.

Managed Care

Managed care was introduced as a response to rising health care costs, and has succeeded in slowing the rate at which health care costs rise. Thus, the trend toward managed care will probably continue. Although managed care is often thought to be synonymous with Health Maintenance Organizations (HMO), an HMO is, in fact, just one of many systems for managing care.[7]

Managed care usually involves set monthly premiums that are lower than those in fee-for-service plans, and this makes those paying the premiums (usually the employers) happy. How do managed care organizations keep their premiums down? By keeping their financial outlays down. Under managed care, expenditures are typically controlled through several mechanisms:

- Participants in a managed care plan agree to use doctors and hospitals that are part of the plan, and these providers are either paid yearly salaries or charge reduced fees for services rendered.
- Primary care physicians serve as "gatekeepers" in limiting the use of expensive medical specialists.
- Guidelines/regulations are implemented that attempt to limit the use of expensive tests and equipment in unnecessary situations.

[7] HMOs specify the doctors and hospitals that participants must use. Another example of a managed care organization is a Preferred Provider Organization (PPO). PPOs encourage the use of certain providers ("preferred providers") but will also cover part of the cost of doctors and hospitals outside of the preferred provider network.

- Inpatient care is reduced, and there is more emphasis on outpatient services (care that does not involve an overnight hospital stay). Associated with the movement toward outpatient care, hospitals are filling fewer of their beds and are seeing a decline in length of stay (LOS) for hospital patients.

Managed care has generated some discontent among some patients and providers in the past. Over the years the distinction between managed care and health insurance has greatly diminished because most insurance companies (and all the larger ones) now provide HMOs, PPOs, and other managed care services. For better or for worse, being a doctor in the twenty-first century is likely to involve practicing in a managed care environment of some form.

The Uninsured

This section on health care delivery and payment would be incomplete without discussing the uninsured. Approximately 15 percent of people in the United States have no health insurance. The United States is unique among industrialized nations in that respect, and it is not exactly something to be proud of. Individuals without health insurance tend to seek medical care—typically through an emergency room—only after a health problem has become really serious. This is obviously bad for the patient, who with early treatment might have avoided serious complications. It is also costly to society, because prevention and early treatment are less expensive than late intervention. Most people—physicians and nonphysicians alike—believe that everyone should have access to health care. However, there is less agreement on how universal access should be achieved and funded, as we saw with the recent health care reform legislation. The health care reform bill signed by Congress in 2010 and measures going into effect in late 2013 and early 2014 dramatically expanded access to and financial support for obtaining coverage. This suggests that the problem of uninsureds will be drastically minimized over the next 10 years. But the reform raises new questions about the scope versus efficacy of health care and how the new emphasis on achieving near-universal coverage will impact the quality and availability of care.

PRIMARY AND PREVENTIVE CARE

Most observers predict that as managed care grows, primary care physicians will continue to play a very important role, and the demand for primary care doctors will remain relatively high. Primary care physicians may be either MDs, DOs, or NDs (see page 22 for a description of each degree).

Gatekeepers

Before the days of managed care, if a person discovered an odd-looking spot on his skin, he could go directly to a dermatologist and be reimbursed by his insurance company for the visit. An important tenet of managed care has been the requirement that enrollees see a primary care physician prior to visiting a specialist. Family practice, pediatrics, internal medicine, and ob/gyn are typically considered primary care fields. The primary care physician serves as a "gatekeeper," presumably reducing unnecessary visits to expensive specialists.

Without the training of a specialist (a dermatologist in our example above), the primary care physician may not be equipped to judge the seriousness of some conditions. Missing a pre-cancerous skin lesion, for example, may cause hardship for the patient later on. On the other hand, if a primary care doctor refers *all* patients with skin lesions to the dermatologist, the system has failed because each patient required two doctor visits rather than one.

Integrated Approach

A benefit of this emphasis on primary care is that, in theory, patients develop a long-term relationship with their primary care doctor who is better able to understand the social, economic, and community-related issues associated with their health. The primary care doctor presumably has an understanding of all physiologic systems. This comprehensive knowledge facilitates diagnosis or at least allows the physician to make the initial decision about what next steps will lead to diagnosis. Primary care physicians are well-positioned to address behavioral changes, such as exercise programs, that aid in the prevention of disease.

Prevention

Several of the major causes of morbidity (illness) and mortality (death) in the United States are preventable. Emphysema, for example, is often the result of heavy smoking. The most common type of diabetes is linked with obesity. We have learned that the spread of HIV can be reduced through educational programs and behavioral interventions. The high death rate in this country due to violent crime is often attributed to the prevalence of handguns, a situation that could be addressed through legislation. Advances in genetics could potentially revolutionize preventive medicine by allowing physicians to identify people who are going to get sick before they show any symptoms of disease.

Prevention is preferable to treatment for the obvious reason that, with prevention, illness is reduced or eliminated altogether. Whether prevention efforts are cost-effective depends upon the disease, its prevalence, and the technology employed. For example, mammography is helpful in detecting breast cancer at a treatable stage and can potentially prevent mortality and reduce the high costs associated with treating end-stage cancer. It is sensible and cost-effective to offer mammograms to women above a certain age. However, it is probably unreasonable to encourage women in their 20s to have annual mammograms because breast cancer at this age is rare and, furthermore, can be difficult to spot on a mammogram from a woman of this age.

GUIDELINES FOR PATIENT CARE

Fundamental to medicine are the doctor-patient relationship, the belief that each patient must be considered individually, and the principle that doctors should be allowed to use their best judgment when providing care. Do these ideals conflict with the recent trend of using guidelines in clinical medicine?

Evidenced-Based Medicine or Cookbook Medicine?

Doctors vary tremendously in their approaches to medicine and disease treatment. This is why, in cases of serious illness, a second opinion is usually recommended. In recent years, there has been increased use of evidenced-based medicine (EBM) in clinical practice. EBM employs *scientific evidence* for the purpose of standardizing and improving patient care. Quantitative indicators such as rate of reduction of disease are typically used to evaluate procedures and treatments. The goal of EBM is to establish guidelines for clinical decision making based on the results of studies, particularly randomized clinical trials (these are generally considered the most accurate type of study).

Some doctors worry that the trend towards EBM de-emphasizes physician judgment, results in strict guidelines for treatment, and amounts to "cookbook medicine." On the other hand, EBM's supporters say that its population-based approach actually complements the one-on-one tradition of medicine by allowing doctors to defend their decisions with data. However, there are many diseases and clinical situations for which the EBM literature fails to provide clear evidence. In some cases, the risks and benefits of a particular therapy may differ depending on the study examined.

Cost Consciousness

Occasionally, guidelines that dictate clinical care are based on cost-cutting objectives rather than on sound medical evidence. Such "guidelines" may compromise patient care. Going back to our mammogram example, an HMO might encourage physicians to recommend mammograms to all women over 50, when research suggests that mammograms are highly beneficial for women in their 40s as well. It is the physician's ethical responsibility to give his patient honest and up-to-date medical advice (in this case, to recommend mammograms after age 40). At the same time, the physician may want to support the cost-cutting goals of his employer. This is the type of conflict that doctors face in the current era of cost-consciousness. There are no easy answers. However, familiarity with medical evidence and the rules of the organization will at least allow you to make informed decisions.

PHYSICIAN SURPLUS OR PHYSICIAN SHORTAGE?

From 1970 to 1990 there was a sharp increase in the number of residency positions in the U.S., largely as a result of government policy encouraging such growth. During the same period, there was a much less dramatic increase in the patient population. Some said that we were training too many doctors and that we would see a surplus. Since 1990, however, the number of residency programs has remained relatively stable, while the patient population has grown (partially as a result of an aging population). The surplus never occured; now some experts predict a shortage.

Whether we have a physician surplus, shortage, or neither, there will always be rural and inner-city areas that are in need of doctors. To combat this problem, federal and state-funded programs offer financial incentives to doctors who agree to work in under-served areas. There is also a shortage of physicians from certain ethnic backgrounds. It is important to have a physician population that represents the population that it serves. Most medical schools attempt to recruit students of ethnic backgrounds that are underrepresented in medicine.

DIVERSITY AMONG PHYSICIANS

Increased diversity among physicians is a positive trend and may result in better pa-tient care.

Women

Approximately 49 percent of entering medical students are women. This is remarkable considering that just 20 years ago, women accounted for about 30 percent of medical students, and in 1960, less than 7 percent of medical students were women. Today, about 25 percent of practicing physicians are women, and this percentage will continue to rise. There are outstanding women physicians in every imaginable medical field. However, women are especially well represented in fields like pediatrics and ob/gyn, and less represented in other fields like surgical subspecialties. Several theories and generaliza-tions have been put forth to help explain why women are attracted to some fields more than others. One such theory is that once there is a critical mass of women within a field, it becomes a more welcoming environment for other women. Also, people tend to be interested in fields that have personal relevance. Finally, many women tend to avoid fields with the very longest residencies (only 10 percent of neurosurgery residents, for example, are women).

Minorities

The medical profession is slowly becoming more ethnically diverse, as increased numbers of non-White medical school graduates enter the work force. This increase in diversity reflects the changing demographics of the U.S. population, better and more widely available educational opportunities, and active minority recruitment on the part of medical schools. If this trend continues, we will someday have a physician work force that is representative of the population at large, including African Americans, Mexican Americans, Puerto Ricans, other Hispanics, Native Americans, and other underrepresented minorities.

AGING POPULATION

In 2020, the median age in the U.S. will be 40 years, up from 36 in 2000 and 30 in 1960. As the population ages, the demand for medical care increases: The average number of doctor visits per year is three for the population at large, but is six for those over 74 years old. The aging of the American population contributes to rising health care costs. Because 99 percent of individuals over 65 are covered by Medicare, government expenditures on health care are expected to rise. The paperwork involved in treating a patient with Medicare is notoriously time consuming.

An older population will cause growth within certain fields, such as geriatrics, internal medicine, orthopedics, and cardiovascular medicine. The incidence of chronic disease, meaning disease that is long-lasting and often incurable, will increase. Thus, physicians will often be called upon to provide palliative care that addresses symptoms when the underlying disease cannot be cured. Physician-researchers will be encouraged to find treatments for conditions that afflict the elderly, such as Alzheimer's Disease.

ETHICAL ISSUES

Physicians have always dealt with important ethical issues related to life and death. As a physician in the twenty-first century, some of your ethical dilemmas are likely to involve the conflict between saving money and saving lives. Consider the following scenario:

> *You are a pediatrician, seeing a patient you have never seen before. The patient is a very ill six-year-old without health insurance. Do you treat her, knowing that you will hear about it later? Or do you send her to the free clinic across town, even though it will entail a long bus ride for the sick girl?*

Ethical issues surrounding end-of-life care will become increasingly relevant because of an older patient population. For example:

> *Your patient is 80 years old and suffers from terminal lung cancer, which has spread to his brain. There are no cures for this man at this stage, so your care has been focused on keeping him comfortable. He can't breathe on his own, is incoherent, and has been more or less motionless in the hospital for one week. His daughter does not want you to remove life support. What do you do?*

The rule of doctor-patient confidentiality can also be the basis for ethical issues. Consider this situation:

> You have been treating a young man in the hospital for a lung infection. During his hospital stay, he was tested for HIV, and the test results were positive. He is unwilling to discuss the matter, does not want medications that will help his HIV symptoms, and appears to be in denial. Do you have a responsibility to alert the man's wife?

Unfortunately, some medical schools barely address ethics, leaving you on your own to learn about and think through important ethical issues. A mentor, someone whose opinion you respect, can serve as a resource for sorting out ethical questions. If you feel strongly about a particular issue, you should consider getting involved—through writing, attending conferences, or engaging in dialogue.

CHANGES IN ACADEMIC MEDICINE AND MEDICAL EDUCATION

Most medical schools are directly affiliated with teaching hospitals. Three advantages to this arrangement are the following:

- Medical students have the opportunity for hands-on learning.
- Patients are treated by expert physicians and benefit from the latest technology.
- The academic environment coupled with the clinical facilities provide an ideal setting for research that ultimately pushes medicine forward and improves care.

Academic medical centers throughout the country are having a tough time financially, leading some experts to question their future viability. Although medical school tuition seems incredibly high, it does not cover the actual cost of medical education; academic medical centers have historically depended on income from clinical activities to subsidize medical education, research activities, and management of a teaching hospital. As discussed, the shift toward outpatient medicine has resulted in reduced earnings for hospitals. For academic medical centers, this means less revenue to cover their high costs. As more and more academic medical centers face financial crisis, there will be pressure to cut costs and/or raise revenue significantly. We might see academic medical centers restrict their patients to those who can pay higher fees, or perhaps we'll see an increase in government funding and/or medical school tuition.

In response to these changes in medicine and health care, most medical schools are attempting to revise their curricula. Some of the revisions we see are the following:

- Less time spent in lecture. Educators recognize that in this age of technology and information, there are simply too many facts to learn. Rather than inundate students with a massive amount of information, some medical schools hope to teach students general concepts that will prepare them for a lifetime of learning.

- More clinical problem solving during the first two years. With all that we know and all the treatment options available today, physicians must be thinkers and problem solvers.

- Greater emphasis on health economics, health care management, and public health. Doctors should understand the interdisciplinary nature of health care and the forces that affect medicine.

- Better training in outpatient medicine, with the use of outpatient clinics and doctors' offices for clinical rotations of outpatient facilities.

With the requirement of at least 11 years of post–high school training, becoming a physician takes longer in the United States than anywhere else in the world. This amount of required education is costly to society. Some people predict that as a result of financial pressures, the amount of schooling required to become a doctor will be reduced. For the time being, however, you have a long (but exciting) road ahead of you.

CONCLUSION: IS MEDICINE YOUR CALLING?

Whether you will be able to work effectively amidst all these changes depends in part on your flexibility. The medical field is in constant flux as technology advances forward and the government initiates new policies.

Apart from flexibility, what other traits will help you succeed and find job satisfaction as a physician in the twenty-first century?

What It Takes to Be a Doctor in the Twenty-First Century

Compassion—a critical part of healing.

Advocacy—for your patients and for those without health care.

Leadership—in improving health care at the team, hospital, and policy level.

Lifelong learning—there will always be more to know.

Interpersonal skills—communication with patients and among providers is key.

Negotiation—ability to work around bureaucratic constraints.

Grasp—of increasing amounts of medical knowledge and of a health care system in flux.

Ask yourself: Is medicine your **calling**?

3 So You Still Want to Be a Doctor . . .

Congratulations! The good news is that you are on your way to entering one of the most rewarding and respected fields, one of the few altruistic careers that pays a livable wage. The bad news is that, even armed with all the information we can give you and the help of a premed advisor, the application process is still tough. The painful reality is that there are more than 45,000 applicants for approximately 19,500 spots.[8] The good news, however, is that if you are persistent and have worked hard for the past several years to make yourself a competitive candidate, you have a good chance of obtaining a certified letter and a career that will keep you challenged and fulfilled for the rest of your life.

WHAT MAKES A COMPETITIVE APPLICANT?

Well, that's the $166,750 question (average debt of current medical school graduates). In 2012, the average matriculated (accepted) medical student had an undergraduate science GPA of 3.31, a non-science GPA of 3.75, and an overall GPA of 3.8; the average matriculated (accepted) medical student had average Medical College Admission Test Computer-Besed Test (MCAT) scores of 9.8 Verbal Reasoning, 10.5 Physical Science, 10.9 Biological Sciences, and a Q on the Writing Sample. But while GPA and MCAT scores will play a large role in the admissions decision, they aren't everything. Solid numbers are a good start, but medical schools are also quite interested in who you are, why you want to be a physician, and whether or not you have a clue about what being a doctor is like. Therefore, in addition to strong grades and scores, you will strengthen your application by having volunteer activities listed, some experience in scientific academic research, practice in leadership roles, extracurricular activities, a well-written personal statement, excellent communication skills, and solid recommendation letters. All these application pieces will provide the admissions committee with a comprehensive picture of who you are, which is more than mere numbers can convey.

Also, keep in mind that, despite the odds, there are always large numbers of normal, sane people who actually didn't get straight A's or perfect MCATs who still manage to get into medical school. You can be one of them, and this book can help you to package yourself and to target schools that are likely to appreciate your unique strengths. If

---

[8] AAMC. U.S. Medical School Applications and Matriculants by School, State of Legal Residence, and Sex, 2012. www.aamc.org/download/321442/data/2012factstable1.pdf. Accessed June 24, 2013.

you have a hunch that your set of qualifications is not what traditional medical school admissions committees are looking for, consider a few alternate career paths. This book covers allopathic (MD) programs in the United States, Puerto Rico, and Canada (many Canadian schools accept only Canadians), osteopathic (DO) programs, and includes a section on naturopathic (ND) programs. Don't rule out programs or schools in other health fields, such as dental school, nursing school, and physician assistant programs.

ALLOPATHIC MEDICINE

Allopathic schools confer the MD on their graduates, and allopathic training is by far the most widely available and recognized type of medical training. There are 150 accredited MD schools in the United States, Puerto Rico, and Canada. The Canadian and Puerto Rican medical schools in this book are part of the American Association of Medical Colleges (AAMC). Teaching methodology varies among schools. The *traditional* model consists of two years of basic science followed by clinical rotations. The *systems-based* program is organized around physiologic systems, such as the lung or kidney. The *case-based* model teaches through clinical vignettes. There are also schools offering hybrids of these approaches. Most schools have made a concerted effort to get students together with patients at a much earlier stage in their education—it used to be that medical students might not come in contact with any patients until they'd already been through two years of school. At most schools, the last two years are spent doing clinical rotations. Even if you're sure that your calling in life is plastic surgery, you're going to have to do a pediatrics rotation. Most medical students really enjoy having a chance to delve into the various specialties, and this structure provides an excellent opportunity to learn about the areas you hope to pursue.

Allopathic training will give you the option to practice in any of the medical specialties, and the MD is universally recognized worldwide as a medical degree. For an abundance of information on all aspects of allopathic training and practice, visit the AAMC website (AAMC.org).

OSTEOPATHIC MEDICINE

Osteopathic medicine in the United States got its start in the late 1800s. Its founding father was Dr. Andrew Taylor Still, who established the American School of Osteopathy in Kirksville, Missouri, in 1892. The various regulatory bodies (osteopathic versions of AAMC and the AMA) were well underway by the early 1900s, and are now the American Osteopathic Association (AOA) and the American Association of Colleges of Osteopathic Medicine (AACOM). The DO is only issued in the United States Visit the AOA's website at Do-Online.org and the AACOM's website at AACOM.org to find out more about these organizations.

Osteopathic medicine has an interesting history; until fairly recently, its focus on preventive care, communication with the patient, and a holistic approach to health was considered to be somewhat radical. Now, of course, much of what osteopathic medicine has always espoused is rapidly becoming part of all medical training. In addition to a philosophical difference in approach, an important distinction between osteopathic and allopathic training is that osteopaths are taught an additional modality of treatment called manipulation (not to be confused with chiropractic manipulation, which has an entirely different system of education and is not recognized as a fully licensed medical degree). The osteopathic philosophy posits that there is a unity between a living organism's anatomy and physiology. Osteopathic science includes "the behavioral, chemical, physical, spiritual, and biological knowledge related to the establishment and maintenance of health as well as the prevention and alleviation of disease." Osteopathic concepts emphasize the following principles[9]:

1. The human being is a dynamic unit of function.

2. The body possesses self-regulatory mechanisms that are self-healing in nature.

3. Structure and function are interrelated at all levels.

4. Rational treatment is based on these principles.

What this means to the average osteopathic student is that he or she has to learn all of the same science as his or her allopathic counterpart, plus osteopathic diagnosis and treatment, in the same amount of time. Practicing osteopaths have another way of helping their patients that allopaths do not. Osteopaths achieved full-practice rights in 1973, although some states certified osteopaths to practice in all public hospitals as complete physicians and surgeons much earlier.

As you might guess from their philosophy and training, many osteopathic doctors choose to become primary care physicians. Most work in family practice, internal medicine, pediatrics, ob/gyn, and general surgery. In the words of one osteopathic dean, they tend to be generalists first and specialists second. However, there are DOs in just about every area of modern medical practice, from neurological surgery to psychiatry, oncology, and emergency medicine. Although the DO was not traditionally considered a research degree, the DO/PhD combination is becoming more common, and the AOA is becoming much more active in encouraging research activities, particularly in primary care.

At most osteopathic schools, matriculates have undergrad GPAs of about a 3.39 and combined MCAT CBT scores of just over 26. For the class entering in fall 2012, there were 14,945 applicants for approximately 5,327 seats.[10] However, osteopathic schools do have a reputation for "looking past the numbers and place a strong emphasis on the whole picture of the candidate." This often makes osteopathic school an attractive choice for nontraditional, older students whose GPAs from their first trek through undergraduate school prove prohibitive in most allopathic programs. If you have a few

[9] *AOA Yearbook of Osteopathic Physicians.* American Osteopathic Association. Chicago: AOA, 1996. 732.
[10] "Osteopathic Medical College Applicant and Matriculant Profile." American Association of Colleges of Osteopathic Medicine. www.aacom.org/data/applicantsmatriculants/Documents/2012-Applicant-Matriculant-Report.pdf. Accessed June 24, 2013.

blemishes on your academic record but a life that suggests you'll make a dedicated physician, you should consider applying to osteopathic schools.

Most premeds trying to decide whether or not to apply to osteopathic schools worry about what will happen to them after they graduate and apply for a residency. Osteopathic graduates participate along with allopaths and foreign medical graduates (both American and nonresident) in the National Resident Matching Program (NRMP), known as "the Match." DOs can apply for either osteopathic or allopathic residencies, and for that reason, many take both the United State Medical Licensing Examination (USMLE) and the Comprehensive Osteopathic Medical Licensing Examination (COMPLEX), which is a series of exams administered by the National Board of Osteopathic Medical Examiners and is now accepted in all 50 states. The best way to decide which path is right for you is to spend time with MDs and DOs and to talk to them at length about their practices.

NATUROPATHIC PROGRAMS

Students enrolled in a school of naturopathic medicine are conferred the doctor of naturopathic medicine (ND) degree upon graduation. The program in naturopathic medicine consists of two years of classroom instruction in standard medical school sciences and two years of clinical training under the supervision of a licensed ND. Graduates of naturopathic medical school programs are licensed as primary care physicians who can use natural therapies such as nutrition, homeopathy, acupuncture, hydrotherapy, and lifestyle modification to treat disease and combine these therapies with conventional medical treatments when appropriate.

Naturopathic physicians (NDs) take a holistic approach to healing and aim to cure disease by taking advantage of the body's self-regenerative powers and harnessing the restorative power of nature. Like osteopaths, naturopathic physicians endeavor to treat the whole person by taking into account the emotional, genetic, and environmental factors that have influenced their state of health. Unlike osteopaths, however, naturopathic physicians emphasize natural remedies. NDs also differ from allopaths (MDs); rather than limiting treatment to synthetic drugs and invasive procedures, NDs predominantly utilize natural medicines and procedures. Naturopathic physicians work to identify and eliminate the *cause* of disease using six basic principles:

1. Do no harm.

2. Utilize the healing power of nature.

3. Identify and treat the causes.

4. Treat the whole person.

5. Focus on preventive medicine.

6. Practice doctor-as-teacher.

Naturopathic medicine gained major visibility in the United States in the late 1800s, when Dr. Benedict Lust opened the nation's first health food stores and helped put the spotlight on diet and nutrition as the primary means to staying healthy. Naturopathic medicine was hugely popular until WWII when rapid advancements in medicine and technology caused it to lose ground to more high-tech forms of treatment, leading to a near-monopoly in health care practices by the chemical and drug industries. Today, a new crop of scientifically focused proponents of naturopathy largely guided by the principles of EBM, have been able to prove that diet and lifestyle have a significant impact on health, placing naturopathic medicine in the spotlight once more.

Students considering a naturopathic medical program should know that the ND license to practice medicine is valid in only 15 U.S. states (including Washington, DC, Puerto Rico, the U.S. Virgin Islands), and 5 Canadian provinces, and graduates are subject to passing national licensing exams. However, legal provisions do allow for the practice of naturopathic medicine in several of the unlicensed states. (See AANMC.org for a list of states and provinces.) NDs may also practice in countries outside of the United States, based on requirements specific to each country. Each of the Association of Accredited Naturopathic Medical Colleges (AANMC) schools is accredited by the Council on Naturopathic Medical Education (CNME) and prepares graduates to sit for board examinations with the North American Board of Naturopathic Examiners (NPLEX). Naturopathic medical schools are looking for applicants who are thoroughly committed to the efficacy of natural therapies and are flexible enough to deal with the challenge of formulating personalized treatment plans. Some opportunities for specialization include dermatology and allergies, women's medicine, pediatrics, diabetes and blood pressure treatment, and cancer treatment and research, to name a few. In order to figure out whether an ND career is right for you, talk to other NDs. Compare their experiences with those of the MDs and DOs you know.

FOREIGN MEDICAL SCHOOLS

If you are seriously considering attending a foreign school but want to practice in the United States, make sure you research the prospective school's USMLE pass rate and residency placement rate. Although foreign schools are much easier to get into, they will put you in just as much debt as U.S. schools, without the same assurance of a career after graduation that will enable you to pay it off.

THE NUMBERS GAME

Because of the sheer volume of applications they have to wade through, admissions officers have to make some initial screening decisions based largely on GPA and MCAT scores—deceptively simple acronyms for the arcane processes they represent.

Your GPA, for the purposes of applying to medical school, consists of your science GPA (biology, chemistry, physics, and math), your non-science GPA (every other class you ever suffered through), and your cumulative GPA. These are calculated for your undergraduate career, any nondegree-seeking postsecondary work, and any degree-seeking postsecondary programs. In other words, you could conceivably have nine GPAs. Each medical school has its own policies for deciding which GPA means the most to them when they're choosing which applicants to interview and/or to matriculate. The average GPA of all applicants (not necessarily accepted) in 2010 was a 3.43 science, a 3.65 non-science, and a 3.53 overall. It is extremely difficult to get into medical school with a cumulative GPA of less than 3.0. Your GPA is the single most important element of your application because it is the best predictor of your academic readiness.

Although community college classes may count as part of your GPA, they may not always be acceptable as prerequisite premedical course work. If you are planning to take some of your core premed courses (biology, chemistry, physics) at a community college, it's an extremely good idea to do some advance planning and call some of the schools that you're interested in to make sure that they have no qualms about community college credit. Similarly, if you took an AP class in high school and then tested out of a core class, such as physics, you may run into trouble when you apply unless you've taken upper-division course work in that subject. Again, it is very much to your advantage to check with a few medical schools and your pre-health advisor to make sure that your academic record doesn't have any holes in it.

Your GPA and MCAT score are interrelated. The MCAT is an immensely important part of your application, but it's not as important as your GPA. As a standardized test, it provides only a snapshot of your academic readiness. Your MCAT score is made up of four separate marks: Verbal Reasoning, Physical Sciences, Biological Sciences, and the Writing sample. Verbal Reasoning and the Science sections are scored from 1 to 15. The Writing portion of the MCAT requires that you write two essays, which generate a single score. This score is reported as a letter J–T, where J is low and T is high. The average score for all applicants on each section in 2012 was 9.8 Verbal Reasoning, 9.5 Physical Sciences, 9.9 Biological Sciences, and a P on the writing sample.

The Writing sample, added to the MCAT a few years ago in an attempt to ensure the applicant's ability to communicate, is largely ignored by Admissions Committees. Virtually the only time the Writing sample is looked at very carefully is in the case of a disconnected application—a beautifully written personal statement with low Verbal scores and/or a low Writing sample score. Some schools will also consider the Writing score if they are evaluating the English ability of English as a Second Language applicants. This does not mean that you can take a nap during the Writing sample. You should make every effort to answer the questions in a coherent and focused way on the off-chance that the committee decides to closely examine your score.

THE SUM OF YOUR EXPERIENCE

Although your GPA and MCAT score play a large role in your application, Admissions Committees are also looking for several other attributes. They are quite interested in who you are, why you want to be a physician, and whether or not you have a clue about what being a doctor is really like.

EXPOSURE TO THE HEALTH CARE FIELD

Although students with no discernible exposure to health care still matriculate, the vast majority of successful premeds have some experience, usually volunteer work, in a hospital, clinic, hospice, or other health care setting. Some premeds are qualified enough to find part-time paying positions as emergency medical technicians (EMTs), nurse's aids, or organ and blood bank workers, while other nontraditional applicants may have had full-time careers in health care. Your goal should be to hold a volunteer or paid position for at least six months. Many premedical programs have specific classes you can take that include organized volunteer time as part of their course work—even if you are a returning adult student and not officially registered as premed. You can often get college credit for community-service work in the medical field. Although it may seem difficult to find the time to volunteer, it will make a huge difference as you work on your personal statement and get through your interviews. You will have stories to tell, and you will be able to speak far more effectively about why you want to become a physician.

LEADERSHIP EXPERIENCE AND COMMUNITY SERVICE

Leadership can mean many things, and being a leader, say, within your family, can be as important as being class president. One of the simpler ways to prove your abilities is to join a club or campus organization and get elected to office. You can also lead youth- or religiously affiliated organizations or participate in a variety of community-service organizations such as food banks, literacy programs, and mentor program. The key is to demonstrate sincere commitment and to have some longevity with whatever cause you decide to embrace, so that you can achieve a measure of responsibility. If you are serious about practicing primary care medicine, for example, this is your chance to build your resume and to start proving yourself. Find a clinic that needs a dedicated volunteer, and get your feet wet.

RESEARCH

Academic research is quite a bit easier to get involved with than you might think. Research labs are always looking for drones—basically undergrads—to help with the unlovely business of test-tube cleaning and organism counting. With any luck, however, you should be able to find a program in which you will actually conduct experiments and write about the results. If you are considering a career in academic medicine, you should try to get involved in research projects as early in your undergraduate career as you can convince someone to take you. One way to find out about cool research projects is to sit down with a teaching and research assistant over a cup of coffee and ask about the various projects going on in their departments. Alternatively, check out the Science Department websites at your university for information on current research.

HUMANITY

Medical schools are interested in training bright, empathetic, communicative people who have a strong interest in science and a wide-ranging intellect. They are not interested in students with perfect grades who have clearly never done anything else with their lives than try to break the curve in chemistry class. The schools want to graduate physicians who will listen to their patients and be able to effectively use the myriad tools available to heal them. What this means is that there is no magic system that will create an unbroken path into medical school. You can major in art history, modern dance, or biochemistry—it doesn't matter, as long as you take the classes you need to fulfill medical school requirements. You can take a few years off and join the Peace Corps or go straight to med school upon college graduation. Admissions committees will be trying to discern what you have learned from your experiences and how the things you have seen and done nurtured the values that have led you to pursue a medical career.

THE Z FACTOR IN MEDICAL SCHOOL ADMISSIONS

Although many medical schools will claim not to use a formula when it comes to evaluating an applicant, in actuality, almost all employ an initial screening process that weeds out applicants based on a cut-off score. While the formula used to arrive at this score varies from institution to institution, it's sure to involve the following three elements: GPA, MCAT score, and a Z *factor*. The Z factor represents the bonus points an institution will award based on an applicant's ethnicity, participation in varsity athletics, and any other extraordinary activity and/or circumstance that the applicant may have experienced. Keep in mind that each medical school has its own target score. In order to maximize your rating, focus on improving your GPA and MCAT numbers so that you don't have to rely on bonus points awarded for the Z factor to achieve the school's cut-off score.

THE APPLICATION PROCESS

There are many factors to consider when applying to medical schools. The first rule of thumb is to apply broadly and include safety schools where you will most likely be accepted. Besides the obvious clinical and scholastic goals, it is important to look for a school in a location that suits you. Although you may think that you won't see the light of day for four years, you should apply to schools that are in geographic areas that appeal to you and that will provide outlets for your hobbies and interests.

APPLYING TO ALLOPATHIC MEDICAL SCHOOLS

Most allopathic medical schools use the American Medical Colleges Application Service (AMCAS), which is a centralized and standardized application that is handled by the Association of American Medical Colleges (AAMC). In the spring of 2001, the AAMC switched to an entirely web-based AMCAS application. The online application is available directly from AAMC.org. The AMCAS application costs $160 for the first school; the fee is $32 for each additional school. If you have significant financial hardship, you can apply directly to AMCAS for a fee waiver on their services. You will also need to prepare transcript requests for every postsecondary school you ever attended, even if you only took one class there or the credits transferred elsewhere. Undergraduate colleges will send your transcripts to AMCAS, who forwards them to all medical schools to which you are applying. AMCAS begins accepting transcripts on May 5 each year and completed applications are due by August 1. It will take a couple of weeks for AAMC to process everything, at which point you'll receive a "transmittal notification." You can call and use AAMC's voice mail to check your status (you can reach AAMC on the Web at AAMC.org or by phone at 202-828-0400). At most universities and colleges, your pre-health advisor will help you navigate the AMCAS application, which can be fairly baffling. One of the toughest parts of the application is the personal comments page, where you have exactly one typewritten, single-spaced page to explain your life and to convince them that you should be one of the chosen few. Needless to say, this part of the application takes time and patience—be sure to read through the suggestions and advice for working on it that are included later in this chapter. Please note that the seven public medical schools in Texas have their own application service called TMDSAS (Texas Medical Dental Schools Application Service). In addition, one U.S. allopathic medical school—the University of North Dakota School of Medicine and Health Sciences—does not participate in any application service at all. If you're interested in attending this school, or any of the 17 accredited Canadian medical schools, you'll need to contact each school directly to obtain an application.

When you are choosing which schools to apply to, make sure you check their in-state residency requirements. Although many allopathic schools are private, there are quite a few public schools that receive free money every year from out-of-state applicants they are prohibited from accepting into their programs. It doesn't matter how qualified you are; if you aren't a state resident, you can't get in.

APPLYING TO OSTEOPATHIC SCHOOLS

Osteopathic schools use their own internal system, called AACOMAS, which in many ways works exactly the same way as AMCAS. Both paper and online applications are available from AACOM. You can request an application from their website at AACOM. org, or call 301-968-4190. Like the AMCAS application, AACOMAS takes some time to fill out, so make sure you get started early. It also includes a personal statement, but it's even shorter than AMCAS's—you have only half of a page to explain why you want to be an osteopathic physician. You will also need to get a recommendation from a DO, a fact that takes some applicants by surprise. If you are serious about osteopathic school, search for a mentor DO as early as possible. One of the nice things about AACOMAS is that all osteopathic schools use it—you don't have to worry about tracking down additional applications. Because osteopathic schools are private institutions, they don't have residency requirements (although some may have tuition breaks for residents of particular states). If you are interested in going to an osteopathic school, investigate all of your options and choose one based on your interest in the program and living conditions in the area.

APPLYING TO NATUROPATHIC SCHOOLS

The admission process varies slightly at each of the seven AANMC schools. In general, naturopathic medical schools require a bachelor's degree and a base of undergraduate science courses that include physics, biology, and general and organic chemistry for an applicant to be considered. Math and psychology courses may also be specified. Admission into most of the naturopathic medicine programs requires students to have completed three years of premedical training. The duration of an ND program is the same as that of an MD program, with residency period optional. Check with each school you are considering in order to make sure that you've met all prerequisites and that you fully understand the school's application procedures. It is worth noting that the MCAT is not required for admission to a naturopathic medical school.

WHEN TO APPLY TO MEDICAL SCHOOL

Whether you're applying to osteopathic, allopathic, or naturopathic medical schools, you need to apply as early as you can in the process. In general, premedical students begin the application process in the spring semester of their junior year, or approximately a year and a half before they want to enter medical school. The vast majority of medical schools engage in some type of rolling admissions, which means that they read and evaluate applications as the folders arrive. Admissions officers are only human. Even though they make every effort to give the same consideration to applicant number 6,005 as they give to applicant number one, the sheer volume of applications takes its toll on their patience and enthusiasm. In practical terms, this means that if you take the April MCAT and get your applications in by late June, you will have a distinct advantage over someone taking the August test. Even if you turn in your AMCAS or AACOMAS application early, many medical schools will not look closely at your application until they have a copy of your MCAT scores. Each year, students are accepted with August test scores and applications that arrived late in the process. Unfortunately, there are also large numbers of students who are not accepted but would have had a decent chance had they applied earlier. Basically, you should try for every possible advantage. Turning in your application early can certainly help to give you an edge. Also, procrastinators take note: AMCAS is serious about its deadlines. If an application or transcript is late, you'll get it back.

Nota Bene: The MCAT is changing in 2015. The natural sciences sections will be updated to cover changes in medical education; the Verbal Reasoning section will become Critical Analysis and Reasoning Skills, and a new section will cover Psychological, Social, and Biological Foundations of Behavior. Be sure to visit www.aamc.org for the most up-to-date information on upcoming test changes.

INFORMATION ABOUT THE MCAT

The MCAT is administered by the AAMC and is an admissions requirement for most allopathic and osteopathic medical school programs. More than 60,000 students take the test each year. The test is broken up into four sections: Physical Sciences, Biological Sciences, Verbal Reasoning, and a Writing sample. All of the questions (with the exception of the Writing sample) are multiple-choice.

In 2007, the AAMC adopted a CBT (computer-based test) format for the MCAT and reduced the number of questions on the test by nearly one-third. The test structure, content, and scoring system did not change.

The MCAT, has four components:

1 Scientific Reasoning: The Physical Sciences

2. Verbal Reasoning

3. Writing Sample

4. Scientific Reasoning: The Biological Sciences

The current test is structured as follows:

Test Section	Questions	Time
Tutorial (optional)		10 minutes
Physical Sciences	52	70 minutes
Break (optional)		10 minutes
Verbal Reasoning	40	60 minutes
Break (optional)		10 minutes
Void Option		5 minutes
Survey		10 minutes
Total Test Content Time		4 hours, 20 minutes

You should arrive at the test center at least one half-hour before testing begins. The entire test day is approximately five and a half hours long.

You will receive four scores, one for each component. The Verbal Reasoning component and the two Scientific Reasoning components (Biological and Physical Sciences) are scored on a scale of 1 to 15 in which 1 is low and 15 is high. The Writing sample component is scored on a scale of J to T in which J is low and T is high. With the new CBT format, scores will be released approximately 30 days after you complete the exam.

WHEN TO TAKE THE MCAT

You should try to take the MCAT on one of the April test dates, at least one year prior to the date you wish to begin medical school. Completing the exam earlier will allow you to complete your application early, and the earlier you submit your application, the better. Of course, not all applicants' academic schedules realistically allow them to take the April test. The new MCAT enables greater flexibility in scheduling by providing students with 22 test dates to choose from throughout the year. To register for the MCAT online, visit the AAMC website.

If you have not finished most of the prerequisites for the test—two semesters each of biology, physics, general chemistry, and organic chemistry—you probably should not sit for the exam. If you are determined to try the test without being fully prepared, take advantage of the fact that you can take a practice test at any Princeton Review office. It is much, much better to find out precisely what your current scoring levels are on a practice exam than to have to explain a woefully low score on a later medical school application.

It is possible, although it's certainly not the best idea, to take the last semester of one of the required science courses concurrently with studying for the MCAT. If you find yourself in this situation, it is vitally important to lighten your course load so that you will be able to adequately study for the exam while maintaining good grades in your courses. Thoroughly studying for the MCAT is not a small task.

HOW TO STUDY FOR THE MCAT

You are correct in assuming that since you're reading a book published by The Princeton Review, we're a little biased as to how we think you should study for the MCAT. The short answer here is that for most people, taking a course to prepare for the MCAT is worth the investment in both time and money. This is simply because MCAT scores are as important as your GPA in terms of admissions criteria. The MCAT is a tedious and wretched business, and having a class full of fellow sufferers at least makes you feel less alone in your pain. A class also forces you to study in a reasonable way, to cover the material effectively, and to get plenty of practice, and the class gives you the resources to fill any gaps in your academic preparation.

There are some people who do not need much preparation for the MCAT, and you'll meet them in medical school. They'll be getting honors designations in all of their classes while maintaining their world rankings as premier ice climbers / Sanskrit poets / master chefs. Unless you're pretty sure you're one of them (you might qualify if you're reading this while skydiving), you'll need some help with the test.

First, assume that you will be spending about 20 hours a week for several months studying for the MCAT. Although it doesn't test everything you've learned in school, it will feel that way. And, if you're rusty or haven't studied one of the subjects in a while—physics, general chemistry, organic chemistry, and biology—you're going to have to do some in-depth review. At the same time, you have to keep in mind that this is a standardized test, and even though it's one of the better ones available, it still suffers from the same flaws as all other standardized tests, which you can use to your advantage.

The key to doing well on the exam is to know the material and then to know the test. The MCAT consists of four timed sections administered over a period of more than five hours.

The MCAT tests basic sciences—but don't assume that the exam is a science test similar to the kind you have learned to take as an undergraduate. Fundamentally, the MCAT is a verbal test, which is why on average, humanities majors tend to get slightly better scores in all of the sections than any other major. They are seeing a test format that they are used to: passages and questions. Science majors, on the other hand, are generally used to manipulating formulas and answering questions that may have a setup but are not embedded in a long series of paragraphs.

In practice, it is much easier to raise your score if you start with low science numbers but a high verbal score. Unfortunately, most examinees are in exactly the opposite position. This is of real concern because more and more medical schools have come to regard scores that are out of balance as undesirable. They will often look more favorably on a candidate with three 10s than someone with an 8 Verbal and two 12s. In order to change your Verbal score, you will have to practice the type of causal, linear logic that it tests. AAMC releases five previous MCATs, including one that is free, and a couple of books of practice items (any formal test preparation course should give you reams of additional practice material). If you don't have access to test preparation courses, you will probably find yourself rapidly running out of verbal practice material, although most college bookstores are reasonably well stocked with practice materials relating to the science portions of the MCAT. You can use reading comprehension sections from other graduate-level standardized tests such as the GRE or LSAT to supplement your verbal study, but keep in mind that the passages in these tests were not written to be read under the same time constraints as were the MCAT passages. In addition, you may want to consider using online training materials.

MCAT SCORE REPORTING—FULL DISCLOSURE

Gone are the days when prospective med students could choose whether or not to release their MCAT scores to schools before seeing them. The MCAT is, in fact, moving toward a full disclosure policy, whereby scores from any MCAT taken in 2003 or later will automatically be reported as part of the examinee's test history. AMCAS and the medical schools to which you're applying will always receive your MCAT Testing History Report, or THx Report (previously known as the Additional Score Report). If you took the MCAT between 1991 and 2002, those scores will be released unless you request that they not be released. Still, the dates of those tests will appear on the THx Report.

Although you'll no longer have the option to withhold MCAT scores except in the case of older test dates, this isn't necessarily a bad thing. In the past, schools knew when you withheld your scores, and as you might imagine, they could interpret this in many different ways. Although some schools told us that they did not hold it against you if you withheld your scores, others said they were inclined to look negatively on withheld scores and would rather see your entire test history. Problem solved! Seriously though, these issues may still come into play if you choose to withhold test scores from 2002 or earlier.

There are a few perks to the new THx Report online system too: The reports are free, and you can check out your score online much earlier—as soon as it's available to the AAMC.

Check out PrincetonReview.com for more information on the MCAT, including a detailed discussion of changes to the test.

YOUR BUDDING CAREER AS A NOVELIST

If you've ever harbored any fantasies of becoming a writer, now is your chance. If you've ever harbored fantasies of wiping the art of composition from human memory in retaliation for the suffering you endured in your freshman English class, you're going to have to find a way to cope. The personal comments section of the ACOMAS and AMCAS application is your chance to convince the committee that you are more than the sum of your numbers and that you deserve a chance at an interview.

Idea Generators

It is extremely difficult to write about anything important in a page or less, so assume that you will be spending some quality time with your computer. To get started, you can try a couple of different approaches to get your fingers moving:

Clustering

You may remember this from freshman Composition. You probably thought it was silly back then, but it just might save you now. Get a large blank piece of paper, and write down a few words to describe some of the experiences that have led you to pursue medical school. Or jot down some interesting, sad, or memorable experiences and later link them to your interest in medicine. You don't have to write them down in any particular order, just scatter your thoughts across the page. After you have several topics to work with, see if you can spot any patterns. Some of them will probably be interrelated. Next, generate longer descriptions of the words you wrote. For example, try to explain what you mean by "intellectual challenge." Was there a particular class you took? A paper you wrote? After you have some ideas on paper, try pulling them together based on the patterns of relationships you see between the topics. For example, telling a story about helping to clean a wound while volunteering in the ER might be a good way of letting the reader know that compassion is one of your qualities. It is often more effective to let the reader draw conclusions rather than spelling them out. For example, relate how you felt while treating a patient, and let the reader see that you are compassionate. Don't write, "That experience demonstrates my compassion."

Free Writing

This is particularly helpful if you find that you are having trouble figuring out where to start. All you have to do is sit down and force yourself to write about anything that comes into your mind. Don't worry about punctuation or grammar—just write for several pages. Take a break and look back at what you wrote. Most of the time, you'll be surprised to discover the beginnings of an idea. Keep a notepad with you and by your bed. Jot down ideas as they come to you.

Talk, Talk, Talk

One way to avoid writer's block is to talk into a tape recorder or to bribe a friend to write as you speak. Sometimes an empty screen or page can be intimidating. You can get started on your essay by telling your story to a tape recorder, or by having a friend write down what he or she thinks is interesting or important as you explain why you want to go to medical school. Don't expect to have suddenly generated your essay in this way. However, you can generate some material with which to start writing.

Three Basic Approaches

There are many different ways to structure the personal essay, but there are three basic approaches that can be used alone or in combination.

"My History in School"

This essay focuses on college experiences. It works well for people whose grades are fairly high and who want to emphasize their growth during the college years. The essay should be about your development, specialties, and strengths. The best essays usually have specific examples. It helps to have a specific class, professor, paper, or experience that crystallizes your experiences and ties into your goals. One of the benefits of this essay is a built-in chronology and organizational structure.

"My Life History"

In this essay, focus on a few events or main ideas that illustrate the qualities you can bring to medicine. If your whole life clearly leads up to being a physician (even if it might not have seemed that way at the time), this can be a good choice. One of the pitfalls of this structure is that it can let you ramble and lose coherency. Although you need to give a brief overview of your life, you also need focus your paragraphs around individual ideas.

"The Story"

This is often the most effective essay if it's done correctly. Focus on one or two stories that illustrate some of the points listed above. The story essay is the most fun for admissions officers to read, and is the most likely to be coherent and cohesive. You don't have to go overboard with adjectives and turns of phrase to write effective narrative. Just pick a few moments that most clearly define why you want to be a physician.

Key Bragging Points

No matter the subject you plan to focus on, the following are points that you should consider incorporating into the finished essay:

Academic Strength

You can discuss this generally, or with a specific example of a class, an assignment, or a moment in which you enjoyed an intellectual challenge. Medical school will require a lot of hard work. What demonstrates your love of hard work?

Commitment to Ideals

No one expects you to be Mother Teresa, but most good physicians have a streak of empathy and altruism.

Balance

What makes you whole? What balances the hardworking academic powerhouse that you are?

Careful, Complex Thinking

It is very difficult to explain something as complicated as your motivation to be a physician. Most people, when writing about a defining moment in their lives, assume that the audience is right there with them. This is not the case. You have to explain what you think and feel after you describe the event. Don't assume that the Admissions Committee is going to fill in the blanks for you.

Why You Want to Be a Doctor

The question you should ask yourself is why—when many other people who've had similar life/career/academic experiences take one look at the horrendous hours involved in medical training and decide that teaching or counseling would be a perfectly good alternative—you want to be a doctor. For instance, although many physicians decide to be doctors because of an early experience with the illness of a family member, there are far greater numbers of people with the same background who never consider medicine—but would still describe themselves as compassionate and moved to help people. You have to force yourself to ascertain what odd mixture of qualities—intellectual and emotional—have convinced you that going more than $150,000 in debt in the era of HMOs is a good idea.

Reasons, Not Excuses, for Weakness

Do not attempt to cover up or gloss over any deficiency, academic or otherwise. You will earn yourself points by honestly and openly dealing with your less-than-sterling qualities. If you have a couple of low grades or if you had a bad semester, briefly explain what happened, discuss what the experience taught you, and move on.

Good, Clever, Interesting Writing

Translation: Lots and lots and lots of drafts. Everybody has a distinct voice, and you're not going to survive medical school without a sense of humor. Find a way to get both qualities across without resorting to clichés. Prohibited phrases include: Lifelong learning, challenge of a lifetime, healing the mind as well as the body, childlike wonder, frail hands, quiet desperation, and any variations on these overused terms.

Overall Conservative Tone

Shock value doesn't work, despite the tales you might have heard about cartoons and poems. Admissions committees expect you to take the exercise seriously and to treat the process with respect. Humor is fine, but it needs to be subtle.

Show, Don't Tell

One of the traps of the personal statement is to rewrite your resume in prose. Instead of listing your accomplishments, explain what they mean to you and show how they have affected your life. For example, if you really want to practice primary care, it is far more effective for you to explain in detail what motivates you than to simply state your goal.

The Evolution of the Essay

Good essays tend to evolve and often bear very little resemblance to rough drafts. Don't be afraid to start over or to let the essay build on itself. If you write something that doesn't use any of the forms described above but that you feel gets across the points you want to make, then that is the essay you should stick with. Don't force yourself into a mold.

No matter what your essay looks like, however, there are a few general issues that you should think about.

Focus

Your essay must communicate specific points clearly and effectively. This means that every time you write a sentence that could be used in any other essay, you need to cross it out and start over. For example, "I truly enjoy working with people" could be the opening line in an application for fry guy at McDonald's just as easily as it could be a statement about the profound impact you want to have on your patients' health.

Editing

No mistakes. If you are not one of those people who goes around making a pest of themselves by correcting everyone else's grammatical errors, you need to find one. Most colleges and universities have writing centers with free editorial assistance, or you can check the local college paper for teaching assistants who are willing to edit for food. No matter what, make sure someone else reads your essay.

Interest

Everyone has a compelling style, and you need to write until you find yours. You are who you are for a reason; you have to write until that reason becomes apparent to anyone reading the essay.

Relevance

At some point, the reader will need a clear sense of why they should let you into medical school. Don't get so caught up in explaining your inner child that you forget to write about your desire to become a doctor.

Coherence

Make sure your essay fits together. You shouldn't be able to move a paragraph or a sentence when you're finished.

Remember that your entire personality is not going to be reflected in this essay, nor can you entirely offset an otherwise weak application. But this is your big chance to talk to the committee, so make the most of it. Spend the necessary time to draft and rework your essay until it is the best measure of your writing ability and candidacy for medical school.

SECONDARIES AND LETTERS OF RECOMMENDATION

After medical schools receive your application, they will send you what's called a *secondary*. Some schools send all of their applicants a secondary, while others go through an initial cut (usually based totally on GPA and MCAT scores). One of the reasons that schools like to send out secondaries is that they usually charge you about $50 for the privilege of filling them out. Secondaries usually include a variety of essay topics that are slightly more directed than the personal comments in either the ACOMAS or AMCAS. The following are some typical secondary questions:

- What is your favorite novel?

- What are your hobbies?

- Where do you see yourself in 10 years?

- Name a leadership role that you've taken and what it taught you about yourself.

- What has been your greatest academic achievement? What has been your greatest academic failure?

- What type of medicine do you think you might want to practice?

As you can see, most of these essays seem fairly simple, but that doesn't mean you shouldn't spend time thoughtfully filling them out. Many secondaries are quite lengthy, so it's a good idea to fill them out as you get them, unless you've decided for some reason not to continue with your application to the school. If you find that the cost of sending back secondaries rapidly becomes prohibitive, you can call the individual schools and request a fee waiver. If you were eligible for a waiver from AMCAS, for example, you will probably be able to have most of your secondary fees waived.

You should also take care of your letters of recommendation at the secondary stage. If you are a student who is still in school and you have access to pre-health advising, your letters will probably be handled by that office, and at least one of your letters will probably be from the pre-health advisor. Usually, your recommenders will write one letter that the Advising Office will copy and send to your list of schools. If you are a returning adult, you may have to take care of all the requests and letters yourself.

Letters of recommendation for medical school work in much the same way as any other such letters; you will have much better luck if you approach your potential recommender with a copy of your resume, transcript, and personal statement. Try to make an appointment to speak to the person to discuss the various schools to which you are applying—and to make your case. Even if you have been out of school for a while, you should try to get at least one letter from a former professor. Medical schools are interested in your character, your desire to be a physician, your academic preparedness, and your intellectual ability. Although most employers could attest to some of those qualities, you will probably need a letter from a professor that discusses your academic abilities. As an undergrad or in your postbacc program, try to build relationships with faculty members so they can write something meaningful about you. Don't ask for a letter from someone famous unless they know you pretty well. Name-dropping is not considered to be particularly attractive in a prospective medical student.

Although many returning adults feel awkward approaching professors they might not have spoken with in several years, most are pleasantly surprised to discover that for the most part, professors do tend to remember their students, and most are happy to write them letters of recommendation. Both current and former students should also consider asking for letters from doctors with whom they have worked or volunteered—and remember that if you're applying to an osteopathic school, you need a letter from a DO.

Once you discover how painless it really is to get a letter of recommendation, you may be tempted to go into overdrive on the theory that inundating the committee with reams of stationary will force them to recognize your worthiness. Resist this! Do not send more letters than the school asks for. The committee will not read them, and you will not have done yourself any favors. The only time you might consider sending extra letters is if you are placed on hold after an interview and have been working in the meantime with someone who you feel would be able to contribute some additional information about your abilities.

Minority Recruitment

Minority status refers to ethnicities that are *underrepresented* in medicine, such as Native Americans, African Americans, Latinos, Native Hawaiians, and some other specific groups. If you are not sure whether you qualify as a minority in this sense, you should contact AMCAS. Many public and private medical schools recognize the value of educating physicians who may choose to work in underserved areas and communities. Some committees look favorably on a candidate with a background that suggests he or she will fill this need. In some cases, this amounts to a preference for candidates with specific ethnic backgrounds—but it is a preference that occurs after a field of equally qualified applicants is generated from the initial pool. Medical schools are simply too competitive to accept candidates who are not up to the intellectual challenge of medicine. This selectivity advantage often extends to people of any ethnicity who come from underserved rural areas and seem inclined to return there to practice medicine.

There is also a type of minority status that AMCAS recognizes that deals only with economic factors and does not take into account ethnicity or country of origin. To be considered a "financially disadvantaged" minority, you need to have been under financial strain for a long period of time, and to have been the recipient of federal aid in the form of AFDC, welfare, food stamps, or other such programs. Your financial situation needs to have had an ongoing and persistent negative effect on your ability to procure education, housing, food, etc. In other words, the average two-job-struggling-to-make-ends-meet college student does not qualify. This minority status is reserved for those who have struggled uphill their entire lives and have somehow managed to make it through undergraduate school. The basic rule of thumb here is: If you are a financially disadvantaged minority, you probably know it. If you're in doubt, you probably aren't.

Medical schools are faced with a problem that is actually a boon for the quality of health care in the United States: They literally have more good applicants than they can take. This means that medical schools can easily fill their classes with students who are academically qualified. Medical schools have the opportunity to select from this pool those students who are most likely to improve underserved communities and to help those with the most need. The AAMC has sought to increase enrollment of underrepresented minorities in recent years. AOA has recently instituted a minority scholarship, the Sherry R. Arnstein Minority Student Award, to boost minority recruitment at osteopathic schools.

WHAT HAPPENS AFTER YOU'VE BEEN ACCEPTED

So you've achieved the impossible, the best-case scenario: multiple acceptances. First, congratulations. Second, it's probably not a good idea to share your good fortune with too many of your premed friends, unless you don't particularly want to keep them, and you've first removed all the sharp objects from the room.

BACK TO REALITY

After the giddiness wears off, you will have to deal with the best problem you will ever have: choosing which school to attend. Remember that you have lots of time to choose the medical school that best fits your goals and lifestyle. You can hang on to your acceptances until May 15, at which point schools will begin dropping your name off of their acceptance lists if you have not committed. Remember, however, that most of your fellow premeds do not share your enviable position. If you are accepted by a school that you know you will not attend, notify them before the deadline so that they can offer the seat to someone else. If you are on the wait list for a school you really want, don't hesitate to write a short note letting the committee know that their school is your first choice.

Factors to Consider

So while you are basking in your acceptance, think seriously about the following factors, but don't selfishly hold onto too many acceptances while you are deliberating:

How much does the school emphasize and reward teaching?

This is a huge concern and often overlooked. Look into how much the school values teaching versus how much they emphasize research. This can be the difference between being taught and being forced to teach yourself. The best way to determine teaching quality is to ask current students for their opinions.

What are community, social life, and support systems like?

Talk to current students to determine the overall community of the school. You'll be there for four years, and you certainly won't be studying all—okay, most, but not all—of the time. Are the students accepting the rigors of med school with a positive attitude or do they waste all of their extra energy complaining? What is the quality of life in general like at this school? Do students study together? Is it a community or commuter lifestyle?

What's the quality of the residents?

The residents are the ones who will be teaching you when you're a med student, so of course you want them to be good. You should presumably be able to approximate the quality of the residents based on the quality of postgraduate training programs (residency programs) at the hospitals affiliated with the school.

How family friendly are the school and its surroundings?

If you're a returning adult student with a family, look into the spouse/partner support services available at the schools you're considering. Getting through medical school will be hard on you and your family, and many places have begun programs that allow spouses/partners to attend special seminars and support groups that acclimate you to the pressures of your chosen educational and career path. Will your partner be able to find work/activities he or she enjoys?

Where will you be living?

Believe it or not, you will occasionally escape to the outside world. Make sure that the activities and hobbies you enjoy are available somewhere in the general vicinity. If you come from one climate and are moving to another, consider how that will affect you. Also, find out how close the clinical facilities are to the school and housing. The closer, the better.

What kind of research opportunities are available?

Some schools are much better equipped than others, and it's not always the high-profile schools that are doing the most cutting-edge research. Different schools have different specialties, and some benefit from affiliated schools of public health, business, or law. Other schools offer paid research opportunities.

Traditional or systems-based?

Teaching methodologies include traditional (two years of science plus two years of rotations), organ-based (learn everything about the liver), case-based (learn science by delving into patient histories), and everything in between. Which method will be best for you? It is difficult to know. It is also likely that other issues are more important for you to consider, such as the school's regard for education, commitment to teaching, and responsiveness to student input and overall academic climate. These issues may prove more important than the curricular grid (i.e., when you take anatomy), in terms of how much you learn and how much you enjoy learning.

What kind of financial aid offer are they making?
Is the offer good for all four years? In comparing offers between schools, consider cost of living differences and variation in the terms of loans.

How much will you owe?
This is the most important financial aid statistic a school can offer because it encompasses tuition, expenses, and financial aid. No matter what kind of financial package you get, you will most likely owe a staggering sum when you graduate, and it all has to be paid back eventually. As an intern and resident, you won't be making much in the way of a salary (about $38,000 to $49,000). Although most physicians eventually achieve a comfortable living (average of approximately $263,000 annual salary in 2011), the practice of medicine is in such a state of flux that it is impossible to predict what kinds of jobs and compensation will be available 10 years from now. A public university education, while perhaps not carrying quite the cachet as a private school, may save you tens of thousands of dollars and relieve some of the stress associated with gargantuan debt.

BEHIND DOOR NUMBER 1 . . . MORE STANDARDIZED TESTS!

Most medical students take the USMLE Step 1 (and/or the first COMLEX—the COMLEX exams go in the same order as the USMLEs) at the end of the second year of medical school. Osteopathic students must pass the USMLE to obtain allopathic residency spots. Step 1 is often used to determine whether or not a student has passed their pre-clinical course work and can continue into their third and fourth years of training. Step 2 is usually taken during the third or fourth year of school during clerkships. At this point, the vast majority of senior U.S. medical students go through the Match in order to obtain residency positions. Very few contract privately for their first year of graduate medical training. Most programs in the Match now use ERAS (Electronic Residency Application Service), which is administered by AAMC, rather than a traditional paper application. Step 3 is usually taken after at least one year of residency (most physicians do at least three years of residency, but still take the test after the first year). The USMLE is written and scored by the National Board of Medical Examiners, which administers Steps 1 and 2. Step 3 is administered by the state. The state confers the license; the USMLE is a prerequisite.

INTERNATIONAL MEDICAL GRADUATES

International medical graduates (IMG) go through a special process to be granted licensure in the United States. Before you can start a residency program, you need to be certified by the Education Commission for Foreign Medical Graduates (ECFMG). To be certified, an IMG must complete the following five steps:

- Take USMLE Steps 1 and 2.

- Send medical credentials and fill out the paperwork necessary to show proof of medical education.

- Take the English test administered by the ECFMG.
- If you don't pass the English test, you can take the Test of English as a Foreign Language instead.
- Take the Clinical Skills Assessment, which is a live standardized patient exam.

After this, contact the board of the state in which you want to practice for the Step 3 requirements (each state determines its own passing score). You can get a residency through the NRMP Match or through a private contract. After passing Step 3 and following any other state guidelines, you are granted a temporary license to practice in that state.

If you are currently in a medical program abroad and are thinking about transferring to a U.S. medical school, you need to contact the school and ask about its transfer policies. In general, it is extremely difficult to transfer into a U.S. medical school.

HIGH SCHOOL STUDENTS

If you've picked up this book and you're still in high school, you're very much ahead of the game. You can get started on the road to medical school by participating in volunteer activities and researching potential college choices to learn about their premedical training. Remember, you can major in any subject that interests you as long as you complete your premedical courses. Choose a subject you enjoy, and you are more likely to earn good grades and get into medical school. A few schools have special programs that funnel students through their undergraduate education directly into medical school. If you are interested in these programs, you should contact the following schools directly for more information:

Boston University

Brown University

Case Western University

East Tennessee State University

George Washington University

Howard University

Louisiana State University—New Orleans

Louisiana State University—Shreveport

Michigan State University

New York University

Northwestern University

University of Alabama

University of Miami

University of Michigan

University of Missouri—Kansas City

University of Rochester

University of South Alabama

University of Southern California

University of Wisconsin

IMPORTANT CONTACT ORGANIZATIONS

AMERICAN ASSOCIATION OF COLLEGES OF OSTEOPATHIC MEDICINE (AACOM)
5550 Friendship Boulevard
Suite 310
Chevy Chase, MD 20815-7231
301-968-4100
301-968-4101 (fax)
www.aacom.org

AMERICAN ASSOCIATION OF MEDICAL COLLEGES (AAMC)
2450 N Street, Northwest
Washington, DC 20037-1126
202-828-0400
202-828-1125 (fax)
www.aamc.org

ASSOCIATION OF ACCREDITED NATUROPATHIC MEDICAL COLLEGES
4435 Wisconsin Avenue, Northwest Suite 403
Washington, DC 20016
202-237-8150 or 866-538-2267 (toll-free)
202-237-8152 (fax)
www.aanmc.org

AMERICAN OSTEOPATHIC ASSOCIATION (AOA)
142 East Ontario Street
Chicago, IL 60611-2864
800-621-1773
312-202-8200 (fax)
www.osteopathic.org, www.do-online.org

EDUCATIONAL COMMISSION FOR FOREIGN MEDICAL GRADUATES
3624 Market Street
Philadelphia, PA 19104-2685
215-386-5900
215-386-9196 (fax)
www.ecfmg.org

FEDERATION OF STATE MEDICAL BOARDS
PO Box 619850
Dallas, TX 75261-9850
817-868-4000
817-868-4099 (fax)
www.fsmb.org

NATIONAL BOARD OF MEDICAL EXAMINERS
3750 Market Street
Philadelphia, PA 19104-3102
215-590-9500
215-590-9457 (fax)
www.nbme.org

TEXAS MEDICAL AND DENTAL SCHOOLS APPLICATION SERVICE
702 Colorado, Suite 6400
Austin, TX 78701
512-499-4785
512-499-4786
www.utsystem.edu/tmdsas

(Texas public schools do not use AMCAS)

4 Advice for the "Nontraditional" Applicant

Forty years ago, most medical school applicants shared certain traits. The "traditional" medical school applicant was white, male, and just older than 20. Most likely, he majored in biology or chemistry while in college. Although he knew that medical school would be difficult and that his career would be challenging, he looked forward to choosing from a wide range of medical specialties and being financially secure. As a trained professional, he would possess real skills and expertise and, as a result, could expect to enjoy authority and autonomy.

The past few decades have seen substantial changes in the composition of the medical school applicant pool and in the professional opportunities available to medical school graduates. Based on the previous idea of the traditional medical student, women and minority applicants could be considered "nontraditional," but the term is currently used to describe applicants who are older than most med students. The average age of applicants is 25, but a significant and increasing proportion of applicants are several years older.

Some of these older applicants, always intending to apply to medical school, completed premedical requirements during their years as undergraduates and simply postponed medical school to work, travel, or start a family. Others were unsuccessful at gaining admission directly out of college and are attempting a second or third time. Another group considered medical school in college but did not complete requirements or the application process. Some older applicants never seriously considered medicine until after they graduated college and were involved in another occupation. Whatever the reason for postponing, older applicants now represent a significant proportion of the medical school candidate pool.

Aspiring doctors who did not take the prerequisite science courses in college or did not excel in them face a formidable challenge. These individuals have a minimum of seven years of medical school and residency on the horizon and, in addition, must complete (and do well in) one to two years of basic science courses before even applying to medical school. Nonetheless, thousands of adults, despite the arduous path ahead of them, decide to tackle this challenge. This chapter is intended as a source of information and support for nontraditional applicants at all stages of the application process. It is written by a nontraditional applicant and includes input from others who are or were in the same category. Follow eight nontraditional applicants through the entire process—from decision making, to postbacc training, to MCAT preparation, and acceptance. The group is composed of real individuals[11] coming from a wide range of backgrounds, some elements of which will hopefully resemble aspects of your own situation. When these people decided that medical school was their goal, this is who they were and what they were doing:

- Becky, a 28-year-old who completed two years of college and had worked as a medical assistant for 10 years.

- Pete, a 28-year-old with a law degree who was unhappy in his field.

- Tina, a 27-year-old art history major who was working in a gallery and dating a medical student.

- Bob, a 35-year-old chemistry professor at a small college.

- Mitch, a 30-year-old former Peace Corps volunteer who was working in international development.

- Jacob, a 24-year-old volunteer firefighter. A car accident and subsequent hospitalization kept him from completing organic chemistry while in college. Discouraged, he dropped out of the premedical track.

- Eve, a 42-year-old wife and mother of three who graduated college 20 years ago, and had little experience working outside of the home.

- Donald, an engineering graduate student who decided that he needed more human contact in his work.

[11] Names have been changed.

DECIDING THAT MEDICINE—AND MEDICAL SCHOOL—IS WHAT YOU WANT

Some of these people were absolutely sure about going to medical school. Jacob, for example, had always known. Tina, who was fascinated by what her boyfriend studied in medical school, had a strong hunch. Donald imagined that being a physician would give him what he felt was missing from his career, but he had limited contact with the medical field and had not fully considered other options that would give him more personal interaction.

Being reasonably sure about medicine is important because you will invest time, money, and energy into the medical school preparation and application process. It is also important because admissions officers will look for indications of your commitment. If you are sure of it, your commitment is more likely to come through in your personal statement and your interview.

If you have never worked or volunteered in a medical setting, you should explore opportunities to do so. You might arrange to informally shadow a physician or to volunteer in a hospital that has a formal program. Some volunteers find that they are given more responsibility at a small clinic than they are in a large hospital, so look into clinic programs as well. Explore opportunities to volunteer in overseas medical projects. Of our eight subjects, those who had more than one medically related experience felt that it was beneficial because they were exposed to the variation that exists within the field. Not only are volunteer activities helpful in your decision-making process, but they will become significant resume builders should you decide to apply to medical school. In addition, they are likely to be valuable and, hopefully, enjoyable experiences.

One way to help determine if medicine is the right career for you is to talk to others who have made the choice. Interview as many people as you can. Talk to practicing physicians, residents, medical students, and those involved in academic medicine such as researchers. Find out what they love and hate about their work. Ask questions that will help you put their comments about medicine in perspective. For example, if you come across someone who positively hated medical school and dislikes being a physician, ask him what part of medical school he hated the least. If his favorite part of the experience was the relaxing cruise-ship vacation he took after his first year, he probably could have made a better career choice for himself. His views of medical school may not be an indication of what the experience will be like for you.

If possible, talk to medical students, practicing physicians, and resident physicians who are or were nontraditional. Find out whether they feel that they made the right decision. What were the biggest sacrifices they had to make? Visit the premedical and medical student discussion pages online where many nontraditional applicants and students share their thoughts.

Bob's decision to apply to medical school was influenced by his sister-in-law. She works in medical equipment sales and is five years older than Bob. She encouraged him to follow his dream, saying that she, too, had entertained the idea of becoming a physician when she was 30. She decided against it and at 40 still dreams about doing it today. But with two young children, she feels that it would be too difficult. Bob decided that it would be more painful to spend his life wondering if he should have gone to medical school than to go and—in the worst-case scenario—drop out and return to teaching.

Mitch also found it helpful to talk to people working in totally unrelated fields. He had worked for two years in a clinic in rural Africa and thought that he wanted to become a pediatrician. However, he became discouraged while talking to his friends who were medical students, residents, or newly graduated practicing physicians because it seemed that few people loved everything about what they were doing. Many of his friends warned him of the burden of debt and the prospect of having little free time. One friend told him that in comparison to Mitch's current job, which involved traveling around the world, he would be *bored* in medicine. Mitch then took an informal poll of all his friends who included teachers, writers, business owners, software designers, lawyers, and full-time parents. He found that people in all occupations both love *and* hate certain things about their work.

Although medical students and physicians complain about debt, teachers complain about low salaries, and business owners complain about financial insecurity. All of Mitch's friends in their early 30s complain about working too hard and about the difficulty of balancing their personal and family lives with their careers. Mitch concluded that despite the initial discouragement he got from friends in the medical profession, people in medicine are among the *most* professionally fulfilled. Although medical students and physicians had complaints, they were engaged in their work, and most couldn't imagine a better career. He also noticed that a significant number of non-physicians he spoke to, although unhappy with their own jobs, still discouraged him from going into medicine. He realized that some of these people had, at one point in their lives, entertained the idea of becoming a doctor. They had successfully talked themselves out of medical school and were sold on all the reasons why *not* to go into medicine. As far as his friend's comment about being bored, Mitch realized that others tended to glamorize his current work because it involved travel. He knew that being a pediatrician would, on a day-to-day basis, be more interesting than the paperwork he dealt with in his current job. Furthermore, he could probably work overseas as a physician if he found himself yearning for travel.

After you follow Mitch's example and grill everyone you know, ask yourself some serious questions. What jobs and experiences have you loved most in your life? Do you foresee medicine providing similar satisfaction? Have you enjoyed some aspects of your medically related work? Do you have the skills it takes to become a physician? To be fulfilled as one? Whether or not to pursue a career in medicine is an important decision that will affect many years of your life. Give yourself time, both for information gathering and personal reflection. Write down your thoughts on what is influencing your decision. Whether or not you decide to go for it, if you carefully weigh the decision now, you will be less likely to doubt it later on.

Resist feeling that because you are older, you should make your decision to enter medical school as quickly as possible. Medical school, internship, and residency require at least seven years to complete. Moreover, medicine is a career of lifelong learning. Start finding things to enjoy about the process of becoming a doctor now. Deciding to go to medical school is part of the process. Try not to stress too much about the decision, and find some satisfaction in your information gathering and self-reflection.

GETTING INTO MEDICAL SCHOOL AS A NONTRADITIONAL APPLICANT

If you are reading this, you have probably decided to move forward with your plan to become an MD, DO, or ND. Hopefully, your level of maturity and your life experience have allowed you to make a well-informed decision that a student just out of college may not be in a position to make. Between 20 percent and 30 percent of applicants in the 24- to 37-year-old age range are admitted to medical school, while approximately 45 percent of 21- to 23-year-olds are admitted. Although these statistics suggest that the odds are against older applicants, age itself is not regarded as a disadvantage, and may in some cases be a plus. Even the most exciting and unique older applicant must have a competitive GPA and MCAT score.

The timing of the admissions process is often an issue for nontraditional applicants. Donald started thinking about medical school midway through his first year of graduate school. We will call this January of Year one. He realized that he had prerequisites to fulfill and that he wouldn't be eligible to enter medical school the following fall, but thought he would be able to matriculate in the fall of Year three. Donald quit his graduate program and entered an intensive premedical curriculum, completing his requirements by January, Year two. He took the MCAT in April, Year two. If Donald had taken premedical courses part-time rather than full-time, he could not have adhered to this schedule. Had he done poorly on the MCAT the first time, he could have been delayed an entire year and postponed entrance until Year four. As a result of the timing of the admissions process, it takes two to four years to matriculate after deciding to pursue medical school. The following are the important dates to remember as you think about timeframe and requirements:

- April: MCAT is given. You should have completed all prerequisite science courses by this date.

- June: AMCAS (preliminary) applications are accepted. Filling out the AMCAS application requires all undergraduate, graduate, and post bacc transcripts (they accept transcripts beginning on March 15, but the completed application isn't accepted until June 1). You will need your own copies, and you will need to have copies sent directly to AMCAS. It is important to submit AMCAS applications as soon as possible because most schools offer rolling admissions.

- August: MCAT is given. Use this test date only if you need to improve your scores from the April test. You will indicate on your AMCAS application whether you intend to take (or retake) the test on this date. If so, many schools will not look at your application until August scores are available (some time in October). The penalty for this delay may very well outweigh your score improvement. Thus, unless you anticipate *significant* score improvement, the August MCAT is not advised.

- August: Medical schools to which AMCAS applications have been submitted begin sending secondary applications. Some schools will review AMCAS applications closely and will send secondary ones to a limited number of applicants. Others send them to everyone who applies through AMCAS. There is usually an additional fee. In some cases, secondary applications require essays or short-answer questions that focus on motivation, personal characteristics, values, and experiences. In other cases, the application is very simple and similar to the AMCAS application. Thus, receiving a secondary application *may* be an indication that a school is interested in you. When you return the application and fee, you demonstrate your interest in the school. Schools often want these back within two to four weeks. You will also need to submit recommendations at this time. Some schools ask for a photo.

- August–May: Based on AMCAS and secondary applications and recommendations, applicants are invited to interview during this period. Some schools conduct all their interviews during one or two months, while others spread them out. Most schools accept 25–50-plus percent of interviewed candidates. Thus, getting an interview is an excellent sign. Most admissions decisions are also made during this period, with the exception of applicants who fall into a "hold" or "wait list" category.

- June–August: Wait listed candidates may be accepted.

ACADEMIC REQUIREMENTS

Most medical schools require or strongly prefer that applicants have a BA or BS degree from a four-year accredited college or university. All medical schools require a minimum level of science preparation that includes approximately one year each of biology, chemistry, organic chemistry, and physics. Some nontraditional candidates meet these requirements by taking night courses while simultaneously working part- or full-time. Others enroll full-time at private or public undergraduate institutions. Some choose to enroll in special *postbaccalaureate premedical* programs (we call them postbacc programs) offered by a surprisingly large number of colleges and universities (see Chapter 10 for a comprehensive listing of postbacc programs). Postbacc programs vary widely in terms of cost, rigor of course work, grading system, percentage of graduates admitted to medical school, structure and flexibility of curriculum, duration, size, and class composition. Unlike medical schools, postbacc programs are neither accredited as such, nor ranked.

Becky needed to complete her BA in addition to fulfilling science prerequisites. When she decided it was time to take a shot at fulfilling her long-time dream of becoming a physician, she lived and worked in California, which has some of the most selective state-affiliated medical schools in the country. Becky decided to move to another state and complete her BA there so that she would be qualified for admission to the state's medical school. Becky enrolled full-time for three years to complete her BA—not all of her previous college credits transferred—and fulfill all her science requirements.

Becky's strategy is interesting and may be advisable for others in similar situations who are prepared to relocate. Before moving across the country, be sure that you understand your new state's criteria for determining residency. In some states, being a full-time student does not ensure resident status. Becky might have saved herself a year of schooling had she looked at more colleges and possibly uncovered schools willing to award her credit for all her previous college work.

Tina graduated from a prestigious college but had taken neither science nor math classes while in school. She was also concerned about her undergraduate GPA, which was 2.9. To make herself a more competitive applicant, she wanted to demonstrate both competence in the sciences and overall improved study skills. Some postbaccalaureate premedical programs are quite structured and involve only the minimum science prerequisites; Tina felt that she needed more than this to make up for her undergrad GPA. One of Tina's options was to apply to a postbacc program that allows participants to take additional courses beyond those in the required scientific disciplines. This type of program tends to be somewhat flexible, allowing students to spend as much time as needed to fulfill requirements and take any additional courses. Students get the opportunity to learn foreign languages, improve writing or math skills, or take courses often recommended—but not required—by medical schools such as biochemistry or statistics. Other postbacc programs apply students' course work toward a master's degree.

Tina decided not to enter an organized postbacc program. Instead, she enrolled full-time as a nondegree candidate at a local, private university. This gave her access to larger course offerings. One of the advantages of postbacc programs is that they are compact, scheduling courses and labs so students may complete all requirements within a year. Tina was less worried about speed and more interested in earning excellent grades. Another important consideration for Tina was letters of recommendation. Medical schools usually prefer that applicants submit a composite letter from their premedical advisor who is typically an administrator or dean, a department head, a specified faculty member, or some type of counselor. The letter discusses the student's qualifications and incorporates comments from his or her premedical professors. Because Tina chose a small school, she had the opportunity to get to know her professors and, presumably, to secure meaningful comments from them. At some colleges, only degree-earning students have full access to premedical and other advisors, but Tina was able to identify one who agreed to write a letter for her. One advantage to true postbacc programs is that the premedical advisors are able to write appropriate letters of recommendation for nontraditional applicants.

Some premedical candidates are highly concerned with getting through the application process quickly and have no interest in prolonging premedical course work. Pete had a 3.7 GPA in college and an excellent record in law school. He had no need to prove himself scholastically, but just wanted to "get the sciences out of the way." He was a good candidate for a highly selective postbacc program. To be admitted to one of these programs, applicants must submit detailed information including personal statements, prior standardized test scores, and several recommendations. Interviews are often required. These programs seek to admit students who will not only complete the course work, but who are likely to be accepted to medical school. Often, the brochures for these programs boast the percentage of graduates who have been admitted into medical school. Although a high acceptance rate is partially a reflection of the quality and resources of the program itself, it also indicates that they accept well-qualified students. In one year, Pete was able to complete all his sciences and study for and take the MCAT.

Pete took advantage of an arrangement between his postbacc program and a medical school, allowing him to enter medical school in the fall following completion of premedical course work. Thus, he avoided an "in between" year generally devoted to the medical school application process. Several selective postbacc programs offer this type of arrangement, affiliation, or linkage with a number of medical schools. In some cases, the medical school and the postbacc program are part of the same university. Many nontraditional candidates are disappointed to discover that top medical schools such as Harvard, University of Pennsylvania, and Columbia do not offer these arrangements with their own university's postbacc program.

Pete took the shortest path possible to medical school. In the fall, he left the law firm where he was working, and the following fall, he was beginning medical school. He was happy to skip the long and stressful medical school application process, having been through a similar experience with law school. While ideal for some, Pete's path is neither available nor advisable for everyone. The short, intensive postbacc programs are grueling and may be too fast paced for some people. Graduates of these programs often claim that their postbacc work was more demanding than medical school itself. Although these programs can serve as excellent preparation for medical school, they may discourage people who could have succeeded had they enrolled in a more relaxed program.

Earning acceptance to a postbacc program with affiliated medical schools does not assure your acceptance to medical schools. Postbacc students in these programs usually apply to the affiliated schools, but acceptances are only provisional, and conditional upon securing a minimum GPA and MCAT score. Only a handful of medical schools participate in these linkages, and each school limits the number of positions available through the direct admissions route. Pete chose his postbacc program in part because one of the linked medical schools interested him. If none of the medical schools that allow admission through this route appeal to you, saving one year now is probably not worth spending four years someplace you don't want to be. Generally, medical schools agree to these arrangements as a means of enrolling students who they would otherwise not attract. Thus, if you are accepted as a postbacc student to one of these schools, you are not likely to be accepted to other schools if you apply through the regular admissions process. Another disadvantage to these arrangements is that they are usually binding: if you get in, you must go. If you earn a perfect score on the MCAT, you cannot withdraw and apply to your dream school for the following year. Additionally, you have no opportunity to compare financial aid packages.

While Donald, Tina, Pete, and Becky quit their jobs to enter premedical studies full-time, Mitch, Jacob, and Eve opted for part-time schooling. Eve wanted to ease into school, and decided to take one course at a time. She enrolled in a general chemistry class through the extension office of a local public university. Her children spent summers at camp and with relatives, allowing her to take a compact organic chemistry course during the summer. The following school year, she enrolled in a two-semester biology course, and she took an intensive physics course the next summer. Eve was concerned that her age would hurt her chances of being accepted to medical school. However, had she crammed all of the required science courses into just one year, she would have been only one year younger when she applied to med school, but a whole lot more frustrated and perhaps not as appealing a candidate because her grades could have suffered. In retrospect, Eve's only regret about taking courses on her own is that she missed the camaraderie and support that she might have had in a postbacc program. An advantage to postbacc programs is that you will meet people facing challenges similar to your own.

Most medical schools advise nontraditional applicants to demonstrate success in *recent* course work. Bob had fulfilled all the prerequisites in college about 15 years earlier. Since Bob had a graduate degree in science and remained active in an academic environment, the fact that he completed his prerequisite courses years earlier did not hurt him. His hurdle was the MCAT, for which he reviewed intensely.

The grading systems vary tremendously among undergraduate institutions and post-bacc programs. Some material that you learn as a premed, such as the basic biochemical processes, will serve you in medical school. Other topics, like whether your rowboat sinks or rises if you fall into the water, might not. As a premedical student, your goals should be to figure out whether you enjoy studying science, to learn the material for the MCAT, and to get good grades.

Some colleges and universities with postbacc programs assign nontraditional students to regular, undergraduate science courses. You attend lectures, labs, and exams along-side undergraduates and may or may not be graded on the same curve as your younger classmates. Most likely, the mean score of postbacc students is somewhat higher than that of the rest of the class. Undergraduates shouldn't be penalized by your presence since, after all, you already have your BA. Thus, schools with significant numbers of postbacc students are likely to separate them from the undergraduates for grading purposes. Unfortunately, this practice could hurt you because you may be competing with your undergraduate classmates for positions in medical schools. Your cumulative test score of 90 percent put you in the middle of the postbacc curve and earned you a C, while your classmate's 90 percent put him at the front end of the undergraduate curve and earned him an A. Although a letter of recommendation could explain that you did in fact maintain a 90 percent average, a C is still a C.

Some postbacc programs address this issue by setting the postbacc curve higher. The mean score will represent a B grade rather than a C grade. Highly selective postbacc programs usually recognize that all their students were strong in college and will set the mean somewhere in the A-minus or B-plus range. If a college that does not have a formal postbacc program allows you to enroll in science courses, your GPA might be slightly higher because you will be graded with your classmates, many of whom are probably less focused and less serious than you about maintaining excellent grades. Note, how-ever, that many medical schools consider the caliber of undergraduate institutions when evaluating GPAs. This applies to traditional and nontraditional applicants alike.

THE MCAT

The MCAT takes about 4.5 hours and is currently offered 28 times yearly at locations throughout the country. It is composed of four sections. An individual's raw score (number wrong out of number possible) on each section is compared with those of test-takers nationwide and is converted to a scaled score. Many find the experience a test of endurance and concentration as much as a test of knowledge (see page 31 for more information on the MCAT).

Virtually all medical schools require the MCAT. Schools evaluate MCAT scores in dif-ferent ways. Some have devised formulas that incorporate MCAT results and GPAs and produce numerical scores to assign to candidates. In some cases, if an applicant's score falls above a cutoff, he will receive a secondary application or perhaps be invited to interview. Although certain sections of the MCAT may be weighted more heavily than others by some admissions offices, most schools regard all sections except the essay as equally important. In some formulas, the MCAT and GPA carry roughly equal weight, while in others one is weighted more heavily. A number of schools claim that GPA is more important than MCAT. Although this may be true, consider such statements in light of the recent outcry against standardized tests. A school that admits to using test scores as its primary means of weeding out applicants could be regarded as lazy and discriminatory.

Most schools claim not to use specified formulas or cutoff points and indicate that they might consider an applicant with a very low MCAT score if other aspects of his application are extraordinary. But generally, admissions committees rely heavily on MCAT scores because they are considered a strong indicator of success in the first two years of medical school, and because they are the easiest part of an application to judge. Examining the average MCAT scores of accepted students at a school gives you a rough idea of what score you will need to gain admission there.

The MCAT is important for all applicants but may be especially so for nontraditional applicants. Eve's college grades were 20 years old. Over the years, colleges and universities have made changes and adjustments to grading scales and curricular requirements. Thus, her GPA might not be comparable to that of someone who graduated from the same school in 2010. Furthermore, how she performed in college 20 years ago is probably not a great indicator of how she will fare in medical school today. Grades in postbacc courses are important, but as mentioned earlier, there is wide variation in grading policies among postbacc programs and between regular undergraduate courses and the same courses within postbacc programs. The benefit of the MCAT is that it is standardized, supposedly allowing admissions committees to compare the aptitude of people with different backgrounds.

When preparing for the MCAT, consider that the results of that one day of work are nearly as important as all your other academic achievements. Beyond striving for a sound academic background, most medical school applicants—both traditional and nontraditional—take some sort of MCAT preparation course like the ones offered by The Princeton Review. For some, a test-prep course teaches material never learned, or never absorbed, in class. For others, it relieves some anxiety associated with standardized tests, allowing for an improved performance. For those lacking self-motivation, taking a course is a good way to encourage studying.

Some postbacc programs offer an MCAT review along with premedical courses. Usually, such a review will be much less intensive than a course offered by an outside organization. In Pete's postbacc program, most students enrolled in a private course that met twice weekly for three months prior to the April MCAT. Since the postbacc program itself was so intensive and required many hours per day of studying, the students needed to be pushed to devote time to MCAT preparation. Pete did not take the course because he felt confident that he would enter medical school the following fall through the arrangement he had made with an affiliated medical school. The medical school required Pete to take the MCAT and to score at least a 9 in all subjects. By January of his postbacc year, Pete was scoring 8's or higher in all sections, and reasoned that, by finishing his premedical courses and studying for the MCAT on his own, he could score 9s.

Formal MCAT courses typically include three or four practice, full-length MCATs. The exams are scored, giving students an idea of their strengths, weaknesses, and overall progress throughout the course. Pete obtained practice MCATs through the Association of American Medical Colleges (AAMC) and set aside three Saturdays prior to the April exam to take them. For those who do not take a course, it is important to order these practice exams and to be disciplined about taking them.[12] The exams come with tables that allow you to convert your raw score to the scaled score that gives you an accurate idea of how you'll score on an actual MCAT. There are a number of books available that review important MCAT topics and offer tips for taking the exam.

Review books and courses are a good idea for nontraditional and traditional students, although nontraditional students who have been out of the standardized test scene for many years may particularly need the help. For example, when Becky took her first practice exam, she was discouraged because she was barely able to complete half of the questions in the science sections. MCAT questions are not arranged in order of difficulty, and Becky was spending too much time on really tough passages that appeared early in the sections. She improved her score significantly on the science sections just by training herself to skip and go back to difficult passages.

Some nontraditional applicants have an advantage on the verbal section. By just being older, you may have had more time than a college student to read a wide variety of books. Eve loves reading and found the verbal section to be a confidence builder. Becky, who did not read extensively for work or pleasure, found the verbal section very difficult. Donald, who learned English as his second language, studied more for the verbal section than for both science sections combined. Becky improved her verbal score by focusing on concentration skills. One way to do this is to read slightly complicated or technical magazine and journal articles every day for several months before the MCAT. Force yourself to concentrate for an extended period of time each day.

[12] Practice exams are real MCATs from years past. Visit AAMC.org/students/MCAT.

THE PERSONAL STATEMENT AND INTERVIEW

Health care has changed dramatically in the United States, and some experts argue that physicians in the twenty-first century will have to possess a wider range of skills than was previously considered adequate (see Chapter 2). Not only must physicians be experts in their respective fields, but it is advantageous to understand the financial, legal, ethical, and political issues surrounding health care provision. Medical schools recognize the need for well-rounded physicians. The schools now offer revised curriculums that include non-science courses, and they admit more and more non-science majors.

As a nontraditional applicant, you have unique experiences and skills. These will help differentiate you from other applicants and can be an important strength. The AMCAS personal statement, essays for secondary applications, and the interview are opportunities for you to shine. Although you are probably tired of being asked why you want to become a doctor, you will have to figure out how to answer the question with sincerity and enthusiasm. As a nontraditional applicant, your motivation for pursuing a career in medicine is an extremely important consideration for Admissions Committees.

Despite recognizing the value of nontraditional students, admissions committees may be skeptical of applicants who are embarking on their second or third career. Essays and interviews are also opportunities for you to address their concerns and doubts about your motivation. In interviews, Donald was often asked what made him so sure he wouldn't drop out of medical school as he had engineering school. The school's concern is that poor judgment with respect to your first career choice may suggest the possibility of poor judgment in your decision to apply to medical school. Or perhaps the worry is that some people are eternally unfulfilled and will therefore be unfulfilled by a career in medicine. Many people believe that if you are good at something, you enjoy it. Thus, not liking your previous job suggests to some that you were bad at it and that you may possess some hidden faults.

All medical school applicants—both traditional and nontraditional—must figure out how to package themselves. Like wrapping a present that is oddly sized, some nontraditional applicants have to be creative in their packaging. Donald's strategy was to maintain a positive attitude. He told interviewers that some of the things that attracted him to engineering, such as the analytic thinking required, also applies to medicine. He asked interviewers whether some of the principles in engineering would translate to physiological issues. He emphasized his excellent academic record, his success in science courses, and his demonstrated willingness to work hard in school. He also stressed how much he enjoyed volunteering at a clinic. He did his best to be personable and talkative, thereby showing off his people skills rather than restating what was written in his essay—that he was switching fields because he wanted to work directly with people.

Tina's story—that she was bored working in an art gallery and envious of her boyfriend's career—would not get her into medical school without clarification. Tina enjoyed certain aspects of her job, such as interacting with artists and clients. She loved much of the art with which she worked, particularly the pieces that were highly expressive and revealed human emotion. On the other hand, she missed a sense of social purpose in her gallery work, and she felt that she wasn't being intellectually challenged. Tina packaged herself as passionate, people-oriented, and interested in helping others. She was good at her job but knew that it would not engage her for life. Through her work, she came to know what she liked and disliked, what fulfilled her and what did not. Unlike children of physicians who are likely to consider medicine as a potential career from an early age, Tina never thought about it as a realistic pursuit until her 20s when her boyfriend entered medical school. Now that she had an idea of what medical school and medicine were like, and now that she knew herself better, she was ready to commit to the career. Because she enjoyed working with people, she envisioned a career in primary care. She believed that as a result of her studies and work in the art world, she had good insight into the mental capacity and emotions of people. She wondered if psychiatry was the field for her.

Packaging Jacob was relatively straightforward. He had a reasonably consistent interest in medicine, demonstrated by earlier premedical courses and more recent firefighting work that involved some emergency medical skills. In Jacob's personal statement, he needed to address the reasons he dropped out of the premedical track in college. Jacob had been hospitalized, and this experience was emotionally difficult for him. Being in a hospital and being around sick and dying people was enough to make him question whether he really could be a physician. When he returned to school, he was less committed to going to medical school and decided to focus on completing his major and general requirements with good grades. After graduation, he fully recovered and had regained his interest in medicine. He took several first aid courses, volunteered in an emergency room, trained to become a fireman, and looked around for postbacc programs. In his essay, Jacob brought up the doubts that he had about becoming a physician, and discussed how he overcame them. Had he glossed over his hospital experience and the fact that he only took one semester of organic chemistry in college, admissions committees may have concluded that he "just couldn't cut it" as a premed. By addressing the situation, he presented himself as someone who matured and grew from a difficult experience.

Some medical schools read the essays and personal statements of all applicants and use them, along with grades and scores, for initial screening. Others only read essays after some applications have been weeded out. If you are filling out applications, you are at the point where you can't do much about your grades or scores. However, you can write an excellent personal statement. Enlist a friend, relative, advisor, or coworker who is well read and writes well to review your statement and make suggestions. Have someone who really knows you read it to be sure that you have conveyed your strengths. On the AMCAS application, exactly one page is provided for an applicant's personal statement. The resume of a nontraditional applicant is probably longer than that of a college senior, and limiting your statement to one page may seem difficult. However, you need not mention all of your accomplishments, experiences, or reasons for pursuing medicine. Choose your most impressive accomplishments, your most meaningful experiences, and your most compelling reasons for pursuing medicine (see page 34 for more advice on how to compose a good essay).

There are countless approaches to writing a personal statement. Becky wrote about learning. By focusing on a concept, she subtly brought up her relevant accomplishments and experiences and explained her motivation for wanting to go to medical school. During her career as a nurse, she learned a tremendous amount from doctors, other nurses, patients, and families. She loved applying her knowledge to her daily work and seeing her work pay off in the people she helped. However, she felt that her formal education did not enable her to really understand disease, treatments, and the healing process. Having worked closely with physicians, she understood that they didn't always know everything. She felt, however, that they had the tools to ask the right questions. Asking and answering questions, addressing problems and solving them, and observing others and analyzing their techniques are among the activities Becky looked forward to in medical school.

Eve concentrated on the doctor-patient relationship, discussing vivid memories of her own pediatrician and comparing the relationship she had with him to that of her children and their current pediatrician. She was able to elaborate on her accomplishment of raising three well-adjusted children, a feat that involved serving as caretaker, healer, friend, manager, teacher, advisor, and so on. Mitch described a few of his work experiences in Africa and Latin America, focusing on the ones that were most directly related to health care issues. He wrote that although he enjoyed working overseas, he felt that he would be able to contribute more as a physician than as a project manager. Jacob's prose included personal accounts of saving peoples' lives as a firefighter and how fulfilling he found that aspect of his work.

The secondary application may have general questions that allow you to elaborate on topics mentioned in the AMCAS essay. Some secondaries contain questions about particular experiences that you may have had, such as research, community service, or employment. Some questions focus on your values and personal experiences. Chapter 7 of this book includes a profile of each allopathic medical school. In the "Application Process" section of each description, we give the percentage of AMCAS applicants who generally receive secondaries. Some schools send secondary applications to a very limited number of applicants, and receiving a secondary from these schools means that you made it through a significant screening.

All schools limit the number of applicants they interview. If you have been invited to interview, it is a sign that you are a competitive applicant and you should be pleased. If you receive several interview invitations, the odds are that you will get into medical school. Nontraditional applicants who have interesting life experiences have an advantage in interviews because there is more to talk about than college courses or summer jobs: In addition, you may have had more experience interviewing for jobs and other educational programs than a college student. Hopefully, this will allow you to be more relaxed during the interview process.

In writing a personal statement, you can edit, rewrite, rethink, and start over. In an interview, you don't have this luxury. Being relaxed is important, but so is being prepared. Interviewers may ask about courses you have taken. Before going into an interview, review your academic transcripts. Which courses were your favorites? Your least favorite? Why? How do your preferences relate to your desire to go to medical school? If there are any particularly low or high grades, be prepared to discuss what went on in those classes. Review your AMCAS and secondary applications. Be sure that you can discuss every experience you have listed or discussed. Think of some sort of interesting, impressive, (tastefully) funny, or meaningful comment for each experience. Be prepared to answer questions about your childhood. What aspect of yourself do you really hate talking about? Be ready to talk about it or figure out a good way to divert the conversation from it. What (of relevance) do you know about and enjoy talking about? Think about ways to introduce this subject into your interview.

Although most interviews are one-on-one, some schools use panels of more than one interviewer. Some schools offer group interviews where you interview alongside other applicants. Interviewers may be faculty members, administrators, medical students, or members of the community. Older applicants may find that interviewing with current students, who could be somewhat younger, is challenging. An important part of being a physician is the ability to communicate and to get along with all types of people in all types of positions. The interview is an opportunity to demonstrate your skills in this area.

There are predictable interview questions, such as, "Why do you want to go to medical school?" Others are much less predictable and may even be surprising or shocking. You may be asked about your strategy for balancing personal/family life and medical school or whether you intend to have children. These questions might seem to be inappropriate, particularly to women. However you choose to answer such questions, it is probably best *not* to get defensive. It is reasonable to have concerns about these issues. Tina found that she got a good response when she turned the questions around and asked the interviewer whether *he* felt being a medical student/resident/physician was stressful on a marriage and what *he* felt about having children while in medical school. For more advice on interviewing techniques, turn to Chapter 6.

CHOOSING YOUR MEDICAL SCHOOL

Due to the intense competition in medical school admissions, most premedical advisors recommend that applicants apply to at least 10 schools. Some applicants, particularly those from states with competitive state-affiliated medical schools and whose grades and test scores are below average, should apply to 30 or more schools. In deciding which and how many schools to apply to, it is valuable to talk to a premedical advisor. They will help you determine how strong your application is.

The average MCAT scores of students at a particular school are an indicator of how difficult it is to get in. Be sure to apply to a few safety schools to which you have a better chance of being admitted. Medical school admission and rejection decisions don't always make sense. Donald was accepted to some of the most prestigious schools in the country, but not to his own state school. This element of chance is one reason it's better to apply to a number of schools and not to set your hopes on a single school.

For legal reasons, most schools claim that "age is not a factor in admissions." One way to evaluate a school's attitude toward nontraditional students is to look at its student body. Are there a significant number of nontraditional students? What is the average age of incoming students, and what is the age range? Typically, a school's student body reflects its applicant pool, and some schools with fewer nontraditional students simply have fewer nontraditional applicants. If a school that interests you has few nontraditional students, you may want to ask why. It is possible that the school is looking to diversify its student population and will be particularly interested in your application. Medical schools that have arrangements with postbacc programs are clearly interested in nontraditional students. You should explore them carefully.

Some people argue that all the medical schools in the United States are very good and that there is no particular reason to aspire toward a "top" school. An important difference between medical school and many other graduate or professional degree programs is that medical training does not end at graduation. Rather, a physician's formal education continues during internship, residency, and possibly into fellowship experiences. In terms of job opportunities, where you do your residency could be more important than where you go to school. While attending a well-reputed school will help in residency placement, doing well at a lesser-known school will also allow you to secure a desirable residency. On the other hand, an advantage to attending a well-reputed school is the comfort of knowing that you don't necessarily have to graduate at the top of the class in order to be competitive after graduation.

For those who want to practice strictly clinical medicine, there are factors to consider that may be as important as, if not more important, than a school's general reputation, which is often based largely on the research associated with the institution. When evaluating the training you will receive, some of the issues to consider are the school's location, the patient population to which students are exposed, the extent to which first- and second-year students learn clinical medicine, the format of the basic science curriculum,[13] interdisciplinary aspects of the curriculum,[14] the learning resources available to students, the school's role in the community and as a health care provider, the emphasis on primary care, the grading system, and the accessibility of faculty. Even if you are uninterested in a career in medical research, there are educational benefits to becoming involved in research efforts while in medical school, and you may be interested in schools that facilitate faculty/student collaboration and encourage student participation in research.

Rather than focusing on prestige or a published ranking,[15] concentrate on what you want from a school. Among other features, Mitch wanted access to a school of public health so that he could continue working in public and international health issues. Eve looked for schools that devoted significant resources to primary care. Donald looked for more structured programs, while Becky was interested in programs that allowed flexibility. Jacob applied primarily to schools with strong reputations for emergency medicine. Bob hoped to continue teaching part-time or during summers while in school. He looked for schools that would allow this.

Beyond academic features, there are lifestyle issues to consider that may be quite different from those faced by recent college graduates. In college, Mitch enjoyed being part of a cohesive student body at a small, remote, private school. As a 30-year-old who had spent significant time overseas, he wanted to live in a more multicultural environment. He hoped to have a social life that, to some degree, involved people other than his medical school classmates. Most of the schools he applied to were either in urban areas or were closely associated with a larger university. Tina wanted to remain near her boyfriend and decided to limit her applications to schools in the region of the country where he was studying. Because of her family, Eve had location issues as well. As a nontraditional student, you are likely to have more responsibilities and complexities in your life than a recent college graduate. As a result, you may find that lifestyle issues play a more important role in determining where you apply and where you go to school.

The day of your interview affords a rare opportunity to hear firsthand what it is like to be a student at a particular medical school. During the course of the day, you will probably speak with current students, either formally or informally. Ask the students you meet for the names of nontraditional students within the class. If you have a spouse and/or children, ask for the names of students in similar situations. While interviewing, you will be focused on making a good impression and getting in. Later, however, you might have some choices to make and you may be desperately trying to differentiate one school from the next. Input from current students, particularly those with backgrounds similar to your own, will be invaluable (for more advice on how to choose a school, turn to page 40).

[13] Some schools use lectures and labs while others have an entirely case-based approach. A number of schools fall somewhere in the middle, incorporating some of each educational methodology. There is no evidence that a particular curriculum is "best." You need to consider your own learning style.

[14] Presumably, nontraditional students bring an interdisciplinary perspective and benefit from this approach.

[15] There is no definitive ranking. *U.S. News & World Report* publishes a yearly report ranking graduate schools. Be sure to understand the methodology used when reading their findings.

FINANCIAL ISSUES

The cost of a medical education is daunting for traditional and nontraditional students alike. With the exception of those who have accrued savings in former careers, financing medical school as a nontraditional student involves challenges. Nontraditional students often have higher living expenses associated with off-campus housing, dependents, debt, and other financial responsibilities. With few exceptions, financial aid offices will look at your parents' income and assets in determining assistance packages. This applies to all students, regardless of their age and whether they themselves are parents. If you are married, medical schools will expect your spouse to contribute to the extent that he or she can. If your parents and/or spouse are less than thrilled about supporting you in this endeavor, financial questions can translate to personal/emotional issues. Older medical students will have less time in the workforce to pay off educational debt, and it is unclear whether financial aid offices consider this in making awards (for more information on financial issues, turn to Chapter 5).

You should carefully consider the financial implications of going to medical school and try to come up with a strategy for dealing with them. If your heart is set on going, financial issues alone should probably not stop you. When deciding where to apply, add to your list of considerations the average debt of graduating students. Even if this figure is not published, financial aid offices will probably provide it if you ask. Look very closely at your state-affiliated medical school because in-state tuition is typically much less than private school costs. Ask financial aid offices about loan repayment programs. Think about ways to trim your budget, such as living with relatives or giving up your car. The material possessions you forego now, and the loan payments you make in the future, should be weighed against the value of having a truly fulfilling career.

5 Financing Medical School

HOW MUCH IS ALL OF THIS GOING TO COST?

There's no doubt that med school is expensive. The average first-year tuition for a U.S. private medical school is upwards of $39,000, and the average tuition at public schools is upwards of $20,000 for in-state residents. When planning for the cost of attending medical school, however, tuition is only part of the picture. You must also pay for books, equipment, housing, utilities, food, insurance, transportation, and miscellaneous costs. All of these expenses add up quickly; depending on where you attend school, they may equal or exceed the price of tuition and can add up to an additional $20,000. Note that tuition is 30 percent higher during second and third years to cover the cost of year-round education.

The cost of a medical education is daunting, but once in practice, physicians are among the most highly paid professionals. In recent years, the difference in pay across specialties has made it difficult to assess physician pay as an overall average. The many options available to current doctors in the way they practice have further complicated this analysis. While all doctors may look forward to earning a comfortable salary, some will be better compensated than others. For example, in 2008 a typical family practitioner made $186,000, while the average for all specialists was close to $340,000. Although it will be years before today's first-year students make that kind of money, they can assume the financial burden of their education with the confidence that they will one day make enough money to justify the investment.

AND HOW CAN I PAY FOR IT?

Since the medical student of today will be the well-paid physician of tomorrow, medical schools expect the students and their families to be responsible for the cost of their education. Except in cases in which a student has exceptional financial resources, it is essential to rely on outside sources of financial assistance to pay the bill.

FINANCIAL AID PROGRAMS

There are two general types of financial assistance available: loans and scholarships/grants. Loans must be repaid and have varying interest rates, deferment options, and repayment periods. Many subsidized loans will be available to you only if you have documented need, while other funds are available regardless of your financial situation. Most medical students borrow heavily, relying on the prospect of a generous salary once they begin practice. For 2010 med school graduates, the average debt was $157,990 for students from private schools, and by all indications, these amounts will continue to increase. Scholarships and grants are gifts that need not be repaid. They can be awarded on the basis of several factors—financial need, outstanding academic merit, specific criteria such as gender, or a promise of future service—or a combination of those factors. Note that the financial aid offices of the schools you are accepted to should provide you with a package that covers all costs somehow. The question is how much of the package comes from you or your parents or from high-interest loans.

Loans

Anyone with good credit can borrow enough money to finance a medical education. Borrowing is simplified if you take advantage of federal lending programs. Qualifications are as follows:

- American citizenship or permanent U.S. resident status.

- If you are a male 18 years of age or older, you are registered for Selective Service, or you have documentation proving that you are not required to register.

- You have a good credit history, including good standing on prior student loans.

- You are an active, enrolled student in good academic standing.

If you have financial resources that disqualify you for some types of need-based aid, but you meet the above requirements, you are still eligible for federal loans (unsubsidized and private loans). The loans for which you qualify may have higher interest rates and offer less favorable repayment schedules than the subsidized loans that are aimed at those with financial need.

Following is a description of five basic types of loans: federal, state, private, charitable, and institutional.

Federal

Federal loan programs are funded by the federal government or are funded by banks and guaranteed by the federal government. Federal loans, particularly the Stafford Loan, are usually the "first resort" for medical student borrowers. Some federal loans such as Perkins or Stafford subsidized loans are need-based, but some higher-interest loans are available to students or their families regardless of financial circumstance.

State

Students who are residents of the state in which they attend medical school may be eligible for state loan programs. Eligibility is often based on need and may be further tied to specific segments of the population (e.g., minority or disadvantaged students, or students who are interested in practicing family medicine in underserved areas of the state). Individual schools can provide you with information about state loan programs.

Private

Privately funded, commercial loans are available from banks and other financial institutions. It is important to research your options intensely because you will want to fully understand the interest that you will accrue as well as the repayment terms before signing on the dotted line.

Charitable

Charity loans are funded by contributions from foundations, corporations, and associations. A number of private loans are targeted to aid particular segments of the population (e.g., minority or disadvantaged students, women, or students who are interested in practicing family medicine in underserved areas of the state). You may have to investigate to identify all of the charitable loans for which you qualify. The best place to begin your search is in public, undergraduate, and med school libraries. There are also a number of commercial financial aid search services available, but beware—financial aid officers warn that search services sometimes charge hefty fees for information that, in the majority of cases, students can obtain themselves. Private financial aid resources are also available online. Visit the Financial Center at PrincetonReview.com to get information on many of them.

Institutional

The amount of loan money available, and the method by which it is disbursed, varies greatly from one school to another. As part of the shift toward emphasizing primary care, some schools offer assistance to students who are committed to providing primary care after graduation. To find out about the resources available at a particular school, refer to its catalog or contact its Financial Aid Office.

In the chart on pages 70 and 71, we have compiled a table of the most commonly used loan programs. Included in this table is information about the characteristics of each loan. The following characteristics are discussed:

Name: The full name of the loan and the acronym, if applicable, by which it is most commonly known.

Source: Information about the organization that funds and administers each loan.

Eligibility: Whether the loans are need-based. Others are open to people regardless of their financial situation. A few federal and private schools require that a student fit a specific demographic profile. Note that regardless of your age or how long you have been independent of your parents, their income is considered in calculating your need in almost all cases.

TABLE OF LOANS

NAME OF LOAN	SOURCE	ELIGIBILITY	MAXIMUM ALLOCATION
Federal Stafford Unsubsidized Loan Studentaid.ed.gov/students/publications/student_guide/index.html	Federal, administered by school		The total Stafford loan limit is $20,500. The maximum aggregate total of Stafford loans is $138,500, including undergraduate loans.
Health Professions Student Loan/Primary Care Loan (HPSL) Contact school for more information	Federal, administered by school	Exceptional financial need; commitment to primary care	For first- and second-year students, the maximum allocation is the cost of attendance (including tuition, educational expenses, and reasonable living expenses). Third and fourth-year students may receive allocations beyond this amount.
Federal PLUS Loans	Federal, administered by school	Not need-based.	The maximum allocation is the cost of attendance (including tuition, educational expenses, and reasonable living expenses as determined by the school).
Perkins Loan (formerly NDSL) Contact school for more information	Federal, administered by school	Exceptional financial need.	$8,000/year, with aggregate of $60,000. Aggregate amount includes undergraduate loans.

TABLE OF LOANS (continued)	
REPAYMENT AND DEFERRAL OPTIONS	**INTEREST RATE**
10–30 years to repay. Interest begins to accrue from day loan is disbursed; you can pay the interest or have it capitalized (added to the principal). Begin repayment 6 months after graduation.	Fixed, 6.8%
10–30 years to repay. Interest begins to accrue from day loan is disbursed; you can pay the interest or have it capitalized (added to principal). Begin repayment 6 months after graduation. Forbearance possible for up to 3 years of residency training.	Fixed, 5%
10 years to repay, beginning 1 year after graduation. Deferrable during residency and under special circumstances.	Fixed, 7.9%.
10 years to repay. Begin repayment 9 months after graduation.	Fixed, 5%.

Maximum Allocation: The maximum amount of money you can borrow from any one program. Many medical students find it necessary to borrow from more than one source. Most loans have both maximum yearly and aggregate loan amounts. Amounts you borrowed from the same loan program for your college education are deducted, in some cases, from the aggregate amount you can borrow in medical school.

Repayment and Deferral Options: Information about the repayment period and deferral options for each loan. Important considerations in structuring your educational debt are how long you have to pay back loans and whether principal and/or interest may be deferred until you have completed your education. It is important to remember that, no matter what the source of a loan, the responsibility for keeping track of loan activity is yours.

Interest Rate: Information about the current interest rate of the loan. Fixed-rate loans use the same interest rate throughout the life of the loan. Variable-rate loans base their interest rate on established financial values, usually 91-day Treasury Bills (T-Bills) or the prime lending rate. Since these rates fluctuate greatly, you should check with a bank to find out the exact interest rate.

Pros: Factors that make this an attractive loan source. Attractive features include long repayment terms, deferral policies that waive interest and principal throughout medical school and all or part of residency training, and low, fixed-rate interest.

Cons: Factors that make a particular loan unattractive. Such features include short repayment times, limited deferral options, or variable, high-interest rates.

Scholarships/Grants

Some grant, or gift money, comes with no strings attached; these are nonobligatory scholarships. Although such scholarships may be available on the basis of outstanding academic merit alone, others are based on a combination of merit and need. In fact, all federal, nonobligatory scholarships are based on need and may also require that you fit a particular demographic profile. Scholarship amounts vary, and they are administered by the same groups as loans: federal and state governments, private foundations, and institutions. For more information about private, state, and institutional scholarships, contact the financial aid offices at some of the schools to which you are going to apply, or visit the Scholarships & Aid section of PrincetonReview.com.

Obligatory Scholarships

Some federal scholarships are available to students who agree to practice at the Public Health Service, at the Veterans Administration, or in the Armed Forces. These scholarships provide full tuition, some or all expenses, and a monthly stipend. Service-based scholarships, which are not based on need, all carry an obligation to serve at least one year for every year of support.

TABLE OF GRANTS				
NAME OF GRANT	**SOURCE**	**ELIGIBILITY**	**SERVICE OF OBLIGATION**	**AMOUNT OF GRANT**
National Health Service Corps (NHSC)	Federal	Need-based; former EFN recipients and students with interest in primary care are preferred.	Two- to four-year contract. Years spent in residency do not count toward fulfilling obligation.	Maximum amount is full tuition and fees plus stipend.
National Medical Fellowship Scholarship (NMF)	Private	First- or second-year underrepresented minority, female, rural, or disadvantaged background with documented financial need.	None	Varies. Awards have ranged from $500–$10,000.
Scholarships for Disadvantaged Students (SDS)	Federal, administered through school	Full-time, financially needy students from disadvantaged backgrounds, enrolled in health professions and nursing programs. U.S. citizens only.	None	Varies; tuition and other educational expenses.
Armed For Health Professions Scholarship Program (HPSP)	U.S. Army, U.S. Navy, and U.S. Air Force	Able to serve in military; age restrictions; U.S. citizens only.	One year for every year of support. Years spent in residency do not count toward fulfilling obligation.	Full tuition, "reasonable" fees, and stipend. Student becomes officer in service branch upon matriculation and receives all benefits of rank.

The advantage—a "free" medical education—is obvious, but this is not an option to take lightly. Time spent in residency—which is often restricted to only military residencies—does not count toward your service debt, so you may be out of medical school for 7 to 12 years before you're free of your obligation. Some states and counties also offer service-based scholarship programs or tuition remission programs. Despite their lengthy obligations, service-based scholarships are in high demand. To increase your chances of obtaining one, apply as early as possible. Ask the financial aid offices of schools in which you are interested whom to contact locally for more information. There are also loan repayment programs available to which you apply after you have accrued debt and when you are ready to start working in an underserved area.

THE FINANCIAL AID PROCESS

PREPARING TO APPLY

Many students miss out on potential assistance by making some basic, avoidable mistakes. Top financial aid officers supplied the following common errors and their remedies.

Missing Deadlines and Keeping Poor Records

Like your applications for admission, your financial aid applications should be submitted as early as possible. File your income tax forms early and encourage your parents (all med students are considered dependent by med schools, even if they have been independent for years) to do the same. Photocopy all forms that you submit and note the date you send them. File these forms along with any material related to the decisions of the financial aid committees of the schools to which you apply. Keep careful track of deadlines, which are strongly enforced.

Submitting Information to the Wrong Needs Analysis Service

There are several third-party organizations that assist medical schools in determining the financial need of entering and continuing students. Many applicants assume that because they have submitted information to one of the services for one school, they have done everything they need to do for all the schools they are considering. Making this assumption can have serious repercussions. Until the proper service completes the needs analysis, the financial aid office cannot package your financial aid. To avoid making this mistake, check with the financial aid offices of all the schools to which you are applying to see which service they use. Submit the proper materials to the appropriate service. More detailed information on the needs analysis services and their function can be found under Calculating Your Expected Family Contribution.

Having a Poor Credit History

People are often unpleasantly surprised when they see their credit histories. Even relatively minor financial problems, like making a couple of late payments on loans or credit cards, can lower your credit rating. Also, credit bureaus sometimes make mistakes, causing negative, but false, information to show up on your record. Since a bad credit history will make you ineligible for many, if not all, loan programs, it is a good idea to check your credit history before you apply for financial aid. Recent federal legislation has made it possible to get a copy of your credit report free of charge once a year from any of the major credit bureaus. You can visit them online at Equifax.com, Experian.com, or TransUnion.com to obtain a copy of your free report.

Defaulting on Undergraduate Student Loans

If you have not kept up with your student loan payments, you will have a very hard time qualifying for loans, especially those funded by the federal government. Clear up any problems with prior student loans well before applying for additional assistance. If you are still in school and have not yet begun repaying your loans, talk to your undergraduate Financial Aid Officer to clarify repayment and deferral options on your loans. Remember that the burden of keeping track of your loan activity is on you, and that once you start medical school, you must keep the lenders apprised of your whereabouts.

APPLYING FOR AID

Schools' policies may vary somewhat, but they all follow the same general lines. To determine whether you qualify and for how much, schools must first determine how much it will cost for you to attend, and then how much of that cost you and your family can absorb.

HOW SCHOOLS DETERMINE THEIR COST

Each medical school prepares a student budget that reflects the expenses associated with being a first-year medical student. Included in this budget are items such as tuition and fees, books, equipment, housing, utilities, food, insurance, transportation, and personal expenses. To some degree, schools customize expenses if a student has particular needs. For example, projected costs may increase if you live off campus.

CALCULATING YOUR CONTRIBUTION

To determine how much you and your family can contribute, medical schools use a needs analysis service. Refer to the financial aid guidelines of the schools you are considering attending. Some schools use more than one service to calculate need, and many ultimately use their own formulas to determine institutional assistance. To make sure you have all the information required to fill out the forms completely, file your previous year's income tax returns early. Because some federal loan programs and some institutions require parental information even from independent or married students, your parents should also file their income tax forms as early as possible.

On the basis of the information you give them, the needs analysis calculates your financial need by subtracting your expected personal and family contribution from the total student budget furnished by the school. If expenses are higher than the estimated contribution, you show financial need.

YOUR TENTATIVE FINANCIAL AID PACKAGE

Most schools will prepare a financial aid package for accepted students only. Once you have been accepted to a school, be on the lookout for a financial aid package. The package can include loans, scholarships, grants, or a combination of these elements. If financial aid is an important consideration in deciding between schools, be sure that you have estimates from all schools by the applicant decision deadline.

ACCEPTING YOUR FINANCIAL AID PACKAGE

Once you matriculate at a school, the Financial Aid Office will put together your actual financial aid package. In most cases, loans will make up a portion of the package. Remember, loans must be repaid—with interest—and the amount of this debt will affect your lifestyle far beyond medical school and residency. For instance, if you borrow a large sum of money for medical school, you may have trouble later obtaining a loan for a large purchase like a car or a house. You are not required to accept all the aid you are offered, so it is in your best interest to borrow only what you need to meet your expenses.

CUTTING COSTS

Medical schools formulate their student budgets by using average expenses for everything except tuition. By making some adjustments to your lifestyle, it is usually possible to undercut this budget and therefore decrease the amount of money you borrow. Following are some strategies recommended by financial aid professionals to reduce debt.

BOOKS AND EQUIPMENT

Buy good-quality used textbooks and equipment whenever possible. Selling books and equipment you no longer need is a good way to earn extra cash.

TRANSPORTATION

Automobile loan payments, insurance premiums, licensing fees, fuel, and maintenance really add up. Evaluate your need for a car before taking one to medical school. If you attend school in a place where public transportation is available or where you can bike or walk to school, leave the car behind. If you must have a car, you can save by raising insurance deductibles and carpooling with fellow students.

INSURANCE

Most medical schools require you to carry medical and, in some cases, disability insurance. Before you buy into the school's plan, check your existing coverage. If your parents still claim you as a dependent, or if you have a spouse whose medical benefits extend to you, you may already have adequate coverage.

OTHER EXPENSES

Millions of Americans find themselves in dire financial straits each year because of revolving credit. Medical students are no exception. If you find that you have trouble avoiding the temptation to pull out the plastic for purchases you can't afford, cut up your cards. Remember, if you can't afford to pay for something with cash or a check, you probably can't afford to charge it either. To keep discretionary expenses from getting out of hand, set up a detailed budget and stick to it. If you've never used a budget before and need help, there are many computer programs that will help you set up a budget, track expenses, and give you reports on how you're doing.

A FINAL WORD

YOUR FINANCIAL AID RIGHTS

- You have the right to expect that the Financial Aid Office will assist you in obtaining financial aid and information about financial aid opportunities.

- Financial Aid Officers to whom you give information about your/your family's financial profile cannot publicize this information.

- You have the right to accept or decline all or part of the aid offered.

- You have the right to appeal your financial aid package if your financial aid picture changes for the worse. (This does not necessarily mean, however, that the amount of aid will increase.)

- You have the right to examine your financial aid file at any time.

- You are entitled to treatment that does not discriminate on the basis of race, creed, age, handicap, gender, or national origin.

YOUR FINANCIAL AID RESPONSIBILITIES

- You are responsible for meeting the expenses related to attending medical school.

- You are responsible for reading and understanding the conditions and terms of all of the elements in your financial aid package.

- You are responsible for submitting financial aid applications on time.

- You are responsible for obtaining and filling out financial aid forms and supplying accurate and complete information on these forms.

- You are responsible for reporting to your Financial Aid Office any outside scholarships or loans that may affect your amount of need.

- You are responsible for using loan funds to pay tuition.

- You are responsible for repaying all loans.

- You are responsible for notifying all lenders of all changes of address during and after medical school.

- You are responsible for keeping accurate and complete records of all financial aid applications and transactions.

6 The Interview:

Separating the Merely Qualified from the Truly Worthy

Be proud if you're invited to an interview. You've made it through two initial screenings, one before and one after the supplemental application. Usually, this means that the Admissions Committee thinks you're qualified to attend their school. Unfortunately, they also invite a lot of other qualified people, and they don't have space to admit all of you. Therefore, your objective is to convince everyone who interviews you that the school would be a better place with you in it. Easy to say, a little harder to do. It is important to realize that the weight of the interview varies from school to school. At some schools it is the key to admission, while at others it is mainly a formality—more for you than for them.

Because almost everyone has heard horror stories about someone else's interview, most people start to worry about the interview before they even submit their applications. Try to relax. A good interview begins with good preparation. You can start by becoming familiar with the interview process.

WHO CONDUCTS INTERVIEWS?

Different schools have different policies about who conducts the actual interview. In general, schools have a Medical Selection Committee made up of professional admissions or student affairs people and faculty members. Often, especially in more progressive schools, upper-level med students also participate. At some schools, you'll have a couple of separate, one-on-one interviews; at others, you'll be interviewed by a panel. You may be the only applicant in front of a panel (this really seems more like an inquisition), or you may be joined by other candidates.

At many schools, the person or people you speak with become your advocates in the final selection process. When all the interviews in a certain time period are finished and the selection committee meets, these people share their observations about you and sometimes recommend a particular action. The final decision, of course, is up to the entire committee.

WHAT CAN I EXPECT?

Expect some interviews to go well and others to go poorly. In the vast majority of cases, the interviewers are trying to build an honest picture of you beyond the numbers, and most try to reduce stress during the interviews. Despite this, you will probably experience one or two bad interviews with interviewers who have not read your file and therefore seem disinterested, are insecure or awkward themselves, or are simply having a bad day. Keep this in mind as your interview dates approach.

HOW SHOULD I ACT?

The golden rule for interviews is "be yourself." Interviewers have been through all of this before, and they're pretty good at spotting people who are putting on an act or reading from a mental script. What they're trying to find out from this interview is what kind of person you are and how you relate to others. Up until now, you've been only a few sheets of paper, a bunch of numbers, and a (probably horrible) photograph. Now's the time to show them your stuff. But remember: no lying and no BS.

BE PREPARED

You should be ready to answer questions about your motivation to become a physician, your academic background, your extracurricular and leisure activities, your job or research experience, and your views on medical problems and ethical issues. Later in this chapter is a sample of questions that current medical students were asked in their interviews. Some of them are typical; others are truly strange. As you get ready to interview, try to answer some of these questions on your own, and then ask a friend, parent, or professor to grill you. In addition, you may want to audio or video record mock interviews to see how you sound and look. When you choose a guinea pig to be your surrogate interviewer, select someone who will be honest with you about the strengths and weaknesses of your responses. Don't try to memorize answers word for word; canned responses, no matter how valid, are stiff and unconvincing (just look at a video of a presidential debate). It is a good idea, however, to enter an interview with several anecdotes or points in mind. Questions are often open-ended, giving you the chance to direct the conversation toward your strengths and away from your weaknesses.

APPROACH WITH CONFIDENCE

Like dogs, interviewers seem to smell fear. The tone of your interview is often set in the first few seconds, so approach with confidence. Greet your interviewer with a firm handshake and look him or her in the eye. During the interview, be positive. Think of it as a pleasant conversation with someone you'd like to get to know better. A good interview is a dialogue, where there is considerable give and take. Unless your interviewer brings them up, avoid controversial or emotionally charged subjects like abortion. If you're asked your views, state them and move on.

TAKE YOUR TIME

In the course of your interviews, you may be asked scores of questions, some on issues to which you haven't given a great deal of thought. Your interviewers don't expect you to have a ready answer for every one of these questions, but they do expect you to come up with a coherent, well-thought-out response. Many applicants are afraid that if they hesitate, it will seem that they are unprepared. Not so. Good physicians don't rush to a conclusion without considering the facts; rather, they think through a problem before they decide how to act. If a question catches you off guard, take a second to think it through. If it seems ambiguous, don't be afraid to ask for clarification. If you don't know, admit it and ask the interviewer to share the answer. By taking the time to make sure that your response is well conceived and well spoken, you will impress the interviewers as thoughtful and articulate—two characteristics essential in a good doctor.

ASK QUESTIONS

Although the interview is the time for medical schools to find out about you, it is also an excellent opportunity for you to find out more about the school. Before you go to an interview, make sure you've studied the school's information packet and are ready to ask intelligent questions about the program. Search the archives at your undergraduate or public library to see if the school has been in the news and, if so, for what. Remember that most people love to talk about themselves. Ask the interviewer about his work or impressions of the curriculum.

BE ON TIME

Make sure that you get detailed directions before you make the trip and arrive with enough time to park and find the office. If you are invited to interview at several schools in the same geographic region, you might save on travel costs and time by making an interview circuit, visiting several schools on the same trip. This can mean that you have several interviews in the same week or even the same day. Give yourself as much time as possible at each, so that you have time to make the transition, both physically and mentally, from one school to the next. If you can, try to get to each campus early enough to walk around, talk to students, and formulate questions that are specific to the school.

DRESS FOR SUCCESS

Like it or not, looks count. No matter what your usual mode of dress, you should dress conservatively and professionally for your interviews. For men, this means a suit or a blazer and nice pants (and, of course, a tie); for women, a suit, blazer and skirt or dress pants, or a business-style dress is appropriate. Regardless of your gender, pay attention to detail; even the most beautiful suit looks shabby if your shoes are scuffed and worn, and the effect of a great-looking blazer is ruined by a ragged backpack. Polish your shoes, invest in a nice portfolio or case for your papers, and by all means, iron your clothes. If you are generally somewhat less than conservative in your dress, you may want to tone it down: men, replace the big hoop earring with a stud; women, take off the gold glitter polish and paint on clear. After all, you don't want to be asked, as one of the respondents to our survey was, "Why are you dressed the way you are? Why did you come here looking the way you do?"

CONDUCT YOURSELF PROFESSIONALLY

Admissions committees can see from your application that you are smart, accomplished, and highly regarded by your professors. The interview is an opportunity for them to gauge things that are not so easily conveyed on paper. Medical schools are looking for students with maturity, empathy, and superior interpersonal skills. All of these things come through in the interview. In a group setting, where the committee talks with more than one candidate at a time, you will be observed not only when you answer a question, but also when your fellow applicants are speaking. Keep alert, and show interest. After all, you never know what you may learn that you can use in your next interview.

HOW AND WHEN TO FOLLOW UP ON YOUR INTERVIEWS

First, don't forget to send a thank-you note after each set of interviews. You can write several different notes to each of your interviewers, or send just one addressed generally to the interview committee. Don't write a novella in your thank-you note. It's fine to mention a particular question or topic you found interesting during your interview, but you should limit yourself to only a few lines. As you might have guessed, it's a good idea to take a few brief notes, such as the interviewer's names and some of the topics they covered, right after you leave the interview. For the thank-you notes themselves, you can use any nice stationery paper.

If the school is not entirely certain of the strength of your application relative to other candidates after your interviews, you may be placed on a hold list. Don't despair. You made it as far as the interview process, which (except in the case of some public schools who interview every candidate) means that you have survived some of the initial cuts. Sometimes being put on hold simply means that the school has already accepted enough students that month. You can, however, send supplementary information to further support your application. For example, if you have been doing research, volunteer work, or taking classes that didn't appear on your initial application, and if you didn't get a chance to talk about your new activities during the interview, you can write a short—less than one page—letter outlining your recent accomplishments and send it to the school. This shows that you are still working hard to better your chances of acceptance into medical school.

WHAT ARE THEY GOING TO ASK?

The sample interview questions in this section come from various sources. Although the following list of questions is by no means exhaustive, it is a good sampling of questions that were asked in real interviews in the recent past. Get ready, because while some of the questions are pretty standard, others are truly bizarre.

SO YOU WANT TO BE A DOCTOR?

Some students are often unprepared for questions like the ones that follow, thinking them so mundane that they wouldn't be asked. However, if you're granted even one interview, you're almost sure to be asked several questions about your motivation and suitability for medical school.

- Why do you want to be a doctor?

- The future of medicine looks bleak. Why do you want to go into it?

- What articles have you read recently that relate to the reasons you want to become a doctor?

- What do you see yourself doing with a medical degree?

- Were you influenced by relatives to pursue a career in medicine?

- Why do you want to attend [name of school]?

- Why should we accept you?

- How are your accomplishments better than those of the other candidates in this interview?

- Evaluate yourself based on the required evaluation of the interviewer.

- Do you think you are motivated enough for medical school?

- When you don't get into medical school, what will you do?

- What career path would you follow if all the medical schools closed today?

- You've taken an odd, nontraditional path to get here. Why are you interested in medicine?

- What disadvantages do you see in being an older student?

- Can you afford to come here?

- How will you finance your medical education?

- Describe what you believe to be the financial rewards of medicine.

- If doctors were paid a teacher's salary, would you still want to be a doctor?

TELL ME A LITTLE BIT ABOUT YOURSELF . . .

Selection committees use the interview as an opportunity to find out what makes you tick. Prepare yourself for personal questions about your character traits, your coping mechanisms, and your life experiences. You may also be asked to comment on your interpersonal relationships. Always be honest.

- What is your worst quality?

- If you could change anything about yourself, what would it be?

- Are you aggressive?

- What makes you a fun person?

- What makes you angry?

- What makes you sad?

- What scares you?

- Do you like sick people?

- Are you afraid of death?

- What are you the most proud of?

- One of the people who wrote a letter of recommendation for you described you as [adjective]. Do you agree with that description?

- Was there a time in your life when you had tremendous responsibility?

- What is the wackiest thing you've ever done?

- What was the biggest mistake you ever made?

- What is the worst thing that has happened to you in the past four years?

- Tell me something you wanted to achieve but did not, or something you've failed at. How did you cope with failure?

- What role has stress played in your life?

- How could you prove to me that you can perform well under stress?

- What do you do to alleviate stress?

- Tell me about your family.

- What role do you play in your family dynamic?

- How is your relationship with your parents?

- What is the physical health of your parents, and how would you handle an illness of theirs while attending school?

- Who is the person in the world to whom you are closest?

- Describe your best friend.

- What does your closest friend think about your relationship with him or her?

- Give one word that a friend would use to describe you.

It's All Academic

Grades, MCAT scores, and courses are fair game for the inquisitive interviewer. You may be asked to explain your performance in a course or to tell what you learned. A hint: To be better prepared for questions of this type, get a copy of your transcript and take a look at it. Look for things that might cause an interviewer to ask a question. Lower-than-normal grades stick out, as do courses with funny names (like Rocks for Jocks). Then again, be honest.

- What do you think of the GPA as a valid method of categorizing students?

- Why were your first-year grades so bad?

- Why do you have so many C grades on your transcript?

- Explain your low math grade.

- Why are your grades high compared to your MCAT scores?

- Do you realize that your MCAT scores aren't anything special?

- Tell me about your research.

- Have you taken any humanities classes, and what papers did you write in them?

- What did you learn in [name of course]? (It's worth noting that some people were asked about normal courses like "Philosophy 101" and others were asked about bizarre courses like "The Art of Murder," "Fairy Tales," and "Play, Games, Toys, and Sports.")

- Who was the author of your biochemistry textbook?

Extra, Extra, Read All About It!

Whatever your extracurricular activities and work experiences, you will most likely be asked how they relate to your commitment to and preparedness for studying medicine. Think about your extracurricular experiences and what you learned about yourself, the medical field, and/or working with people as a result of participating in these activities. If you've been out of school for a while and have worked extensively in another field, be ready for questions about why you decided to change fields. Scientific or medical research experience is a plus, but it can be a real liability if you're not able to discuss it in detail.

- What are your hobbies?

- How does your hobby relate to being a doctor?

- Have you taught yourself to do anything, and if so, what?

- How has working as a [name of job] made you a better candidate for medical school?

- What volunteer work contributed to your commitment to become a doctor?

- What did you do with your job earnings?

MEDICAL ISSUES AND ETHICS: WHERE DO YOU STAND?

Interviewers love to ask students about a medical issue or about an ethical dilemma related to medicine. In general, there are no wrong answers to these questions. You should know the terminology (for example, the difference between euthanasia and euthenics) and be aware of some pros and cons for each of these issues. Since the health care crisis and attendant problems in reforming the health care delivery system have been grabbing headlines, you should be prepared to discuss the issues intelligently. No one expects you to be an expert on this or any other issue, but you should do some research before your interviews. Don't be surprised if an interviewer challenges your view on an issue; usually, he or she is trying to see how well you support your argument.

- What is the greatest problem facing medicine today?

- What do you consider the most important thing medicine has done for humanity?

- What do you think will be the most significant scientific breakthrough in the next 10 years?

- If you could find a cure for AIDS or for cancer, which would you choose and why?

- If you were the U.S. Surgeon General, what is the first thing you would do?

- If you were the health commissioner of [a large city], what would you do?

- What is preventive medicine?

- What is the biggest problem family practitioners face?

- What are your views on euthanasia?

- What do you think about euthenics (not euthanasia)?

- What would you do about the alcoholism problem in this country?

- What do you think about condoms being distributed in high schools?

- What are your views on mandatory HIV testing for doctors and patients?

- Current AIDS education programs aren't working; what should we do?

- Why will organ rationing be the problem of the future in medicine?

- Should people have the right to sell their own organs?

- Do you think it's ethical to take the life of a fetus for a cell line to save the life of a sibling with cancer?

- Should we spend so much time and effort trying to keep premature infants alive?

- If a cure were invented for aging, what repercussions would it have on society in general and the medical profession in particular?

- How do you feel about animal research?

- What role should politics play in medicine?

- Is health care a right or a privilege?

- What is your opinion of socialized medicine?

- How would you organize health care in an ideal world?

- Discuss the health care system of Australia.

- What do you think should be done about patients who can't pay for treatment?

- What is the difference between Medicare and Medicaid?

- What is your opinion of HMOs and PPOs?

- How will you react to the death of your first patient?

- Who would you go to if your mom needed surgery: a surgeon with good hands and a bland personality or a surgeon with not as good hands with a great personality?

- How would you tell your best friend's wife (who is your patient) that she has cancer? What would you do if she then refused to tell her family?

- You have to amputate one of the legs of an eight-year-old child. How would you tell him?

- Would you give a transfusion to a child whose parents were Jehovah's Witnesses?

- If a Hindu, for example, comes in and refuses surgery on the basis of religion, and the surgery is his only hope, what would you do? What if the patient was this man or woman's child?

- If you diagnosed a patient with a terminal illness as having only two months to live and the family and the patient wanted to end the turmoil ("pull the plug"), would you allow it or strongly disagree?

- What would you do if you saw a bleeding child on the side of the road?

- What would you do if you had a female patient who was trying to conceive, and your colleague had that patient's husband, and the husband was HIV positive?

- If one of your colleagues refused to treat a patient with AIDS, how would you address that colleague?

- How would you react if a fellow medical student had AIDS and entered surgery with you?

- Would you let a surgeon with AIDS operate on you?

- Would you treat a white supremacist, and should physicians be forced to treat such a patient?

- If you made a mistake as a physician, how would you handle it?

To Choose or Not to Choose

Abortion is not only a hot political topic, it also seems to be a hot topic for interviews. Some schools are affiliated with hospitals where abortions are performed; some are not. Don't try to guess if the interviewer is hoping you will espouse a particular position; honesty seems the best policy on this issue. If you are asked about your willingness to perform an abortion (as a large number of those we surveyed were), you may want to mention that it is not only your beliefs but also the rules of the hospital or laws of the land that you must consider.

- What should a physician's role be in the politics of abortion?

- What would you do as a physician if you were asked to do something contrary to your stand on abortion?

- Would you perform an abortion for a teenager, and would you tell her parents?

- How would you justify being a Catholic and going to an institution that allows abortion?

Have You Heard the News?

Good doctors are aware of, and involved in, the world around them. You may be asked about current events, even things completely unrelated to medicine. The questions that follow are only examples; in most cases, these events are no longer current. To prepare for questions like these, keep up with what's happening. If you get most of your news from the television or radio, start reading newspapers and news magazines for more in-depth coverage.

- Who is the U.S. Secretary of State?

- What do you think about the political situation in Iraq and surrounding countries?

- Do you think the Israelis beat up on the Palestinians?

Philosophy 101

From the serious to the silly, questions interviewers ask can make you stop and think. (And for some of these questions, one of the things you might think is, "What does this have to do with med school?")

- What are the top five priorities of society?

- Do you see any parallels between medicine and the priesthood?

- What is Zen Buddhism?

- Explain Hinduism.

- Are you a racist?

- Do you believe that racism still exists?

- How do you feel about affirmative action?

- Would you move to Canada to avoid serving active duty during a military conflict abroad?

- What is your view on censorship in the arts?

- What would you do if you saw a classmate cheating on a test?

- Do you believe in drug legalization?

- Do you believe that volunteerism could help eliminate greed from society's social structure?

- Is altruism ever pure, without some kind of motive?

- Do you believe in life after death?

- What is your opinion about natural law ethics?

- Explain the mind-body problem.

- Are you a vertical or horizontal thinker?

- If you could be any cell in the human body, what would you be?

- If you were to build a human being, what would you include and exclude?

- Define hope.

TRIED AND TRUE

Some questions sound more like pickup lines than med school interview questions. Although none of those surveyed was asked, "What's your sign?" there were plenty of old favorites that you may as well be prepared for.

- Are you a person who thinks a glass is half empty or half full?

- If you could go back in history and meet anyone, who would it be and why?

- If you could talk to someone from the future, what would you ask him or her?

- If a genie were able to grant you three wishes, what would they be?

- If you were stranded on a desert island, what five books would you want?

- If your house was burning down and you could save only one thing, what would it be?

- If you could be any vegetable, what would you be?

- If you could be any kind of fruit, what would you be?

- If you could be any kind of animal, what would you be?

- What is your favorite color?

- What was the last book you read, and how did it influence your life?

- What was the last good movie you saw?

- Tell me what you see when you look in the mirror.

- What was the most embarrassing moment in your life?

- Who is your hero?

- If you could invite three role models to dinner, who would they be and why, and what would you serve them?

- When you die, what would you like your tombstone to read?

I'LL TAKE "POTPOURRI" FOR $500, ALEX

The students we surveyed were asked some trivia worthy of "Final Jeopardy." The bad news is that because of the very nature of these questions, you can't prepare for them. The good news is that a simple "I don't know" seemed to satisfy the interviewers. For bonus points, ask for the answer or, as one student did, tell them you'll check and get back to them. He did, and subsequently, he got in.

- What is the largest lobbyist group in the United States?

- Which state first had women's suffrage?

- What language did Abraham (of the Bible) speak?

- When did Iraq become an independent nation?

- How many numbers that contain 9 are there between 1 and 100?

- What is the capital of Vietnam?

- When and how was Pakistan formed?

- Who won the 1969 World Series?

- What is the difference between European and American eighteenth-century poetry?

- Why was the Civil War fought?

- What is the origin of the name "Cincinnati"?

- What do the e's in e.e. cummings' name stand for?

- When and why was the March of Dimes founded?

- When did Istanbul become Istanbul?

- Name the four non-Arabic-speaking countries in the Middle East.

- What was Thomas Aquinas famous for?

- Who was the architect who built the Great Wall of China?

- Where was Millard Filmore born?

- Give a brief history of the Jesuit order.

- Define the Apollonian and the Dionysian as they figure in the philosophy of Nietzsche.

- Who was the head of NATO during World War II?

- What size tippets do you use on your fly lines with a 14X fly?

A Corollary: I'll Take "Science & Medicine" for $1,000, Alex

A few interviewees were asked trivia questions that actually related to science and medicine. For the most part, they knew the answers. When they didn't, and the question was obscure, it didn't seem to hurt their chances of getting in. Your undergraduate course work and MCAT review should be preparation enough for a lot of these questions.

- What was the first industrialized country to practice socialized medicine? The second?

- How much does the United States spend each year on medical care?

- How does a lightbulb work?

- Why don't fish die in winter?

- Why does ice float on the top of water?

- How do you make a protein?

- So what is Alzheimer's disease, anyway?

- Where is your hamstring region?

- Tell me what you know about DNA.

- What is the Grignard Reaction?

- What is Poisson's equation?

- Describe protein structure.

- What is PKU?

CAN YOU SAY "INAPPROPRIATE"?

Despite the media attention that issues of gender discrimination and sexual harassment receive, medical school interviewers are still asking questions that, if they were asked in a job interview, would be deemed inappropriate or illegal. These kinds of questions are more common than you would expect. The students who told us they'd been asked these questions (and there were lots of them, mostly female) expressed emotions from confusion to outrage. Still, most admitted to being afraid that they would be rejected if they did anything but reply calmly, and therefore they answered honestly and without additional comment. How you handle a question like this is up to you. At this point, you too might feel that there is too much at stake to make waves, but on the other hand, it is certainly within your rights to ask how the question is relevant or even to politely decline to answer.

- How did you get such a high score in math? I've never seen such a high score from a woman!

- Do you know that you have extraordinarily good looks?

- Why do you want to be a doctor rather than a nurse?

- Will you faint if I take you into surgery?

- Would you feel uncomfortable being alone with a male patient?

- How did taking a nude art class make you feel?

- What would your ideal date be?

- Do you find it hard to find educated black men to date?

- Why don't you like men?

- How does your boyfriend feel about your going to medical school?

- Would having a boyfriend affect your decision in choosing a medical school and career?

- Are you prepared to handle possibly losing your boyfriend/girlfriend over the stress and distance?

- Are you married?

- What kind of person would you like to marry?

- Do you plan to marry while in medical school?

- Why aren't you married?

- How will you deal with being married while in medical school?

- What does your husband do?

- Why did you get divorced?

- Do you plan to remarry?

- Do you expect to have a family? If so, why are you applying to medical school?

- If you become pregnant, what will you do?

- How do you plan to manage a family and a career? After all, you are a woman.

- How would you raise your children if you were a doctor?

- What would you do if you were sexually harassed at any time during school, residency, or your career?

- Are you prepared for the sexual discrimination you will most likely face as a student, resident, intern, and so on?

EXPECT THE UNEXPECTED

Although most of the questions fall into one of the previous categories, some of the questions are just plain off the wall. Some of the following questions were logical from the perspective of the candidates' background, so be prepared to answer questions about the leisure activities you listed on your application or the experiences you related in your essays. Other questions came straight out of left field. These are unlikely to be repeated, but they give you an idea of the kind of things interviewers ask to catch you off balance. If you're asked a question like this, take your time and think it through. If all else fails, remember, it's better to say "I don't know" than to try to baffle 'em with bull. As one of those surveyed said after an unsuccessful attempt at bluffing, "It doesn't work—they've heard it all before."

- What would you do if I dropped unconscious right now?

- What would you say if you smashed your finger with a hammer?

- How tall are you?

- How did you get your hair to do that?

- Is that your natural hair color?

- Why are you dressed the way you are? Why did you come here looking the way you do?

- Do you think that anyone can become a singer?

- Do you know how to play an instrument?

- Who is your favorite classical music composer?

- What's your favorite Beatles album?

- What is your favorite college football team?

- What do you think the chances are that the [team name] will make the playoffs?
- Why are the majority of NBA players black?
- How much can you bench press?
- If you're accepted, will you play on our softball team?
- What was your opinion of the rich, yuppie Greek students on your undergraduate campus?
- How much do you drink?
- Have you ever cheated?
- Have you ever tried an illegal substance?
- Have you ever stolen a car?
- What kind of car do you drive?
- What is your opinion of Charlie Brown?
- Do you prefer the old Star Trek or the new one?
- Why didn't you take Latin?
- Do you dream in Chinese or English?
- Do you know how to surf?
- Are you most like Madonna, Margaret Thatcher, or Mother Teresa, and why?
- What is your favorite card game?
- Do you play bingo?
- Does your mother know where you are?

7 Allopathic Profiles

ALBANY MEDICAL COLLEGE

ALBANY MEDICAL COLLEGE

47 NEW SCOTLAND AVENUE, MAIL CODE 3, ALBANY, NY 12208 • ADMISSION: 518-262-5521 • FAX: 518-262-5887
E-MAIL: ADMISSIONS@MAIL.AMC.EDU • WEBSITE: WWW.AMC.EDU

STUDENT BODY

Type	Private
Enrollment of medical school	571
% male/female	54/46
% underrepresented minorities	4
% out-of-state	78
% international	9
# countries represented	6
Average age of entering class	24

FACULTY

Total faculty	1,522
% female faculty	24
% minority faculty	7
% part-time faculty	64
Student-faculty ratio	3.0:1

ADMISSIONS

# applied	7,658
% accepted	5
% enrolled	27

Average GPA and MCAT Scores

Overall GPA	3.6
MCAT Bio	11.2
MCAT Phys	10.8
MCAT Verbal	9.9
MCAT Essay	P

Application Information

Regular application	11/15
Regular notification	12/1
Are transfers accepted?	Yes
Admissions may be deferred?	Yes
Admissions need-blind?	No
Application fee	$110

Academics

Albany Medical College responded to the changing health care needs in the United States by restructuring its curriculum in 1993 to better address contemporary issues in health care, while simultaneously providing a solid clinical and scientific education. The curriculum focuses specifically on the principles and practices of comprehensive care—health care that addresses the full spectrum of patient needs from medical and preventive to palliative and psychosocial. Grades of honors, excellent, good, marginal, and unsatisfactory are used to evaluate student performance. In the clinical years narrative assessments of performance are also used as an important evaluation tool. Graduation requirements include passing Step 1 of the USMLE and taking Step 2, including the clinical skills exam.

BASIC SCIENCES: Basic science education is coordinated and integrated in a manner that spans all four years of medical school, systematically increasing basic science knowledge within the context of clinical medicine. By teaching within a clinical context, the college offers a learning environment that focuses on developing problem-solving skills. Basic science concepts are divided into themes or modules that are most often organ based. Taught in conjunction with clinical case experience, these modules come together to form the foundation for the clinical education. In the first year students combine basic science instruction with clinical cases to focus on normal function. In the second year students further expand their knowledge and focus primarily on abnormal function and the disease state. Students learn clinical skills beginning in their first year by working within small groups and interacting with standardized patients who are trained to simulate actual illness. Students explore legal, ethical, and humanistic concerns in a four-year module called Health Care and Society. Systems of health care, epidemiology, biostatistics, and the principals of evidence based medicine are concurrently studied in a four-year module called Evidence Based Healthcare. Fundamental knowledge of nutrition also begins in year one and is integrated in all four years of the curriculum. Managing information is a key component throughout all thematic modules. The Schaffer Library of Health Sciences houses more than 144,000 volumes, 974 journals in print and 8500 available on-line, contains 3,900 multimedia programs and has 40 computer stations in the independent learning center. Throughout their medical education, students rely on these resources as well as the support of the library faculty.

CLINICAL TRAINING

An innovative experience, Orientation Clerkship, transitions students from the first two years of the curriculum to the clinical and rotation requirements of the final two years. This two-week clerkship occurs during the summer prior to year three. These learning opportunities on standardized patients enable medical students to develop, practice, and enhance their clinical skills and abilities. Students participate in mock preceptor rounds, assess their own clinical skills and perform basic medical procedures. The third year required clinical clerkships are a combination of hospital-based experiences to hospital- and ambulatory-based experiences. The third-year required clerkships are Medicine (12 weeks); Surgery (8 weeks); Ob/Gyn (6 weeks); Pediatrics (8 weeks); Family Practice (6 weeks); and Psychiatry (6 weeks). Fourth-year rotation requirements are Emergency Medicine (4 weeks); Neuro/Opthomology (4 weeks); Critical Care (4 weeks); and an elective in either Family Practice, Medicine, Surgery, or Pediatrics (4 weeks). Required rotations take place primarily at Albany Medical Center Hospital as well as other regional and local community hospitals, community health centers, psychiatric inpatient units, nursing homes, adult homes, and in patients' homes. The remainder of fourth year includes electives chosen by the students.

Students

STUDENT LIFE

The student community is very active both on and off campus. There are about thirty campus clubs and organizations, including a student newspaper, outdoor and athletic clubs, support groups for students with similar backgrounds or situations, and groups focused on community activities. For example, one student organization arranges activities for the Medical Center's pediatric cancer patients, while another brings AIDS education programs to local schools.

Admissions

REQUIREMENTS

Requirements are six semester hours each or nine quarter hours of Biology, General Chemistry, Organic Chemistry, and Physics each of which must include associated labs. When assessing GPAs, the Admissions Committee considers the intensity of each student's course load as well as his or her undergraduate institution. The MCAT is required of all applicants. For those who have retaken the exam, the best set of scores is considered most important, though all scores should be submitted.

SUGGESTIONS

Community service and medically related activities are valued. College courses should be varied, and demonstrate breadth and depth. There is no preference for New York State residents.

PROCESS

All AMCAS applicants are sent secondary applications. About 25 percent of those completing secondaries are interviewed. Interviews take place from September through April, and are conducted by faculty, students, administrators and local physicians. The interview day also features a group orientation and the opportunity to meet with deans, faculty, and students. Candidates are notified on a rolling basis, and are either accepted, rejected, or under consideration. Albany Medical College offers combined degree programs with Siena College, Union College, and Rensselaer Polytechnic Institute with a special focus on community service, business management or research, respectively. Interested students should apply during their senior year in high school. The MCAT is waived for students admitted through these joint programs. Students admitted to the programs earn both degrees in seven or eight years depending on the undergraduate institution.

Admissions Requirements (Required)

MCAT Scores, Essays, Science GPA, Non-Science GPA, Recommendation, Interview

Admissions Requirements (Optional)

Extracurricular activities, Exposure to medical profession, State Residency

COSTS AND AID

Tuition & Fees

Annual tuition	$52,160
Room & board	$11,529
Cost of books	$956
Fees (in-state out-of-state)	$140/$140

Financial Aid

% students receiving any aid	90
% students receiving grants	6
% students receiving loans	76
% aid that is merit-based	0
Average grant	$9,193
Average loan	$60,914
Average total aid package	$77,036
Average debt	$177,367

BAYLOR COLLEGE OF MEDICINE

BAYLOR COLLEGE OF MEDICINE

OFFICE OF ADMISSIONS INFORMATION, ONE BAYLOR PLAZA, HOUSTON, TX 77030 • **ADMISSION:** 713-798-4842
FAX: 713-798-55637 • **E-MAIL:** ADMISSIONS@BCM.EDU • **WEBSITE:** WWW.BCM.EDU

STUDENT BODY

Type	Private
Enrollment of medical school	678
% male/female	52/48
% out-of-state	25
% international	19
Average age of entering class	23

FACULTY

Total faculty	2,111
% part-time faculty	18
Student-faculty ratio	· 3.0:1

ADMISSIONS

# applied	4,285
% accepted	7
% enrolled	59

Average GPA and MCAT Scores

Overall GPA	3.8

Application Information

Regular application	11/1
Early application	6/1
Early notification	10/1
Are transfers accepted?	Yes
Admissions may be deferred?	Yes
Admissions need-blind?	No
Application fee	$70

Academics

Students enjoy a flexible curriculum with various opportunities for individualized experiences. For all students, grading in basic science courses is Honors, Pass, Marginal Pass, and Fail. During clinical training, students are evaluated with Honors, High Pass, Pass, Marginal Pass, and Fail. The USMLE is not a specified academic requirement. About 12 students each year enter a combined M.D./Ph.D. program, earning the doctorate degree in Biochemistry and Molecular Biology, Cardiovascular Sciences, Molecular and Cellular Biology, Developmental Biology, Immunology, Molecular and Human Genetics, Molecular Physiology and Biophysics, Molecular Virology and Microbiology, Neuroscience, or Pharmacology. Interdisciplinary programs at Baylor and the University of Houston, and an engineering program with Rice University are also options. Nineteen M.D./Ph.D. students are funded annually by the NIH M.S.T.P. training grant. Other students are supported by private or institutional sources.

BASIC SCIENCES: Complementing basic science courses are clinical experiences, behavioral sciences, and social/ethical perspectives. Throughout the first year and a half, students take Integrated Problem Solving (IPS) and Patient, Physician, and Society (PPS). The IPS course develops lifelong learning skills by focusing on problem-solving and the use of modern informational systems. The PPS course introduces, basic clinical skills such as the physical diagnosis and examination along with principles of patient care. Other first-year subjects are organized into blocks. Courses are: Gross Anatomy and Embryology; Cell Biology and Histology; Biochemistry; Physiology; Immunology; General Pharmacology; Bioethics; Nervous System; Behavioral Sciences; Infectious Disease; and General Pathology. The first semester of the second year is organized around body/organ systems: Immunology/Rheumatology; Cardiology; Genetics; Respiratory; Gastroenterology; Dermatology; Renal; Genitourinary/Gynecology; Endocrinology; Age-related Topics; and Hematology/Oncology. Both faculty and student tutors are available for additional instruction outside of the classroom. Basic sciences are taught primarily at the DeBakey Biomedical Research Building. The Learning Resources Center provides study areas and educational aids such as computers with medical software and Internet access, videotapes, and interactive learning programs. The Houston Academy of Medicine—Texas Medical Center Library contains more than 260,000 volumes, making it one of the largest medical libraries in the country.

CLINICAL TRAINING

Clinical rotations begin in January of year two. Required clerkships are: Pediatrics (8 weeks); Ob/Gyn (8 weeks); Psychiatry (8 weeks); Family and Community Medicine (4 weeks); Medicine (12 weeks); Surgery (12 weeks); Surgical Subspecialties (4 weeks); and Neurology (4 weeks). Throughout year three, students participate in Longitudinal Ambulatory Care Experience (LACE) that requires one half-day each week. Other requirements include four weeks of Selectives and 20 weeks of Electives in addition to a year-long course on the Mechanisms and Management of Disease (MM.D.). The MM.D. course is comprised of modules that correlate basic science principles with clinical concepts. At the end of the fourth year, students may elect a two-week course in Integrated Clinical Experiences (ICE), which serves as a transition to post-graduate training. Students train in the Baylor Affiliated Teaching Hospitals in the Texas Medical Center complex and at other sites around the city. In total, Baylor's teaching facilities hold approximately 5,000 beds. Elective credits may be earned at institutions throughout the United States as well as overseas.

Students

Approximately 70–75 percent of students are Texas residents. Students in the class that entered in 1999 came from 64 undergraduate institutions. About 16–20 percent of students are underrepresented minorities, and a wide age range is seen within the student body. Entering class size is 168.

STUDENT LIFE

A two-day orientation introduces entering students to the school's academic and nonacademic resources and promotes a supportive atmosphere from the beginning. First-year students also benefit from peer counseling groups and professional advising. Numerous organizations promote extracurricular, professional, community service, and religious interests, or offer support for minority or other groups of medical students. Some examples include the Family Practice Club, the Texas Medical Association Medical Student Section, and the Baylor Association of Minority Medical Students. An athletic center with exercise equipment and weights, basketball, racquetball, aerobics, and volleyball is available to medical students. Houston is home to almost two million people and is a center for commerce, industry, arts, and recreation. A dormitory operated by the Texas Medical Center is located near Baylor, although most medical students opt to live off campus in nearby residential areas.

GRADUATES

Graduates are successful in securing residencies in all generalist and specialty areas. Baylor also administers post-graduate programs.

Admissions

REQUIREMENTS

Prerequisites are one year each of Biology, Chemistry, Organic Chemistry, and English. Science courses must include associated labs. The MCAT is required and must be from within the past five years. For applicants who have taken the exam on more than one occasion, the most recent set of scores is weighted most heavily.

SUGGESTIONS

Approximately 70–75 percent of the positions in each class are reserved for Texas residents, making non-resident positions highly competitive. The April, rather than August, MCAT is recommended. Beyond intellectual ability, Baylor is interested in personal integrity and demonstrated interest in medicine.

PROCESS

Baylor does not participate in AMCAS. Institutional applications are available in June preceding the year of anticipated entrance. Approximately 15 percent of applicants are interviewed between September and February. Interviews usually consist of three 30-minute sessions each with a faculty member or medical student. The interview weekend features a group orientation session, a campus tour, and the opportunity to meet informally with students and faculty members. Of interviewed candidates, about 40 percent are accepted on a rolling basis.

Admissions Requirements (Required)
MCAT Scores, Essays, Science GPA, Non-Science GPA, Recommendation, Interview

Admissions Requirements (Optional)
Extracurricular activities, Exposure to medical profession, State Residency

COSTS AND AID

Tuition & Fees

Annual tuition (in-state out-of-state)	$6,550/$19,650
Room & board	$13,365
Cost of books	$5,775
Fees	$11,968

Financial Aid

% students receiving any aid	81
% students receiving loans	75
% aid that is merit-based	1
Average grant	$8,823
Average loan	$21,557
Average total aid package	$18,820
Average debt	$67,679

BOSTON UNIVERSITY
SCHOOL OF MEDICINE

72 EAST CONCORD STREET, BOSTON, MA 02118 • ADMISSION: 617-638-4630 • FAX: 617-638-4718
E-MAIL: MEDADMS@BU.EDU • WEBSITE: WWW.BUMC.BU.EDU

STUDENT BODY

Type	Private
Enrollment of parent institution	32,897
Enrollment of medical school	713
% male/female	50/50
% underrepresented minorities	4
% out-of-state	82
% international	49
# countries represented	130
Average age of entering class	22

FACULTY

Total faculty	2,324
% female faculty	42
% minority faculty	5
% part-time faculty	8
Student-faculty ratio	0.5:1

ADMISSIONS

# applied	9,665
% accepted	5
% enrolled	37

Average GPA and MCAT Scores

Overall GPA	3.7
MCAT Bio	11.8
MCAT Phys	11.7
MCAT Verbal	10.7
MCAT Essay	P

Application Information

Regular application	11/1
Early application	8/1
Early notification	10/1
Are transfers accepted?	No
Admissions may be deferred?	No
Admissions need-blind?	No
Application fee	$110

Academics

Several combined degree programs are offered, including the MD/MPH, MD/MBA, and MD/MACI, to which all students accepted into the medical school may apply. Qualified students may pursue a joint MD/PhD program, earning the doctorate degree in Anatomy, Biochemistry, Biomedical Engineering, Biophysics, Behavioral Neuroscience, Cell Biology, Genetics, Immunology, Microbiology, Molecular Biology, Pathology, Pharmacology, or Physiology. Most students take part in a four-year curriculum of foundational and clinical science, leading to the MD However, up to ten students each year enter an Alternative Curriculum which spreads one year of study over two calendar years, thereby freeing up time for academic or personal interests. The evaluation of students is Pass/Fail in the foundational science curriculum in the first two years and Honors, High Pass, Pass/Fail, in the third and fourth year clinical clerkships, during which the evaluations also include narrative reports. Passing the USMLE Step 1 is a requirement for promotion to year three.

BASIC SCIENCES: An Integrated Problems course supplements the traditional lecture/lab/small group discussion format of first- and second-year courses. Integrated Problems meets in small groups, and uses an interdisciplinary, faculty-facilitated approach to tackle case studies that relate to subjects discussed in other courses. First-year courses are: Anatomy; Histology; Biochemistry and Cell Biology; Physiology; Endocrinology; Neuroscience; Human Behavior in Medicine; Essentials of Public Health; Immunology; Genetics; and Introduction to Clinical Medicine I (ICM I). ICM I develops an understanding of the doctor-patient relationship and discusses sociocultural issues related to it. The second year consists of a two-semester course, Disease and Therapy, which integrates the study of disease including pathophysiology, infectious etiologies, and pharmacologic management in an organ-based context; ICM II; and Integrated Problems. In ICM II, students learn to conduct patient interviews and physical examinations. The ICM continuum involves mentorships with practicing physicians, often in primary care settings. Most foundational science instruction takes place in the Instructional Building, which has classrooms, teaching laboratories, the Clinical Skills and Simulation Center, and administrative offices for key faculty members. The Alumni Medical Library (http://medlib.bu.edu) provides 7,341 electronic journals, 7,069 electronic books, 328 databases, and 121 Subject pages. Print collections consist of 136,232 volumes, including 29,421 monograph volumes. In addition to the resources of the Medical Library, students, faculty, and staff have access to the University libraries' collections located at the Mugar, Science/Engineering, and other BU libraries. Alumni Medical Library Computing Services staff provide student laptop support and manage 188 computers in the Library, and in Computer Labs and Classrooms in the Library and in the McNary Learning Center.

CLINICAL TRAINING

Required third-year clerkships are: Family Medicine (6 weeks); Internal Medicine (8 weeks); Surgery (8 weeks); Ob/Gyn (6 weeks); Pediatrics (6 weeks); and Psychiatry (6 weeks). Third-year students also choose two of the following three options: Radiology (4 weeks), Neurology (4 weeks); and/or an elective (4 weeks). More than half of the fourth year is reserved for advanced clinical electives and many of our students complete one or more blocks in International Health. Required fourth-year clerkships are: Geriatrics (4 weeks); Ambulatory Medicine (4 weeks); Surgical Subspecialties (4 weeks); and a

Sub-internship (4 weeks). Clinical training takes place at the Boston Medical Center (508 beds), the Veterans Affairs Administration Medical Center (180 beds), and at twenty other affiliated hospitals and ambulatory health centers. Several research facilities are part of the Medical Center, and many BUSM students pursue basic science, public health, or clinical research.

Students

Under-represented minorities account for approximately 20 percent of the student body. The average age of entering students is 22, with a very broad range. A large number of colleges are represented, students come from many states and countries of origin, and entering students have pursued a diverse set of programs of study prior to medical school.

STUDENT LIFE

Students are involved in a large number of student organizations, both professional and cultural. These activities range from the Creative Arts Society to volunteer efforts like the Domestic Violence Awareness Project or the Outreach Van Project that provides food, clothing and medical care to the poor and homeless, as well as interest groups in the most clinical specialties. Housing is convenient to the health sciences campus, with a new on-campus Residence Hall available to all members of the entering class. Medical students have access to the academic and athletic facilities of the medical campus as well as those on the Charles River Campus, including the student union and fitness center. There is a comprehensive advising system through the Academies of Advisors which includes peer advising as well as carefully selected faculty known for their mentoring and teaching skills. As part of the Introduction to Clinical Medicine courses and the clinical rotations, medical students travel around Boston, giving them a chance to explore diverse neighborhoods and communities, one of the exceptional features of a medical education at Boston University School of Medicine.

GRADUATES

In the 2012 graduating class, the most popular specialties were Internal Medicine (27%), Pediatrics (12.5%), Family Medicine (6%), Obstetrics/Gynecology (5%), Emergency Medicine (4.5%), and General Surgery (3%), but virtually every specialty was represented among the graduates.

Admissions

REQUIREMENTS

Pre-requisites include one year each of English, Humanities, General Chemistry with lab, Organic Chemistry with lab, Biology with lab, and Physics. Applicants may substitute Biochemistry for the second semester of Organic Chemistry. In evaluating the academic record, factors such as the intensity of the undergraduate workload and the trajectory of performance are considered. The MCAT is required and must be taken within four years of the anticipated date of matriculation. Applicants using Advanced Placement courses and community or junior college courses in fulfilling pre-requisites are encouraged to take higher level courses in those disciplines.

SUGGESTIONS

In addition to requirements, college level mathematics (preferably Statistics), Biochemistry and Genetics are recommended, as is a broad background in the Humanities and Social Sciences. For applicants who have been out of college for a period of time some recent course work in the biological or physical sciences is advised.

PROCESS

BUSM utilizes a comprehensive, holistic review program throughout the admissions process. In this model, all aspects of the applicant portfolio are considered in a balanced manner.

Admissions Requirements (Required)

MCAT Scores, Essays, Science GPA, Extracurricular activities, Non-Science GPA, Exposure to medical profession, Recommendation, Interview

Admissions Requirements (Optional)

State Residency

COSTS AND AID

Tuition & Fees

Annual tuition	$52,426
Room & board	$10,500
Cost of books	$2,979
Fees	$760

Financial Aid

% students receiving any aid	79
% students receiving grants	53
% students receiving loans	64
% aid that is merit-based	20
Average debt	$188,193

BROWN UNIVERSITY
THE WARREN ALPERT MEDICAL SCHOOL

222 RICHMOND STREET, BOX G-M, PROVIDENCE, RI 02912 • **ADMISSION:** 401-863-2149 • **FAX:** 401-863-50967
E-MAIL: MEDSCHOOL_ADMISSIONS@BROWN.EDU • **WEBSITE:** BROWN.EDU / ACADEMICS / MEDICAL

STUDENT BODY

Type	Private
Enrollment of parent institution	8,400
Enrollment of medical school	452
% male/female	45/55
% underrepresented minorities	2
% out-of-state	94
% international	50
# countries represented	100
Average age of entering class	24

FACULTY

Total faculty	2,121
% female faculty	39
% minority faculty	14
% part-time faculty	61
Student-faculty ratio	6.0:1

ADMISSIONS

# applied	6,782
% accepted	3
% enrolled	53

Average GPA and MCAT Scores

Overall GPA	3.7
MCAT Bio	11.1
MCAT Phys	11.1
MCAT Verbal	10.5
MCAT Essay	Q

Application Information

Regular application	11/1
Are transfers accepted?	No
Admissions may be deferred?	Yes
Admissions need-blind?	No
Application fee	$100

Academics

The Warren Alpert Medical School of Brown University continues to update and revise its medical curriculum. This curriculum renewal aims to achieve several goals: the integration of science content between disciplines, the integration of science content with clinical medicine through the Doctoring course, and the promotion of scholarship and opportunities for creativity in the medical curriculum. The latter is being pursued through a Scholarly Concentrations Program that allows students to pursue academic and career goals both within and beyond the traditional areas of medical education. Students are encouraged to develop independent study options either at Brown or sites in the US or overseas. The Warren Alpert Medical School admits students through several routes of admissions: AMCAS (standard premedical); Program in Liberal Medical Education (PLME), an eight-year bachelors/MD combined degree program; Postbaccalaureate Linkages; and an Early Identification Program.

BASIC SCIENCES: Principles of patient care and the social and behavioral aspects of medicine are integrated into the basic science curriculum. The first two years are organized into semesters. During the fall semester of year one, students participate in two courses: Integrated Medical Sciences (IMS) and Doctoring. IMS sections include the Scientific Foundations of Medicine, Histology, Anatomy, and Pathology. During the spring semester, the IMS sections include Brain Sciences, Integrated Endocrine Sciences and Microbiology/Infectious Diseases, which again are coordinated with the content of Doctoring. The basic science courses are taught primarily through lectures and labs but also utilizing small-group teaching and clinical correlations. The Integrated Pathophysiology/Pathology/Pharmacology/Epidemiology course provides the structure for year two, which is organized around organ systems such as: Cardiovascular, Renal, Hematology, Pulmonary, Human Reproduction, Gastroenterology, Supporting Structures, and Endocrine. Doctoring II rounds out the second-year curriculum. Preclinical instruction takes place primarily in the new Medical Education Building, situated between Brown's campus and the primary teaching hospitals. The Science Library is fully computerized, with access to 250 online database systems. Medical students have access to all of Brown's academic facilities, including the main library, housing two million volumes. Grading in the first two years is primarily Satisfactory/No Credit, with Honors awarded in some IMS sections.

CLINICAL TRAINING

Patient contact begins in the first year with Doctoring, a two-year clinical skills course. In each semester of Doctoring, students spend one half-day per week at a community site with a physician-mentor, where theoretical concepts are applied to a real-world setting. Formal clinical training, consisting of required core rotations and electives, occupies years three and four. In total, 50 weeks are devoted to core clerkships and 30 weeks to electives. Requirements are: Medicine (12 weeks); Surgery (6 weeks); Pediatrics (6 weeks); Ob/Gyn (6 weeks); Family Medicine (6 weeks); Psychiatry (6 weeks); Community Health (6 weeks); Subinternship (4 weeks); and a Longitudinal Ambulatory Clerkship (one half-day per week for 26 weeks). Clinical training takes place at seven affiliated teaching hospitals in the Providence area: Bradley Hospital; Butler Hospital; The Miriam Hospital; Memorial Hospital of Rhode Island; Rhode Island Hospital; Hasbro Children's Hospital; V.A. Medical Center; and Women & Infants Hospital. The hospitals attract an ethnically and socioeconomically diverse population. Noteworthy areas of clinical care and research include Child/Adolescent Medicine, Psychiatric

Care, Global Health, Cancer, AIDS/HIV, Artificial Organs, and Diabetes Treatment and Management. Evaluation of clinical performance uses an Honors/Satisfactory/No Credit scale supplemented by narratives. Students are required to take the USMLE Steps 1 and Step 2 (CK and CS) prior to graduation.

Students

The medical student body is a heterogenous group admitted through several routes. In 2012, the range of matriculants' ages was 20–32 years, resulting in an active enrollment with diverse life experiences. About 75% of medical students participate in a community-based activity before graduation, while more than 80% of the graduates collaborate on a research project with a faculty sponsor. The American Medical Student Association (AMSA) chapter has a long tradition of service and advocacy; three Brown students have been served as president of the national organization during the past 30 years.

STUDENT LIFE
Medical students have full access to the school's recreational activities and facilities. Brown University has over 200 student clubs and organizations that unite students. Although most students choose to live off campus, residence halls and housing co-ops are available.

GRADUATES
In recent years, 14.5% of graduates entered residency programs at hospitals affiliated with Brown. About 40% of each graduating class enters primary care residencies.

Admissions

REQUIREMENTS
Students admitted to Alpert Medical School must attain competence in the sciences basic to medicine and sufficient to provide adequate preparation for medical school. Applicants are expected to demonstrate competence by successfully completing courses in the following areas of study: Biology (at least two courses); Chemistry (two courses in general inorganic chemistry and one course in organic chemistry); Physics (a two-course sequence for coverage of topics in mechanics, heat, electricity, optics, and radiation physics); and Social and Behavioral Sciences (at least two courses, preferably in anthropology, sociology, psychology, economics or political science). The MCAT is required for students applying to the standard route of admission. All applicants are selected on the basis of academic achievement, faculty evaluations, evidence of maturity, motivation, leadership, integrity, and compassion. In order to be eligible for consideration, candidates generally must present a minimum cumulative grade point average of 3.00 (on a 4.00 scale) in courses taken as a matriculated student at an undergraduate college. Applicants who have attended graduate school generally must achieve a cumulative grade point average of 3.00 (on a 4.00 scale) in courses taken in graduate school. In addition, applicants must have completed the requirements for a baccalaureate degree prior to matriculation into medical school.

SUGGESTIONS
A new medical education building allows for an increase in class size to 120 students for MD Class of 2016.

PROCESS
Brown accepts applications from qualified graduates of accredited colleges or universities through the AMCAS admissions route. Students are also admitted through the PLME, the Postbaccalaureate pathway, and the Early Identification Program (EIP). Those interested in applying for the standard route of admission must file an application with the American Medical College Application Service (AMCAS) by November 1 and submit a secondary application with required documents before December 31. The PLME application is part of the undergraduate application package. Students enrolled in premedical, postbaccalaureate programs at Bryn Mawr College, Columbia University, Goucher College, and Johns Hopkins University apply through the Postbaccalaureate pathway. Students attending schools that are part of the EIP program in Rhode Island should contact their premedical advisors for application procedures. Interviews are required of most applicant groups.

CASE WESTERN RESERVE UNIVERSITY
SCHOOL OF MEDICINE

OFFICE OF ADMISSIONS, T-308, 10900 EUCLID AVENUE CLEVELAND, OH 44106 • ADMISSION: 216-368-3450
FAX: 216-368-60117 • E-MAIL: CASEMED-ADMISSIONS@CASE.EDU • WEBSITE: CASEMED.CASE.EDU

STUDENT BODY

Type	Private
Enrollment of medical school	823
% male/female	54/46
% underrepresented minorities	4
% out-of-state	73
% international	12
# countries represented	10
Average age of entering class	24

FACULTY

Total faculty	2,023

ADMISSIONS

# applied	5,947
% accepted	9
% enrolled	37

Average GPA and MCAT Scores

Overall GPA	3.7
MCAT Bio	12.2
MCAT Phys	12.3
MCAT Verbal	11.1
MCAT Essay	Q

Application Information

Regular application	11/1
Early notification	10/16
Are transfers accepted?	No
Admissions may be deferred?	Yes
Admissions need-blind?	No
Application fee	$85

Academics

In 1952, the School of Medicine at CWRU (then known as Western Reserve University) implemented the innovative curriculum widely credited with initiating changes in medical education throughout the country and around the world. Our education program continues to receive accolades; in 2002, the School of Medicine became only the third institution in history to receive the best review possible by the authority that grants accreditation to U.S. and Canadian medical degree programs, the Liaison Committee on Medical Education.

CLINICAL TRAINING

We provide students with the chance to learn and practice in multiple clinical settings at some of the best teaching hospitals in the region and country. Affiliated teaching hospitals are viewed as an extension of the School's academic and research expertise. Our Affiliates include University Hospitals Case Medical Center, Rainbow Babies and Children's Hospital, Cleveland Clinic, MetroHealth Medical Center, and the Louis Stokes Cleveland Veterans Medical Center.

Students

CWRU does not have an in-state admissions quota and accepts regardless of state of legal residence. 85% of the classes are not from the state of Ohio.

STUDENT LIFE

Most students choose to live off campus and most rely on cars for transportation to and from school. The University does not provide graduate housing. Student groups are involved in both community and social activities. The structure of the academic program allows time for extra-curricular activities, and students participate in both University and community events. The cost of living on a student budget is very affordable in Cleveland.

GRADUATES

Our graduates go onto some of the top residency programs in Ohio and across the country.

Admissions

REQUIREMENTS

1 year of inorganic chemistry with labs, 1 semester of organic chemistry with lab, 1 semester of Biochemistry, 1 semester of English/Writing course. Other science coursework is recommended. Recent academic performance is more heavily weighted, and although many older students are admitted, most have taken some relevant courses within the past two years. The MCAT is required, and the most recent set of scores is considered. Due to the rolling admissions process, applicants are encouraged to submit materials as soon as possible. http://casemed.case.edu/admissions/process/requirements.cfm

SUGGESTIONS

Any additional upper level science courses would help prepare a student for medical school. CWRU accepts students of all undergraduate majors.

PROCESS

All applicants with a verified AMCAS application receive a secondary application. Secondaries should be completed within 2 weeks of receipt and are due by December 15 at the latest. Interviews are held from September to March. University Track applicants have two interviews: 1 with a faculty member, 1 with a medical student. College Track applicants have three interviews: 2 faculty, 1 with a medical student. Those interviewed are notified shortly afterward of their status: accept, reject, or wait-list. The wait-list is not ranked. Wait-listed candidates may submit updates and indicate a continued interest in the School.

Admissions Requirements (Required)

MCAT Scores, Essays, Science GPA, Extracurricular activities, Non-Science GPA, Exposure to medical profession, Recommendation, Interview

Admissions Requirements (Optional)

State Residency

COSTS AND AID

Tuition & Fees

Annual tuition	$53,320
Room & board	$20,600
Cost of books	$4,300
Fees	$20

Financial Aid

Average debt	$180,184

COLUMBIA UNIVERSITY
COLLEGE OF PHYSICIANS AND SURGEONS

ADMISSIONS OFFICE, ROOM 1-416, 630 WEST 168TH STREET BOX 41, NEW YORK, NY 10032 • ADMISSION: 212-305-3595
FAX: 212-305-36017 • E-MAIL: PSADMISSIONS@COLUMBIA.EDU • WEBSITE: CUMC.COLUMBIA.EDU/DEPT/PS

STUDENT BODY

Type	Private
Enrollment of medical school	624

ADMISSIONS

# applied	4,595
% accepted	6
% enrolled	57

Average GPA and MCAT Scores

Overall GPA	3.8
MCAT Bio	12.1
MCAT Phys	12.1
MCAT Verbal	11.2
MCAT Essay	Q

Application Information

Regular application	11/15
Regular notification	3/1
Are transfers accepted?	Yes
Admissions may be deferred?	Yes
Admissions need-blind?	No
Application fee	$75

ACADEMICS

The Columbia curriculum is multidisciplinary and integrated-it focuses on not only understanding the science, skills, and techniques of medicine, but also appreciating the art and ethics involved. Several joint-degree programs, such as the M.D./M.P.H. and M.D./M.B.A. are offered in conjunction with other schools and departments at Columbia. Qualified students interested in careers in scientific research may pursue a combined M.D./Ph.D., earning the doctorate in fields such as Anatomy, Biochemistry, Biophysics, Cell Biology, Genetics, Immunology, Microbiology, Molecular Biology, Neuroscience, Pathology, Pharmacology, and Physiology. Medical students are evaluated with an Honors/Pass/Fail system. Successful completion of Steps 1 and 2 of the USMLE are required for graduation.

BASIC SCIENCES: The first two years provides information and experiences essential for all physicians. The majority of instruction is conducted in lectures and lab, but small-group teaching is increasingly emphasized. Students spend approximately 25 hours per week in scheduled activity. The first year (42 weeks) includes Gross Anatomy, Neural Science, Clinical Practice and an integrated course that covers Biochemistry, Cell Biology, Genetics, Human Development, and Physiology. The majority of the second year (40 weeks) is devoted to a multidisciplinary course that examines the basic concepts of Immunology, Pathology, Microbiology, and Pharmacology. Physical Diagnosis, Basic Psychiatry, and Clinical Practice are also taught. Columbia has extensive laboratory, informational, and computer facilities that enhance classroom learning. The Augustus C. Long Health Sciences Library houses nearly 450,000 volumes and is one of the largest medical center libraries in the nation.

CLINICAL TRAINING

In the third year, students complete required rotations in the following: Medicine (10 weeks); Surgery (5 weeks); Pediatrics (5 weeks); Ob/Gyn (5 weeks); Primary Care (5 weeks); Psychiatry (5 weeks); Neurology (5 weeks); Anesthesiology (2 weeks); Orthopedics (2 weeks); Urology (2 weeks); Otolaryngology (1 week); and Ophthalmology (1 week). The fourth year consists of one- and two-month-long electives drawn from a large number of offerings and student-designed experiences. There are extensive opportunities for clinical electives abroad. Each student is also required to complete a "back-to-basic science" elective. These include one-month seminars in Advanced Pathophysiology, Clinical Pharmacology, or Clinical Pathology. Rotations are conducted at various medical centers and hospitals throughout the metropolitan area. Columbia-Presbyterian Medical Center, Harlem Hospital Center, Roosevelt Hospital, St. Luke's Hospital, and other institutions combine for a comprehensive clinical experience.

Students

Columbia attracts an extremely diverse, nationally represented student body. About 10 percent of students are underrepresented minorities. There is a wide age range among incoming students, with significant numbers of students in their late 20s and 30s.

STUDENT LIFE

Despite the rigorous schedule, student life abounds at Columbia. Medical students have access to the recreational and athletic facilities of Columbia University and to university-sponsored cultural events. The P&S Club, the oldest student organization of its kind at any medical school in America, provides a variety of extracurricular activities. Students have opportunities in the fine arts, athletics, and service-oriented projects. In addition, Manhattan offers unparalleled access to museums, concerts, and every imaginable type of dining. Most students live in on-campus housing, which helps make New York affordable. Both residential halls and apartments buildings are available. Newly accepted married students are guaranteed married-student housing.

GRADUATES

Graduates gain acceptance to the most competitive residency programs in the nation. A Columbia education allows students to emphasize academic medicine, research, or primary care.

Admissions

REQUIREMENTS

One year each of English, Biology, Physics, Chemistry, and Organic Chemistry are required for admission along with the MCAT. For those students who have taken the MCAT more than once, the most recent scores are weighed most heavily. Thus, there is no advantage in withholding scores. Columbia does not admit students on a rolling basis. Therefore, submitting MCAT scores from the fall of the admission year does not place applicants at a disadvantage.

SUGGESTIONS

The Admissions Committee is interested in the depth and breadth of an applicant's extracurricular experiences. Community service, artistic activities, athletics and medically related experiences are all valuable. It is valuable to denote that Columbia is an applicant's first choice for medical school, particularly for those who have been placed on the wait list.

PROCESS

Columbia is a participant in the AMCAS application. All applicants are invited to fill out the P&S secondary application which can be accessed through the Columbia website. Between Labor Day and early March, approximately 25 percent of applicants are invited for an interview. The interview day consists of one session with a faculty member who is a member of the Admissions Committee. Applicants also have lunch and tour the facilities with a current medical student. About 15 percent of interviewed applicants are accepted, with notification occurring in early March. A wait-list is also created at this time. Wait-listed applicants may send additional information to update their files.

Admissions Requirements (Required)

MCAT Scores, Essays, Science GPA, Extracurricular activities, Non-Science GPA, Exposure to medical profession, Recommendation, Interview

Admissions Requirements (Optional)

State Residency

COSTS AND AID

Tuition & Fees

Annual tuition	$53,543
Room & board	$20,058
Cost of books	$2,534
Fees	$6,602

Financial Aid

Average grant	$0
Average loan	$0

CORNELL UNIVERSITY

JOAN & SANFORD I. WEILL MEDICAL COLLEGE

OFFICE OF ADMISSIONS, 445 EAST 69TH STREET, NEW YORK, NY 10021 • ADMISSION: 212-746-1067
FAX: 212-746-80527 • E-MAIL: CUMC-ADMISSIONS@MED.CORNELL.EDU • WEBSITE: WWW.MED.CORNELL.EDU

STUDENT BODY

Type	Private
Enrollment of medical school	405
% male/female	50/50
Average age of entering class	24

FACULTY

Total faculty	2,340

ADMISSIONS

# applied	5,235
% accepted	5
% enrolled	37

Average GPA and MCAT Scores

Overall GPA	3.7
MCAT Bio	11.8
MCAT Phys	11.6
MCAT Verbal	10.8
MCAT Essay	Q

Application Information

Regular application	10/15
Regular notification	3/10
Are transfers accepted?	Yes
Admissions may be deferred?	Yes
Admissions need-blind?	No
Application fee	$75

Academics

A revised curriculum strives to limit the time students spend in lectures, thereby promoting independent and interactive learning and research. The curriculum integrates basic and clinical sciences, utilizes problem-based learning, includes principles of public health, and encourages student research efforts. Joint M.D./Ph.D. programs can be pursued in conjunction with the Weill Graduate School of Medical Sciences, Rockefeller University, and the Sloan-Kettering Institute in the following fields: Biochemistry, Cell Biology, Immunology, Molecular Biology and Genetics; Molecular Pharmacology, Neuroscience, Physiology; and Microbiology. Fifteen students per year may enter joint programs.

BASIC SCIENCES: The curriculum was completely revised in 1996 and has been both highly successful and widely emulated. The first and second years of study consist of five basic science courses and Medicine, Patients, and Society. In the first year, the basic science courses are Molecules to Cells and Genetics, Human Structure and Function, and Host Defenses. In the second year, they are Brain and Mind and Basis of Disease. The core basic science courses are sequential, integrated, interdisciplinary block courses that employ problem-based learning (PBL) in small groups. PBL emphasizes active learning and requires the student first to identify issues needed to solve a medical problem, then to seek out the information needed to solve the problem, and then to reconvene in small groups with the faculty to apply the information learned. Lectures are few and emphasize the conceptual framework of a field. Anatomic dissection and experimental laboratories complete the learning experience. The course Medicine, Patients, and Society approaches the doctor-patient relationship from both the conceptual and practical perspectives. For one day each week throughout each year, students spend the morning in seminar and the afternoon in physicians offices. Areas treated include medical interviewing, physical diagnosis, human behavior in illness, medical ethics, public health, biostatistics, clinical epidemiology, and others. Thus, students learn these vital topics in a patient-centered context. The evaluation system uses an Honor/Pass/Fail scale.

CLINICAL TRAINING

Upon completion of the second year students take three Introductory Clinical Courses: Clinical Pharmacology, Anesthesia, and the Introductory Clerkship. The third year is dedicated to clinical learning and emphasizes the core clerkships, including Medicine, Surgery, Pediatrics, Obstetrics-Gynecology, Psychiatry, Neurology, and Primary Care. In these courses, students are assigned to clinical inpatient and outpatient services at New York-Presbyterian Medical Center and throughout the network of clinical affiliates. Clinical affiliates include the Hospital for Special Surgery, a leader in the fields of orthopedics, rheumatology, and sports medicine; Memorial Sloan-Kettering Cancer Center, one the premier facilities in the world devoted to the study and treatment of cancer; The New York Methodist Hospital; and others throughout the city. Students are integral members of the health care team and actively care for patients, under the supervision of the faculty. The fourth year centers on completion of clinical requirements, a subinternship, and electives. While electives can be taken at any time in the third or fourth years, most students focus on three major types of electives in the fourth year: clinical electives, often in subspecialty areas; research; and international electives. Each year up to half of the fourth-year class spends time abroad, typically in Cornell-funded programs that combine clinical care and research in the third world: South America, the Caribbean, Africa, and Asia. In the month before graduation, eight weeks of advanced basic science allow students to study leading-edge biomedical science in depth.

Students

In a typical class, students graduated from over 40 different undergraduate institutions and came from over 25 different states. Class size is 101.

STUDENT LIFE

Despite the urban environment, students are cohesive and student life is apparent around the Medical College. Ninety-five percent of students live within three blocks of campus, generally in college-owned dorms or apartments. The rent is subsidized and competitive for New York. In the residence halls, there are athletic facilities for student use. Student organizations, including those that support women and minority students, are active. Parks, including Central Park, are accessible, as are countless museums, theaters, shops, and restaurants. Students do not own cars.

GRADUATES

Graduates gain acceptance to the nations top residency programs. Many stay in New York City for post-graduate training.

Admissions

REQUIREMENTS

Weill/Cornell requires 24 semester credit hours in science courses, including 2 semesters each of Biology, General Chemistry, Organic Chemistry, and Physics. In addition, six semester hours of English are required. The science GPA is given considerable weight. The MCAT is required and is used to assist the Admissions Committee in assessing the GPAs of applicants who typically come from a wide range of undergraduate backgrounds. If an applicant has repeated the MCAT, the both scores are considered.

SUGGESTIONS

Beyond required courses, Weill/Cornell recommends one to two additional upper division Biology courses for nonscience majors. For students who graduated college several years ago, recent science course work is suggested. The Medical College is interested in the extracurricular activities of applicants, particularly if they demonstrate commitment and dedication. Some exposure to the field of medicine is also desirable. Biomedical research is recommended.

PROCESS

All AMCAS applicants receive secondary applications. About 13 percent of applicants who complete secondaries are invited to interview, and about 30 percent of those who interview are offered a place in the first-year class. Interviews are held from October through February and consist of two 30-minute sessions, each with a member of the Admissions Committee. Decisions are announced by March 15. For a wait-listed candidate, submitting supplemental material can serve to strengthen his or her application and is also helpful in that it indicates interest in attending Weill/Cornell.

Admissions Requirements (Required)

MCAT Scores, Essays, Science GPA, Extracurricular activities, Non-Science GPA, Exposure to medical profession, Recommendation, Interview

Admissions Requirements (Optional)

State Residency

COSTS AND AID

Tuition & Fees

Annual tuition	$51,338
Room & board	$23,555
Cost of books	$1,800

Financial Aid

% students receiving any aid	83
% students receiving grants	58
% students receiving loans	65
% aid that is merit-based	0

CREIGHTON UNIVERSITY
CREIGHTON UNIVERSITY SCHOOL OF MEDICINE

OFFICE OF MEDICAL ADMISSIONS, 2500 CALIFORNIA PLAZA OMAHA, NE 68178 • ADMISSION: 402-280-2799
FAX: 402-280-12417 • E-MAIL: MEDSCHADM@CREIGHTON.EDU • WEBSITE: WWW2.CREIGHTON.EDU/MEDSCHOOL

STUDENT BODY

Type	Private
Enrollment of parent institution	6,891
Enrollment of medical school	582
% male/female	51/49
% underrepresented minorities	7.3
% out-of-state	68

FACULTY

Total faculty	288
% female faculty	30
% part-time faculty	11
Student-faculty ratio	2.0:1

ADMISSIONS

# applied	6,206
% accepted	6.8
% enrolled	35.9

Average GPA and MCAT Scores

Overall GPA	3.7
MCAT Bio	10.2
MCAT Phys	9.7
MCAT Verbal	9.8
MCAT Essay	P

Application Information

Regular application	11/1
Are transfers accepted?	Yes
Admissions may be deferred?	Yes
Admissions need-blind?	No
Application fee	$75

Academics

The educational program is divided into four years based on: (1) biomedical fundamentals; (2) organ- and disease-based concepts; (3) clinical clerkships; and (4) elective clinical experiences. Students may apply to Ph.D. programs in several areas of biomedical science medical microbiology, or pharmacology and pursue the degree jointly with the M.D. The grading system at Creighton uses Honors/Pass/Fail supplemented with written, narrative evaluations. Students are not ranked against their peers.

BASIC SCIENCES: In some cases, basic sciences are taught using the traditional lecture/lab format and in others, small groups and case-based learning is used. First- and second-year students are in scheduled sessions of some sort for about 25 hours per week. First-year courses, comprising the first unit, are Molecular and Cell Biology, Anatomy, Pharmacology, Microbiology, Host Defense, Neuroscience, Interviewing and Physical Exam, Ethics in Medicine, Evidence Based Medicine, and Human Development in Medicine. Many students use the summer between years one and two for funded research projects. The second component, organized by organ-and disease-based concepts, occurs during year two. Concepts or systems include Cardiovascular, Respiratory, Renal-Urinary Hematology/Oncology, Gastrointestinal, Muscular/Skeletal, Endocrinology Reproductive, Psychiatry, Infectious Disease, and Multi-Systems Courses. Throughout year two, students take Psychological and Social Dimensions of Medical Practice, in which they are exposed to health policy, public health, medical ethics and behavioral science issues. During years one and two, students also participate in clinical activities related to the patient physical and examination. Tutoring and review sessions for the USMLE Step 1 are provided. Creighton's Bio-Information Center houses 200,000 books and maintains extensive multi-media resources, computer teaching laboratories, and computerized literature search facilities. Passing the USMLE Step 1 is a requirement for progression to year three. Students at Creighton benefit from the new on-site computer testing facility for administration of their exams, which is one of eight in the nation.

CLINICAL TRAINING

Second-year students take part in a longitudinal care clerkship, which demands one half-day per week. This allows students to develop longer-term relationships with mentors and patients. Third-year, core clerkships are Primary Care (8 weeks, encompassing Internal Medicine and Family Medicine); Inpatient General Medicine (8 weeks); Psychiatry (8 weeks); Surgery (8 weeks); Pediatrics (8 weeks); and Ob/Gyn (8 weeks). Fourth-year guidelines require that students select one Surgery elective, one Critical Care elective, one Primary Care sub-internship, one Neurology clerkship, and participate in Senior Colloquium. The remaining 28 weeks are reserved for residency interviewing and electives. CUMC (404 beds) is the primary teaching hospital. Other sites for clinical training include Omaha Children's Hospital; Omaha Veterans Medical Center and Bergen Mercy Medical Center. During the summer, Creighton students have the opportunity to gain clinical experience through volunteer efforts in medical settings in the Dominican Republic or in communities closer to home.

Students

Among the 126 students in a recent class, California, Minnesota, and Nebraska accounted for 40 percent of the students' home states, though 30 states were represented. Seventy colleges were represented, with about 17 percent of the class having graduated from Creighton—either with an undergraduate or graduate degree. About 74 percent of the students were science majors. The age range was 20 to 34, with an average of 23. Of the entire class, 50 percent are women, 9 percent are members of underrepresented minority groups (mostly Hispanic and African American), and 6 percent have at least one parent who is an M.D. alumnus/alumna of Creighton.

STUDENT LIFE

The student body is cohesive and supportive, as evidenced by a student-published Wellness Chronicle that offers tips and shares experiences on issues such as exercise, nutrition, mental health, relationships, and spirituality. Through clubs, organizations, and extensive volunteer opportunities, students associate with each other outside of an academic setting. The School of Medicine is part of the main campus of Creighton, allowing medical students to take advantage of programs and facilities of the greater University, and to integrate with students from other programs. The Physical Fitness Center, the Student Center, and graduate student housing are all convenient to the School of Medicine. Omaha is a comfortable, friendly, and inexpensive city, allowing students to meet their own lifestyle needs. Affordable off-campus housing is widely available.

GRADUATES

Our students have gained entrance into virtually all available specialty areas and prestigious programs throughout the United States. Over the last three years an average of 52 percent of the graduates enter primary care specialties, defined as Internal Medicine, Family Practice, or Pediatrics. This is well above the national average of 48 percent. Creighton alumni are found in every state, but are more numerous in the Midwest and Western regions.

Admissions

REQUIREMENTS

Requirements are Biology (8 semester hours); Chemistry (8 hours); Organic Chemistry (8 hours); Physics (8 hours); and English (6 hours). The MCAT is required, and scores must be from within the past three years. For applicants who have retaken the exam, the best set of scores is considered.

SUGGESTIONS

No particular courses or majors are recommended beyond requirements, but advanced courses including Biochemistry and/or Molecular Biology are a plus. Studying overseas is encouraged, as are volunteer and community activities that demonstrate motivation and character.

PROCESS

All AMCAS applicants receive a secondary application, and about 15 percent of those returning secondaries are invited to interview. Interviews are held from September through the spring and consist of one 30-minute session with a faculty or alumnus member of the admissions committee, and one session with a medical student who is usually a committee member. A tour of the campus and lunch with current medical students are also provided. About half the interviewed candidates are initially offered a place in the class, with notification occurring on a rolling basis. Wait-listed candidates may send supplementary information, such as grades and updates on extracurricular activities.

Admissions Requirements (Required)

MCAT Scores, Essays, Science GPA, Extracurricular activities, Non-Science GPA, Exposure to medical profession, Recommendation, Interview

Admissions Requirements (Optional)

State Residency

COSTS AND AID

Tuition & Fees

Annual tuition	$50,348
Room & board	$14,400
Cost of books	$1,730
Fees	$1,518

Financial Aid

% students receiving any aid	94
% students receiving grants	18
% students receiving loans	94
Average grant	$9,229
Average loan	$45,388
Average total aid package	$61,828
Average debt	$192,292

DALHOUSIE UNIVERSITY

DALHOUSIE UNIVERSITY FACULTY OF MEDICINE

5849 UNIVERSITY AVENUE, HALIFAX, NS B3H 4H7 • ADMISSION: 902-494-1874 • FAX: 902-494-63697
E-MAIL: MEDICINE.ADMISSIONS@DAL.CA • WEBSITE: WWW.MEDICINE.DAL.CA

STUDENT BODY

Type	Public
Enrollment of medical school	91
% male/female	44/56
% international	37
Average age of entering class	24

FACULTY

Total faculty	1,311
% female faculty	30
% part-time faculty	32

ADMISSIONS

# applied	990

Average GPA and MCAT Scores

Overall GPA	3.8
MCAT Bio	10.0
MCAT Phys	10.0
MCAT Verbal	9.0
MCAT Essay	0

Application Information

Regular application	10/31
Regular notification	3/1
Are transfers accepted?	No
Admissions may be deferred?	No
Admissions need-blind?	Yes
Application fee	$70

Academics

The progressive Case-Oriented Problem-Stimulated (COPS) curriculum, which was introduced in 1992, prepares students for the pressures and problems facing physicians today. The COPS curriculum uses real-life patient cases and is based on a tutorial system that emphasizes group learning, contextual learning, communication skills, and clinical interaction with patients. In addition to the M.D. curriculum, programs leading to Masters and Ph.D. degrees are offered. Some students opt for a combined degree program, earning both an M.D. and a graduate degree in a biomedical or related field.

BASIC SCIENCES: In their first two years, students are organized into small groups and build their basic science knowledge by examining matter relevant to patient cases. Faculty/staff tutors guide the group's learning process. Students also choose specific areas of medicine for an elective period and begin to acquire clinical skills in the first month of school. The first academic period lasts 40 weeks and covers the following subjects: Human Body; Metabolism and Function; Pathology, Immunology and Microbiology; Genetics, Embryology and Reproduction; Pharmacology; and Clinical Epidemiology and Critical Thinking. During the second academic period, students learn Brain and Behavior; Skin, Glands, and Blood; Respiratory and Cardiovascular; Genitourinary, Gastrointestinal, and Musculoskeletal; and Population Health, Community Service and Critical Thinking. Throughout the first and second years, students have ongoing patient contact through the Patient-Doctor unit and have the opportunity to take elective courses. Teaching, research, and administration take place within two buildings, the Sir Charles Tupper Medical Building and the Clinical Research Center. The Patient-Doctor sessions are organized within the hospitals and pair the students with a clinical preceptor each week. Additionally, students attend the Learning resource centre weekly where they participate in small groups in hands on Skills & Procedures, such as casting, blood gases, tubes and wires, etc. Each student also completes case practice sessions which support each unit and use simulated patients. The students gain exposure to pediatrics, psychiatry, and various disciplines of medicine. The Kellogg Health Sciences Library houses more than 150,000 books and journals. The library is fully computerized and provides links to other libraries on campus.

CLINICAL TRAINING

The clerkship is organized into two phases, each of which has a central theme. All clerks will begin in a one-month Introduction to Clerkship unit in which clinical skills, procedures, history-taking, and physical-taking skills will be reviewed for all students. Phase 1 includes Medicine, Surgery, Obstetrics and Gynecology, Pediatrics, Family Medicine, Emergency Medicine, and Psychiatry. Each unit will be accountable for integrating objectives from other disciplines, and ambulatory and community experiences will be expected. Phase 2 begins with elective rotations offering the clerks maximum choice or remediation depending on their performance. In the final unit, Continuing and Preventive Care, clerks are required to complete three-week rotations in Long Term Care and care of the Elderly and again have an opportunity for a choice of rotations. Clerks will be evaluated frequently to receive feedback on their progress to guide self-directed learning. The major teaching hospitals are within walking distance of the school. They include a 202-bed pediatric hospital, a 254-bed obstetrics hospital, a psychiatric hospital, a rehabilitation center, and two large tertiary care adult hospitals. Other affiliated hospitals, clinics, and outpatient facilities also provide important training sites for medical students.

Students

Each entering class has 90 students. In a recent class, 81 students were from the Maritime provinces and 9 were from non-Maritime regions. At least 50 percent of students are women.

STUDENT LIFE

Although the academic workload is heavy, students are encouraged to pursue nonacademic interests. All students belong to the Dalhousie Medical School Society (DMSS), which promotes the interests of medical undergraduates. The DMSS organizes social and sporting events and raises money to support various nonprofit organizations. Through the Student Advisory, students have access to informal counseling, activities, and organized discussions that are coordinated and sponsored by other students. Dalhousie offers a variety of housing options on campus including residencies, singles rooms, and shared apartments. Outside of the campus, the city of Halifax offers a wide variety of entertainment, leisure, and shopping activities.

GRADUATES

Many graduates choose to enter postgraduate training at Dalhousie. Areas of training include Family Practice, numerous surgical and medical specialties, and laboratory medicine.

Admissions

REQUIREMENTS

The MCAT is required, and scores cannot be more than five years old. A baccalaureate degree is required for entrance to Dalhousie Medicine. There are no absolute prerequisite courses, though a minimal science background is advisable for success on the MCAT. Maritime applicants (those from Nova Scotia, New Brunswick, and Prince Edward Island) should have a minimum academic average of a B+, while non-Maritime applicants should have at least an A average.

SUGGESTIONS

Applicants from non-Maritime provinces and countries other than Canada should be exceptionally qualified. In addition to place of residence and academic credentials, the Admissions Committee reviews recommendations, results of personal interviews, and the applicant's extracurricular interests and activities.

PROCESS

For applications and details on the admissions cycle, view the website at www.admissions.medicine.dal.ca or contact the Admissions office at the phone number and/or address above. Applications are available on line only beginning September 1st of each year.

Admissions Requirements (Required)

MCAT Scores, Essays, Extracurricular activities, Non-Science GPA, Exposure to medical profession, Recommendation, Interview

Admissions Requirements (Optional)

Science GPA, State Residency

COSTS AND AID

Tuition & Fees

Annual tuition	$17,430/$
Cost of books	$2,000
Fees	$674/$674

Financial Aid

Average grant	$4,000
Average loan	$12,000

DARTMOUTH COLLEGE
GEISEL SCHOOL OF MEDICINE AT DARTMOUTH

3 ROPE FERRY ROAD, HANOVER, NH 03755-1404 • ADMISSION: 603-650-1505 • FAX: 603-650-15607
E-MAIL: GEISEL.ADMISSIONS@DARTMOUTH.EDU • WEBSITE: WWW.GEISELMED.DARTMOUTH.EDU

STUDENT BODY

Type	Private
Enrollment of parent institution	6,277
Enrollment of medical school	395
% male/female	47/53
% underrepresented minorities	12
% out-of-state	92
Average age of entering class	25

FACULTY

Total faculty	1,556
% female faculty	33
% minority faculty	7
Student-faculty ratio	0.2:1

ADMISSIONS

# applied	5,236
% accepted	5
% enrolled	33

Average GPA and MCAT Scores

Overall GPA	3.8
MCAT Bio	12.0
MCAT Phys	12.0
MCAT Verbal	11.0
MCAT Essay	Q

Application Information

Regular application	11/1
Are transfers accepted?	Yes
Admissions may be deferred?	Yes
Admissions need-blind?	No
Application fee	$130

Academics

Founded in 1797, the Geisel School of Medicine at Dartmouth strives to improve the lives of the people it serves; students, patients, and global and local communities. The School builds healthier communities through innovations in research, education, and patient care. As one of America's top medical schools, the Geisel School of Medicine at Dartmouth is committed to creating physician leaders who will help solve our most vexing challenges in health care. Well-known for its commitment to teaching, excellence in clinical care, and strong sense of collegiality, the Geisel School of Medicine is also an important research institution. In the past decade, annual research grants and contracts awarded to the Medical School more than doubled. Today, the total research funding at the Geisel School of Medicine is $137 million. The Geisel School of Medicine maintains a smaller student class size, representing a national and global student body, where individual attention from and opportunities for collaboration with world-renowned faculty abound. The curriculum integrates study of the basic and clinical sciences throughout the four years of medical school and combines small-group discussions, problem-based learning, independent study, and traditional classroom presentations in the right mix to supply focus and support without hindering individual learning and creativity. Our curriculum at the Geisel School of Medicine is as dynamic as the world of medicine itself. Each year, the school reviews and updates each of our required courses and clerkships to keep pace with medicine's rapid advances and complexities, and to assure that each student develops competency in six broad areas: medical knowledge; clinical skills; interpersonal and communications skills; professionalism; personal assessment and improvement in the practice environment; and managing patient care in a complex health care system. When you leave the Geisel School of Medicine, you will have the tools, the skills, and the attitudes necessary for a lifetime of learning—one of the realities and rewards of practicing medicine in the 21st century.

BASIC SCIENCES: In Year One, students gain a strong basic science grounding through coursework in human gross anatomy and embryology, microscopic anatomy, microbiology, immunology, neuroscience, pathology, and physiology. The year also includes an integrated course called "The Biochemical and Genetic Basis of Medicine." Topics in biostatistics and epidemiology are introduced, as well as biochemistry and metabolism. The major component of Year Two is an interdisciplinary pathophysiology course called "The Scientific Basis of Medicine," as students begin their transition to the clinical years.

CLINICAL TRAINING
Clinical training begins at the start of the first year when students are paired with a faculty preceptor in the "On Doctoring" course. "On Doctoring" continues through Year Two. Clinical rotations take place in a range of major medical centers such as the highly ranked Dartmouth-Hitchcock Medical Center, and in the White River Junction VA Medical Center. The White River Junction VA has been awarded the Robert W. Carey Quality Achievement Award, the Department of Veteran's Affairs' highest quality award, nine years in a row. The Geisel School also has an educational affiliation with California Pacific Medical Center in San Francisco, where Third Year students can get clinical experience in a large, urban academic medical center. In addition to other teaching sites in New Hampshire, students can complete clinical clerkships in Dartmouth-affiliated teaching hospitals in Alaska, Arizona, California, Connecticut, Maine, New Mexico, and Rhode Island. Fellowships from the Dartmouth International Health Group have made

it possible for Geisel medical students to explore health care opportunities throughout the world. The newly established Center for Health Equity brings the medical school's innovative student programs and experiences in urban, rural, and global health under one roof, providing focused, rewarding community, cultural and clinical training for students at the Geisel School.

Students

The Geisel School of Medicine is located on the campus of Dartmouth College, an Ivy-League institution with an international student body and reputation. Geisel medical students participate fully in the life of the Institution and have access to the facilities, events, activities, and society that are part of the academic community. Students may enjoy national performing arts groups, professional theater, and high-quality films at Dartmouth's Hopkins Center. The Hood Museum of Art, the new Black Family Visual Arts Center, the Berry Sports Center, Thompson Arena, and Alumni Gymnasium are other focal points of interest. Dartmouth's athletic facilities include a ski area, golf course, horse farm, boathouses, approximately 5,000 acres on Mt. Moosilauke, and 27,000 acres in the Second College Grant in northern New Hampshire. Many medical students volunteer in the community through such organizations as Planned Parenthood, the Good Neighbor Health Clinic, UVWRT (Upper Valley Wilderness Response Team), and the Dermatones, a singing ensemble. There are several medical interest groups at the Medical School. On-campus housing is available, though the majority of students live off-campus.

STUDENT LIFE

Student life at the Geisel School is marked by a strong sense of community and collaborative spirit. In an entering class of 87 individuals, approximately 56 different undergraduate institutions are represented along with every region of the country and several foreign countries. Minority and international students comprise approximately one-half of the student body. Though medical education is demanding, students here do not typically view medical school as four years "set aside." The environment is rich in opportunities for intellectual and personal growth.

GRADUATES

Graduates are successful in securing residencies in all fields at top-ranked academic medical centers across the country. The Dartmouth-Hitchcock Medical Center sponsors 48 ACGME accredited residency and fellowship training programs.

Admissions

REQUIREMENTS

One year (eight semester hours) each of general biology, and physics, along with one-half year of calculus or statistics, are required. Two years (16 semester hours or equivalent) of chemistry, which must include one semester (or equivalent) of organic chemistry and one semester (or equivalent) of biochemistry. Facility in written and spoken English is also required. MCAT results are strongly recommended and must be no more than 3 years old as of date of admission.

SUGGESTIONS

In addition to scientific acumen, applicants should demonstrate motivation and interest in their chosen major, which need not be science. Relevant research, medical experience, social service, and other co-curricular activities are important evidence of commitment.

PROCESS

All AMCAS applicants to the Geisel School of Medicine receive a secondary application, which must be completed by January 2, 2014. Approximately 800 applicants are invited to interview from a pool of over 4,500 completed applications. Interviews occur from September to April and take place on the Dartmouth campus.

Admissions Requirements (Required)

Essays, Science GPA, Extracurricular activities, Non-Science GPA, Exposure to medical profession, Recommendation, Interview

Admissions Requirements (Optional)

StandardizedTest, State Residency

COSTS AND AID

Tuition & Fees

Annual tuition	$50,646
Room & board	$10,750
Cost of books	$1,500
Fees	$1,755

Financial Aid

% students receiving any aid	78
% students receiving grants	52
% students receiving loans	79
% aid that is merit-based	0
Average grant	$22,600
Average loan	$38,243
Average total aid package	$48,401
Average debt	$133,000

DREXEL UNIVERSITY

DREXEL UNIVERSITY COLLEGE OF MEDICINE

2900 QUEEN LANE, PHILADELPHIA, PA 19129 • ADMISSION: 215-991-8202 • FAX: 215-843-17667
E-MAIL: MEDADMIS@DREXEL.EDU • WEBSITE: WWW.DREXELMED.EDU

STUDENT BODY

Type	Private
Enrollment of parent institution	24,860
Enrollment of medical school	1,064
% male/female	51/50
% out-of-state	67
% international	44
# countries represented	135
Average age of entering class	24

FACULTY

Total faculty	641
% female faculty	43
% minority faculty	28
% part-time faculty	16
Student-faculty ratio	2.3:1

ADMISSIONS

# applied	10,443
% accepted	6
% enrolled	40

Average GPA and MCAT Scores

Overall GPA	3.6
MCAT Bio	10.6
MCAT Phys	10.2
MCAT Verbal	9.5
MCAT Essay	P

Application Information

Regular application	12/1
Regular notification	10/15
Early application	8/1
Early notification	10/1
Are transfers accepted?	Yes
Admissions may be deferred?	Yes
Admissions need-blind?	No
Application fee	$100

Academics

With its dedication to academic and clinical excellence and a historic commitment to diversity, Drexel University College of Medicine has earned national recognition as an institution that provides innovation in medical education. Medical students are trained to consider each patient's case and needs in a comprehensive, integrated manner, taking into account more factors than the presenting physiological condition. Students learn to think like physicians from their first days on campus. First-year students are introduced very early on in the academic year to clinical experiences and community service. Standardized patients and model examination rooms are used to enhance clinical instruction. Students also have access to our state-of-the-art Medical Simulation Center for simulated learning in a hospital-like OR and ER setting in all four years of medical school. Students also spend time in primary care physician's offices, gaining firsthand experience with patient care. Students can gain research experience in the laboratory of a participating mentor through the Summer Research Fellowship Program. Combined MD/MPH, MD/MBA, and MD/MS programs are available, as are MD/PhD programs through which students may earn graduate degrees in bioengineering; microbiology and immunology; molecular and cell biology and genetics; molecular pathobiology; neuroscience; pharmacology and physiology; and biochemistry. The Medical Humanities Program and the Women's Health Program allow students who are particularly interested in these areas to graduate with the designation of Humanities Scholar or Women's Health Scholar. The Women's Health Education Program incorporates women's health into all aspects of medical education. Medical students are evaluated using the grades of Honors/Highly Satisfactory/Satisfactory/Unsatisfactory. Passing Step 1 of the USMLE is required for promotion to year 3, and passing Step 2 (CS and CK) of the USMLE is required for graduation.

BASIC SCIENCES: College of Medicine students choose between two innovative academic curricula for their first two years of study. Interdisciplinary Foundations of Medicine (IFM) integrates the basic science courses and presents them through clinical symptom-based modules. Students learn in lectures, labs, and small group settings. The Program for Integrated Learning (PIL), a problem-based curriculum, teaches the basic sciences primarily in small groups, supervised and facilitated by faculty. Laboratories and resource sessions complement the case studies.

CLINICAL TRAINING
Required rotations, most of which are completed in the third year, are medicine (12 weeks), surgery (12 weeks), pediatrics (6 weeks), ob/gyn (6 weeks), psychiatry (6 weeks), and family medicine (6 weeks). Neurology and a sub-internship in medicine are required in the fourth year; as well as a unique Pathway System in the fourth year for career planning and advising. Drexel University College of Medicine has many affiliated hospitals to accommodate students who wish to work in large tertiary care hospitals and those who prefer small community hospitals. Our academic campuses include leading hospitals in Pennsylvania and New Jersey. A sampling of our clinical sites includes: Hahnemann University Hospital, St. Christopher's Hospital for Children, Abington Memorial Hospital, Allegheny General Hospital, Saint Peter's University Hospital, Friends Hospital, Mercy Catholic Medical Center, York Hospital, Monmouth Medical Center, Pinnacle Health, and our new affiliation with Kaiser Permanente Hospitals in Sacramento, CA.

Students

Thirty-eight percent of students are underrepresented minorities, 50 percent are women, and at least 25 percent of students are nontraditional, having pursued other interests or careers in between college and medical school.

STUDENT LIFE

Students are a cohesive group and are supportive of each other despite the relatively large class size. Drexel University College of Medicine offers a variety of clubs and activities that are both academically and socially oriented. Many students are involved in community outreach activities in local public schools, health clinics, and rehabilitation centers. Students have access to an on-site fitness center at the College of Medicine. Philadelphia, a diverse and interesting city with a large student population, is replete with history, culture, sports, clubs, and restaurants. Affordable and attractive housing surrounds the Queen Lane campus. For additional attractions, New York City and other urban areas can be easily reached by train or car.

GRADUATES

Drexel graduates do very well in the residency matching program, both in primary care and in more specialized fields. Matches for the past two years can be viewed on the school's website.

Admissions

REQUIREMENTS

Applicants are required to have two semesters each of biology, English, general chemistry, organic chemistry, and physics. Science courses must include associated labs. The MCAT is required, and scores must be from within the past three years. For applicants who have retaken the exam, the most recent set of scores is weighted most heavily.

SUGGESTIONS

Beyond prerequisites, recommended courses include ethics, history, philosophy, psychology, and other social science and humanities courses. An advanced course in molecular biology or genetics is strongly encouraged. Drexel University College of Medicine seeks highly qualified and motivated students who demonstrate the desire, intelligence, integrity, and emotional maturity to become excellent physicians. The College encourages nontraditional applicants and is committed to a diverse student body. Students who have demonstrated a commitment to the service of others are given strong consideration. In accordance with this institution's historic commitments, women, students interested in careers as generalist physicians, those who come from Pennsylvania, non-traditional students, and those who come from populations that are underrepresented in medicine are particularly encouraged to apply. Applicants must be U.S. citizens or permanent residents.

PROCESS

All AMCAS applicants receive secondary applications. Of those returning secondaries, about 11 percent are interviewed between September and April. The interview typically consists of two sessions, one with a faculty member or administrator, which is open file, and one with a student, which is closed file. Of interviewed candidates, about half are accepted on a rolling basis. Wait-listed candidates may send transcripts or other material to update their files. An alternate route to admissions is through BA/MD and BS/MD (3+4) programs in conjunction with Lehigh, Drexel, and Villanova Universities, and Rosemont College. We also have early assurance programs with Monmouth University, Muhlenberg College, Kean University, Robert Morris University, Franklin and Marshall College, Grove City College, Rutgers University, Ursinus College, and West Chester University for students interested in 4+4 programs. For highly qualified post-baccalaureate students at participating institutions, a provisional acceptance to Drexel University College of Medicine may be granted, contingent on successful completion of the premedical curriculum. Post-baccalaureate programs through which this type of arrangement is possible are offered at Drexel University, Bryn Mawr College, the University of Pennsylvania, Scripps College, and West Chester University.

Admissions Requirements (Required)

MCAT Scores, Essays, Science GPA, Non-Science GPA, Recommendation, Interview

Admissions Requirements (Optional)

Extracurricular activities, Exposure to medical profession, State Residency

COSTS AND AID

Tuition & Fees

Annual tuition	$49,870
Room & board	$16,500
Cost of books	$4,979
Fees	$1,582

Financial Aid

% students receiving any aid	79
% students receiving grants	11
% students receiving loans	78
% aid that is merit-based	0
Average grant	$15,386
Average loan	$57,713
Average total aid package	$58,847
Average debt	$211,040

DUKE UNIVERSITY
SCHOOL OF MEDICINE

COMMITTEE ON ADMISSIONS, P.O. BOX 3710, DUMC, DURHAM, NC 27710 • **ADMISSION:** 919-684-2985
FAX: 919-684-88937 • **E-MAIL:** MEDADM@MC.DUKE.EDU • **WEBSITE:** WWW.DUKEMED.DUKE.EDU

STUDENT BODY

Type	Private
Enrollment of medical school	402
% male/female	50/50
% underrepresented minorities	9
% out-of-state	75
% international	20

ADMISSIONS

# applied	2,566
% accepted	7
% enrolled	56

Average GPA and MCAT Scores

Overall GPA	3.8
MCAT Bio	12.0
MCAT Phys	12.0
MCAT Verbal	11.0
MCAT Essay	Q

Application Information

Regular application	12/1
Regular notification	3/1
Are transfers accepted?	No
Admissions may be deferred?	Yes
Admissions need-blind?	No
Application fee	$80

Academics

By condensing the basic sciences into the first year, and scheduling required clinical clerkships for the second year, Duke allows medical students additional opportunities for research, clinical, or other enriching experiences during their third year. Those who are particularly interested in research may apply for joint M.D./Ph.D. programs in fields such as Anatomy, Biochemistry, Biomedical Engineering, Cell Biology, Genetics, Immunology, Microbiology, Molecular Biology, Neuroscience, Pathology, Pharmacology, and Physiology. Other joint degree programs are the M.D./J.D., M.D./M.B.A., M.D./M.P.H., M.D./M.P.P., and the Medical Historian Program, which leads to an M.D. and either an M.A. or Ph.D. in History. In most courses, medical students are evaluated by the grades Pass with Honors, Pass, Incomplete, or Fail. The USMLE is not required for graduation, though most students opt to take it, and virtually all pass each section with scores in the 90th percentile or higher.

BASIC SCIENCES: A new Introduction to Critical Care course meets weekly during the first and second years, and integrates clinical and basic science concepts. Each week during the first year, Practice alternates between the classroom, where students meet in small groups, and the clinics, so that shortly after lessons are learned, they are applied. Computers are issued to all students to be used in the Practice course for informational and instructional purposes. Also, part of the course is an intensive three-week "Preparation for Year II" segment, which prepares students for clinical rotations. Other first-year courses, taught primarily in a lecture/lab format, are organized into five blocks, so that no more than three subjects are tackled at a time. Courses are Biochemistry, Cell Biology, Genetics, Gross Anatomy, Microanatomy, Physiology, Neurobiology, Microbiology, Immunology, Pathology I, Pharmacology, and Pathology II. In total, first-year students are in class or scheduled sessions for approximately 30 hours per week. Classes are held in buildings central to the medical complex. The Medical Center Library houses 276,000 books, including a renowned medical history collection. The Medical Library Education Center has electronic classroom and multimedia areas. Basic science concepts are reinforced during clinical rotations in year two.

CLINICAL TRAINING

Preparation for and exposure to clinical medicine begins during the first year, as part of the Introduction to Critical Care course. The year-long preparation for clinical clerkships provides students with significant experience in clinical settings before the beginning of their formal clerkships in year two. Clerkship requirements are fulfilled in the second year. They are: Medicine (8 weeks); Ob/Gyn (8 weeks); Pediatrics (8 weeks); Psychiatry (6 weeks); Cost-Effective Care (2 weeks); Surgery (8 weeks); and Family Medicine (8 weeks, or Neurology and Family Medicine, 4 weeks each). Clinical training takes place at Duke Hospital (1,124 beds), Durham Veterans Affairs Medical Center (455 beds), Lenox Baker Children's Hospital, Durham Regional Hospital (451 beds), and at multiple affiliated hospitals and clinics. The third year is spent in research as part of an independent scholarship project, which may be in Behavioral Neuroscience; Biomedical Engineering; Biometry; Biophysics; Cancer Biology; Cardiovascular Studies; Cell and Regulatory Biology; Epidemiology Health Services and Health Policy; Immunology; Infectious Diseases; Neurobiology; Ophthalmology and Visual Studies; and Pathology. Third-year students may design a year of mentored research at Duke or at approved extramural sites, e.g. NIH, or students may begin the dual-degree curricula. During their fourth year, students complete clinical training through elective clerkships. There are more than 150 electives offered at Duke. In addition, students may spend up to two months in rotations at other institutions.

Students

In the most recent class, 22 percent of the students are underrepresented minorities, most of whom are African American. Women account for 49 percent of the class, and the average age is 22, with an age range of 19–42. Forty-three undergraduate institutions are represented, the top six being Duke, Harvard, North Carolina State, Johns Hopkins, UNC at Chapel Hill, and Yale. Twenty-eight states are represented, and the top five are North Carolina, California, New York, Ohio, and Virginia. Class size is 100.

STUDENT LIFE

Students, faculty, and administrators come together for events that promote a sense of community, congeniality, and friendship within the medical school. For example, the Dean hosts five "Dean's Desserts" for medical students to interact with teaching, research, and clinical faculty during the year. Organizations based on volunteer work, professional goals, or extracurricular interests are numerous. Medical students have access to all of Duke's athletic and recreational facilities. Durham is popular with students, offering parks, shopping districts, restaurants, and museums. Mountains and beaches are just a few hours away. Convenient campus-owned apartments, some of which have athletic facilities, are available on a limited basis. Social events sponsored by various medical school-based organizations provide opportunities for students to interact together. A fitness facility located with the major hospital complex for medial students and house staff only has recently opened.

GRADUATES

Graduates enter top residency programs, in primary and specialty fields. Most students get their top choice for residency appointment.

Admissions

REQUIREMENTS

Prerequisites are one year each of English, Inorganic Chemistry, Organic Chemistry, Physics, Biology, and Calculus. The MCAT is required, and scores must be from within the past four years. If the exam has been taken on multiple occasions, the most recent set of scores is generally considered. For those who have taken time off after college, science work must have been completed not more than seven years before matriculation at Duke.

SUGGESTIONS

An introductory course in Biochemistry is recommended. The character, motivation, and dedication of applicants is considered along with academic merits. Extracurricular activities, particularly those that are medically related, community service, volunteer experience, research exposure, and work experience are all considered in admission.

PROCESS

About 60 percent of AMCAS applicants receive secondary applications. Of those returning secondaries, about 30 percent are interviewed. Interviews are conducted from September through February, and consist of two half-hour sessions with members of the Admissions Committee. On interview day, students also receive a campus tour, and have the opportunity to eat lunch and speak with students. About one-third of interviewees will be considered for admission.

Admissions Requirements (Required)

MCAT Scores, Essays, Science GPA, Extracurricular activities, Non-Science GPA, Exposure to medical profession, Recommendation, Interview

Admissions Requirements (Optional)

State Residency

COSTS AND AID

Tuition & Fees

Annual tuition	$51,888
Room & board	$16,440
Cost of books	$2,480
Fees	$2,290

Financial Aid

% students receiving any aid	85
% students receiving grants	63
% students receiving loans	66
% aid that is merit-based	18
Average grant	$21,110
Average loan	$24,500
Average total aid package	$41,846
Average debt	$68,848

EAST CAROLINA UNIVERSITY
BRODY SCHOOL OF MEDICINE

OFFICE OF ADMISSIONS, BRODY SCHOOL OF MEDICINE AT ECU, 600 MOYE BLVD., BRODY 2N-49 GREENVILLE, NC 27834
ADMISSION: 252-744-2202 • **FAX:** 252-744-19267
E-MAIL: SOMADMISSIONS@ECU.EDU • **WEBSITE:** WWW.ECU.EDU/BSOMADMISSIONS

STUDENT BODY

Type	Public
Enrollment of parent institution	27,386
Enrollment of medical school	320
% male/female	50/50
% out-of-state	0
% international	33
Average age of entering class	24

FACULTY

Total faculty	482
% female faculty	30
% minority faculty	6
% part-time faculty	13

ADMISSIONS

# applied	884
% accepted	15
% enrolled	60

Average GPA and MCAT Scores

Overall GPA	3.7
MCAT Bio	10.0
MCAT Phys	10.0
MCAT Verbal	10.0
MCAT Essay	P

Application Information

Regular application	11/1
Early application	8/1
Early notification	10/1
Are transfers accepted?	No
Admissions may be deferred?	No
Admissions need-blind?	No
Application fee	$70

Academics

All first- and second-year students are paired with community physician mentors, and have the opportunity for ongoing patient contact and exposure to primary health care settings. Grading uses A, B, C and F. In addition, Honors may be awarded in some instances. Passing the USMLE Step 1 is a requirement for promotion to year three, and passing the USMLE Step 2 is a requirement for graduation. Joint Ph.D./M.D. programs can be arranged on a case-by-case basis.

BASIC SCIENCES: During the first two years, students spend about 28 hours per week in classes, most of which are taught in a lecture/lab format. Small group discussions, problem-based learning, and an introduction to clinical medicine are also part of the basic science curriculum. First-year courses are Microbiology and Immunology; Biochemistry; Behavioral Science; Primary Care Preceptorship; Genetics; Gross Anatomy; Histology; Embryology; Neurobiology; Ethical and Social Issues in Medicine; Physiology; and Clinical Skills I. Second-year courses are Introduction to Medicine; Primary Care Preceptorship; Psychopathology and Human Sexuality; Introduction to Child Development; Pathogenic Microbiology; Pathology; Pharmacology; Ethical Social Issues in Medicine; Clinical Skills II and Clinical Aspects of Lifestyle Abuse, which addresses behavioral aspects of health maintenance both for patients and physicians. The Academic Support and Counseling Services Office assists students in a variety of ways, including enrichment sessions and tutorials. Most classes take place in the Brody Medical Sciences Building, a modern facility that has classrooms with computer and video technology, large laboratories, auditoriums, and a clinical Outpatient Center. The presence of a clinical facility in this classroom structure suggests the importance of integrating basic and clinical sciences at East Carolina. Another building used frequently by first- and second-year students is the W.E. Laupus Health Sciences Library, which has 52,900 volumes and 1,550 subscriptions in addition to computer and audiovisual learning aids.

CLINICAL TRAINING

Required clerkships are Family Medicine (8 weeks); Internal Medicine (8 weeks); Ob/Gyn (6 weeks); Pediatrics (8 weeks); Psychiatry (6 weeks); Surgery (8 weeks); Cardiovascular (2 weeks), and an elective (2 weeks). At least 10 of these 48 weeks are spent in an ambulatory setting. Fourth-year students make selections from specified categories: Primary Care (1 months); Emergency Medicine (1 month); Intensive Care (1 month); Acting Internship; Transition to Residency (1 month); and Electives (4 months). Clinical training takes place at sites throughout Eastern North Carolina, with the cooperation of the School's extended faculty members, some of whom practice in remote, rural areas. Training also takes place at: the Developmental Evaluation Clinic; Eastern Carolina Family Practice Center; Vidant Medical Center (861 beds); specialized research institutes; and at rural affiliated hospitals throughout the state.

Students

All students are North Carolina residents, many of whom attended college outside of the state. More than 20 percent of students are underrepresented minorities, mostly African Americans. Almost half of entering students have taken some time off between undergraduate and medical school. In a recent entering class, the mean age at matriculation was 24. Class size is 80.

STUDENT LIFE

The University has an active student union, and facilities such as student lounges, theaters, concert halls, museums, and an athletic center. Medical students are integrated into the greater campus community, but also have a cohesive social life among themselves. Medical student groups are organized around volunteer efforts, professional interests, support groups, and religious affiliations, among other themes. Examples are the Generalist Physicians in Training Interest Group, the Medical Student Council, Peer Counseling, the Christian Medical/Dental Fellowship, and the Greenville Community Shelter Clinic. Greenville is known for its gentle climate and low cost of living, both assets for medical students. There are plenty of housing options, both on and off campus, for married or single students.

GRADUATES

There are at 13 residency programs and 17 fellowship programs offered at Vidant Medical Center, with the majority of positions in Internal Medicine, Family Medicine, and Emergency Medicine.

Admissions

REQUIREMENTS

One year each of Physics, Biology, General Chemistry, Organic Chemistry, and English are all required. Laboratories are required with all science courses. The MCAT is required and must be no more than three years old. For those who have retaken the exam, the most recent set of scores is generally considered. State residency is a requirement for admission.

SUGGESTIONS

While not required, courses in genetics, biostatistics, humanities, social science, and an additional year of English are strongly recommended. Taking classes that are part of the medical school curriculum is not recommended. Extracurricular activities that involve exposure to the medical practice are important. The Admissions Committee looks for applicants who are likely to contribute to meeting the health care needs of North Carolina.

PROCESS

All AMCAS applicants who are state residents are sent secondary applications. Over 50 percent of those returning secondaries are interviewed, with interviews taking place between August and March. The interview consists of two 30 minute sessions with faculty or student members of the committee. On interview day, applicants have an opportunity to meet with students and to tour the campus. About 15–20 percent of interviewed candidates are accepted, while others are rejected or wait-listed. Candidates awaiting a decision may send additional information to enhance their files.

Admissions Requirements (Required)

MCAT Scores, Essays, Science GPA, Extracurricular activities, Non-Science GPA, Exposure to medical profession, Recommendation, Interview, State Residency

COSTS AND AID

Tuition & Fees

Annual tuition	$12,534
Room & board	$14,876
Cost of books	$2,000
Fees	$3,133

Financial Aid

% students receiving any aid	93
% students receiving grants	75
% students receiving loans	90
Average grant	$1,500
Average loan	$20,000
Average total aid package	$30,000
Average debt	$85,000

EAST TENNESSEE STATE UNIVERSITY
JAMES H. QUILLEN COLLEGE OF MEDICINE

JAMES H. QUILLEN COLLEGE OF MEDICINE, BOX 70580 JOHNSON CITY, TN 37614-1708
ADMISSION: 423-439-2033 • FAX: 423-439-21107 • E-MAIL: SACOM@ETSU.EDU • WEBSITE: COM.ETSU.EDU

STUDENT BODY

Type	Public

ADMISSIONS

# applied	1,225
% accepted	11

Application Information

Regular application	11/15
Regular notification	7/1
Early application	8/1
Early notification	10/1
Are transfers accepted?	Yes
Admissions may be deferred?	Yes
Admissions need-blind?	Yes
Application fee	$50

Academics

Quillen College of Medicine offers the following degrees of study: Doctor of Medicine, Master of Science, and Doctor of Philosophy. Most Students earn an M.D. in four years, through either the traditional track or the Rural Primary Care Track. Quillen admits a medical class of 60 each fall. Quillen's major educational emphasis is primary care and rural medicine. The Biomedical Science Graduate Program offers study leading to the Doctor of Philosophy and Master of Science in Biomedical Science. The purpose of the program is to prepare students for careers in research and education in the life sciences. Students receive their degrees in Biomedical Science with a concentration in one of these five areas of basic science: Anatomy and Cell Biology, Biochemistry and Molecular Biology, Microbiology, Pharmacology, and Physiology.

BASIC SCIENCES: With the exception of clinical work, basic science courses are taught primarily in a lecture/lab format. Students are in scheduled sessions for about 24 hours per week. First-year courses for all students are Anatomy, Biochemistry, Biostatistics and Epidemiology, Communication Skills for Health Professionals, Cell and Tissue Biology, Physiology, Geriatrics, Behavorial Science and Lifespan Development, and Human Development Biology and Genetics. Traditional students also take Case Oriented Learning, while RPCT students take Introduction to Rural Health, Rural and Community Health, and Health Assessment/Examination. Patient contact begins in Case Oriented Learning for traditional track students and as part of weekly visits to rural health providers for RPCT students. The second-year curriculum for all students is Geriatrics, Neuroscience, Microbiology, Practicing Medicine, Immunology, Pathology, Psychiatry, and Pharmacology. Traditional track students take Clinical Skills and Clinical Preceptorship while RPCT students take Rural Health Needs, Health Assessment, and Patient/Client Assessment. Instructional facilities are located in a newly constructed, multi-million dollar Basic Sciences building on the grounds of the Mountain Home Veterans Affairs facility. The Medical Library, also located on the same databases, has almost 100,000 volumes, several online medical databases, educational software programs, computerized access to the University library system, computers for student use, and rooms for audiovisual study, reading, and conferences. Evaluation uses an A-F grading system. Students must pass Step 1 of the USMLE for promotion to year three.

CLINICAL TRAINING

Third-year required rotations for traditional track students are Family Medicine (8 weeks); Ob/Gyn (8 weeks); Pediatrics (8 weeks); Psychiatry (8 weeks); Internal Medicine (8 weeks); and Surgery (8 weeks). RPCT students take part in shorter rotations in the same specialties, and are required to complete a 16-week primary care clerkship in a rural area. During the fourth year, all students complete a minimum of 16 weeks of electives. RPCT students have additional rural, primary care requirements, and traditional tract students must take Internal Medicine and Senior Surgery. Clinical training takes place in three cities, Bristol, Kingsport, and Johnson City, and in neighboring rural towns. Affiliated hospitals are The Johnson City Medical Center; VA Medical Center, Woodridge Psychiatric Hospital, Johnson City Specialty Hospital; Northside Hospital, The Holston Valley Hospital, Indian Path Medical Center, Bristol Regional Medical Center, and Hawkins County Hospital. In total, these hospitals provide 3,000 patient beds. Evaluation uses an A-F grading system, and the USMLE Step 2 is required for graduation.

Students

Almost all students are from Tennessee or the immediately surrounding areas. Most students went to college in Tennessee, although undergraduate institutions from around the country are represented in the medical student body. About 15 percent of students are underrepresented minorities, most of them African American. Class size is 60.

STUDENT LIFE

Medical students take advantage of the extracurricular opportunities at ETSU, such as its theater, films, intramural sports, and athletic and recreational facilities. They are active in a wide variety of special interest and service organizations. Housing options include campus housing as well as a selection of apartments, townhouses, condominiums and houses for rent or sale. As an urban area, Johnson City offers many services and attractions.

GRADUATES

More than 60% of Quillen graduates pursue careers in primary care medicine and 22% practice in rural settings. Quillen provides a strong background in both the art and science of medicine, and graduates who wish to pursue advanced training in specialty areas have a high degree of success getting into residency programs of their choice.

Admissions

REQUIREMENTS

Applicants must complete Chemistry (8 semester hours); Organic Chemistry (8 hours); Physics (8 hours); Biology (8 hours); and Communication Skills (9 hours). An additional 49 hours of course work is required. The MCAT is required and should be no more than two years old. The April MCAT is advised as the August exam will delay application processing.

SUGGESTIONS

Other recommended courses are Comparative Vertebrate Anatomy, Histology, Mammalian Anatomy, Advanced Mathematics, Statistics, Biochemistry, Microbiology, Public Speaking, History, Economics, Philosophy, Psychology, Social Science, and Foreign Languages. For those who have been out of school for a significant period of time, recent course work is helpful. The Admissions Committee looks for traits and experiences that are consistent with primary care practice. Admissions is particularly competitive for out-of-state residents, and with the exception of applicants from the contiguous Appalachian region who are interested in primary care, out-of-state applicants must have extremely strong qualifications to be considered.

PROCESS

About one-third of AMCAS applicants are sent secondary applications. Of those submitting secondaries, the majority of Tennessee residents and about 10 percent of out-of-state residents are invited to interview between September and March. Applicants receive two one-hour interviews with faculty, medical students, administrators, or community members. Of interviewed candidates, about 40 percent of Tennessee residents and 15 percent of out-of-state residents are accepted on a rolling basis. Others are either rejected or wait-listed. Generally, only a few students are accepted off of the wait list.

Admissions Requirements (Required)

MCAT Scores, Essays, Science GPA, Extracurricular activities, Non-Science GPA, Exposure to medical profession, Recommendation, Interview, State Residency

COSTS AND AID

Tuition & Fees

Annual tuition (in-state out-of-state)	$19,034/$38,798
Room & board	$12,000
Cost of books	$1,360
Fees	$847

Financial Aid

% students receiving any aid	91
% students receiving grants	36
% students receiving loans	89
% aid that is merit-based	1
Average grant	$8,000
Average loan	$28,000
Average total aid package	$32,650
Average debt	$94,000

EASTERN VIRGINIA MEDICAL SCHOOL

EASTERN VIRGINIA MEDICAL SCHOOL

OFFICE OF ADMISSIONS, 721 FAIRFAX AVENUE, NORFOLK, VA 23507-2000 • ADMISSION: 757-446-5812
FAX: 757-446-58967 • E-MAIL: NANEZKF@EVMS.EDU • WEBSITE: WWW.EVMS.EDU

STUDENT BODY

Type	Private
Enrollment of medical school	432
% male/female	47/53
% out-of-state	30
% international	12

ADMISSIONS

# applied	2,565
% accepted	13
% enrolled	33

Average GPA and MCAT Scores

Overall GPA	3.5
MCAT Bio	10.0
MCAT Phys	9.8
MCAT Verbal	9.5

Application Information

Regular application	11/15
Early application	8/1
Early notification	10/1
Are transfers accepted?	Yes
Admissions may be deferred?	Yes
Admissions need-blind?	No
Application fee	$90

Academics

The curriculum is designed to help students master both the science of medicine and the art of clinical problem solving. A combined M.D./Ph.D. program is available for qualified students, leading to the doctorate degree in one of the biomedical science fields. For medical students interested in medical research, summer research projects are available. Medical students are evaluated with Honors, High Pass, Pass, and Fail.

BASIC SCIENCES: The first two years are devoted to basic sciences that are fundamental to the practice of medicine. Students also learn the clinical skills of physical diagnosis and interviewing. Throughout the first two years, students are in class or other scheduled sessions for about 25 hours per week. Lectures, labs, and small-group discussions are the instructional modalities used. First-year courses are the following: Biochemistry; Gross Anatomy; Histology; Human Development; Introduction to the Patient/Longitudinal Generalist Mentorship; Medical Ethics; Medical Molecular and Cellular Biology; Neuroscience; Physiology; and The Doctor, The Patient. Second-year courses are the following: Biostatistics; Epidemiology; Introduction to the Patient/Longitudinal Mentorship; Medical Ethics; Microbiology/Immunology; Pathology; Pathophysiology; Pharmacology; and Psychopathology.

CLINICAL TRAINING

Required third-year clerkships are: Family Medicine (6 weeks); Internal Medicine (12 weeks); Ob/Gyn (8 weeks); Pediatrics (8 weeks); Psychiatry (6 weeks); and Surgery (8 weeks). Fourth-year required clerkships include four weeks of Surgical Specialties, two weeks of Geriatrics, one week of Substance Abuse, and 25 weeks of electives, which may be selected from basic science and clinical offerings. For clinical training, students have access to a wide range of facilities including the East Coast's largest naval hospital, full-service community hospitals, interdisciplinary primary care centers, one of the largest Level I shock trauma centers in the state, private hospitals, a prestigious children's hospital, and clinics built for the medically underserved.

Students

At least 70 percent of students are Virginia residents. The student body has a number of older or "nontraditional" students, and the average age of incoming students is often around 26. Underrepresented minorities account for approximately 7 percent of the student body. Class size is 105.

STUDENT LIFE

EVMS supports students' non-academic lives and puts significant resources into the well-being of its students. Each fall, students and faculty members convene at a nearby resort for the orientation retreat sponsored by the school's Human Values in Medicine Program. The retreat provides a relaxed and informal atmosphere and allows incoming students the chance to interact before classes begin. Throughout the year, students are involved in a number of organizations and events, including ongoing community-service projects and a monthly Friday-night social hour. In general, the school's location in the Hampton Roads area is ideal for medical students, offering urban conveniences, the friendliness of a small town, and the attractions of a beach community. Most medical students live in the section of Norfolk near the medical school known as Ghent, a beautiful neighborhood of tree-lined streets and Victorian houses. EVMS also owns and operates an apartment complex near the school that offers housing for both married and single students. Washington, D.C., with its many attractions and recreational opportunities, is only a four-hour drive.

GRADUATES

From 20 percent to 25 percent of graduates are accepted into one of the many residency programs sponsored by the Eastern Virginia Graduate School. Other graduating students are successful in securing residency positions at institutions throughout the state and at locations around the country.

Admissions

REQUIREMENTS

Required courses are one year each of Biology, Chemistry, Organic Chemistry, and Physics all with associated labs. Applicants are expected to have a B or better in these courses. The MCAT is required, and scores should be from no more than two years prior to the date of application. For applicants who have retaken the exam, the best set of scores is weighed most heavily. Thus, there is no advantage in withholding scores.

SUGGESTIONS

In addition to academic transcripts, an applicant's experiences and background are examined. Personal characteristics are evaluated during the interviews, and honesty and spontaneity are considered essential qualities. Interviewers are interested in an applicant's concept of a physician's role, motivation, sensitivity to the needs of others, and communication skills.

PROCESS

After an initial screening of academic credentials, state residency, and other factors, about 50 percent of AMCAS applicants are sent secondary applications. A slightly larger percentage of state-resident applicants are asked to submit secondaries. Of those returning secondaries, about one-third are interviewed between September and March. Interviews consist of one session with a small panel of faculty members and medical students. On interview day, candidates also have the opportunity to meet with current students, tour the campus, and attend group information presentations. About one-third of interviewed candidates are accepted on a rolling basis. Alternate paths to admission are possible for students at schools that have special arrangements with EVMS. These are Old Dominion University, The College of William and Mary, Norfolk State University, Hampton University, and Hampden-Sydney College.

Admissions Requirements (Required)

MCAT Scores, Science GPA, Extracurricular activities, Non-Science GPA, Exposure to medical profession, Recommendation, Interview

Admissions Requirements (Optional)

Essays, State Residency

COSTS AND AID

Tuition & Fees

Annual tuition (in-state out-of-state)	$23,396/$56,382
Cost of books	$1,000
Fees	$1,446

Financial Aid

% students receiving any aid	90

EMORY UNIVERSITY

EMORY UNIVERSITY SCHOOL OF MEDICINE

1648 PIERCE DRIVE NE SUITE 231, ATLANTA, GA 30322-4510 • ADMISSION: 404-727-5660 • FAX: 404-727-54567
E-MAIL: MEDADMISS@EMORY.EDU • WEBSITE: WWW.MED.EMORY.EDU

STUDENT BODY

Type	Private
Enrollment of parent institution	13,893
Enrollment of medical school	531
% male/female	46/54
% underrepresented minorities	3
% out-of-state	66
% international	29
# countries represented	116
Average age of entering class	23

FACULTY

Total faculty	2,374
% female faculty	39
% minority faculty	14
% part-time faculty	9
Student-faculty ratio	0.2:1

ADMISSIONS

# applied	4,926
% accepted	7
% enrolled	42

Average GPA and MCAT Scores

Overall GPA	3.7
MCAT Bio	11.8
MCAT Phys	11.4
MCAT Verbal	10.8
MCAT Essay	Q

Application Information

Regular application	10/15
Are transfers accepted?	No
Admissions may be deferred?	Yes
Admissions need-blind?	No
Application fee	$100

Academics

In 2007, Emory School of Medicine opened a new Medical Education Building and began a new curriculum. Costing in excess of $55 million, this 162,000 square-foot environmentally "green" structure incorporates the historic facades of the school's original Anatomy and Physiology Buildings, but also contains state-of-the-art classroom, laboratory, and study space. The new MD curriculum reflects the extraordinary advances taking place in biomedical science; meets the needs of an ever-changing local and global healthcare environment; takes advantage of the unique educational resources in Atlanta; and respects the intellectually-gifted and highly-motivated students who choose to come to Emory. The new curriculum stresses early clinical exposure, an interweaving of basic and clinical science, close faculty-student interactions, and a discovery phase.

CLINICAL TRAINING

An Emory medical education is now anchored in a Society system. Every student is assigned to a Society small group during the first week of their medical education. A practicing physician serves as the small group leader and oversees the holistic development of students throughout the four years of medical education. The society small group advisor meets with students in small group and individually on a regular basis, serving as a teacher of clinical skills and medical science. The Foundations Phase begins with a four-month section on the "Healthy Human," a section designed around the human life cycle and emphasizing healthy human activities: Development, Neural Function (including cognition), Exercise, Nutrition, and Aging. Basic science concepts including cell biology, genetics, biochemistry, physiology, embryology, histology, reproduction, and human development are covered during the Healthy Human section. By beginning with the "Healthy Human" approach, the curriculum emphasizes: 1) the important role that behavior plays in health and disease; 2) that the approach to the patient must include consideration of the community, environment, family, and the "whole" of the person; and 3) the importance of healthy human activities, such as exercise, nutrition, procreation, and cognition/creativity as foundational to human well-being. The Healthy Human is followed by Prologue II, a section designed to prepare students for the Human Disease Section. Prologue II introduces the principles of microbiology, pathology, immunology, and pharmacology. The Human Disease section consists of organ block sections. Human Anatomy, including cadaveric dissection, is completed during the first five months of the Human Disease Section, and where possible, correlates with the organ system being taught. The organ system blocks begin each week with a simulated or real case presentation. Approximately two hours of class and two hours of small group each morning are augmented with longer small groups/skills sessions on Tuesday afternoons; each student attends a primary care clinic one half day every other week. Normal human function is taught simultaneously with the disease process where appropriate. Clinical cases drive the week's learning objectives, including social topics such as cultural competency, addiction, homelessness, etc. The Foundations Phase and Step I of the USMLE are completed within 19 months, allowing students to begin the Applications Phase during the middle of Year 2. Students complete the Applications Phase in the middle of Year 3, at which time an individual student may move directly into five months of Discovery, or may choose to take clinical electives in sub-specialty fields. This will afford students the opportunity to choose their research area within their expected field of residency, if desired. The Applications Phase includes "clerkship" training in the core clinical areas of medicine, including Ambulatory Care, Internal Medicine, Surgery, Obstetrics/Gynecology, Pediatrics, Psychiatry, and Neurology. During clinical rotations, students operate as full members of a medical care team. While core clinical knowledge is learned, patient-directed learning is emphasized. This patient-directed learning is the best preparation for the engaged life of a practicing, inquisitive physician/learner. The mandatory Discovery Phase is new for Emory and coincides with an enormous growth in research at the University level. Approximately 80 percent of Emory medical students have participated in a research project in past years, the majority of those experiences occurring between the first and second year and lasting 8-10 weeks. When designing the new curriculum, faculty and students strongly supported the concept of a longer, more in-depth 5-month Discovery Phase. The Discovery Phase may be spent in any field, but must be related to medicine, closely mentored, and result in a final product approved by the mentor. The time period for this phase may be extended to 9 months by using elective months available during the Translations Phase. Alternatively, students may choose to spend an extra year in research, either at Emory (tuition-free) or at another institution (e.g. CDC or NIH). The new curriculum provides extra time for projects and field experiences for the MD/MPH dual degree program. While it is anticipated that most students will spend their Discovery Phase in a basic science lab or on a clinical science or public health project, students may also choose to spend this time in matters of the medical humanities, medical anthropology, medical sociology, etc. The Translation Phase includes four required rotations: Intensive Care Unit (ICU); Emergency Medicine; a Senior Clerkship in Medicine, Surgery, or Pediatrics; and a Capstone Course. The ICU month reinforces essential basic science concepts and ethical precepts. The Capstone month occurs the final month as an Emory medical student and will include team training, standardized patient cases, instruction in the art of clinical teaching for "soon-to-be" residents, and important didactic material relevant to medical-legal, ethical, and communication issues.

Students

Students at Emory are encouraged to engage in a wide variety of non-academic pursuits. Medical students participate in a broad range of athletic, artistic, and service activities. The medical campus is situated adjacent to the main University campus, affording students the opportunity to attend outstanding events sponsored by Emory University.

STUDENT LIFE

Medical students have access to the organizations, events, and facilities of the medical school, as well as the other professional graduate and undergraduate schools on campus. The campus includes two state-of-the-art athletic centers, nine libraries, a museum, a performing arts center, and a park—just across the street from the medical school—featuring wooded trails and paved walkways for running, rollerblading, walking, and biking. Medical students also participate in intramural sports. Medical students organize community service projects and participate in local and national medical student organizations, which serve to integrate students into the greater community and often provide additional clinical exposure. Atlanta is an excellent city for students since it is affordable and offers many cultural, recreational, and entertainment opportunities. Almost all students live off campus; nearby apartments and houses are plentiful and affordable. In addition, Georgia's climate is conducive to many outdoor recreational amenities, offering both urban and rural opportunities year around.

GRADUATES

Graduates and Undergraduates intermingle at the dining facilities, athletic center, and campus wide activities.

Admissions

REQUIREMENTS

In addition to the traditional requirements of one year each of Biology, Chemistry, Physics, and Organic Chemistry, Emory also requires six semester hours of English and 18 semester hours of Humanities and Behavioral/Social Science course work. The MCAT is required. For applicants who have retaken the exam, the most recent set of scores is typically weighted most heavily. Emory operates on a rolling admissions cycle, making it beneficial for the applicant to submit MCAT scores and application materials early in the summer.

Admissions Requirements (Required)

MCAT Scores, Essays, Science GPA, Extracurricular activities, Non-Science GPA, Exposure to medical profession, Recommendation, Interview

Admissions Requirements (Optional)

State Residency

COSTS AND AID

Tuition & Fees

Annual tuition	$45,000
Room & board	$27,824
Cost of books	$3,166
Fees	$798

Financial Aid

% students receiving any aid	84
% students receiving grants	67
% students receiving loans	71
% aid that is merit-based	13
Average grant	$20,809
Average loan	$37,965
Average total aid package	$48,877
Average debt	$138,088

FLORIDA STATE UNIVERSITY

FLORIDA STATE UNIVERSITY COLLEGE OF MEDICINE

1115 WEST CALL STREET, TALLAHASSEE, FL 32306-4300 • ADMISSION: 850-644-7904 • FAX: 850-645-28467
E-MAIL: MEDADMISSIONS@MED.FSU.EDU • WEBSITE: MED.FSU.EDU

STUDENT BODY

Type	Public
Enrollment of parent institution	40,838
Enrollment of medical school	475
% male/female	52/48
% out-of-state	1
% international	42
# countries represented	130
Average age of entering class	22

FACULTY

Total faculty	2,212
% female faculty	42
% minority faculty	24
% part-time faculty	94
Student-faculty ratio	1.0:1

ADMISSIONS

# applied	2,256
% accepted	8
% enrolled	66

Average GPA and MCAT Scores

Overall GPA	3.7
MCAT Bio	9.9
MCAT Phys	9.2
MCAT Verbal	8.8
MCAT Essay	O

Application Information

Regular application	12/1
Regular notification	4/15
Early application	8/1
Early notification	10/1
Are transfers accepted?	No
Admissions may be deferred?	Yes
Admissions need-blind?	Yes
Application fee	$0

Academics

The FSU College of Medicine is truly a 21st century medical school. Created in June of 2000 by the Florida Legislature, it is the first new medical school to open in the United States since 1982, and as such it is charting a new course for medical education.

BASIC SCIENCES: The basic science component of the training program takes place on the FSU campus and is integrated into the culture and value system of the liberal arts university. The curriculum is based on a biopsychosocial foundation that balances biomedicine, medical humanities and social sciences. Basic science faculty responsible for the first two years of the medical education program are chosen to provide a diverse range of background and experience across all specialties. Some faculty are responsible for research and are valued contributors to medical education for first- and second-year students. The majority of the basic science faculty are positioned to make medical education their primary focus, producing a climate of innovative teaching methods and individual attention rarely found in medical education in the United States today. In this faculty-scholar model, highly skilled faculty present a well-structured continuum of education in biomedical, behavioral and clinical sciences utilizing problem-based and small-group learning experiences.

CLINICAL TRAINING

Clinical training begins in the first week with introduction to working with standardized patients in a state-of-the-art Clinical Skills and Simulation Center. Numerous opportunities to work with community physicians in Tallahassee and at area health clinics also are available during the first two years. From a clinical training standpoint, students especially reap the rewards of the College of Medicine's community-based model during the third and fourth years. All clinical training from that point takes place on the front lines of the health care delivery system throughout Florida. The emphasis is on ambulatory care settings such as hospitals, physicians' clinics, HMOs, and chronic care facilities in rural, urban and suburban areas. Because the College of Medicine partners with existing medical facilities and practitioners throughout the state rather than operating a teaching hospital, students have the opportunity to learn under the direct supervision of physicians throughout Florida. More than 1,900 of the state's top physicians, carefully chosen for their ability to provide high quality and personalized educational experiences, are part of the College of Medicine faculty. Community campuses are located in Daytona Beach, Ft. Pierce, Orlando, Pensacola, Sarasota and Tallahassee.

Students

In partnership with Florida communities, the FSU College of Medicine is creating a new model of medical education and research that uses interdisciplinary teams and emerging technologies. Building upon the FSU Program in Medical Sciences, a first-year medical school program begun in 1971, the college's educational program is designed to produce compassionate physicians who will practice patient-centered medicine and who are prepared to practice in a rapidly changing healthcare environment. FSU trains the physicians of tomorrow in such a way that they will become lifelong learners equipped to teach themselves what they need to know in an era of tremendous innovation in knowledge management and information technology.

STUDENT LIFE

The Florida State University College of Medicine carefully selects students who are outstanding academically and are committed to the college's mission of service to Florida's medically underserved populations. FSU medical students are culturally diverse and many come from small towns and rural areas, but the state's major metropolitan areas are also well represented. A number of students are older than average for medical school and bring a broad range of professional and life experiences, while others come straight out of undergraduate programs. Most are active in student organizations, community service projects and medical outreach programs.

GRADUATES

The College of Medicine's seven graduating classes to date have produced 450 physicians currently either in residency training or practicing medicine. Eighty-one alumni have completed residency and are practicing physicians—51 of those in Florida and more than 70 percent of those in Florida in primary care. The college's residency success is well documented and can be viewed at http://med.fsu.edu/index.cfm?page=alumniFriends.whereTheyMatched

Admissions

REQUIREMENTS

Applications are accepted through the AMCAS and invited applicants submit a secondary application before being invited for a personal interview at the main campus in Tallahassee. The College of Medicine accepts 120 students a year and, as an early-start program, classes begin in June. Applicants should meet academic standards predictive of success in medical school through academic grade point average and MCAT (Medical College Aptitude Test) score. An applicant's MCAT score should be dated no more than three years prior to the beginning of the year of the application cycle. If an applicant is currently enrolled in a degree program, the program must be completed and final transcripts provided to the College of Medicine Admissions Office prior to the beginning of classes. Non-U.S. citizens must possess a permanent resident visa. Applicants are assessed on their qualifications without discrimination in regard to gender, sexual orientation, color, age, disability, race, religion, veteran status, or national origin. Applicants may begin to certify and submit their AMCAS application beginning June 1. The deadline for submitting applications to AMCAS is December 1.

PROCESS

We seek students who have demonstrated a commitment of service to others and we encourage applications from traditional and nontraditional students, as well as students from rural, inner city or other medically underserved areas. An applicant should have completed prerequisite courses in English, biology, chemistry, organic chemistry, physics and biochemistry. While grades and test scores are important, a great deal of emphasis is placed on finding students committed to service and to the ideals of compassionate medical care. Personal interviews, conducted between September and March, provide an excellent opportunity for applicants to exhibit the personal qualities such as motivation, sensitivity to the needs of others, oral communication skills and maturity that the College of Medicine is looking for. In addition, personal attributes such as compassion and altruism are, in the view of the admissions committee, essential to the art of good medical practice and are of special interest in the selection process.

Admissions Requirements (Required)

MCAT Scores, Essays, Science GPA, Extracurricular activities, Non-Science GPA, Exposure to medical profession, Recommendation, Interview

Admissions Requirements (Optional)

State Residency

COSTS AND AID

Tuition & Fees

Annual tuition (in-state out-of-state)	$23,043/$68,619
Room & board	$15,104
Cost of books	$2,320

Financial Aid

% students receiving any aid	84
% students receiving grants	38
% students receiving loans	81
% aid that is merit-based	0
Average grant	$1,225
Average loan	$35,694
Average total aid package	$36,919
Average debt	$123,277

THE GEORGE WASHINGTON UNIVERSITY
SCHOOL OF MEDICINE AND HEALTH SCIENCES

OFFICE OF ADMISSIONS; 2300 I STREET, NW, ROSS HALL 106 WASHINGTON, DC 20037 • ADMISSION: 202-994-3506
FAX: 202-994-17537 • E-MAIL: MEDADMIT@GWU.EDU • WEBSITE: WWW.SMHS.GWUMC.EDU/MDPROGRAMS/ADMISSIONS

STUDENT BODY

Type	Private
Enrollment of parent institution	25,000
Enrollment of medical school	716
% male/female	47/53
% underrepresented minorities	2
% international	40
Average age of entering class	23

ADMISSIONS

# applied	10,493
% accepted	3
% enrolled	52

Average GPA and MCAT Scores

Overall GPA	3.7
MCAT Bio	10.7
MCAT Phys	10.2
MCAT Verbal	9.6
MCAT Essay	P

Application Information

Regular application	12/1
Early application	8/15
Early notification	10/1
Are transfers accepted?	Yes
Admissions may be deferred?	Yes
Admissions need-blind?	No
Application fee	$125

Academics

The George Washington University School of Medicine and Health Sciences (SMHS) is steps away from the White House in the heart of the nation's capital. This unique location provides students the opportunity to participate in internships with prestigious scientific, professional, and government agencies and organizations that serve the community, shape health policy, or make a difference in the world. There is an exciting range of opportunities for students to pursue their dreams through study, research, and the practice of medicine under the guidance of nationally and internationally recognized faculty and physicians.

BASIC SCIENCES: The George Washington University MD curriculum prepares well-trained physicians to complete residencies in primary care or specialized areas of concentration. Our medical school also stresses education through cooperation and collaboration rather than competition and emphasizes working with groups of colleagues and co-workers. Courses in gross anatomy, microscopic anatomy, Practice of Medicine I, medical biochemistry, immunology, neurobiology, psychopathology, and physiology constitute the first year study. The second-year curriculum focuses on abnormal human biology through courses in microbiology, pathology, pharmacology, an interdisciplinary, organ-system course titled Introduction to Clinical Medicine, and Practice of Medicine II.

CLINICAL TRAINING

The School of Medicine curriculum contains a unique course titled, "The Practice of Medicine (POM)." This revolutionary course, spanning all four years, allows students to begin clinical training during their first year of medical school while at the same time learning the traditional basic sciences. During POM, students learn about the doctor-patient relationship, essential communication skills, basic clinical assessment skills of interviewing and physical examination, professionalism, ethics, and many issues of the medicine-society interface. In addition to the early clinical training is two-year continuum of clinical clerkships in Year 3 including eight-week clerkships in each of the six major clinical disciplines conducted at the GW hospital and affiliated institutions. In Year 4 there is a four-week "acting internship" in Medicine, Pediatrics, or Family Medicine. The GW Clinical Learning and Simulation Skills (CLASS) Center is housed on the 6th floor of the GW Hospital. Dedicated to education and research, the Center features cutting edge technology in a setting that is among the most innovative in the nation. It is in this setting that students gain the comprehensive clinical exposure, feedback, and evaluation they need to become both technically adept and humane caregivers for their patients. We have other affiliates and our pediatrics faculty practice at the Children's National Medical Center.

Students

The Fall 2012 entering class hailed from 25 different states, spanning the United States from Oregon to Florida and matriculating from 79 different undergraduate institutions. Thirty-two percent of incoming students were non-science majors and twelve percent held various graduate degrees. Last year's entering class ranged in age from twenty to forty-seven years old.

STUDENT LIFE

The GW campus is nestled in the Foggy Bottom area of Washington D.C. and is within walking distance of the White House and many other governmental, historical, and cultural landmarks. The campus is subway accessible; the Foggy Bottom/GWU metro stop sits immediately outside the School of Medicine. A state-of-the-art Health and Wellness Center, also two blocks from Ross Hall, is an 188,000 square foot facility that hosts a wide variety of fitness and instructional classes; walk-in recreation; and sport club, intramural, and wellness programs and services.

GRADUATES

The GW SMHS maintains a national reputation for placing qualified graduates into quality residency programs. Many students choose to continue their postgraduate work at GW and be a part of our state-of-the-art hospital. In fact, of the graduating class of 2012, 21 members remained at GW to complete their residencies. Some of the other institutions at which members of the class of 2012 were placed include: Yale-New Haven Hospital, Mt. Sinai Hospital, Stanford University, and Johns Hopkins Hospital. The following list indicates some of the specialties and/or programs that were most highly matched by GW graduates: Anesthesiology, Emergency Medicine, Surgery, Internal Medicine, Pediatrics, Radiology, Family Practice, OB/GYN, and Psychiatry.

Admissions

REQUIREMENTS

Have completed or plan to complete a minimum of 90 semester hours at an accredited American or Canadian college or university prior to matriculation. A completed bachelors degree before the start of your first year of medical school is preferred. Transfer coursework from foreign schools is not acceptable. Online coursework is not acceptable. Have completed or plan to complete 6 credits of English and 6 credits of lecture and 2 credits of lab in each of the following sciences: Biology (not Botany or Ecology courses), General Chemistry, Organic Chemistry, and Physics Taken or plan to take the Medical College Admission Test (MCAT) by no later than September 30, 2012. No MCAT scores prior to April 2010 will be accepted for consideration.For more information about the changes to the MCAT which will go into effect in 2015, please visit: https://www.aamc.org/students/applying/mcat/mcat2015/ Meet our technical standards requirements Those without U.S. citizenship, Canadian citizenship, or U.S. permanent residency must apply to the International Medicine Program.

SUGGESTIONS

We strongly urge you to complete your file as early as possible.

PROCESS

Once the Admissions Office receives an AMCAS application, the secondary application is sent to the applicant. GW requires three letters of recommendation (one from science faculty and one familiar with your personal traits), a pre-medical advisor letter or committee advisory letter. Applicants have letters sent directly to AMCAS. It will take several weeks to process your application and letters of recommendation after AMCAS has confirmed receipt of all letters. The application process is very competitive, as there are over 13,000 applicants for approximately 177 seats. Interviews and acceptances are offered on a rolling admissions basis. Please note the following deadlines: AMCAS: December 1 GW Secondary Application: January 1 (postmarked) Letters of Recommendation: must be received by AMCAS by January 1 (postmarked) Each year the Admissions Office offers approximately 1,000 interviews to selected applicants. These interviews are "blind" (the interviewers do not read the applicant's file prior to the interview). Interviews are from September to March. Acceptances into the class may be offered from 10/15 until early August.

Admissions Requirements (Required)

MCAT Scores, Essays, Science GPA, Extracurricular activities, Non-Science GPA, Exposure to medical profession, Recommendation, Interview

Admissions Requirements (Optional)

State Residency

COSTS AND AID

Tuition & Fees

Annual tuition	$50,903
Room & board	$17,937
Cost of books	$4,976
Fees	$375

Financial Aid

% students receiving any aid	78
% students receiving grants	38
% students receiving loans	76
% aid that is merit-based	14
Average grant	$10,725
Average loan	$43,275
Average total aid package	$79,028
Average debt	$197,485

HARVARD UNIVERSITY

HARVARD MEDICAL SCHOOL

OFFICE OF ADMISSIONS, 210 GORDON HALL, 25 SHATTUCK STREET, BOSTON, MA 02115 • **ADMISSION:** 617-432-1550
FAX: 617-432-33077 • **E-MAIL:** ADMISSIONS_OFFICE@HMS.HARVARD.EDU • **WEBSITE:** WWW.HMS.HARVARD.EDU

STUDENT BODY

Type	Private
Enrollment of medical school	735
% male/female	46/54
% underrepresented minorities	19
Average age of entering class	23

FACULTY

Total faculty	9,352

ADMISSIONS

# applied	5,779
% accepted	3.8
% enrolled	76

Average GPA and MCAT Scores

Overall GPA	3.8
MCAT Bio	12.0
MCAT Phys	12.0
MCAT Verbal	11.0
MCAT Essay	Q

Application Information

Regular application	10/15
Regular notification	3/7
Are transfers accepted?	No
Admissions may be deferred?	Yes
Admissions need-blind?	No
Application fee	$85

Academics

Two distinct programs are available at Harvard—the New Pathway and the Health Science and Technology (HST) Program. All entering students are assigned to one of five Societies, organizational units used both to structure academic activities and to facilitate interaction among students and between faculty and students. Joint Degree opportunities include the M.S.T.P.; other M.D./Ph.D. programs designed in collaboration with science and nonscience graduate departments; the combined M.D./M.P.H.; and an M.D./M.P.P. with the Kennedy School of Government. More than half of the students take at least five years to complete their education in order to take full advantage of scholastic and research opportunities, some of which are actually off campus and perhaps overseas.

BASIC SCIENCES: Students in the first year of the New Pathway concentrate on Biomedical and Social Sciences. The year is divided into six sections: The Human Body, Chemistry and Biology of the Cell, Physiology, Pharmacology, Genetics, and Immunology. Students are also introduced to clinical medicine in their first year. Year two has four segments: Human Nervous System, Pathology, Human Systems I, and Human Systems II. Concepts of behavioral and community health are integrated into the basic science studies. During the first two years, lectures are scheduled for only one hour out of each day. Lectures are enhanced with tutorials and labs, but most learning takes place outside of the classroom environment. Students are responsible for addressing specific clinical challenges through independent and small-group research and analysis. Participants in HST also manage their own learning but pose questions to answer through research rather than answering questions that arise through case presentations. During the Fall Semester of year one, H.S.T. students take the following: Functional Human Anatomy, Human Pathology, Cellular and Molecular Immunology, Molecular Biology, and Genetics. During Spring Semester students take Endocrinology; Cardiovascular, Renal, and Respiratory Pathophysiology; and Research. Electives in Social and Clinical Medicine are taken throughout the year. During Year Two, Students take Neuroscience, Microbial Pathogenesis, Research, Reproductive Biology, and Gastroenterology during the first semester and Pharmacology, Clinical Medicine, Hematology, and Psychopathology during the second semester. HST students complete a thesis as part of their requirements. Computers, loaded with curriculum-related software and linked with online data sources, are considered an important information management tool and are accessible in the Educational Center, the library, and the residence hall. The Countway Library of Medicine has one of the largest biomedical collections in the country. Grading is Satisfactory/Unsatisfactory for all courses. Passing Step 1 of the USMLE is required prior to graduation.

CLINICAL TRAINING
Patient contact begins in year one, when students learn to take histories and become familiar with basic elements of the physical exam. Formal clinical instruction begins in year three, when H.S.T. and New Pathway students join for required clerkships. These are Medicine (4 months); Neurology (1 month); Women's and Children's Health (3 months); Psychiatry (1 month); Radiology (1 month); and Surgery (3 months). Throughout years three and four, students take part in ongoing, part-time primary care training. Year four is composed mostly of electives, which can be clinical and/or research oriented. Elective credit may be earned from several departments at Harvard

University or from MIT. Clinical training takes place at Harvard-affiliated hospitals, which are Beth Israel Medical Center; Brigham and Women's Hospital; Cambridge Hospital; The Center for Blood Research; The Children's Hospital; The Dana-Farber Cancer Institute; DVA Medical Center; Harvard Pilgrim Health Care; Joslin Diabetes Center; Judge Baker Children's Center; Mass. Eye and Ear; Mass. General; Mass. Mental Health Center; McLean Hospital; Mount Auburn Hospital; Schepens Eye Research; and Spaulding Rehab Hospital. Evaluation of student performance in clinical settings uses a High Honors/Honors/Satisfactory/Unsatisfactory scale. Narrative comments accompany these marks. In addition to formal rotations, students can gain experience in clinical environments through volunteer activities such as the Urban Health Project, which provides preventive and curative care to community health centers and underserved populations. Students must pass the USMLE Step 2 in order to graduate.

Students

About 75 percent of students were science majors in college. About 20 percent of the members of a typical class are underrepresented minorities, and about 30 percent took significant time off between college and medical school. Students are from all around the country. Class size is 165, of which 30 are H.S.T. and 135 are New Pathway participants.

STUDENT LIFE

The compact class schedule allows students to take part in activities of the Medical School, the greater University, and the city of Boston. About 50 percent of medical students live in Vanderbilt Hall, a renovated building adjacent to the Medical School. Married students live either off campus or in university-owned apartments. Students are active in organizations focused on topics ranging from support for various minority groups, to abortion rights, to soccer.

GRADUATES

Approximately half of each graduating class remains at Harvard for their residencies. The University of California at San Francisco also appears to be a popular choice. Of the 1997 graduating class, the most common specialty choices were Internal Medicine (34%); Pediatrics (13%); General Surgery (9%); and Orthopedic Surgery (7%).

Admissions

REQUIREMENTS

Requirements include one year of Biology with lab; Physics with lab; Expository Writing; and college-level Calculus. Two years of Chemistry are required, both of which should involve laboratory experience. For New Pathway applicants, at least 16 additional credit hours in nonscience courses are required. For HST applicants, Calculus through differential equations and Calculus-based Physics are required. The quality of an applicant's undergraduate institution is assessed in evaluating his or her GPA. The MCAT is required, and all scores are considered.

SUGGESTIONS

Unlike many schools with rolling admissions, decisions at Harvard are made after all interviews are complete. Thus, applicants submitting scores from the August MCAT are not penalized. There is no preference for particular undergraduate majors, but demonstration of academic excellence is expected. In addition, most successful applicants have impressive professional, volunteer, community service, or other extracurricular achievements.

PROCESS

Interviews take place from September through January and consist of two one-hour sessions each with a member of the Admissions Committee. Decisions are made in late February, and all applicants are notified at once. A wait-list is established at that time, but usually only a few candidates are ultimately accepted from the list.

Admissions Requirements (Required)

MCAT Scores, Essays, Science GPA, Extracurricular activities, Non-Science GPA, Recommendation, Interview

Admissions Requirements (Optional)

Exposure to medical profession, State Residency

COSTS AND AID

Tuition & Fees

Annual tuition	$52,100
Room & board (on-campus off-campus)	$11,525/$10,180
Cost of books	$2,064
Fees	$3,671

Financial Aid

% students receiving any aid	74
% students receiving grants	46
% students receiving loans	74
% aid that is merit-based	0
Average grant	$40,675
Average loan	$25,950
Average debt	$104,107

Hofstra University

Hofstra North Shore - LIJ School of Medicine

500 Hofstra University, Hempstead, NY 11549 • **Admission:** 516-463-7519 • **Fax:** 516-463-75437
E-mail: Medicine.admissions@hofstra.edu • **Website:** medicine.hofstra.edu

STUDENT BODY

Type	Private
Enrollment of parent institution	11,023
Enrollment of medical school	175
% male/female	51/49
% out-of-state	48
% international	14
Average age of entering class	24

FACULTY

Total faculty	1,542
% female faculty	29
% minority faculty	6
% part-time faculty	0
Student-faculty ratio	0.1:1

ADMISSIONS

# applied	5,585
% accepted	4
% enrolled	34

Average GPA and MCAT Scores

Overall GPA	3.7
MCAT Bio	11.0
MCAT Phys	11.0
MCAT Verbal	10.0

Application Information

Regular application	11/15
Are transfers accepted?	No
Admissions may be deferred?	Yes
Admissions need-blind?	No
Application fee	$100

Academics

Hofstra's educational program is innovative and stresses translation of knowledge and understanding into action. Science and clinical medicine are wrapped together throughout all four years of the curriculum in an interactive format that emphasizes critical evaluation and application of basic and clinical scientific information to socially contextualized patient care. The School of Medicine offers educational programs for the MD, PhD and MD/PhD degrees, as well as a combined MD/MPH. The program for the MD degree is intentionally designed to provide a general, interdisciplinary medical education that prepares students for all career options in medicine. The PhD program trains individuals in biomedical, translational and clinical research, culminating in awarding of the PhD in The Molecular Basis of Medicine. MD/PhD students complete the entire MD educational program, three longitudinal seminar courses, and significant, original scholarly activity.

BASIC SCIENCES: Like the Departments of Molecular Medicine and Science Education, the natural and social science curricula are intentionally designed to be cross-disciplinary. In the first 100 weeks of the program, basic science and clinical content are interwoven through case-based inquiry sessions, or PEARLS (Patient-Centered Explorations in Active Reasoning, Learning and Synthesis). PEARLS cases are the "spools" around which the learning objectives are threaded and from which all learning sessions are derived; they are specifically designed to ensure that students developmentally acquire the skills needed to solve clinical problems by critically evaluating and applying basic and clinical scientific knowledge to socially contextualized patient care.

CLINICAL TRAINING

Students learn clinical medicine within the North Shore-LIJ Health System, the country's third largest non-profit, secular healthcare system and home to over 100 accredited post-graduate residency and fellowship training programs. During the first half of their training, students engage in longitudinal, one-on-one, active, initial clinical learning experiences with a panel of patients and preceptors in each of five core disciplines. In the advanced clinical experiences during the second half of their training, students move ahead in their competency-based learning program in preparation for residency. Throughout their training, students are coached and assessed as they advance toward acquisition of developmentally appropriate competencies.

Students

The Medical Education Center of the Hofstra North Shore—LIJ School of Medicine is located on the Hofstra University campus. Located 25 miles from New York City, the 240 acre campus offers the best of both the urban and suburban environment. Additionally, being located on the campus allows medical students the opportunity to interact with the other graduate and undergraduate students on campus.

STUDENT LIFE

Students in the Hofstra North Shore—LIJ School of Medicine have the option to reside on campus in the graduate resident hall. There is an array of dining options, including the School of Medicine's own eatery. In addition, Hofstra boasts extensive and recently renovated fitness and athletic facilities, including an indoor pool and gymnasium, as well as outstanding entertainment such as concerts, films, lectures, sporting events and an art museum. In addition, medical students have the unique opportunity to create and participate in experiences that shape the culture of the school.

Admissions

REQUIREMENTS

In addition to an AMCAS application, applicants are required to submit a supplemental application to the School of Medicine. The Admissions Committee uses a holistic approach to evaluate each application. The Committee considers an applicant's individual attributes and experiences, as well as academic metrics. Competitive applicants are asked to visit the school for an interview; all students are required to interview prior to matriculation.

SUGGESTIONS

Prospective students are encouraged to learn more about our selection process by reading the materials posted for prospective students on our website, http://medicine.hofstra.edu.

PROCESS

Applicants can apply through the AMCAS in July for the following year. Through AMCAS, applicants submit a committee letter of recommendation or three individual letters of recommendation, as well as an MCAT score from an examination taken within the previous three years.

Admissions Requirements (Required)

MCAT Scores, Essays, Science GPA, Extracurricular activities, Non-Science GPA, Exposure to medical profession, Recommendation, Interview

COSTS AND AID

Tuition & Fees

Annual tuition	$45,000
Room & board (on-campus off-campus)	$17,551/$19,725
Cost of books	$7,797
Fees	$1,500

Financial Aid

% students receiving any aid	83
% students receiving grants	83
% students receiving loans	78
Average grant	$20,285
Average loan	$47,266
Average total aid package	$67,551

HOWARD UNIVERSITY
COLLEGE OF MEDICINE

ADMISSIONS OFFICE, 520 WEST STREET, NW, WASHINGTON, DC 20059 • ADMISSION: 202-806-6270
FAX: 202-806-79347 • E-MAIL: BHLOGAN@ACCESS.HOWARD.EDU • WEBSITE: WWW.MED.HOWARD.EDU

STUDENT BODY	
Type	Private
Enrollment of medical school	454
% male/female	51/49
% international	59

ADMISSIONS	
# applied	5,505

Application Information	
Regular application	12/15
Are transfers accepted?	No
Admissions may be deferred?	Yes
Admissions need-blind?	Yes
Application fee	$45

Academics

Although most students earn their M.D. in four years, some are given permission to complete requirements over a five-year period. The College of Medicine and the Graduate School of Arts and Sciences offer a joint M.D./Ph.D. program. The departments that award the Ph.D. are the following: Anatomy, Biochemistry, Biology, Chemistry, Genetics, Microbiology, Pharmacology, and Physiology.

BASIC SCIENCES: Basic sciences are presented primarily in a lecture/lab format. Students are in scheduled classes from 25 to 30 hours per week. First-year courses are: Anatomy; Biochemistry; Psychiatry; Histology; Microbiology; Immunology; Physiology; Neuroscience; Introduction to Patient Care, in which students visit clinics and interact with physicians; and Introduction to Psychodynamic Thinking, which discusses healthy and pathological mental mechanisms. Second-year courses are the following: Microbiology, Immunology, Pathology, Genetics, Physiology, Physical Diagnosis, Pathophysiology, Pharmacology, Psychopathology, and Epidemiology. Grading is Honors/Satisfactory and Unsatisfactory, and academic support services such as workshops, tutorials, and summer sessions are available. The USMLE Step 1 is required for promotion to year three. Instruction takes place in the Seeley G. Mudd Building, which features auditoriums, laboratories, and audiovisual and computer-assisted study areas. The Health Sciences Library has 260,000 volumes and journals, video equipment, and a computer linkage with the National Library of Medicine.

CLINICAL TRAINING
Patient contact begins in the first year, in Introduction to Patient Care. Throughout medical school, students have the opportunity to gain clinical experience by volunteering and participating in community outreach programs. Others gain research experience through work at NIH or other prominent institutions. Formal clinical training begins in year three (or year four for those in a five-year course of study), with the following required clerkships: Medicine (12 weeks); Surgery (8 weeks); Ob/Gyn (8 weeks); Pediatrics (8 weeks); Psychiatry (6 weeks); Rehabilitation and Neurological Disease (4 weeks); and Family Practice (4 weeks). For two hours per week, during one semester, third-year students attend lectures on ethical and legal issues in health care. Senior-year requirements are Medicine (4 weeks) and Surgery (4 weeks). In addition, students take 20-24 weeks of electives in four-week blocks. Evaluation of clinical performance uses Honors/Satisfactory/Unsatisfactory, and the USMLE Step 2 is required for graduation. Clinical training takes place largely at Howard University Hospital (300 beds). Other sites used are Howard University Cancer Center; Center for Sickle Cell Disease; Walter Reed Army and National Naval Medical Centers; D.C. General Hospital; St. Elizabeth's Hospital; VA Medical Center; Providence Hospital; Greater Southeast Community Hospital; Prince George's Hospital Center; Washington Hospital Center; and National Rehabilitation Hospital.

Students

About 60 percent of the students are African American, and about 10 percent are from African or Caribbean countries. An average of thirty states and several foreign countries are usually represented. From 10 percent to 20 percent of the students in each entering class attended Howard for undergraduate, pre-medical studies. About 20 percent of entrants are considered nontraditional, having taken time off between college and medical school and participated in some sort of post-baccalaureate pre-medical program. Class size is 110.

STUDENT LIFE

Medical students enjoy both an active campus life and involvement in the greater community. They may participate in Howard University activities, such as its radio and television stations, intramural athletic teams and events, conferences, and social or special-interest clubs. Washington, D.C., is a center for cultural, academic, recreational, and obviously, political activities. In addition to being an international city, D.C. has a strong local, predominantly African American community that is highly diverse. The College of Medicine is part of Howard's downtown campus, which is metro accessible and convenient to lively neighborhoods and interesting parts of the city such as the White House and Smithsonian Museums. Housing for graduate students is available in modern, University-owned apartments. However, most students live off campus and either walk or take public transportation to school.

GRADUATES

About 25 percent of African American physicians practicing in the United States are Howard Alumni. Howard graduates secure post-graduate positions at institutions all over the country. Significant numbers enter one of the 16 residency programs at Howard University Hospital or at D.C. General Hospital, where they are also supervised by Howard faculty.

Admissions

REQUIREMENTS

Requirements are the following: Biology (8 hours); Chemistry (8 hours); Organic Chemistry (8 hours); Physics (8 hours); College Math (6 hours); and English (6 hours). The MCAT is required and must have been taken within the past three years

SUGGESTIONS

Beyond required courses, Cell Biology, Biochemistry, and Developmental Biology or Embryology are recommended. For students who have taken time off after college, recent course work is helpful. The Admissions Committee values activities that demonstrate an interest in working with underserved communities.

PROCESS

All AMCAS applicants receive secondary applications. Of those submitting secondaries, about 10 percent are interviewed with faculty or administrators. Others are rejected, advised to retake the MCAT, or put in a hold category and considered for interview later in the year. Of those interviewed, 70 percent are accepted on a rolling basis, and the rest are either rejected or wait-listed. Wait-listed candidates may submit supplementary information and grades. A limited number of high school seniors are accepted into a combined B.S./M.D. program organized with Howard's College of Arts and Sciences that allows students to earn both degrees in a six-year period. Through an Early Entrance Program, a few students nationwide may be admitted to the College of Medicine after their college junior year.

Admissions Requirements (Required)

MCAT Scores, Science GPA, Extracurricular activities, Non-Science GPA, Exposure to medical profession, Recommendation, Interview, State Residency

Admissions Requirements (Optional)

Essays

COSTS AND AID

Tuition & Fees

Annual tuition	$24,055
Room & board	$11,663
Cost of books	$1,240
Fees	$1,636

Financial Aid

% students receiving any aid	85
Average debt	$63,000

ICAHN SCHOOL OF MEDICINE AT MOUNT SINAI

ICAHN SCHOOL OF MEDICINE AT MOUNT SINAI

ANNENBERG 5-04A, BOX 1002, ONE GUSTAVE L. LEVY PLACE, NEW YORK, NY 10029-6574 • ADMISSION: 212-241-6696
FAX: 212-828-41357 • E-MAIL: ADMISSIONS@MSSM.EDU • WEBSITE: WWW.MSSM.EDU/BULLETIN

STUDENT BODY

Type	Private
Enrollment of medical school	505
% male/female	45/55
% underrepresented minorities	33
% out-of-state	60
% international	35
Average age of entering class	24

FACULTY

Total faculty	1,922
% female faculty	36
% minority faculty	25
% part-time faculty	13
Student-faculty ratio	4.0:1

ADMISSIONS

# applied	4,770
% accepted	7
% enrolled	40

Average GPA and MCAT Scores

Overall GPA	3.6
MCAT Bio	11.4
MCAT Phys	10.7
MCAT Verbal	11.7
MCAT Essay	Q

Application Information

Regular application	11/1
Early application	8/1
Early notification	10/1
Are transfers accepted?	Yes
Admissions may be deferred?	Yes
Admissions need-blind?	No
Application fee	$105

Academics

Mount Sinai's approach to medical education emphasizes cooperative rather than competitive learning to prepare students for the lifelong learning that is essential for the modern medical career. Group study, small classes and, for the past 30 years, a Pass/Fail grading system for the first- and second-year students contribute to this emphasis. The majority of the students' time in the first two (pre-clinical) years is focused on the core biomedical knowledge and the basic skills of the doctor-patient relationship. Through direct patient contact during the third and fourth (clinical) years in inpatient and ambulatory settings, students develop the skills necessary for the practice of medicine. We offer the following joint degree programs: M.S./M.D., M.D/M.P.H., M.D./M.B.A. In addition, eight to ten students each year pursue an MSTP-sponsored Ph.D. degree along with the M.D. in conjunction with the Mount Sinai Graduate School of Biological Sciences. The Ph.D. may be earned in Biochemistry, Biomathematical Sciences, Cell Biology and Anatomy, Genetics, Immunobiology, Microbiology, Molecular Biology, Neuroscience, Pharmacology, or Physiology/Biophysics. Evaluation of student performance uses Pass/Fail for the pre-clinical courses and Honor/High Pass/Pass/Fail for clinical training. Students must pass Step 1 of the USMLE for promotion to year three, and Step 2 in order to graduate.

BASIC SCIENCES: Basic sciences are taught through a combination of lectures, small-group discussions, labs, and clinical correlates. Lecture time is kept to two hours per day and students typically have three mornings or afternoons per week study time. Beginning on Day One, The Art and Science of Medicine, taught in both the first and second years, introduces students to the skills needed to care for patients. Throughout both years the emphasis is on case-based learning. Integrated with every course are numerous means for providing clinical relevance for the basic science being studied. Topics—such as ethics, radiology, and palliative care—that overlap many areas are incorporated into the curriculum of all four years through Courses Without Walls. First-year courses are Genetics, First Aid, Embryology, Molecules and Cells, Histology and Physiology, and Pathogenesis and Host Defense Mechanisms. The year ends with an integrative core that focuses on translational topics, allowing students to work with faculty from the bench to the bedside on a selected and structured topic. Extensive study of Mechanisms of Disease and Therapy is the major focus of the second year. This sequence of courses addresses each of the major pathophysiology topics essential to the practice of medicine. Organs and systems covered include respiratory, cardiovascular, renal/genitourinary, breast, skin, gynecologic, hematologic, endocrine, and musculoskeletal. A section on Brain and Behavior encompasses both psychopathology and neurology and at the end of the year the focus shifts to epidemiology and biostatistics.

CLINICAL TRAINING

The curriculum in the third year is composed of four 12-week modules of clinical clerkships. The modules are Pediatrics, Obstetrics, Nursery, and Gynecology; Medicine and Geriatrics; Surgery and Psychiatry; and Neurology, Anesthesia and Family Practice. Four weeks of electives are also offered in the third year. As in the first two years, an integrated case-based curriculum enriches the learning opportunities throughout the year. The fourth year begins with a four-week preparation period for Step 2 of the USMLE followed by an emergency rotation and a subinternship in medicine. A clinical

Translational Fellowship combines the clinical practice of medicine with the relevant basic science. A four-week required Post-Match Integrated Selective addresses issues essential for students to explore before going on to residency. A significant portion of clinical training takes place at The Mount Sinai Hospital, which includes the 625-bed Guggenheim Pavilion and a Primary Care Building with an expansive ambulatory care program. Affiliated teaching facilities include, but are not limited to, Bronx Veterans Affairs Medical Center (561 beds), Elmhurst Hospital Center (Queens, 526 beds), Englewood Hospital and Medical Center (New Jersey, 520 beds), North General Hospital (Central and East Harlem), and Maimonedes Medical Center.

Students

A recent entering class came from 46 different undergraduate institutions and pursued 54 undergraduate majors. Underrepresented minorities accounted for 21 percent of the students. The average age of incoming students was 23.

STUDENT LIFE

Mount Sinai provides a healthy environment and encourages the development of life-long healthy habits. Cultural diversity is respected and supported, both in and out of the classroom. Students are active in a wide range of school-related organizations, particularly those focused on community service activities, and New York City is a rich source of extracurricular life. The Recreation Office provides discounted tickets to theater, movies, sporting events, and concerts. The Aron Residence Hall offers over 600 furnished suites for single students. It is conveniently located, and features a fitness center, among other amenities. School-owned housing for couples is also available.

GRADUATES

Among a recent graduating class, 21 percent entered Internal Medicine, 8 percent entered Pediatrics, 19 percent entered Surgical Specialties, and 5 percent entered Ob/Gyn. The remainder entered a broad range of other post-graduate programs.

Admissions

REQUIREMENTS

Prerequisites are one year each of General Chemistry, Organic Chemistry, Biology, college-level Math, English, and Physics. The MCAT is required, and scores from 2000 onward are acceptable.

SUGGESTIONS

Students who have taken significant time off after college should have some recent course work. No particular extracurricular activities are specified, although successful applicants usually have some community service, research, or medically-related experience.

PROCESS

All AMCAS applicants receive secondary applications. Of those returning secondaries, about 17 percent are interviewed. Interviews are conducted from September through March, and consist of two half-hour sessions, either with two faculty members or a faculty member and a medical student. Candidates are notified of the committee's decision with two to six weeks after the interview. Wait-listed candidates may send supplementary material to update their files. An early assurance program admits a limited number of sophomores with admission contingent upon completing undergraduate requirements.

Admissions Requirements (Required)

MCAT Scores, Essays, Science GPA, Extracurricular activities, Non-Science GPA, Exposure to medical profession, Recommendation, Interview

Admissions Requirements (Optional)

State Residency

COSTS AND AID

Tuition & Fees

Annual tuition	$33,250
Room & board	$13,800
Cost of books	$1,220
Fees	$3,800

Indiana University
School of Medicine

1120 South Drive Fesler Hall 213, Indianapolis, IN 46202 • **Admission:** 317-274-3772 • **Fax:** 317-278-02117
E-mail: INMEDADM@IUPUI.EDU • **Website:** WWW.ADMISSIONS.MEDICINE.IU.EDU

STUDENT BODY

Type	Public
Enrollment of medical school	1,318
% male/female	56/44
% underrepresented minorities	1
% out-of-state	19
% international	27
Average age of entering class	23

FACULTY

Total faculty	1,977
% part-time faculty	7

ADMISSIONS

# applied	4,711
% accepted	11
% enrolled	64

Average GPA and MCAT Scores

Overall GPA	3.7
MCAT Bio	11.1
MCAT Phys	10.9
MCAT Verbal	10.1
MCAT Essay	0

Application Information

Regular application	12/15
Regular notification	10/15
Early application	8/1
Early notification	10/1
Are transfers accepted?	No
Admissions may be deferred?	Yes
Admissions need-blind?	No
Application fee	$50

Academics

The School of Medicine in Indianapolis is part of the Indiana University (IU) Medical Center, which includes schools of Nursing, Dentistry, and Health and Rehabilitation Sciences. The Medical Center complex occupies 85 acres and is situated one mile from downtown Indianapolis. In conjunction with the University Graduate School, The School of Medicine offers selected students an opportunity to pursue the M.S. or Ph.D. degrees along with an M.D. Through this program, degrees may be earned in Anatomy, Biochemistry, Biophysics, Genetics, Neurobiology, Microbiology, Pathology, Pharmacology, Physiology, Toxicology, and in Humanities and Social Studies disciplines.

BASIC SCIENCES: First-year students select one of the following nine locations for their pre-clinical studies: IU Bloomington; IU Indianapolis; Lafayette Center at Purdue; University of Notre Dame; Ball State University; Indiana State University; University of Evansville; Indiana University Northwest; and Fort Wayne Center for Medical Education at Purdue. While the curriculum is essentially the same at each campus, the methods of instruction may differ, with some programs relying more or less on case-based learning. At all schools, the "core" basic science courses are complemented by early clinical correlations. Throughout the first two years, scheduled classes account for 26-28 hours per week. At the Indianapolis campus, 80 percent of class time is devoted to lectures and labs, and 20 percent is used for small-group discussions. First-year courses are the following: Anatomy; Histology; Biochemistry; Physiology; Microbiology; Evidence-Based Medicine; Immunology; Patient/Doctor Relationship; and Concepts of Health and Disease, which teaches students how to apply basic science concepts to clinical problems. Year two courses are: Biostatistics; Pharmacology; Pathology; Clinical Medicine; Medical Genetics; and Neurobiology. With the exception of Clinical Medicine, during which students join medical teams in hospitals, second-year courses use lectures and labs as instructional techniques. The Medical Center offers all modern learning tools, including computers and audiovisual equipment. The Ruth Lilly Medical Library (200,000 volumes) is located in the Medical Research Building in Indianapolis and serves the Schools of Medicine and Nursing. All campuses have affiliated library systems, and all libraries are electronically linked. The libraries have access to 400 databases and online informational resources. Evaluation uses an Honors/High Pass/Pass/Fail system. Passing the USMLE Step 1 is a requirement for promotion to year three.

CLINICAL TRAINING

All students spend their third year at the Medical Center in Indianapolis, rotating through 11 hospitals in the Indianapolis area. The patient population is drawn from both urban and rural areas. Year three is largely composed of required rotations which are the following: Medicine (12 weeks); Surgery (8 weeks); Pediatrics (8 weeks); Ob/Gyn (6 weeks); Psychiatry (6 weeks); and Family Medicine (4 weeks). Required fourth-year clerkships are Surgical Subspecialties (8 weeks), Neurology (4 weeks), and Radiology (4 weeks). Year four is mostly dedicated to elective study, which may be pursued off campus, around the country, or overseas. Evaluation of clinical performance uses an Honors/High Pass/Pass/Fail system, augmented by narratives. Honors students generally take part in departmental research activities. Passing the USMLE Step 2 is a requirement for graduation.

Students

Typically, 85 percent of an entering class are Indiana residents. About 12 percent are underrepresented minorities, most of whom are African Americans. Approximately 5 percent of students are older than 30 at the time of matriculation.

STUDENT LIFE

Students are given a voice in school administration and curriculum development through an elected Student Government. Though student life differs from one campus to another, in general medical students benefit from the social and cultural offerings of a large university system. There is a wide range of lifestyles among students, with some living on campus in residence halls or apartments and others living off campus, perhaps with their families. Medical students have access to all campus recreational facilities and events.

GRADUATES

Slightly less than half of the 2013 graduating class entered residency programs in Indiana. Other popular locations for post-graduate training were Michigan, Ohio, and Illinois. The most common specialty choices were Family Medicine (16% of the class); Internal Medicine (11%); Pediatrics (11%); Surgery (10%); Radiology (9%); Ob/Gyn (8%); and Emergency Medicine (7%); and Anesthesia (7%). About 60% of graduates entered fields considered to be primary care.

Admissions

REQUIREMENTS

Required undergraduate courses are one year each of the following: Chemistry, Organic Chemistry, Biology, Physics, biochemisty, sociology, and psychology. All courses must include labs. Beyond GPA, the quality of an applicant's undergraduate course load is considered rather than the quantity of extra course hours. The MCAT is required, and must be no more than four years old. If an applicant has retaken the MCAT, the most recent score is considered.

SUGGESTIONS

Undergraduate course work in Social Sciences and Humanities is important. For applicants who have taken significant time off after college, some recent course work is useful. The April, rather than August MCAT is strongly recommended. Among out-of-state applicants, those with strong qualifications and some sort of ties to the state are the most likely to be admitted. The School aims to admit candidates who are likely to choose careers in primary care.

PROCESS

Only highly qualified candidates are sent supplmental packets. Interviews take place on Wednesdays, from September through February and are scheduled in the order in which completed applications are received. Interviews consist of a one-hour session with a team of faculty members. Notification occurs on a monthly basis, beginning in October. Applicants are either accepted, rejected, or deferred and re-evaluated later in the year. In the spring, a wait-list is established. Wait-listed candidates may submit supplementary material if it adds new information to his or her file.

Admissions Requirements (Required)

MCAT Scores, Essays, Science GPA, Extracurricular activities, Non-Science GPA, Exposure to medical profession, Recommendation, Interview, State Residency

COSTS AND AID

Tuition & Fees

Annual tuition (in-state out-of-state)	$33,019/$51,888
Room & board	$11,144
Cost of books	$3,610
Fees	$455

Financial Aid

% students receiving any aid	91
% students receiving grants	41
% students receiving loans	86
% aid that is merit-based	14
Average grant	$8,345
Average loan	$45,923
Average total aid package	$46,850
Average debt	$157,212

JOHNS HOPKINS UNIVERSITY
SCHOOL OF MEDICINE

733 N. BROADWAY, SUITE G-49, BALTIMORE, MD 21205 • ADMISSION: 410-955-3182 • FAX: 410-955-74947
E-MAIL: SOMADMISS@JHMI.EDU • WEBSITE: WWW.HOPKINSMEDICINE.ORG

STUDENT BODY	
Type	Private
Enrollment of parent institution	16,000
Enrollment of medical school	473
% out-of-state	83
# countries represented	30
Average age of entering class	23

ADMISSIONS	
# applied	3,655
% accepted	7
% enrolled	49

Average GPA and MCAT Scores	
Overall GPA	3.9
MCAT Bio	12.5
MCAT Phys	12.0
MCAT Verbal	10.9
MCAT Essay	R

Application Information	
Regular application	10/15
Early application	8/1
Early notification	10/1
Are transfers accepted?	No
Admissions may be deferred?	Yes
Admissions need-blind?	No
Application fee	$80

Academics

In 1992 Hopkins implemented a revised curriculum that introduced case-based learning, exposure to clinical settings during the first year, and a Physicians and Society (P&S) course, which integrates social, economic, and ethical perspectives into the four-year basic and clinical science curriculum. Studies leading to both an M.D. and a Ph.D. or M.A./M.S. in the following fields are possible: Biochemistry, Cellular and Molecular Biology, Biological Chemistry, Biomedical Engineering, Biophysics, Biophysics/ Molecular Biophysics, Cell Biology and Anatomy, Cellular and Molecular Medicine, History of Medicine, Genetics, History of Science, Medicine and Technology, Human Genetics and Molecular Biology, Immunology, Medical and Biological Illustration, Neuroscience, Pharmacology, Molecular Sciences, Physiology, and Public Health. The combined M.D./M.P.H. is particularly popular, which is not surprising given the excellent reputation of the School of Public Health.

BASIC SCIENCES: Classroom Learning: Year 1 begins with 7 weeks of Anatomy, followed by 10 weeks of Scientific Foundations (introductory courses in cell biology, molecular biology, genetics, biochemistry, public health and epidemiology). A 45 week course, Genes to Society (GTS), spans the remainder of the Year 1 and Year 2 curriculum. This course is organized into systems blocks, e.g. Cardiovascular, Immunology, etc., and integrates content from molecular biology to public health in presenting each system. Lectures, discussion, case-study, and student presentations are all important components of the GTS curriculum Blocks are separated by Intersession weeks which address integrative aspects of medicine, such as Health Promotion, Pain Care, Global Health, and Patient Safety. Intersessions are directed by multidisciplinary faculty with emphasis on small group discussion and skills acquisition. During the last 2 years of the curriculum, students return to the basic sciences with week-long seminars in topics of Inflammation, Cancer, Infectious Disease and Metabolism, to explore research and translational medicine. For the Scholarly Concentration course, students choose one of five areas of interest, Basic Research, Clinical Research, Public Health and Policy, Medical Humanities and History of Medicine. Students will participate in seminars and complete a mentored project in their Scholarly Concentration. Many students take on research projects during the summer between their first and second years; 60% of students choose to take an additional year of research to complete the curriculum. Grading is Pass/Fail. Faculty members, assigned to incoming students, both advise and monitor student progress.

CLINICAL TRAINING

Clinical Training: Facilities for clinical training include the Johns Hopkins Hospital complex, which is comprised of numerous affiliates, is housed in 37 buildings, and contains over 1,100 beds. In addition to serving the urban population of Baltimore and the surrounding areas, Johns Hopkins Hospitals attract patients from around the country and the world. Students are also encouraged to pursue clinical experiences away from Hopkins, and a significant number do so overseas. The clinical curriculum begins with introduction to the medical interview and physical diagnosis in the first 4 months of Year 1; continues with a Longitudinal Clerkship one half-day per week from mid-Year 1 to mid Year 2. At completion of Year 2, students do a month of Transitions to the Wards with integrative problem based learning and simulations to prepare for hospital based medicine. Each of the 7 required clinical clerkships includes several days of simulation and interdisciplinary team training. Year 4 emphasizes complex and critical care, with required rotations in intensive care unit, chronic care and rehabilitation and a subinternship. A two week course occurs after Match Day to prepare students for internship with ACLS certification, rapid response simulations, advanced communications and reflective exercises. Thirty weeks of the clinical curriculum is elective time. Successful completion of a comprehensive clinical skills examination taken in the fall of Year 4 is required for graduation. Grading is Honors/High Pass/Pass/Fail.

Students

The diversity of the student body reflects the School's national reputation. A typical class has students from 35 different states and 70 or more colleges. As is the case with most top schools, half the entrants are women. Efforts are made to recruit ethnic minorities, and approximately 15 percent of the student body are from Underrepresented Minorities groups. Class size is limited to 120.

STUDENT LIFE

For some, social life revolves around school, where students spend a great deal of time. Others, particularly those from the area or with families, have lives outside of the Medical School. Housing is available for single students or for married students living alone, in Reed Hall dorms adjacent to campus. However, most choose to live in apartments off campus. For those accustomed to New York or Washington, D.C., the housing situation in Baltimore is good. The Housing Office assists students in their apartment searches. Recreational facilities, including a full-size gym, are free to medical students and are located next to Reed Hall. Several medical societies exist, including a Women's Medical Alumni Association, which provides support for women students and physicians. There is also a Student National Medical Association, which is active in both campus and community minority affairs.

GRADUATES

Graduates of Hopkins have their pick of residency programs, even those graduating with GPAs that are at the lower end of their class. About 50 percent of graduates enter Primary Care specialties; 20 percent ultimately enter academic medicine or work primarily in research.

Admissions

REQUIREMENTS

In addition to the typical requirement of one year each, Biology, Chemistry, Organic Chemistry, Physics, and one year of Calculus (or one semester of Calculus and one semester of Statistics is acceptable), and 24 semester hours combined of humanities and social sciences are required. Advanced Placement credits accepted by the applicant's undergraduate institution may be submitted in lieu of taking the required courses for Chemistry, Physics and Calculus. Johns Hopkins does participate in AMCAS. The on-line secondary application may be accessed at anytime after June 1 once the applicant has received an AAMC ID number, but before the December 1 deadlline.

SUGGESTIONS

Hopkins is concerned with both the academic and personal records of applicants and notes that intellectual progress through college is important. Extracurricular activities need not be medically related, but should demonstrate humanistic values and perseverance.

PROCESS

About 15 percent of applicants are invited for interviews, which occur between September and March, and about 29 percent of those interviewed are accepted on a rolling basis. Applicants are interviewed by Admissions Committee Members, and regional interviews may be arranged for applicants living a distance from Baltimore. At Admissions Committee meetings, decisions are made to admit, reject, or wait-list applicants. In April, wait-listed candidates are notified of their position on the list.

Admissions Requirements (Required)

MCAT Scores, Essays, Science GPA, Non-Science GPA, Recommendation, Interview

Admissions Requirements (Optional)

Extracurricular activities, Exposure to medical profession, State Residency

COSTS AND AID

Tuition & Fees

Annual tuition	$38,000
Room & board (on-campus off-campus)	$17,356/$8,960
Cost of books	$7,191
Fees	$3,760

Financial Aid

% students receiving any aid	85
% students receiving grants	80
% students receiving loans	88
% aid that is merit-based	0
Average grant	$25,447
Average loan	$24,376
Average total aid package	$43,008
Average debt	$96,614

LOMA LINDA UNIVERSITY
SCHOOL OF MEDICINE

LOMA LINDA UNIVERSITY SCHOOL OF MEDICINE, LOMA LINDA, CA 92350 • **ADMISSION:** (909) 558-1100
FAX: 909-824-41467 • **E-MAIL:** WEBMASTER@CCMAIL.LLU.EDU • **WEBSITE:** WWW.LLU.EDU/SM1.HTML

Academics

Joint degree programs are offered to qualified students. Along with the M.D., students may earn the M.S. or Ph.D. degree in fields such as Anatomy, Biochemistry, Genetics, Immunology, Microbiology, Neuroscience, Molecular Biology, Pharmacology, and Physiology. Examinations and other methods of evaluation are given percentile scores, but the courses are graded Pass or Fail. Passing the USMLE Step 1 is a requirement for promotion to year three.

BASIC SCIENCES: Although Loma Linda's curriculum covers the basic science topics typical of most medical schools, its religious affiliation adds another dimension. In addition to learning about human biology, the nature of disease, and the appropriate treatment for disease, first- and second-year students participate in a course called Whole Person Formation, which emphasizes Biblical, ethical, and relational aspects of the practice of medicine. Patient contact occurs during the first year, in Physical Diagnosis and Interviewing. Other first-year courses are Biochemistry/Molecular Biology; Cell Structure and Function; Gross Anatomy and Embryology; Human Behavior; Information Sciences and Population-Based Medicine; Medical Applications of the Basic Sciences; and Neuroscience. Second-year courses are HumanBehavior; Microbiology; Pathology; Physiology; Pathophysiology and Applied Physical Diagnosis; and Pharmacology. First- and second-year instruction takes place in facilities located on the Loma Linda campus and close to the Medical Center, giving students access toUniversity resources and clinical activities. Computers are available in a comprehensive computer lab, and are used for instruction and research.

CLINICAL TRAINING

Third-year required rotations are Orientation to Clinical Medicine/Preventive Medicine (4 weeks); Family Medicine (4 weeks); Ob/Gyn (6 weeks); Internal Medicine (12 weeks); Pediatrics (8 weeks); Psychiatry (6 weeks); and Surgery (12 weeks). Half of the fourth year is reserved entirely for basic science and clinical electives, and half of the year is split between required clerkships and selectives. Required clerkships are Subinternship Selectives (8 weeks, selected from Family Medicine, Internal Medicine, Ob/Gyn, Pediatrics, and Surgery); Intensive Care Unit (4 weeks); Neurology (4 weeks); Ambulatory Care (4 weeks); and Electives (16-22 weeks). Training takes place primarily at Loma Linda University Medical Center (500 beds), the Jerry L. Pettis Memorial Veterans Hospital, Riverside General Hospital, and the White Memorial Medical Center in Los Angeles. Other affiliated sites are San Bernardino County General Hospital, Kaiser Foundation Hospital, and Glendale Adventist Medical Center.

Students

Most students are members of the Seventh-Day Adventist Church. About 6 percent of students are underrepresented minorities, most of whom are African American. Generally, there is a wide age range among incoming students, with the average at about 24. Class size is 189.

STUDENT LIFE

For the most part, student life revolves around the medical school and the immediate community. When in need of a change of scenery, Los Angeles and beautiful Southern California beaches are a short drive. Perhaps as a result of a shared religious background, students are cohesive. Alcohol is not a part of the social life, as it is prohibited in the Seventh-Day Adventist Church. Beyond extracurricular activities sponsored by the medical school, students are welcome to participate in University-wide events and organizations. Medical students have access to the University's athletic facilities, and are active in intramural sports. Students live both on and off campus, and virtually all students own cars.

GRADUATES

Graduates are successful in securing residencies in all specialty fields. Loma Linda Medical Center is a popular destination for post-graduate training, offering about 25 residency programs.

Admissions

REQUIREMENTS

Prerequisite course work is eight semester hours each of Biology, General Chemistry, Organic Chemistry, and Physics. Applicants should have met the English and Religion requirements of their respective undergraduate institution. The MCAT is required, and scores should be no more than three years old. For applicants who have **taken the** test more than once, all sets of scores are considered.

SUGGESTIONS

Courses in the Humanities and Social Sciences are recommended, and applicants are urged to take the April rather than August MCAT. For applicants who have taken time off after college, recent course work is important. Some involvement in health care delivery is valued by the Admissions Committee. Preference is given to qualified applicants who are members of the Seventh-Day Adventist Church. However, others who demonstrate a commitment to Christian principles are also considered favorably.

PROCESS

All AMCAS applicants are sent secondary applications. Of those returning secondaries, about 10 percent are invited to interview between November and March. Interviews consist of one or two hour-long sessions with faculty, students, and/or administrators. On interview day, lunch, a campus tour, and the opportunity to meet with current students are all provided. About 40 percent of interviewed candidates are accepted on a rolling basis, while others are rejected or wait-listed. Wait-listed candidates may send updated transcripts.

Admissions Requirements (Required)

MCAT Scores, Science GPA, Extracurricular activities, Non-Science GPA, Exposure to medical profession, Recommendation, State Residency

Admissions Requirements (Optional)

Essays, Interview

COSTS AND AID

Tuition & Fees

Annual tuition	$32,944
Fees	$736

LOUISIANA STATE UNIVERSITY
SCHOOL OF MEDICINE IN NEW ORLEANS

OFFICE OF ADMISSIONS, 1901 PERDIDO STREET BOX P3-4, NEW ORLEANS, LA 70112 • ADMISSION: 504-568-6262 •
FAX: 504-568-77017 • E-MAIL: MS-ADMISSIONS@LSUHSC.EDU • WEBSITE: WWW.MEDSCHOOL.LSUHSC.EDU/ADMISSIONS

STUDENT BODY

Type	Public
Enrollment of medical school	712
% male/female	59/41
% out-of-state	0
% international	15

ADMISSIONS

# applied	1,179
% accepted	20
% enrolled	74

Average GPA and MCAT Scores

Overall GPA	3.5
MCAT Bio	9.5
MCAT Phys	9.0
MCAT Verbal	9.0
MCAT Essay	P

Application Information

Regular application	11/15
Are transfers accepted?	Yes
Admissions may be deferred?	Yes
Admissions need-blind?	Yes

Academics

The course of instruction leading to the M.D. extends over a four-year period. A revised first- and second-year curriculum was introduced in 1995, and changes in the third- and fourth-year clinical curriculum were implemented in 1996. An Honors Program, which involves independent research, challenges the exceptional student and is open to those who excel during their first semester of medical school. For highly qualified students interested in careers in research, a combined M.D./Ph.D. program is available. Medical students are graded with Honors, High Pass, Pass, and Fail. All students are required to pass Step 1 of the USMLE following completion of year two, and fourth-year students must pass Step 2 of the exam.

BASIC SCIENCES: Although most instruction uses a lecture format, small-group discussions and tutorials are also part of the curriculum. First year courses are Anatomy, Human Prenatal Development, Cell Biology and Micro-Anatomy, Biochemistry, Physiology, Clinical Correlation, Neuroscience, Medicine, Medical Ethics, Introduction to Clinical Medicine, Psychiatry, and Social Issues in Medicine. Electives are offered in Geriatrics, Problem Based Learning, Community Service, and Health Promotion and Wellness. Second year courses are Microbiology, Immunology and Parasitology, Pathology, Clinical Pathology, Pharmacology, and Introduction to Clinical Medicine. Basic sciences are taught in a modern building that is part of the medical center complex. Important educational resources are maintained by the LSU Division of Learning Resources, which provides audiovisual and classroom services to the downtown campus of the LSU Health Sciences Center. The medical library in New Orleans has a total of about 188,000 volumes, nearly 4,000 audiovisual titles, and approximately 2,000 periodicals. The library is fully computerized and houses individual computers that are equipped with educational software programs.

CLINICAL TRAINING
The third and fourth years are devoted primarily to clinical rotations. Lectures, conferences, and small-group discussions supplement the hands-on clinical training. Year three consists of eight and one-half days of ophthalmology course work in addition to rotations in: Medicine (12 weeks); General Surgery (8 weeks); Otolaryngology (2 weeks); Urology (2 weeks); Pediatrics (8 weeks); Family Medicine (4 weeks); Ob/Gyn (6 weeks); and Psychiatry (6 weeks). The final year consists of 36 weeks divided into nine four-week blocks, which are Ambulatory care, General Medicine, Neural Sciences, Special Topics, and an Acting Internship. The special-topics block includes Nutrition, Human Sexuality, Geriatrics, Drug and Alcohol Abuse, Office Management, and Financial Planning. The remainder of the year may include electives either in basic or clinical sciences with four weeks allowed for vacation. Most training takes place at LSU-affiliated hospitals including Charity Hospital, which has a total of 2,200 beds. Elective requirements may be fulfilled at any accredited medical school or teaching hospital in the United States or Canada. With approval, electives may also be taken at foreign institutions.

Students

All students are Louisiana residents. Approximately 15 percent of students are under-represented minorities, most of whom are African American. The average age of entering students is about 23, and there are usually a number of students in their late 20s and 30s. Class size is 165.

STUDENT LIFE

Some medical students are active in the student government, which works closely with the faculty and the administration on a range of important issues. Others are involved in the student publication or in any number of professional clubs, honor societies, recreational groups, and community service projects. Extracurricular opportunities in New Orleans abound. The restaurants, music scene, historic and cultural sights, and annual festivals and events are world-renowned. Some students opt to live in the school's residence hall, which has its own student center. Others live off campus where housing is generally reasonably priced.

GRADUATES

The School assists and advises graduating students in obtaining suitable appointments in hospitals. LSU—New Orleans itself offers a comprehensive graduate medical-education program in more than 20 specialty fields.

Admissions

REQUIREMENTS

Louisiana residency is a requirement. Prerequisite courses are 8 semester hours each of Biology, Chemistry, Organic Chemistry, and Physics, all with associated labs. Strength in both written and spoken English is required. The MCAT is required, and scores should be from within the past three years. For applicants who have taken the exam more than once, the most recent set of scores is weighed most heavily.

SUGGESTIONS

A well-rounded undergraduate experience with course work in Humanities, Social Sciences, Math, and English is advised. Community service or medically related work or volunteer activities are valued.

PROCESS

All AMCAS applicants who are Louisiana residents are sent secondary applications. Of those returning secondaries, about 50 percent are invited to interview between October and April. The interview consists of two or three one-on-one sessions, each with a faculty member, student, or administrator. On interview day, candidates also have the opportunity to meet with students, tour the campus, and have lunch. About 60 percent of interviewed candidates are accepted on a rolling basis. Wait-listed candidates may send additional information to update their files.

Admissions Requirements (Required)

MCAT Scores, Science GPA, Extracurricular activities, Non-Science GPA, Exposure to medical profession, Recommendation, Interview, State Residency

Admissions Requirements (Optional)

Essays

COSTS AND AID

Tuition & Fees

Annual tuition (in-state out-of-state)	$11,534/$25,682
Fees	$1,427

Louisiana State University

School of Medicine in Shreveport

Admissions Office, 1501 Kings Highway, P.O. Box 33932, Shreveport, LA 71130-3932 • **Admission:** 318-675-5190
Fax: 318-675-52447 • **E-mail:** SHVADM@LSUMC.EDU • **Website:** WWW.LSUMC.EDU

STUDENT BODY

Type	Public
Enrollment of medical school	391
% male/female	67/33
% out-of-state	0
% international	5

ADMISSIONS

# applied	1,046
% accepted	3

Application Information

Regular application	11/15
Are transfers accepted?	Yes
Admissions may be deferred?	Yes
Admissions need-blind?	No
Application fee	$50

Academics

The first two years are devoted to basic medical sciences with orientation to clinical applications. The second two years are devoted to clinical training and are spent primarily in hospitals and clinics. In addition to the M.D. degree, advanced studies leading to the M.D./Ph.D. are possible. The doctorate may be earned in Anatomy, Biochemistry, Microbiology, Pharmacology, and Physiology. All medical students are encouraged to take advantage of the many research opportunities available during summers and year-round. Special funds are provided for this purpose, and medical students who complete prescribed research activities are awarded diplomas with the special designation "Honors Research Participant." During summer terms, the school offers opportunities for rural, clinical electives. Medical students are evaluated with an A–F scale, with the exception of elective courses, which are Pass/Fail. Passing both steps of the USMLE is a graduation requirement.

BASIC SCIENCES: During the first year, students are in lectures, small-group seminars, labs, or other scheduled sessions for about 25 hours per week. Courses are CPR; Human Anatomy; Biometry; Ethics; Medical Neuroscience; Library Science; Family Medicine and Comprehensive Care; Radiology; Introduction to Computer-Aided Learning; Medical Genetics; Histology; Physiology and Biophysics; Psychiatry; Biochemistry and Molecular Biology; and Human Embryology. The second year is increasingly clinically oriented. Students are in class or other scheduled sessions for about 35 hours per week. Courses are Pathology; Radiology; Perspectives in Medicine; Psychiatry; Family Medicine and Comprehensive Care; Microbiology; Pharmacology; Clinical Neurology; Clinical Diagnosis; Clinical Pathology; and Clinical-Pathological Conference. A note-taking service, organized by and for students, assists with learning and retaining material. Computer-assisted instruction is a critical component of the basic-science education, and all entering students are required to own a computer.

CLINICAL TRAINING

An unusual, longitudinal clerkship called Comprehensive Care spans both the third and fourth years. In it, students work together and serve as the primary caregivers in a functioning clinic. Other third-year required rotations are Medicine (8 weeks); Surgery (4 weeks); Surgery Subspecialties (3 weeks); Pediatrics (4 weeks); Ob/Gyn (8 weeks); Psychiatry (4 weeks); and Family Medicine (8 weeks). A minimum of 16 weeks during the fourth year are reserved for electives. Required clerkships are Medicine (6 weeks), Surgery (3 weeks), Pediatrics (3 weeks), and Neuroscience (3 weeks). Most training takes place at the LSU Hospital (650 beds), the Shreveport Veterans' Administration Hospital, and the Comprehensive Care Clinic.

Students

All students are Louisiana residents. About 5 percent of students are underrepresented minorities. There is a wide age range among entering students, including those in their late twenties or thirties. Class size is 100.

STUDENT LIFE

Outside of class, LSU offers medical students a rich campus life. The University offers more than 60 student organizations in addition to intramural sports, performing arts events, visiting speakers, and social activities. The University Center has dining facilities, a lounge, student activity rooms, and a bookstore, among other student services. Generally, it serves as a meeting place for students. The Health and Physical Education Building houses an indoor swimming pool; handball and racquetball courts; basketball; tennis, volleyball, and badminton courts; a dance studio; and fitness and weight training rooms. Shreveport is a historic Southern city with a population of more than 370,000. Museums, art galleries, parks, gardens, restaurants, bars, and shopping areas are some of its many attractions. The cities of Baton Rouge and New Orleans are easily accessible. Houston, Memphis, Little Rock, and Jackson are also within driving distance. Most medical students live off campus.

GRADUATES

An increasing proportion of graduates are entering primary care fields. The majority of graduates return to Louisiana to practice.

Admissions

REQUIREMENTS

Admission to the School of Medicine is limited to Louisiana residents. Requirements are one year each of Biology, Chemistry, Organic Chemistry, Physics, and English. All science courses must include laboratory work. The MCAT is required, and scores should be from within three years of application. For applicants who have taken the exam more than once, the most recent set of scores is generally weighed most heavily.

SUGGESTIONS

Once prerequisites are fulfilled, perspective applicants are encouraged to pursue their own interests and to develop their own special talents in gaining a broad educational background. In making admissions decisions, a candidate's motivation as well as his or her intellectual ability and preparation are assessed. Applicants must show potential of developing into mature, sensitive physicians who will inspire and deserve trust and confidence.

PROCESS

All AMCAS applicants who are Louisiana residents are sent secondary applications. Of those returning secondaries, about 30 percent are invited to interview between September and March. Interviews are given by members of the Admissions Committee, which is composed of Medical School faculty from the basic and clinical sciences as well as physicians from the community at large. The interview is used to assess personal traits and also allows candidates to see the facilities and to meet current students. Approximately 90 percent of interviewed candidates are accepted on a rolling basis. Others are rejected or wait-listed.

LOYOLA UNIVERSITY CHICAGO
STRITCH SCHOOL OF MEDICINE

2160 SOUTH FIRST AVENUE, MAYWOOD, IL 60153 • ADMISSION: 708-216-3229 • FAX: 708-216-91607
WEBSITE: WWW.MEDDEAN.LUMC.EDU

STUDENT BODY

Type	Private
Enrollment of medical school	559
% male/female	49/51
% out-of-state	55
% international	22
Average age of entering class	23

FACULTY

Total faculty	1,442
% female faculty	30
% minority faculty	24
% part-time faculty	55
Student-faculty ratio	2.0:1

ADMISSIONS

# applied	5,490
% accepted	7
% enrolled	40

Average GPA and MCAT Scores

Overall GPA	3.6
MCAT Bio	10.9
MCAT Phys	10.3
MCAT Verbal	10.2
MCAT Essay	P

Application Information

Regular application	11/15
Regular notification	10/15
Are transfers accepted?	Yes
Admissions may be deferred?	Yes
Admissions need-blind?	No
Application fee	$75

Academics

Students follow a four-year curriculum leading to the M.D. degree. A dual degree M.D./Ph.D. program accepts up to three students each year. In this program, a doctorate degree may be earned in anatomy, biochemistry, cell biology, immunology, microbiology, molecular biology, neuroscience, pathology, pharmacology, or physiology. Evaluation of student performance uses Honors/High Pass/Pass/Fail. Students must pass USMLE Step 1 and USMLE Step 2 in order to graduate.

BASIC SCIENCES: Stritch's curriculum relies on small-group sessions and problem-based learning as much as it does on traditional lectures and labs. Students are in class or other scheduled sessions for approximately 25 hours per week, discussing behavioral science and humanistic perspectives along with basic science concepts. First-year courses are: host defense, molecular cell biology and genetics; structure of the human body; function of the human body; and Patient Centered Medicine I, a two-year continuum that begins with the medical interview and later covers the physical diagnosis, health promotion, medical ethics, healthcare finance, and legal issues in medicine. As part of the course, each student participates in special mentoring programs, participating on hospital rounds with a primary care physician and chaplain. Second-year courses are: neuroscience; mechanisms of human disease; pharmacology and therapeutics; behavioral development, and Patient Centered Medicine II. During years 2, 3 and 4, medical humanities and ethics grand rounds take place. The Stritch facility includes classrooms of many different sizes to accommodate different instructional modalities, labs, video equipment, computer laboratories, lounges, study areas, and other spaces. The Health Sciences Library houses about 170,000 volumes and periodicals.

CLINICAL TRAINING

Required third-year rotations are family medicine (6 weeks); internal medicine (12 weeks); ob/gyn (6 weeks); pediatrics (6 weeks); psychiatry (6 weeks); and surgery (12 weeks). During the fourth year, requirements are neurology (4 weeks); medical humanities (1 week); subinternships (8 weeks); and 26 weeks of electives. Clinical facilities include: Hines Veterans Affairs Hospital; Loyola University Hospital and Loyola Outpatient Center; Cardinal Bernardin Cancer Center; and a variety of community hospitals. Elective credits can be earned at other academic or clinical institutions.

Students

STUDENT LIFE

At Loyola, there is a very strong indentity among each class. Class officers, including social chairs, promote numerous group activities, from small study groups to class specific events to all-school social events. In order to help promote the interaction among classes, students from all classes are assigned to one of three communities. Each student has a wardrobe locker and mailbox within the community and shared study space along with a lounge area and kitchenette. Students also get to know one another through an active student government and almost 30 registered student organizations, which include professional, academic, social, and religious based groups. Each organization has a faculty advisor, who in turn helps the student leaders and student members to direct their own organization. During the first two years, most preclinical courses end early enough to allow time for self-directed learning and extracurricular pursuits. Many students use this time to volunteer for public clinics, homeless shelters, senior centers, hospital based pediatrics, school and reading programs, and to present educational health-related topics at various local schools. On and off-campus events and programs also are sponsored by University Ministry. To help round out the physical well being of the students, there is a 62,000 square foot Health and Fitness Center adjacent to the medical school. The center features various cardio equipment, a state-of-the-art aerobic/exercise studio, free weights and variable resistance equipment, basketball and volleyball court, aquatics area, elevated running track, racquetball courts, and spa and massage services. Off-campus activities are plentiful, as Chicago is easily accessible from the medical center. All students live off-campus and most within the western suburbs of Chicago.

GRADUATES

Graduates are successful in securing residency positions nationwide in primary care and specialized fields. About 56 percent of graduates remain in the Midwest, 20 percent go to the western United States, 17 percent to the east, and 6 percent to the south.

Admissions

REQUIREMENTS

Applicants must be U.S. citizens or hold a permanent resident visa. Prerequisites are one year each of biology, chemistry, organic chemistry, and physics, all with associated labs. One semester of biochemistry may be substituted for a semester of organic chemistry. The MCAT is required and scores should be from within four years of anticipated entrance to medical school.

SUGGESTIONS

Although state residents are given some preference, there are no positions reserved for them. Some recent course work is important for nontraditional applicants who have been out of school for a period of time. Qualities that are sought in applicants are maturity, integrity, the ability to work with diverse populations, dedication to community service, and an awareness of the environment surrounding health care provision.

PROCESS

All applicants who meet minimum qualifications receive secondary applications. Of those returning secondaries, about 12 percent are interviewed between September and April. Interviews consist of two one-hour sessions each with a faculty member administrator or Student Committee on Admissions member. On interview day, candidates also have lunch with current medical students and tour the campus. Among interviewed candidates, about 50 percent are accepted on a rolling basis, with notification beginning in October. Wait-listed candidates, or those in a hold category, may send additional information to update their files and indicate interest in Loyola.

Admissions Requirements (Required)

MCAT Scores, Essays, Science GPA, Extracurricular activities, Non-Science GPA, Exposure to medical profession, Recommendation, Interview

Admissions Requirements (Optional)

State Residency

COSTS AND AID

Tuition & Fees

Annual tuition	$36,600
Room & board	$13,688
Cost of books	$3,544
Fees	$1,108

Financial Aid

% students receiving any aid	95
% students receiving grants	69
% students receiving loans	87
% aid that is merit-based	5
Average grant	$10,608
Average loan	$46,567
Average total aid package	$47,936
Average debt	$169,042

MARSHALL UNIVERSITY

MARSHALL UNIVERSITY JOAN C. EDWARDS SCHOOL OF MEDICINE

OFFICE OF ADMISSIONS, 1600 MEDICAL CENTER DRIVE, HUNTINGTON, WV 25701 • ADMISSION: 800-544-8514
FAX: 304-691-17447 • E-MAIL: WARREN@MARSHALL.EDU • WEBSITE: WWW.MUSOM.MARSHALL.EDU

STUDENT BODY

Type	Public
Enrollment of parent institution	16,000
Enrollment of medical school	290
Average age of entering class	25

FACULTY

Total faculty	228
% female faculty	35
% minority faculty	19
% part-time faculty	16
Student-faculty ratio	1.0:1

ADMISSIONS

# applied	1,382
% accepted	10
% enrolled	49

Average GPA and MCAT Scores

Overall GPA	3.5
MCAT Bio	10.0
MCAT Phys	9.3
MCAT Verbal	9.8
MCAT Essay	Q

Application Information

Regular application	11/1
Regular notification	10/15
Are transfers accepted?	No
Admissions may be deferred?	Yes
Admissions need-blind?	No
Application fee	$75

Academics

The Marshall University Joan C. Edwards School of Medicine is a community-based, Veterans Affairs afflitiated medical school dedicated to providing high quality medical education and postgraduate training programs to foster a skilled physician workforce to meet the unique healthcare needs of West Virginia and Central Appalachia. Although most students complete a four-year course of study leading to the M.D. degree, qualified students interested in research may concurrently pursue an M.S. or Ph.D. in Biomedical Sciences. Evaluation of student performance uses an A-F scale. Passing Step 1 of the USMLE is required for promotion to year three, and passing Step 2 CK & CS is a graduation requirement.

BASIC SCIENCES: Both the Year One and Year Two curriculum are integrated into a systems-based format. Throughout both years students have direct patient contact and learn foundational principles of patient care. Students learn in a variety of settings including didactic, small group, team-base learning, laboratory and independent study as they transition into becoming clinical learners in Year Three.

CLINICAL TRAINING

Third-year students participate in required third-year clerkships. These are: Medicine (8 weeks); Ob/Gyn (8 weeks); Psychiatry (6 weeks); Neurology (2 weeks); Surgery (8 weeks); Pediatrics (8 weeks); Family Practice (8 weeks). During the fourth year, required rotations are Selective Subinternship (Family Medicine, General Surgery, Medicine, Obstetrics, Orthopaedics, or Pediatrics–4 weeks); Selective ICU (MICU, NICU, PICU or SICU–2 weeks); and Emergency Medicine (4 weeks). A full 26 weeks are reserved for elective study. Affiliated clinical teaching sites are numerous and include Cabell Huntington Hospital (300 beds), St. Mary's Medical Center (440 beds) and the Veterans Affairs Medical Center (80 beds).

Students

Among entering students in a recent class, 27 percent graduated from Marshall's undergraduate college. A total of 41 other undergraduate institutions were represented in the class. Thirty-six percent majored in Biology, 18 percent in Chemistry, and the remainder in other disciplines. The average age of incoming students is about 25, with an age range of 21–35. About 12 percent are minorities. Class size is 75.

STUDENT LIFE

The small class size at Marshall contributes to a supportive and friendly environment. Students are active in chapters of national organizations and in groups like the American Medical Women's Association, American Medical Student Association, American Medical Association—Medical Student Section and the Community Service Organization. Huntington is a small city offering the amenities and resources that students need while providing easy access to rural areas. For more recreational and cultural opportunities, the larger cities of Pittsburgh and Cincinnati are each about a four-hour drive. Medical students have access to the athletic and recreational facilities of the main University and take part in University-wide events. Off-campus housing is also affordable and readily available.

GRADUATES

Over 50% of graduates enter primary care fields, which include Internal Medicine, Family Medicine, Pediatrics, and Ob/Gyn. Graduates are successful in securing residencies inside and outside of West Virginia.

Admissions

REQUIREMENTS

Prerequisites are eight semester hours each (with lab) of Biology, Chemistry, Organic Chemistry, and Physics and three semester hours of Biochemistry. Six semester hours each of Social or Behavioral Science and English are also required. An applicant's GPA is evaluated with consideration given to the academic institution and the rigor of courses taken. The MCAT is required and scores must be from within three years of matriculation. For applicants who have retaken the exam, the latest set of scores is weighed most heavily.

SUGGESTIONS

As a state school, Marshall gives preference to West Virginia residents. A maximum of twenty-five positions in each year's class are reserved for residents of Ohio, Kentucky, Virginia, Maryland and Pennsylvania and for candidates with strong ties to the state. A spring MCAT test date is recommended. However, scores from September test dates will be used in the consideration of applications. In addition to the academic record, Marshall considers personal qualities such as judgment, responsibility, altruism, integrity, and sensitivity important. Strong communication skills are valued.

PROCESS

All West Virginia and bordering state AMCAS applicants receive secondary applications. Almost all West Virginia residents are interviewed, while only about 5 percent of out-of-state applicants are interviewed. Interviews take place between September and February and consist of two 30-minute sessions with members of the Admissions Committee. Acceptances are issued on a rolling basis. Wait-listed candidates may send information to update their files as the year progresses.

Admissions Requirements (Required)

MCAT Scores, Science GPA, Extracurricular activities, Non-Science GPA, Recommendation, Interview

Admissions Requirements (Optional)

Essays, Exposure to medical profession, State Residency

COSTS AND AID

Tuition & Fees

Annual tuition (in-state out-of-state)	$19,010/$46,600
Room & board	$14,500
Cost of books	$2,000
Fees	$1,070

Financial Aid

% students receiving any aid	91
% students receiving grants	51
% students receiving loans	91
% aid that is merit-based	12
Average grant	$13,522
Average loan	$42,490
Average total aid package	$51,000
Average debt	$169,793

Mayo Clinic College of Medicine
Mayo Medical School

Mayo Medical School, 200 First Street SW Rochester, MN 55905 • Admission: 507-284-2316
Fax: 507-284-26347 • E-mail: medschooladmissions@mayo.edu • Website: www.mayo.edu/mms

STUDENT BODY

Type	Private
Enrollment of medical school	194
% male/female	51/49
% underrepresented minorities	6
% out-of-state	84
% international	13
Average age of entering class	24

ADMISSIONS

# applied	4,081
% accepted	2
% enrolled	49

Average GPA and MCAT Scores

Overall GPA	3.9
MCAT Essay	P

Application Information

Regular application	10/1
Are transfers accepted?	No
Admissions may be deferred?	Yes
Admissions need-blind?	No
Application fee	$120

Academics

Each year, 42 students begin a four-year curriculum, leading to the M.D. degree, and six students pursue a joint M.D./Ph.D. program in connection with the Mayo Graduate School. Through this program, a Ph.D. may be obtained in: Biochemistry, Biomedical Engineering, Immunology, Cell Biology and Genetics, Molecular Neuroscience, Muloecular Pharmacology and Experimental Therapeutics, Tumor Biology and Virology and Gene Therapy. Two students with D.D.S. degrees are admitted each year for training towards careers in oral and maxillofacial surgery. Courses are grouped into units, which are The Organ, The Patient, Physician and Society, The Scientific Foundation of Medical Practice, The Clinical Experience, and The Research Quarter. All students are required to write a research paper while at Mayo, and 80 percent of these works are published. Evaluation of student performance uses Honors, High Pass, Pass, Marginal Pass, and Fail. Taking the USMLE Steps 1 and 2 is a requirement for graduation.

BASIC SCIENCES: During the first five months of school, students take Molecular Biology and Genetics, Pathology and Cell Biology, Immunology, and Anatomy. The remainder of year one is organized around the following organ and physiological systems: Cutaneous System, Respiratory System, Hematopoietic System, Neuroscience, Growth and Development, Renal System, Cardiovascular System, Digestive System, Endocrine System, Allergy, and Musculoskeletal System. Patient contact begins in year one, in Introduction to the Patient and Continuity of Care. Small groups and problem-based learning enhance the lecture/lab format and account for about one-third of the 28 hours per week of scheduled class time. The second year is split between clinical and basic science education. The first block of year two includes: Microbiology and Infectious Disease, Psychopathology, and ENT, SAR/Sexual Medicine, and Bioethics. In the next block, second-year students attend lectures and seminars and rotate through several clinical departments, evaluating patients under the guidance of a preceptor. Clinical rotations are: Dermatology (3 weeks); Family Medicine (2 weeks); Musculoskeletal Medicine and Rehabilitation (3 weeks); Medicine (9 weeks); Surgery (3 weeks); Pediatrics (6 weeks); and Clinical Skills Aquisition (3 weeks). Tutoring and a wide variety of advising services are available to students, and a formal system is in place to identify and assist students who may be experiencing academic difficulties. Scheduled classes and labs take place on the Mayo campus, while independent and computer-aided instruction is offered in the Learning Resource Center located in the Mitchell Student Center. The Mayo Medical Library houses 353,000 volumes and subscribes to 4,300 journals.

CLINICAL TRAINING

The third year is divided into four quarters. The Research Quarter is a 13-week experience in which students participate in a biomedical research project and produce a related scientific paper. Three quarters are spent in clinical rotations: Family Medicine (2 weeks); Internal Medicine (6 weeks); Neurology (3 weeks); Surgery (6 weeks); Pediatrics (6 weeks); Ob/Gyn (6 weeks); and Psychiatry (4 weeks); and a 3-week elective at Mayo. Training takes place at the Mayo Clinic, Rochester Methodist, and Saint Mary's Hospitals, which together have 2,000 beds.

Students

The student body consists of about 190 students from more than 40 states. About 14 percent of a typical class are underrepresented minorities. Class size is 50.

STUDENT LIFE

The small class size facilitates cohesion among students. Mitchell Student Center, in addition to housing the Learning Resource Center, provides an area for relaxation and communal study. Students are actively involved in medically-related organizations and societies, community service projects, and groups organized around athletic and cultural interests. Students also play an important role in the School's administration, participating in governing committees. Rochester's population is 100,000, offering concerts, theater, museums, golf courses, and parks, among other recreational opportunities. All students live off campus.

GRADUATES

In a class of recent graduates, 37 percent entered residencies in primary care. Specialties selected by more than one student were: Family Medicine (12%); Internal Medicine (12%); Ob/Gyn (5%); Pediatrics (9%); Anesthesiology (14%); Dermatology (5%); Emergency Medicine (7%); Ophthalmology (5%); Psychiatry (9%); Radiation Oncology (7%).

Admissions

REQUIREMENTS

Prerequisites are: Biology with lab (one year); Chemistry with lab (one year); Organic Chemistry with lab (one year); Physics with lab (one year); and Biochemistry (one course). The MCAT is required and must be no more than three years old.

SUGGESTIONS

Mayo is interested in undergraduate course work that demonstrates both aptitude in science and breadth of knowledge in social science and humanities. Substantial experience in community service and leadership are also very important considerations. Additionally, Mayo is committed to matriculating a diverse student body that includes students from racial and ethnic backgrounds which are underrepresented in medicine.

PROCESS

No supplementary application is required. About 50 percent of AMCAS applicants receive a request for letters of recommendation. About 10 percent of those screened applicants are invited to an on-campus interview. The interviews are scheduled between September and December. Applicants have two 30 minute interviews with faculty, students, community members, or administrators. Of interviewed applicants, about 15 percent are accepted on a rolling basis. Others are rejected or wait-listed. Additional material from wait-listed candidates is not encouraged.

Admissions Requirements (Required)

MCAT Scores, Essays, Science GPA, Extracurricular activities, Non-Science GPA, Recommendation, Interview

Admissions Requirements (Optional)

Exposure to medical profession, State Residency

COSTS AND AID

Tuition & Fees

Annual tuition	$35,960
Room & board	$18,588
Cost of books	$2,492
Fees	$0

Financial Aid

% students receiving any aid	100
% students receiving grants	100
% students receiving loans	84
% aid that is merit-based	84
Average grant	$29,000
Average loan	$25,000
Average total aid package	$66,000
Average debt	$75,217

McGill University

McGill University, Faculty of Medicine

3655 Promenade Sir William Osler, Suite 602 Montreal, QC H3G 1Y6 • **Admission:** +1-514-398-3517
Fax: +1-514-398-46317 • **E-mail:** ADMISSIONS.MED@MCGILL.CA • **Website:** WWW.MEDICINE.MCGILL.CA/ADMISSIONS

STUDENT BODY

Type	Public
Enrollment of parent institution	32,500
Enrollment of medical school	172
% male/female	45/55
% underrepresented minorities	5
% out-of-state	4
# countries represented	150
Average age of entering class	22

FACULTY

Total faculty	674
% female faculty	55
% part-time faculty	0

ADMISSIONS

# applied	1,179
% accepted	21
% enrolled	72

Average GPA and MCAT Scores

Overall GPA	3.8
MCAT Bio	11.0
MCAT Phys	11.0
MCAT Verbal	10.0
MCAT Essay	P

Application Information

Regular application	11/15
Regular notification	3/31
Are transfers accepted?	No
Admissions may be deferred?	Yes
Admissions need-blind?	No
Application fee	$80

Academics

The curriculum recognizes the importance of a solid database and a multidisciplinary approach to medical education with integration of clinical and basic science experience. It is designed to permit a variety of teaching and evaluation methods recognizing the importance of small-group teaching and clinical relevance of material. Flexibility in the program permits opportunities for research and for a range of ongoing clinical inpatient and ambulatory care experience. The curriculum is composed of four components entitled Basis of Medicine, Introduction to Clinical Medicine, Practice of Medicine, and Back to Basics. Though most students complete a four-year program leading to the M.D. degree, joint degree programs are also offered. An M.D./Ph.D. program is open to qualified students interested in a research career in academic medicine. For students interested in both medicine and health management, the faculties of Medicine and Management offer a five year program leading to an M.D./M.B.A. degree.

BASIC SCIENCES: The first academic period begins in September and continues through December of the second year. The theme of the first academic period is Basis of Medicine, and courses are organized into blocks. These are: Molecules, Cells, and Tissues (4 weeks); Gas, Fluids, and Electrolytes (9 weeks); Life Cycle (3 weeks); Endocrinology, Metabolism, and Nutrition (7 weeks); Musculoskeletal and Blood (4 weeks); Nervous System and Special Senses (8 weeks); Host Defense and Host Parasite (8 weeks); and Pathobiology, Treatment, and Prevention of Disease.

CLINICAL TRAINING

The second academic period, Introduction to Clinical Medicine (ICM), begins in January of the second year and goes through September of the third year. ICM takes place in hospitals and outpatient clinical settings. Topics covered are Introduction to Clinical Sciences, Medical Ethics, Health Law, Medicine, Family Medicine, Geriatric Medicine, Neurology, Surgery, Emergency Medicine, Anesthesia, Radiology, Introduction to Hospital Practice, Pediatrics, Psychiatry, Ob/Gyn, and an elective. During the third academic period, Practice of Medicine, students rotate through required clerkships. These are Medicine (8 weeks), Surgery (8 weeks), Psychiatry (8 weeks), Psychiatry (8 weeks), Ob/Gyn (8 weeks), Pediatrics (8 weeks), Family Medicine (4 weeks), and Electives/Selectives (16 weeks). The final academic period is Back to Basics. During this 16-week session, students take Medicine and Society, Topics in Medical Science, and Ambulatory Care. Teaching hospitals include Montreal General Hospital, Montreal Children's Hospital, Montreal Neurological Hospital, Sir Mortimer B. Davis-Jewish General Hospital, Douglas Hospital, and Royal Victoria Hospital. Training also takes place at a number of affiliated hospitals and other clinical care centers.

Students

Each entering class has about 110 students. Typically, 25 percent of students are non-Canadians, most of whom are from the U.S. About 50 percent of students are women.

STUDENT LIFE

McGill is a large and active campus that offers social and recreational activities to a diverse student body. In addition, the city of Montreal itself is an interesting and exciting place for students to live. McGill has four co-educational residences and one women's residence located on the main campus, which are open to medical students. Information concerning apartments or flats located in the vicinity of the campus can be obtained from the Off-Campus Housing Office.

Admissions

REQUIREMENTS

The Faculty of Medicine offers a four-year undergraduate medical curriculum. Students are ordinarily admitted into the first year of this program, but admission is also available by means of a Med-P program directly after CEGEP. The faculty does not accept students for part-time medical studies. An M.D.-Ph.D. program is offered for students interested in a research career in academic medicine. For students interested in both medicine and management, the faculties of medicine and management offer a five-year program leading to an M.D.-M.B.A. degree. The language of instruction is English. Requirements: Applicants must have received an undergraduate degree or be in the final year of a course of study at a recognized college or university leading to an undergraduate degree with at least 120 academic credits. Prerequisites include one year with laboratory work in each of General Biology, General Chemistry, Organic Chemistry, and Physics. The MCAT is required and applicants must have taken the exam no later than August 1999.

SUGGESTIONS

In addition to prerequisite science courses, some course work in Biochemistry or Molecular Biology is strongly recommended. Applicants to the four-year program should have undergraduate GPAs of 3.5 or better and a total of 30 or more in the MCAT scores. In a recent entering class, the average GPA was a 3.7 and the average overall MCAT score was 31.10.

PROCESS

The deadline for receipt of applications to the regular M.D. program is January 15 for Quebec residents and November 15 for all others. Applicants with strong academic qualifications submit an application that includes an autobiographical letter used to assess personal qualities and achievements. Selection for interview is based on grades, MCAT scores, letters of reference, and autobiographical letter. Once interviews have been completed, all the components of the application are considered in making admissions decisions. Residents of Quebec will be notified after May 1. Nonresidents will be notified as soon as possible after March 31.

Admissions Requirements (Required)

MCAT Scores, Essays, Science GPA, Extracurricular activities, Non-Science GPA, Exposure to medical profession, Recommendation, Interview

Admissions Requirements (Optional)

State Residency

COSTS AND AID

Tuition & Fees

Annual tuition (in-state out-of-state)	$3,565/$24,846
Cost of books	$213

MEDICAL COLLEGE OF GEORGIA
SCHOOL OF MEDICINE

OFFICE OF ADMISSIONS, AA-2040 AUGUSTA, GA 30912 • **ADMISSION:** 706-721-3186 • **FAX:** 706-721-09597
E-MAIL: STDADMIN@MAIL.MCG.EDU • **WEBSITE:** WWW.MCG.EDU

STUDENT BODY

Type	Public
Enrollment of parent institution	2,227
Enrollment of medical school	734

FACULTY

Total faculty	612
% female faculty	22
% minority faculty	23
% part-time faculty	22

ADMISSIONS

# applied	1,917
% accepted	14
% enrolled	70

Average GPA and MCAT Scores

Overall GPA	3.7
MCAT Bio	10.3
MCAT Phys	9.7
MCAT Verbal	9.9

Application Information

Regular application	11/1
Regular notification	5/1
Early application	8/1
Early notification	10/1
Are transfers accepted?	Yes
Admissions may be deferred?	Yes
Admissions need-blind?	Yes
Application fee	$0

Academics

The School emphasizes early patient contact, uses problem-based learning, and strives to educate physicians who will help meet the health care needs of Georgians. Students and applicants interested in earning both an M.D. and a Ph.D. may apply to combined degree programs arranged with the School of Graduate Studies or with departments of the University of Georgia, Georgia Institute of Technology, or Georgia State University. Areas of doctorate study include, but are not limited to, Biochemistry, Anatomy, Biomedical Engineering, Biophysics, Cell Biology, Genetics, Immunology, Microbiology, Molecular Biology, Neuroscience, Pharmacology, and Physiology.

BASIC SCIENCES: During the two pre-clinical years, students acquire the building blocks of basic science that underlie medical practice and the skills required for clinical decision-making and patient interaction. The modular content of the curriculum is taught in lectures, labs with integrated clinical conferences and small-group activities. In the first semester of year one, the introductory Molecular Cell Biology module provides a foundation for the basic sciences and is followed by the Cellular and Systems Structures module to introduce students to Gross Anatomy, Histology, and Development. In the second semester, Biochemistry and Physiology are taught in the Cellular and Systems Processes module while the Brain and Behavior module, gives students an understanding of the interplay between Psychiatry and Neuroscience. Offered concurrently with the basic science modules, the yearlong Essentials of Clinical Medicine emphasizes family, cultural and population aspects of health care, communication skills, and information retrieval and analysis, health promotion/disease prevention, ethics, history taking with children and adults, and a community project. The Essentials of Clinical Medicine is a two-year sequence that emphasizes skills needed for success in the third year. In year two, Essentials of Clinical Medicine addresses interviewing and physical examination, common medical problems, and interdisciplinary topics such as ethics, nutrition, and the impact of behavior on health while highlighting principles of patient care for each stage of life. Cellular and Systems Disease States is a yearlong module running in parallel so the students are exposed to the topics of Medical Microbiology, Pathology, and Pharmacology as the issues related to patient care throughout the stages of life arise. Teaching strategies, including interactive small groups, preceptor relationships, and lectures are linked to course objectives. On average, students are in scheduled activities for 26 hours per week during the first two years. Classes are held in the modern Research and Education Building and the Medical Student Resource Area, which includes small group rooms with computers and Internet access. Each student is advised to purchase a computer capable of using relevant educational software. The Greenblatt Library maintains more than 1800 current journal subscriptions and provides access to many external databases. Audiovisual learning aids are used in class and are available to the library. Grading is A–F with a C constituting a passing grade. Passing the USMLE Step 1 is a requirement for promotion to the third year.

CLINICAL TRAINING
Patient contact begins during year one in the Essentials Clinical Medicine course, which extends through year two. Year three consists of required core clerkships: Internal Medicine (12 weeks); Pediatrics (6 weeks); Family Medicine (6 weeks); Ob/Gyn (6 weeks); Surgery (8 weeks); Psychiatry (6 weeks); and Neurology (4 weeks). Core clerkships take place at the Medical College of Georgia Hospitals and Clinics the Children's

Medical Center and various affiliated hospitals and community-based teaching sites throughout the state. Students may rotate to affiliated community hospitals for part of the core curriculum. During year four, students must complete four-week rotations in Emergency Medicine, Critical Care, and an acting internship in Medicine, Family Medicine, Pediatrics, Surgery or Obstetrics and Gynecology. The remainder of the fourth year is for elective study, which can include both clinical and research courses. Evaluation during the clinical years is based on assessment of knowledge, clinical skills, and professional behavior, and uses an A-F scale. Passing the USMLE Step 2 is a requirement for graduation.

Students

At least 95 percent of students are Georgia residents. Underrepresented minorities account for about 6 percent of the student body. About one-quarter of each class took time off after college, and there is a wide range or prior experiences within the student body. Class size is 180.

STUDENT LIFE
The campus is close to downtown Augusta, the second-largest metropolitan area in Georgia. Augusta offers a wide range of activities including museums, theater, restaurants, music, shopping, water skiing, sailing, tennis and golf. Students are cohesive, brought together by popular on-campus housing and student groups. Students are involved in organizations focused on professional, social, athletic, and community service activities. Many on-campus housing options are available, including residency halls, one- or two-bedroom apartments, and family housing.

GRADUATES
In the past, the majority of graduates have selected specialized fields. As part of their Generalist Initiative, the Medical College encourages students to explore primary care. The goal of the Initiative is for at least half of the graduates to enter residencies in Family Practice, Internal Medicine, or Pediatrics. Students may remain at the Medical College of Georgia for their post-graduate study while others enter programs elsewhere in the state and the nation.

Admissions

REQUIREMENTS
Undergraduate preparation must include: Biology with lab (1 year); Inorganic Chemistry with lab (1 year); Organic Chemistry with lab (1 semester); additional upper-level Chemistry (1 semester); Physics with lab (1 year); and English (1 year). Transcripts should have grades; Pass/Fail courses are not advised. The MCAT is required and must be no more than three years old.

SUGGESTIONS
The April, rather than August, MCAT is strongly advised. For students who have taken time off after college, recent course work is recommended. Experiences that involve patient contact is valuable. In addition to academic strength and general personal qualities, the Admissions Committee looks for an individual's potential for meeting the health care needs of Georgia.

PROCESS
All Georgia residents who submit AMCAS application are sent secondary applications, while only selected out-of-state residents receive secondaries. About half of in-state residents and less than 5 percent of out of state residents are interviewed. Interviews consist of two one-half hour sessions, with faculty, administrators, or students. One interview is done by a member of the Admissions Committee and the other interview is done by a faculty member who is not a member of the Admissions Commitee. Interviews take place from October through March. Notification is rolling for regular admissions. After enough offers have been made to fill the class, an alternate list is established from which about 40-50 candidates are usually admitted.

Admissions Requirements (Required)

MCAT Scores, Essays, Science GPA, Extracurricular activities, Non-Science GPA, Exposure to medical profession, Recommendation, Interview, State Residency

COSTS AND AID

Tuition & Fees

Annual tuition (in-state out-of-state)	$12,350/$30,976
Fees	$923

MEDICAL COLLEGE OF WISCONSIN

MEDICAL COLLEGE OF WISCONSIN

OFFICE OF ADMISSIONS, 8701 WATERTOWN PLANK ROAD, MILWAUKEE, WI 53226 • ADMISSION: 414-955-8246
FAX: 414-955-65057 • E-MAIL: WWW.MEDSCHOOL@MCW.EDU • WEBSITE: WWW.MCW.EDU

STUDENT BODY

Type	Private
Enrollment of medical school	820
% male/female	55/45
% out-of-state	61
% international	10
Average age of entering class	22

FACULTY

Total faculty	1,400

ADMISSIONS

# applied	6,254
% accepted	8
% enrolled	43

Average GPA and MCAT Scores

Overall GPA	3.7
MCAT Bio	11.0
MCAT Phys	10.7
MCAT Verbal	10.2
MCAT Essay	P

Application Information

Regular application	11/1
Regular notification	10/15
Are transfers accepted?	Yes
Admissions may be deferred?	Yes
Admissions need-blind?	No
Application fee	$70

Academics

The curriculum provides a foundation for a career in any discipline of medicine and is evolving to enhance flexibility, individuality, and early clinical exposure. Currently, students gain exposure to basic science and experience the clinical environment through a mentor course and clinically-related course work in the Clinical Continuum during the first two years. Students rotate through required clinical clerkships and an optional elective experience in the third year. Students are required to take two subinternships, one each in a medically- and surgically-oriented specialty, ambulatory medicine, an Integrated Selective and five one-month electives in the fourth year. Joint degree programs or an Honors in Research program are available to students with specific research interests. To provide students the opportunity to pursue and strengthen their own interests in medicine, five new Pathways have been implemented that include Master Clinician, Urban and Community Health, Physician Scientist, Clinician Educator and Global Health.

Students

MCW is one of the largest free standing medical school in the country. With grants totally more then $145 milllion dollars the College had 3,000 research projects in progess during the past year. As a free standing institution MCW attracts and enrolls students from across the country each year in its class of 204 students. Located on the Milwaukee Regional Medical Center Campus, the Medical College is able to provide all clinical clerkships and rotations at this location or in the metropolitan area.

STUDENT LIFE

Student organizations focus on professional and leadership development, community service, and recreational pursuits. The College is involved in over 30 community service activities, including a student run clinic for the uninsured, an AIDS interventions center, and health education programs in local schools. Organized social events include parties, dinners and ongoing activities such as intramural sports. Along with the College's fitness center, these activities allow students to relax, socialize or exercise between or after class. Located in a suburb seven miles west of downtown Milwaukee, students live and go to school in a safe comfortable environment. At the same time they are also within easy access of the cultural, social and sporting events offered in the metropolitan

GRADUATES

MCW students consistently perform at or better then the national average on the USLME. This coupled with the school's reputation for providing excellent clinical training results in an excellent placement record for graduates.

Admissions

REQUIREMENTS

Eligibility requirements to apply include: Candidates must have completed or are in the process of completing 90 or more undergraduate graded credits, including the prerequisites, at an accredited college/university in the United States or Canada. The MCAT is required and must have been taken no more then three years prior to matriculation. Prerequisites include eight semester hours, two of which must be labs, in biology, inorganic chemistry, and organic chemistry, eight semester hours of physics, four of college algebra and six of English. With the exception of organic chemistry, AP credit is accepted for prerequisites.

SUGGESTIONS

Beyond required courses, applicants are encouraged to present a well rounded academic background with coursework in public speaking, social studies and the humanities. In addition to academic credentials a mature sense of values, motivation, dedication, and a clear understanding of clinical medicine are important factors in the selection process.

PROCESS

Applications are reviewed on rolling basis by the completion date. Applicants are encouraged to apply early. Interviews are an integral part of the selection process and offers are made on a rolling basis until the class is filled.

Admissions Requirements (Required)

MCAT Scores, Essays, Science GPA, Extracurricular activities, Non-Science GPA, Exposure to medical profession, Recommendation, Interview

Admissions Requirements (Optional)

State Residency

MEDICAL UNIVERSITY OF SOUTH CAROLINA
COLLEGE OF MEDICINE

96 JONATHAN LUCAS STREET, SUITE 601, MSC 617, CHARLESTON, SC 29425 • **ADMISSION:** 843-792-2055
FAX: 843-792-02047 • **E-MAIL:** TAYLORWL@MUSC.EDU • **WEBSITE:** WWW.MUSC.EDU / COM1

STUDENT BODY

Type	Public
Enrollment of parent institution	2,731
Enrollment of medical school	706
% male/female	56/44
% underrepresented minorities	1
% out-of-state	14
% international	28
Average age of entering class	24

FACULTY

Total faculty	1,128
% female faculty	41
% minority faculty	6
Student-faculty ratio	2.0:1

ADMISSIONS

# applied	1,973
% accepted	11
% enrolled	74

Average GPA and MCAT Scores

Overall GPA	3.7
MCAT Bio	10.2
MCAT Phys	9.7
MCAT Verbal	9.8
MCAT Essay	O

Application Information

Regular application	12/1
Early application	8/1
Early notification	10/1
Are transfers accepted?	Yes
Admissions may be deferred?	Yes
Admissions need-blind?	No
Application fee	$95

Academics

The goal of the College of Medicine is to produce caring and competent physicians capable of succeeding in their postgraduate career. The four-year program, which leads to an M.D. degree, is divided into two years of preclinical instruction which consists of education in the basic sciences and an introduction into clinical medicine, followed by years of clinical science education. The curriculum during the first two years addresses four major objectives: provision of basic science concepts, acquisition of problem-solving strategies, development of skills which permit the performance of an adequate history and physical examination, and an introduction to the role of the physician in society. Throughout, emphasis is placed on small group instruction. The curriculum was changed in fall, 1999, to expand and improve opportunities for independent, self-directed learning. As a result, students are being exposed earlier to clinical skills.

CLINICAL TRAINING

The junior year consists of eight clinical core clerkships. The clinical core consists of eight weeks each of internal medicine, obstetrics/gynecology, pediatrics, and surgery, as well as four weeks each of family medicine, psychiatry, Dean's Rural Primary Care, and neurology. During the clerkships, emphasis is placed on the development of clinical, interpersonal, and professional competence. In addition, students participate in the Foundations in Clinical Medicine course. This course is designed to integrate basic and clinical sciences utilizing small group discussions and patient case scenarios. During the senior year, students take a minimum of eight four-week rotations. The student is required to take a clinical externship and one month each of surgery, psychiatry, and internal medicine. The remaining four blocks are elective and, depending upon previous academic performance, can be taken at approved sites throughout the state or country. A complete listing of elective courses may be found in the Catalog of Electives at http://academicdepartments.musc.edu/com/UME In addition, students are required to complete and satisfactorily pass the Clinical Practice Exam (CPX).

Students

Over 95 percent of students are South Carolina residents. About 15 percent are underrepresented minorities, most of whom are African American. The average age of incoming students is typically around 25, and usually at least 10 percent of entering classes are over 30 years old. Class size is 165.

STUDENT LIFE

During orientation, incoming students are assigned to groups composed of first- and second-year students and a faculty member. The groups serve as informational resources for both academic and nonacademic matters. Also during the first week of school, the Activities Fair is held and introduces various student activities, groups, and events. Organizations that are popular with medical students include chapters of national medical fraternities, professionally oriented interest groups, and groups focused on health care related community service. Intramural sports are also popular. The Harper Student Center (HSC) houses student service offices, a student lounge, and a comprehensive fitness center with indoor and outdoor tracks, rooftop tennis courts, and a swimming pool, among other features. HSC is also a gathering site for students, offering happy hours and other social events. Beyond the campus, Charleston is a city known for its beauty and charm. Students enjoy the nearby beaches and other outdoor attractions. All students live off campus.

GRADUATES

Graduates are successful in securing residencies in all medical fields, with a significant number entering Family Medicine. MUSC itself offers over 20 post-graduate training programs. More than 95 percent pass USMLE Step 2.

Admissions

REQUIREMENTS

No prerequisites are specified. An applicant's GPA is evaluated with consideration given to the undergraduate institution attended and the difficulty of the course load. The MCAT is required, and scores must be from within the past three years. For applicants who have taken the exam on multiple occasions, the best set of scores is used.

SUGGESTIONS

South Carolina residents are given strong preference. The MCAT requirement suggests that applicants should have a basic science background. However, breadth of course work, including courses in the Humanities and Social Sciences, is also valued. Since the best set of MCAT scores is used, withholding scores has no advantage. Extracurricular activities, specifically those that are medically, community-service, or research related are important. During the interview, non cognitive traits such as emotional stability, integrity, honesty, and enthusiasm are evaluated.

PROCESS

All applicants are asked to submit secondary applications. Of those returning secondaries, about 65 percent of state residents, and 3 percent of out-of-state residents are interviewed if they are academically qualified. Interviews are conducted from September through March, and consist of three sessions each with a faculty member or MUSC alumni. About one-third of interviewees are accepted on a rolling basis. Others are rejected or wait-listed.

Admissions Requirements (Required)

MCAT Scores, Essays, Science GPA, Extracurricular activities, Non-Science GPA, Exposure to medical profession, Recommendation, Interview

Admissions Requirements (Optional)

State Residency

COSTS AND AID

Tuition & Fees

Annual tuition (in-state out-of-state)	$35,654/$62,109
Room & board	$13,340
Fees (in-state out-of-state)	$1,918/$2,257

Financial Aid

% students receiving any aid	87
% students receiving grants	33
% students receiving loans	81
% aid that is merit-based	0
Average grant	$10,419
Average loan	$52,572
Average total aid package	$58,844
Average debt	$155,870

MEHARRY MEDICAL COLLEGE
MEHARRY SCHOOL OF MEDICINE

1005 Dr. D.B. Todd Jr. Boulevard, Nashville, TN 37208-3599 • **Admission:** 615-327-6223 • **Fax:** 615-327-62287
E-mail: ADMISSIONS@MMC.EDU • **Website:** WWW.MMC.EDU

STUDENT BODY

Type	Private
Enrollment of parent institution	730
Enrollment of medical school	380
% male/female	44/56
% underrepresented minorities	2
% out-of-state	78
% international	65
# countries represented	12
Average age of entering class	26

FACULTY

Total faculty	184
Student-faculty ratio	2.0:1

ADMISSIONS

# applied	4,500
% accepted	4
% enrolled	51

Application Information

Regular application	12/15
Regular notification	10/15
Early application	8/1
Early notification	10/1
Are transfers accepted?	Yes
Admissions may be deferred?	Yes
Admissions need-blind?	Yes
Application fee	$60

Academics

Meharry benefits from its proximity to Fisk University and Tennessee State University. The three schools share certain facilities and together provide an active academic community. Most medical students at Meharry complete their studies in four years, although some extend their first year over a longer period of time and complete medical training in five years. A combined M.D./Ph.D. program is offered in Biochemistry, Biomedical Science, Microbiology, Pharmacology, and Physiology. Grades are A, B, C, and F. All medical students must pass Step 1 of the USMLE in order to be promoted to year three, and Step 2 in order to graduate.

BASIC SCIENCES: First-year courses are Anatomy, Biochemistry, Physiology, and Introduction to Clinical Medicine I. Students are in class or other scheduled sessions for 20-25 hours per week. Most instruction uses a lecture format, supplemented by labs and small-group discussions. Second-year courses are Microbiology, General and Clinical Pathology, Behavioral Sciences, Genetics, Pharmacology, and Introduction to Clinical Medicine II. During the second year, students are in class for about 30 hours per week, a significant proportion of which is devoted to small-group discussions. The Teaching and Learning Resource Center is located in the Student Center, serves as a comprehensive academic support unit, and provides tutoring and board review, among other services. The Library, holding over 50,000 volumes and 1,000 journals, is located in the same complex.

CLINICAL TRAINING

Third-year required rotations are Medicine (12 weeks); Surgery (12 weeks); Pediatrics (8 weeks); Ob/Gyn (8 weeks); Family and Preventive Medicine (8 weeks); and Psychiatry (4 weeks). Fourth-year subinternships are Medicine (4 weeks); Surgery (4 weeks); Family and Preventive Medicine (4 weeks); Radiology (4 weeks); and Psychiatry (4 weeks). Twelve weeks are reserved for electives. Major teaching hospitals are Metropolitan Nashville General Hospital, Alvin C. York Veterans Administration Medical Center, and Blanchefield Army Community Hospital. Other affiliated health care institutions are Centennial Medical Center, Vanderbilt Medical Center, Middle Tennessee Mental Health Hospital, and numerous clinics and health centers throughout the state. All students complete an ambulatory rotation in an underserved area.

Students

About 70 percent of students are African American. Students come from around the country, with about 20 percent of students from Tennessee. Class size is 80.

STUDENT LIFE

Students are supportive and cooperative, usually opting to study together in groups. There are a large number of student organizations, including honor societies, medical fraternities, support groups such as the Meharry Wives Club, groups focused on professional interests, such as the Family Practice Club, and societies focused on a common religion or ethnicity. The Daniel T. Rolfe Student Center accommodates student activities and organizations and provides a focal point for extracurricular life. Many students are involved in community activities, such as serving as mentors for high school students. Medical students interact with other Meharry students and also with peers at nearby universities. Nashville offers restaurants, nightlife, outdoor activities, and a generally student-friendly atmosphere. On-campus housing options are residence halls and apartment complexes with both one- and two-bedroom units.

GRADUATES

The College of Medicine has graduated more than 5,000 African American physicians, almost half of the total number of African American physicians who studied and who practice in the United States. About three-quarters of graduates go on to work in medically underserved rural and inner-city areas. Some graduates enter residency programs at Meharry, which has a total of 30 post-graduate positions in Family Practice, Internal Medicine, Occupational Medicine, Preventive Medicine, and Psychiatry.

Admissions

REQUIREMENTS

Required course work is eight semesters hours each of Biology, General Chemistry, Organic Chemistry, and Physics, all with associated labs. Six semester hours of English are also required. The MCAT is required, and scores should be from within the past three years. The April, rather than August, MCAT is strongly advised. For applicants who have taken the exam on multiple occasions, all sets of scores are considered.

SUGGESTIONS

Special consideration is given to underrepresented minority students and students from disadvantaged backgrounds. Meharry is interested in applicants who are dedicated to improving health care for the underserved. In addition to academic credentials, medically related or community service activities are viewed as important.

PROCESS

All qualified AMCAS applicants are sent secondary applications. Of those returning secondaries, about 10 percent are interviewed between September and May. Interviews consist of two sessions, each with a faculty member, administrator, or current medical student. On interview day, applicants also have the opportunity to meet informally with students. About one-third of interviewed candidates are accepted on a rolling basis. Others are rejected or placed on a wait-list. Wait-listed candidates may send additional information if it serves to update their files.

Admissions Requirements (Required)

MCAT Scores, Essays, Science GPA, Extracurricular activities, Non-Science GPA, Exposure to medical profession, Recommendation, Interview

Admissions Requirements (Optional)

State Residency

COSTS AND AID

Tuition & Fees

Annual tuition	$27,957
Room & board	$11,813
Cost of books	$1,185
Fees	$1,435

Financial Aid

% students receiving any aid	79
% students receiving grants	23
% students receiving loans	60
% aid that is merit-based	10
Average grant	$1,000
Average loan	$28,893
Average total aid package	$33,996
Average debt	$125,339

MEMORIAL UNIVERSITY NEWFOUNDLAND

FACULTY OF MEDICINE, MEMORIAL UNIVERSITY

ROOM 1751, HEALTH SCIENCES CENTER, ST. JOHN'S, NF A1B 3V6 • ADMISSION: 709-777-6615 • FAX: 709-777-84227
E-MAIL: MUNMED@MUN.CA • WEBSITE: WWW.MED.MUN.CA/ADMISSIONS

STUDENT BODY

Type	Public
Enrollment of medical school	244
% male/female	48/52
% international	0

FACULTY

Total faculty	186
% female faculty	31
% part-time faculty	60

ADMISSIONS

# applied	648
% accepted	12
% enrolled	78

Average GPA and MCAT Scores

Overall GPA	3.7
MCAT Bio	9.0
MCAT Phys	9.0
MCAT Verbal	9.0
MCAT Essay	0

Application Information

Regular application	11/15
Regular notification	3/1
Are transfers accepted?	No
Admissions may be deferred?	Yes
Admissions need-blind?	Yes
Application fee	$75

Academics

Each of the first two years is organized into three terms. Although the emphasis of the course work is on basic science, clinical medicine is also introduced. During the second two years, students perform clerkships in affiliated hospitals that provide both undergraduate and graduate medical education. In addition to the four-year M.D. degree, M.Sc. and Ph.D. degree programs are also open to qualified students. Areas of academic strength include Endocrinology and Metabolism; Gastroenterology, Human Genetics; Immunology; Molecular Biology; Neurosciences, and Cardiovascular Sciences including Epidemiology; and Community Medicine.

BASIC SCIENCES: An important component of the first year is Basic Science of Medicine. This course introduces students to the biology of the normal human and integrates Biochemistry, Physiology, Immunology, Cell Biology, Genetics, Microbiology, Nutrition, Pharmacology, Pathology, and Anatomy. Teaching methods include lectures, small group sessions, laboratories, seminars, and open discussions. Students have the opportunity to initiate basic science research, which can be pursued throughout medical school. First-year students also take Integrated Study of Disease, which teaches Pathology and Pharmacology through the study of diseases of the major organ systems. In Clinical Skills, students are first introduced to the medical interview and techniques of counseling. The physical exam and important ethical issues are also part of the course. Community Medicine is a unique course, which focuses on the contextual aspects of disease and introduces Preventive Medicine, Biostatistics, Epidemiology, Social and Organizational Factors in Health, Environmental and Occupational Health, Community Nutrition, and Behavioral Sciences. The course includes visits to community-based hospitals and clinics. All courses continue in the second year, building on principles learned during the first year. On average, preclinical students are in class or other scheduled sessions for twenty-three hours per week.

CLINICAL TRAINING

Year three is of twelve months duration beginning in September and continuing to the following Fall. It is composed of the core clerkships and some electives. Core clerkships, typically eight weeks in length, are Internal Medicine, Surgery, Psychiatry, Pediatrics and Ob/Gyn. A four-week Rural Family Medicine rotation is also required. The fourth year consists of electives and selectives, some of which may be completed at institutions other than those affiliated with the University. Teaching hospitals include General Hospital (531 beds), Grace General Hospital, Dr. Charles A Janeway Child Health Centre, St. Clare's Mercy Hospital, Waterford Hospital, and a number of institutions that are not under the Health Care Corporation of St. Johns.

Students

The school's class size is relatively small at 60 students. The male/female ratio within the student body is about 50/50.

STUDENT LIFE

On-campus housing is available for both single and married students. In addition, the University provides assistance in locating off-campus housing. Medical students benefit from an active counseling center, childcare services, learning enhancement programs, a career planning office, and a student health service. The Student's Union promotes artistic, educational, charitable, and social activities, and the graduate student union provides common areas for social and other activities. Medical students have access to the services and resources of the greater university.

GRADUATES

A significant proportion of graduates enter residencies at affiliated hospitals in areas such as Anesthesia, Internal Medicine, Neurology, Ob/Gyn, Orthopedics, Anatomic Pathology, General Pathology, Pediatrics, Psychiatry, Radiology, and Surgery. Most graduates enter clinical medicine, often in primary care fields.

Admissions

REQUIREMENTS

To be eligible for admission, a bachelor's degree is required in almost all circumstances. Requirements include two courses in English. The MCAT is also required, and must be taken prior to the application deadline, which is normally November 15. Transcripts and letters of reference must be submitted by November 29. Interviews are required of some candidates. The majority of places in each class are reserved for applicants who are residents of Newfoundland and Labrador. There are a limited number of places available for applicants from New Brunswick, from other Canadian provinces, and non-Canadians. Non-Canadians pay higher fees.

SUGGESTIONS

There are approximately 650 applications received for 60 places each year. Therefore, competition is high. Material submitted after the stated deadlines will not be considered. Academic achievement, MCAT scores, work or other experiences, and personal traits are all reviewed in admissions decisions. Though age itself is not used as a basis for selection, time away from academic studies may be taken into consideration.

PROCESS

Requests for applications should be directed to the address above. Applications are accepted until November 15 in the year preceding anticipated matriculation. Decisions are made in the spring. Notification of the committee's decision will be made to candidates by letter from the Admissions Committee. Applicants have 14 days in which to confirm that he/she will accept the place offered to them.

Admissions Requirements (Required)

MCAT Scores, Essays, Extracurricular activities, Recommendation, Interview

Admissions Requirements (Optional)

Science GPA, Non-Science GPA, Exposure to medical profession, State Residency

COSTS AND AID

Tuition & Fees

Annual tuition (in-state out-of-state)	$6,250/$30,000
Room & board	$9,000
Cost of books	$1,593
Fees (in-state out-of-state)	$457/$645

Financial Aid

% students receiving any aid	90
% students receiving grants	10
% students receiving loans	90
Average grant	$800
Average total aid package	$39,000
Average debt	$150,000

MERCER UNIVERSITY
MERCER UNIVERSITY SCHOOL OF MEDICINE

1550 COLLEGE STREET, MACON, GA 31207 • ADMISSION: 478-301-2542 • FAX: 478-301-25477
E-MAIL: PUTNAM_MC@MERCER.EDU • WEBSITE: WWW.MERCER.EDU

STUDENT BODY	
Type	Private
Enrollment of medical school	241
% male/female	52/48
Average age of entering class	23

ADMISSIONS	
# applied	738
% accepted	8
% enrolled	100

Average GPA and MCAT Scores	
Overall GPA	3.5
MCAT Bio	8.9
MCAT Phys	8.5
MCAT Verbal	9.1
MCAT Essay	N

Application Information	
Regular application	11/1
Early application	8/1
Early notification	10/1
Are transfers accepted?	Yes
Admissions may be deferred?	Yes
Admissions need-blind?	Yes
Application fee	$50

Academics

Each entering student is assigned to a faculty advisor who assists with the transition to medical school, with strategies for pre-clinical studies, and later with decisions involved in elective and specialty selection. Almost all students complete the M.D. curriculum in four years. Evaluation uses Satisfactory/Unsatisfactory during the first two years, and Honors/Satisfactory/Unsatisfactory during the third and fourth years. Self and Peer Evaluations are also used in some situations. Passing both steps of the USMLE is a requirement for graduation.

BASIC SCIENCES: Basic sciences are presented during the first two years as part of the Biomedical Problems Program, which uses case-based instructional techniques and computer-assisted, self-directed study. The curriculum is organized around physiological systems or "phases," which are Cells and Metabolism, Genetics and Development, Host Defense, Hematology, Neurology, Brain and Behavior, Musculoskeletal, Cardiology, Pulmonology, Gastrointestinal, Renal Endocrinology, Biology of Reproduction, and Infectious Disease. Issues related to Medical Ethics are also discussed in the context of case studies. Community Science is another important part of the first two years. Courses included in this category are Community Epidemiology; Rural Preceptorship; Managed Care and Physician Workforce; Clinical Biostatistics; and Research Design and the Medical Literature. Clinical training begins during the first year, when students learn interviewing and examination skills by working with simulated patients. Actual patient contact occurs through the Community Office Practice Program (COPP) in which students work directly with community physicians. Most basic science instruction takes place in the Medical Education Building, which, in addition to classrooms, houses the Medical Library, Mercer Health Systems (which provides clinical services), the Health Education Center, and the school's administrative offices. This physical arrangement, with basic science and clinical facilities in the same building, guarantees first- and second-year students an integrated educational experience. The library has over 90,000 volumes, 2,500 audiovisuals, and 850 current subscriptions. The Learning Resource Center offers computers and labs.

CLINICAL TRAINING

Third-year required rotations are Internal Medicine (12 weeks); Surgery (8 weeks); Pediatrics (8 weeks); Ob/Gyn (6 weeks); Family Medicine (8 weeks); and Psychiatry (6 weeks). During the fourth year, students choose among fields within Surgical Subspecialities (4 weeks) and also complete clerkships in Community Science (4 weeks); Substance Abuse (2 weeks); and Critical Care (2 weeks). The remainder of the year is reserved for elective study. The primary teaching hospitals are the Medical Center of Central Georgia in Macon (518 beds) and the Memorial Health University Medical Center in Savannah (530 beds). Other major affiliates are Floyd Medical Center in Rome, Phoebe Putney Memorial Hospital in Albany, and the Medical Center in Columbus. Training also takes place outside of major hospitals, at sites such as community hospitals, clinics, and physicians' offices throughout the state.

Students

All students are Georgia residents. About 4 percent are underrepresented minorities. The average age of incoming students is around 24, and at least 20 percent of a typical entering class took significant time off between college and medical school.

STUDENT LIFE

Medical students have access to the facilities of the greater University. These include cafeterias, athletic facilities, and recreational centers. Medical students also have their own student center, which has a snack bar and functions as a meeting place. Students may join chapters of national medical student organizations, including those that focus on the needs of women and minority medical students. Mercer offers conveniently located, campus-owned apartments to medical students on a limited basis. Affordable accommodations are also available in and around Macon. The Office of Admissions and Student Affairs helps students find suitable housing.

GRADUATES

Most graduates enter residency programs in Georgia and go on to practice in primary care fields within the state.

Admissions

REQUIREMENTS

Generally, only residents of Georgia are accepted. Required course work is one year each of Biology, Physics, Chemistry, and Organic Chemistry. The MCAT is required and scores must be no more than two years old.

SUGGESTIONS

In addition to required preparatory courses, Biochemistry is recommended. The April MCAT is strongly advised as files are not reviewed until MCAT scores are available. The Admissions Committee is interested in students who are strongly motivated to work with underserved populations and in rural areas. For applicants who have taken time off after college, some recent course work is important.

PROCESS

Secondary applications are sent to AMCAS applicants who meet minimum requirements. Typically, about 70 percent of Georgia residents who apply receive secondary applications. Of those returning secondaries, about 20 percent are invited to interview. Interviews take place between October and March, and consist of two sessions with faculty. About one-third of interviewees are accepted. All decisions are made before March 30, at which point a wait-list is formed.

Admissions Requirements (Required)

MCAT Scores, Essays, Science GPA, Extracurricular activities, Non-Science GPA, Exposure to medical profession, Recommendation, Interview, State Residency

COSTS AND AID

Tuition & Fees

Annual tuition	$38,885
Room & board	$14,070
Cost of books	$2,900
Fees	$200

Financial Aid

% students receiving any aid	94
% students receiving grants	77
% students receiving loans	91
% aid that is merit-based	0
Average grant	$8,880
Average loan	$27,619
Average total aid package	$44,218
Average debt	$165,823

MICHIGAN STATE UNIVERSITY
COLLEGE OF HUMAN MEDICINE

LIFE SCIENCE BUILDING, 1355 BOGUE STREET, RM A239 EAST LANSING, MI 48824 • **ADMISSION:** 517-353-9620
FAX: 517-432-00217 • **E-MAIL:** MDADMISSIONS@MSU.EDU • **WEBSITE:** MDADMISSIONS.MSU.EDU

STUDENT BODY

Type	Public
Enrollment of parent institution	49,343
Enrollment of medical school	851
% male/female	49/51
% underrepresented minorities	1
% out-of-state	19
% international	13
# countries represented	15
Average age of entering class	24

FACULTY

Total faculty	625
% part-time faculty	3

ADMISSIONS

# applied	6,342
% accepted	5
% enrolled	62

Average GPA and MCAT Scores

Overall GPA	3.6
MCAT Bio	10.0
MCAT Phys	9.0
MCAT Verbal	9.0
MCAT Essay	0

Application Information

Regular application	11/1
Early application	8/1
Early notification	10/1
Are transfers accepted?	No
Admissions may be deferred?	Yes
Admissions need-blind?	No
Application fee	$80

Academics

The four-year curriculum is modern and highly innovative. While the first two years are spent at MSU's main campus in East Lansing, during the third and fourth years, students are assigned to one of six community-based programs for clinical training. These communities are the following: Kalamazoo, Upper Peninsula, Grand Rapids, Flint, Lansing, and Saginaw. Special clinical programs include the Rural Physician Program and Leadership in Medicine for the Underserved. Along with its focus on primary care, the College of Human Medicine welcomes students seeking a dual degree. Fields in which graduate degrees may be earned include: Biochemistry/Molecular Biology, Bioethics/Humanities/Society, Epidemiology, Health Communication, Microbiology/Molecular Genetics, Pharmacology/Toxiocology, and Physiology. Medical students are evaluated with a modified Pass/No Pass system.

BASIC SCIENCES: In addition to mastering basic science concepts, first-year students address the doctor/patient relationship in Clinical Skills. A unique Mentor Program assigns small groups of students to a preceptor, allowing the groups to explore patient care and the complex roles of the physician. Students accompany their mentor for hospital rounds and patient visits. The course Integrative Clinical Correlations, taught by basic science faculty members and clinicians, develops problem-solving skills and allows students to apply basic science concepts to clinical case studies. Other first-year courses are the following: Gross Anatomy, Biochemistry, Neuroscience, Molecular Biology and Genetics, Cell Biology and Physiology, Microbiology and Immunology, Human Developmen and Behavior in Society, Pathology, Biostatistics and Epidemiology, Clinical Skills, Pharmacology, and Radiology. The second year is organized around body systems and general disease categories. These are the following: Infectious Diseases; Disorders of Development and Behavior; Hematopoietic/Neoplasia; Cardiovascular; Urinary Tract; Pulmonary; Metabolic Endocrine Reproductive; Digestive; Neurological/Musculoskeletal; and Major Mental Disorders. In the Social Context of Clinical Decisions, students take part in a series of small-group seminars dealing with the concepts of Medical Ethics; Epidemiology; Biostatistics; Critical Reasoning; Humanities; and Social, Economic, and Organizational Issues in Medicine. The primary mode of instruction during the second year is small-group discussions/tutorials. Students are in scheduled sessions for less than 20 hours per week, allowing ample time for individual and group study. Academic facilities include the Echt Computer Lab, which offers computer-based instructional programs and audio/visual aids, a 24-hour exclusive and comprehensive Student Learning Center, and MSU's main library.

CLINICAL TRAINING

Most clerkship requirements are fulfilled during the third year and the early part of year four. Students move to one of six communities during the summer of their third year. They then rotate through eight weeks of each of the following: Family Practice, Internal Medicine, Pediatrics, Surgery, Ob/Gyn, and Psychiatry. Four weeks of Advanced Medicine and Advanced Surgery are also required. Throughout the period in which students complete required clerkships, students also participate in a Core Competency Seminar, which requires 2 hours per week and provides a forum for discussion of interdisciplinary topics important to the care and health management of patients. A total of 20 weeks are reserved for elective experiences. Students may rotate to other communities in the state, to hospitals and academic centers in other states, and to clinical sites overseas.

Students

At least 80 percent of students are Michigan residents. Class size is 200. In a recent class, the average age of incoming students was 25.

STUDENT LIFE

Students spend their preclinical years (years one and two) at either the East Lansing or the Grand Rapids preclinical campus. The East Lansing preclinical campus is located at one of the largest and most diverse universities in the country, Michigan State University. The Grand Rapids preclinical campus is based at the Secchia Center, located in the rapidly expanding health sciences corridor in downtown Grand Rapids. The two campuses differ greatly in terms of setting. The MSU campus is part of a traditional University setting, while the Secchia Center campus is located in the heart of downtown Grand Rapids. However, the first- and second-year curriculums, calendar, and examinations are the same at both preclinical campuses. The Office of Admissions makes all preclinical campus placement decisions. Students spend their third and fourth year at one of six clinical campuses (Flint, Grand Rapids, Lansing, Midland Region, Traverse City, and the Upper Peninsula Region). The Office of Student Affairs and Services determines where students spend their third and fourth years.

GRADUATES

Students typically score above the national average on the USMLE, contributing to their success in securing top-choice residency positions. A recent three year average of residency choices resolved: Family Practice (27%); Internal Medicine (15%); Ob/Gyn (10 %); Surgery (13%); Pediatrics (15%); Psychiatry (3%), other programs (17%). About 50% of graduates remained in Michigan for residency programs.

Admissions

REQUIREMENTS

Prerequisites are one year each of Biology, Chemistry, and Organic Chemistry, all with one associated lab. One year each in English and Social Science, two upper level Biology courses, and College Algebra or Statistics and Probability are also required. The MCAT is required, and scores must be no more than four years old. For applicants who have retaken the exam, the most recent set of scores is used. Applicants should be United States or Canadian citizens, hold a US permanent resident visa, or have asylum in the United States. A bachelor's degree earned in the US or Canada is also required.

SUGGESTIONS

Though Michigan residents are given preference, about 20 percent of the positions in an entering class are available to highly qualified nonresident applicants. MSU is focused on training generalist physicians and seeks applicants with an interest in primary care and community-based medicine. Applicants should have medical/clinical experience. Important personal traits are excellent interpersonal communication skills, leadership, social responsibility, and compassion. The Self Assessment Guide on the CHM Office of Admissions website is helpful in determining if an applicant is prepared to submit a competitive application to CHM.

PROCESS

About one-third of AMCAS applicants are interviewed. Multiple Mini Interviews (MMI) are conducted on select Fridays in East Lansing and Grand Rapids, from September through March. In addition to the MMI, the applicants have a 20 minute interview with a current medical student. On Interview Day, candidates attend informational sessions and have lunch with medical students. About one-third of interviewees are accepted on a rolling basis.

Admissions Requirements (Required)

MCAT Scores, Essays, Science GPA, Extracurricular activities, Non-Science GPA, Exposure to medical profession, Recommendation, Interview

Admissions Requirements (Optional)

State Residency

COSTS AND AID

Tuition & Fees

Annual tuition (in-state out-of-state)	$30,081/$61,548
Room & board	$14,616
Cost of books	$2,407
Fees	$56

Financial Aid

% students receiving any aid	90
% students receiving grants	48
% students receiving loans	82
% aid that is merit-based	0
Average grant	$6,653
Average loan	$44,605
Average total aid package	$44,424
Average debt	$212,952

MOREHOUSE
SCHOOL OF MEDICINE

ADMISSIONS AND STUDENT AFFAIRS, 720 WESTVIEW DRIVE, SW, ATLANTA, GA 30310 • ADMISSION: 404-752-1650
FAX: 404-752-15127 • E-MAIL: • WEBSITE: WWW.MSM.EDU

Academics

Most students follow a four-year curriculum leading to the M.D., although some pursue joint degree programs of M.D./M.P.H or M.D./Ph.D. To be considered for these programs, applications must be submitted to the appropriate graduate department at the time of application to medical school. Medical students are evaluated on an A-F scale. Passing the USMLE Step 1 is a requirement for promotion to year three, and passing Step 2 is a requirement for graduation.

BASIC SCIENCES: Instruction uses a lecture/lab format, and students are in class or laboratories for about 30 hours per week. First-year courses are Human Morphology, Medical Biochemistry, Neurobiology, Medical Physiology, Fundamentals of Medicine I, Community Health, and a weekly preceptorship with a community physician. Second-year courses are Fundamentals of Medicine II, Pathophysiology, Microbiology and Immunology, Pathology, Pharmacology, and Nutrition. During the second year, students learn patient interview and examination techniques. Instruction takes place in the Basic Medical Sciences Building, which contains classrooms, laboratories, and administrative offices, and in the adjacent Medical Education Building.

CLINICAL TRAINING
Third- and fourth-year required clerkships are Internal Medicine (2 months); Pediatrics (2 months); Ob/Gyn (2 months); Psychiatry (7 weeks); Surgery (2 months); Family Medicine (1 month); Ambulatory Medicine (1 month and a year long Fundamentals of Medicine III Series); Maternal Child Health (1 month); and Rural Primary Care (1 month). Five months are reserved for electives. Third-year rotations take place primarily at Grady Memorial Hospital (1,000 beds), a full-service facility for indigent patients that, for training purposes, is shared with Emory University. A portion of elective credit may be earned at accredited medical schools other than Morehouse, and at a wide range of clinical institutions.

Students

Approximately 67 percent of students are African American. About 51 percent of students are from Georgia, while others are from a wide geographic area. Class size is 52.

STUDENT LIFE
Community service is an important part of student life, and virtually all students are involved in some sort of volunteer activity while in medical school. Students are cohesive both in and out of the classroom. A demonstration of cooperation between students is the large percentage of students who are in study groups. Students participate in local chapters of national medical school organizations and in student groups focused on professional interests. Atlanta is the cultural, financial and industrial hub of the Southeastern United States, and offers a wide range of activities and attractions including arts, sports, recreation, dining, and entertainment. The city is accessible by public transportation. Although there is no school-owned housing, students are able to locate affordable housing off campus.

GRADUATES

Graduates are successful in securing residencies in prestigious programs nationwide. Approximately 75 percent of graduates enter primary care fields, one of the highest percentages among medical schools. Most go on to work with underserved populations, either in inner cities or in rural areas.

Admissions

REQUIREMENTS

Required courses are Biology (one year); General Chemistry (one year); Organic Chemistry (one year); Physics (one year); college-level Math (one year), and English (one year). All science courses must include associated labs. Grades are assessed with consideration given to academic improvement, balance and depth of academic program, difficulty of courses taken, and overall achievement. The MCAT is required, and scores must be from within the past two years. Applicants who have taken the exam on multiple occasions are not penalized, but the most recent set of scores is weighed most heavily.

SUGGESTIONS

Of the 52 spots in a class, at least 20 are reserved for Georgia residents. Thus, competition for out-of-state residents can be intense. For all applicants, the April, rather than August, MCAT is advised. Beyond academic achievement, the committee is interested in extracurricular activities, research projects and experiences, and evidence of pursuing interests and talents in depth. Compassion, honesty, motivation, and perseverance are qualities that are considered important to the practice of medicine.

PROCESS

About 80 percent of AMCAS applicants are sent secondary applications. Of those returning secondaries, about 8 percent are invited to interview between October and March. Of Georgia residents, about 25 percent are invited to interview. Interviews generally consist of one 30-minute session with a faculty member. On interview day, candidates receive a campus tour, group orientation sessions, lunch, and the opportunity to meet with current medical students. About 10-20 percent of interviewees are accepted, with notification beginning in December. Wait-listed candidates may send supplementary material to update or strengthen their files.

Admissions Requirements (Required)

MCAT Scores, Essays, Science GPA, Extracurricular activities, Non-Science GPA, Exposure to medical profession, Recommendation, Interview

Admissions Requirements (Optional)

State Residency

COSTS AND AID

Tuition & Fees

Annual tuition	$26,000
Room & board	$12,470
Cost of books	$11,087
Fees	$6,252

Financial Aid

% students receiving any aid	93
% students receiving grants	31
% students receiving loans	89
% aid that is merit-based	17
Average grant	$11,148
Average loan	$38,817
Average total aid package	$43,700
Average debt	$136,335

NEW YORK MEDICAL COLLEGE

NEW YORK MEDICAL COLLEGE

OFFICE OF ADMISSIONS, ADMINISTRATION BUILDING VALHALLA, NY 10595 • **ADMISSION:** 914-594-4507
FAX: 914-594-49767 • **E-MAIL:** MDADMIT@NYMC.EDU • **WEBSITE:** WWW.NYMC.EDU

STUDENT BODY

Type	Private
Enrollment of parent institution	1,424
Enrollment of medical school	774
% male/female	49/51
% out-of-state	67
% international	4
# countries represented	10
Average age of entering class	24

FACULTY

Total faculty	3,018
% female faculty	30
% minority faculty	32
% part-time faculty	1

ADMISSIONS

# applied	7,559
% accepted	10
% enrolled	26

Average GPA and MCAT Scores

Overall GPA	3.5
MCAT Bio	10.4
MCAT Phys	10.0
MCAT Verbal	9.4
MCAT Essay	Q

Application Information

Regular application	12/15
Early application	8/1
Early notification	10/1
Are transfers accepted?	Yes
Admissions may be deferred?	Yes
Admissions need-blind?	No
Application fee	$100

Academics

Students have an opportunity to earn joint degrees, combining the M.D. with an M.P.H., which is of great value considering the increased awareness of public health issues, or a Ph.D. in the basic medical sciences. Grading is Honors/High Pass/Pass/Fail. Passing Step 1 and 2 of the USMLE is a graduation requirement. In recent years, the pass rate has been at or near 100 percent.

BASIC SCIENCES: The curriculum of the first two years, although focused on the basic sciences, maintains a consistent clinical orientation. The program has been revised to bring clinical relevance and small-group teaching into all courses. The first two years focus on developing a thorough understanding of the sciences basic to clinical medicine. The core of the first-year curriculum—Anatomy, Histology, Biochemistry, Physiology, Neural Science, and Behavioral Science—supplemented by clinical case correlations and courses in Epidemiology and Biostatistics. The second-year curriculum, with its strong focus on Pathology/Pathophysiology, emphasizes small-group discussion, problem-based learning, and self-study, with only 25 percent of class time spent in large lectures. Clinical Skills Training, Pharmacology, and Medical Microbiology prepare students for the clerkship experience of the next two years.

CLINICAL TRAINING

While immersed in the basic science curriculum, all first-year students have ongoing, direct patient contact, working in the office of a primary care physician. This one-on-one placement gives students clinical exposure and a personal mentor relationship. This preceptorship experience continues throughout the second year. Third-year clinical clerkships are the following: Medicine (12 weeks); Surgery (8 weeks); Pediatrics (8 weeks); Ob/Gyn (6 weeks); Psychiatry (6 weeks); Neurology (4 weeks); Family Medicine Clerkship (4 weeks). The school's location in the suburban New York area and large hospital network afford clinical-training opportunities in demographically and clinically diverse settings. About half of the third-year class moves into New York City for their clinical years. Fourth-year requirements are the following: Medicine or Pediatrics Subinternship (4 weeks); Ambulatory Surgical Subspecialties (4 weeks); Geriatrics or Chronic Care Pediatrics (4 weeks); and Anesthesiology/Rehabilitation Medicine (2 weeks). The 18 weeks of electives can be taken anywhere. About 15–20 students take international electives each year.

Students

The school's student body is generally representative of the demographic diversity of the country. The first-year class size is 190 students; in recent years it has been fairly equally divided by gender, with the proportion of females increasing incrementally. About half come from public colleges and universities.

STUDENT LIFE

Most first- and second-year students live on campus in attractive, unfurnished garden apartments or furnished suite-style apartment shares in a suburban setting that encourages a sense of community. Students gather for pick-up football, soccer and basketball games outdoors when weather permits. New York Medical College has an arrangement with Fordham University to allow our students to use recreational facilities at Fordham's Marymount campus in Tarrytown, about 10 minutes away. The facilities include cardio and weight rooms, locker and shower rooms, a pool for lap swimming and a gymnasium for basketball. Students can participate in more than 40 clubs and organizations groups focused on professional, cultural, social, educational and athletic interests. These include The Arrhythmias, a cappella singing group, a chamber music club and other cultural groups. Project Sunshine works to better the lives of children in hospitals, and AMSA, AMA, AMWA, and SMNA—student chapters of major professional organizations—offer students an opportunity to represent the school at regional and national student conferences.

GRADUATES

The School of Medicine encourages students to aim high in applying for residency matches. While a large number of students are choosing to match in primary care disciplines, there are equally impressive matches in highly competitive specialty programs. Matches for the current year can be viewed on the school's website. Some 12,000 alumni are supported by alumni association chapters in major cities. Alumni can track University announcements of upcoming events on the Website, and a special Alumni section allows them to post news and read about other alumni. Alumni can also keep current on their classmates' activities via the University magazine, Chironian, which is mailed to all alumni and is also available for viewing on the web.

Admissions

REQUIREMENTS

All applicants must have taken the MCAT within the last three years and must have completed or have in progress the following prerequisites: two semesters of Biology, Chemistry, Organic Chemistry and Physics. Each of these must have been completed with lab work. Two semesters of English are also required. The most recent MCAT scores are given greatest weight. While most students have majored in the sciences, the school encourages those with strong humanities backgrounds and the necessary science requirements to apply.

SUGGESTIONS

In addition to purely academic factors, we look for students who show clear evidence through their activities of strong motivation toward medicine and a sense of dedication to the service of others. Personal qualities of character and personality are evaluated from letters of recommendation, from the personal statement and from the interview. New York Medical College does not deny admission to any applicant on the basis of race, color, creed, religion, national or ethnic origin, age, sex, sexual orientation or disability.

PROCESS

All AMCAS applicants are requested to complete an online secondary application. After the completed secondary application and all letters of recommendation have been processed, the applicant's file is reviewed for consideration. Interviews are by invitation and are conducted on campus. We generally interview from October through April and decisions are made on a rolling basis.

Admissions Requirements (Required)

MCAT Scores, Essays, Science GPA, Extracurricular activities, Non-Science GPA, Exposure to medical profession, Recommendation, Interview

COSTS AND AID

Tuition & Fees

Annual tuition	$38,500
Room & board (on-campus off-campus)	$17,538/$13,306
Cost of books	$2,028
Fees (in-state out-of-state)	$3,270

Financial Aid

% students receiving any aid	90
% students receiving grants	48
% students receiving loans	85
% aid that is merit-based	20
Average grant	$20,000
Average loan	$45,000
Average total aid package	$45,000
Average debt	$166,000

New York University

New York University School of Medicine

Office of Admissions, 550 First Avenue New York, NY 10016 • Admission: 212-263-5290 • Fax: 212-263-07207
E-mail: ADMISSIONS@MED.NYU.EDU • Website: WWW.MED.NYU.EDU

STUDENT BODY

Type	Private
Enrollment of medical school	711
% male/female	50/50
% underrepresented minorities	1
% out-of-state	50
% international	12
# countries represented	4
Average age of entering class	24

FACULTY

Total faculty	1,344
% female faculty	33
% minority faculty	4
% part-time faculty	22

ADMISSIONS

# applied	7,423
% accepted	6
% enrolled	34

Average GPA and MCAT Scores

Overall GPA	3.8
MCAT Bio	11.2
MCAT Phys	11.2
MCAT Verbal	10.3
MCAT Essay	Q

Application Information

Regular application	10/15
Regular notification	3/1
Are transfers accepted?	No
Admissions may be deferred?	Yes
Admissions need-blind?	No
Application fee	$100

Academics

The goal of the curriculum is to train physician-scholars who will approach the profession of medicine with intellectual rigor and who also understand the humanistic and ethical aspects of the field. Selected students may pursue a curriculum leading to both the M.D. and Ph.D. degrees. The Ph.D. degree is earned in a basic medical science field. The honors program permits students who are following the standard four-year M.D. curriculum to supplement formal class work with summer research or ongoing projects and to receive credit. Grading during the preclinical years is Pass/Fail. Letter grades are given during the clinical clerkship.

BASIC SCIENCES: In the fall of 1997, the School of Medicine implemented a new basic science curriculum organized into interdisciplinary modules. Year one has three modules. The first module is comprised of Molecular Biology/ Genetics and Biochemistry; Anatomy; and Embryology. Module Two includes Cellular Biology; Physiology; Histology; and Immunology. Module Three is Organ Physiology; Histology of Tissues/ Organs; Microbiology; Immunology and Parasitology. Throughout the first year, students take Behavioral Science/Introduction to Clinical Medicine, which addresses the interrelationship among patients, their families, environments, their particular illness, and their care. The first year also includes The Skills and Science of Doctoring. This includes a preceptorship in the office of a practicing physician and serves to integrate basic science concepts with clinical applications. First-semester, second-year courses are the following: Neuroscience, General Pathology, and Psychopathology. In second semester, Pathophysiology; Systemic Pathology; Pharmacology and Biostatistics/ Epidemiology are integrated in a Human Organ System module. During the first two years, class time is divided between lectures and small-group discussions. Laboratory work and computer-assisted instruction enhance learning. In total, first- and second-year students are in class or other scheduled sessions for about 20 hours per week. Our Division of Academic Computing has resulted in increased integration of bioinformatics into the curriculum. Each of the courses has a Web page, and students can access all course materials, including lecture slides, through the Web. Instruction takes place in the Medical Science Building and adjacent facilities, which provide laboratory space, lecture halls, rooms for small-group discussions, and conference rooms. The Frederick L. Ehrman Medical Library occupies three stories in the Medical Science Building and has areas that are open to students 24 hours a day. Its collection includes over 160,000 volumes and 2,000 current serial titles.

CLINICAL TRAINING

Required clerkships must be completed during year three and the first part of year four. These are the following: Medicine (10 weeks); Pediatrics (8 weeks); Surgery (10 weeks); Ob/Gyn (6 weeks); Psychiatry (6 weeks); Neurology (4 weeks); and Ambulatory Care Medicine (4 weeks). During the fourth year, all students take six weeks of advanced medicine. The remainder of the year is reserved for elective study, which typically involves a research project. Clinical training takes place at Bellevue Hospital Center and New York University Medical Center Complex and at affiliated institutions. A portion of electives may be taken at other hospitals in the United States or abroad.

Students

Approximately 50 percent of students are New York residents. Others come from all regions of the country. Though the majority of students are in their early 20s, each class has several nontraditional students who pursued careers or other activities between college and medical school. Class size is 160.

STUDENT LIFE

NYU School of Medicine (SoM) is located in one of the most vibrant and centrally located neighborhoods in New York City. The area's many resources are easily accessible to NYU's campus, so that our students are presented with a vast array of cultural, social, and recreational opportunities. By way of the NYU SoM student ticket office, students are able to take advantage of the city's many cultural events and performances at discounted prices. The NYU SoM is easily accessible to other parts of the city. Midtown and Union Square are within walking distance, and other popular neighborhoods are only a short subway ride away. The SoM operates housing facilities for students, assuring that all NYU medical students afford convenient and comfortable housing. Both residence halls and apartments are available.

GRADUATES

Of the 2005 graduates, the most prevalent fields for post-graduate training were the following: Internal Medicine (18%); Pediatrics (10%); Diagnostic Radiology (10%); and Emergency Medicine (7%). Most graduates enter residency programs at top institutions nationwide.

Admissions

REQUIREMENTS

Prerequisites are six semester hours each: General Chemistry, Organic Chemistry, Physics, Biology, and English. All science courses must include laboratory work. The MCAT is required and must be taken no more than 3 years prior to application. For applicants who have taken the exam more than once, the best set of scores is considered.

SUGGESTIONS

Biochemistry is strongly recommended. Other recommended courses are Calculus, Quantitative and Physical Chemistry, Genetics, Embryology, and Spanish, particularly if the applicant intends to practice in New York City. Experience in health care, research and community service are considered valuable.

PROCESS

NYU Medical School participates in the AMCAS program. About 15 percent of applicants are invited to interview between September and December. Interviews consist of one session with a faculty member. On interview day applicants tour the campus and have lunch with current students. About 35 percent of interviewed candidates are accepted, with notification occurring by late January. Others are either wait-listed or rejected. Wait listed candidates can be selected for admission up until the first day of class in August.

Admissions Requirements (Required)

MCAT Scores, Essays, Science GPA, Extracurricular activities, Non-Science GPA, Exposure to medical profession, Recommendation, Interview

Admissions Requirements (Optional)

State Residency

COSTS AND AID

Tuition & Fees

Annual tuition	$33,200
Room & board	$15,000
Cost of books	$1,200
Fees	$7,550

Financial Aid

% students receiving any aid	69
% students receiving grants	56
% students receiving loans	66
% aid that is merit-based	0
Average grant	$9,960
Average loan	$37,000
Average total aid package	$43,335
Average debt	$128,000

NORTHEASTERN OHIO UNIVERSITIES COLLEGE OF MEDICINE

NORTHEASTERN OHIO UNIVERSITIES COLLEGE OF MEDICINE

P.O. Box 95, ROOTSTOWN, OH 44272-0095 • ADMISSION: 330-325-6270 • FAX: 330-325-83727
E-MAIL: ADMISSION@NEOUCOM.EDU • WEBSITE: WWW.NEOUCOM.EDU

STUDENT BODY

Type	Public
Enrollment of medical school	460
% male/female	51/49
% out-of-state	2
% international	6
Average age of entering class	22

FACULTY

Total faculty	1,905
% female faculty	19
% minority faculty	15
% part-time faculty	86

ADMISSIONS

# applied	2,050
% accepted	8
% enrolled	68

Average GPA and MCAT Scores

Overall GPA	3.7
MCAT Bio	9.6
MCAT Phys	9.0
MCAT Verbal	9.4
MCAT Essay	0

Application Information

Regular application	11/1
Regular notification	3/21
Early application	8/1
Early notification	10/1
Are transfers accepted?	Yes
Admissions may be deferred?	Yes
Admissions need-blind?	No
Application fee	$75

Academics

While most students participate in the 6- or 7-year B.S./M.D. program, about 30-40 students each year enter the four-year M.D. program. A four-year doctor of pharmacy (Pharm.D.) program is offered. A combined M.D./Ph.D. program is offered in collaboration with either Kent State University or The University of Akron, leading to the doctorate degree in biomedical engineering or a number of medically related science fields. A Summer Fellowship Program provides a stipend to selected medical students who undertake research or clinical education projects related to community health. Medical students are evaluated with marks of Honors, Pass, or Fail for most courses. Passing the USMLE Step 1 is a requirement for promotion to year three, passing Step 2CK is a requirement for graduation, and taking Step 2CS is a requirement for graduation.

BASIC SCIENCES: Basic sciences are taught primarily in a lecture/lab format; however, many courses incorporate small-group discussions. On average, students are in class or other scheduled sessions for 22 hours per week. First-year courses focus on gross anatomy, microscopic anatomy, biochemistry, genetics, physiology, and the central nervous system. Second-year courses focus on microbiology, immunology, infectious diseases and pathophysiology.

CLINICAL TRAINING

Third-year required rotations are Internal Medicine, Surgery, Pediatrics, Ob/Gyn, Psychiatry, and Family Medicine. Students are also required to complete four weeks of exploratory experience within six areas (i.e. research, medical specialty, community). During the fourth year, students are required to take six electives along with a Clinical Epilogue and Capstone course that will assist them in the transition to residency. During this course, students are required to complete a service project.

Students

Approximately 95 percent of students are Ohio residents. 105 students in each class are admitted through the B.S./M.D. program, and approximately 25 percent are admitted through the Direct Entry program.

STUDENT LIFE

Rootstown is a small town located about fifteen miles east of Akron. On the Medical School campus are recreation and exercise centers, student lounges, a picnic area, and tennis, basketball, and volleyball courts. Student groups include chapters of national medical student organizations, groups focused on professional interests, student-to-student support groups, and a recreation club.

GRADUATES

NEOUCOM graduates typically complete residency programs in Ohio, with approximately 25 percent completing residencies within our consortium hospitals (Akron, Canton and Youngstown). About half of our graduates complete a residency in primary care.

Admissions

REQUIREMENTS

Prerequisites are one year each of Organic Chemistry and Physics and a semester of Biology. The MCAT is required, and scores must be no more than two years old. For applicants who have retaken the exam, the most recent set of scores is considered. Thus, there is no advantage to withholding scores.

SUGGESTIONS

Ohio residents are given strong preference in the admissions process, and slight preference is given to graduates of consortium schools. Highly qualified applicants are encouraged to apply to the early decision program. Beyond requirements, recommended course work includes Calculus, Community Health, Embryology, General Biology, General Chemistry, Humanities, Microbiology, Molecular Biology, Physiology, Psychology, Sociology, and Statistics. For applicants who have taken time off after college, some recent course work is advised.

PROCESS

High school students interested in the combined B.S./M.D. program apply in the fall of the senior year to NEUOCOM, and complete a condensed undergraduate experience at Kent State University, The University of Akron, or Youngstown State University before arriving at the Rootstown campus. As a result of attrition from this program, a limited number of seats are available for college graduates interested in the four-year M.D. program. These applicants must apply through AMCAS. All AMCAS applicants receive a secondary application. Upon invitation, candidates are interviewed between November and March. On interview day, candidates receive one interview with a panel, a tour of the campus, lunch with current students, and a group informational session. Of interviewed candidates, about 10 percent are accepted on a rolling basis. Wait-listed candidates may update their files with transcripts.

Admissions Requirements (Required)

MCAT Scores, Essays, Science GPA, Non-Science GPA, Recommendation, Interview

Admissions Requirements (Optional)

Extracurricular activities, Exposure to medical profession, State Residency

COSTS AND AID

Tuition & Fees

Annual tuition (in-state out-of-state)	$27,861/$55,722
Room & board	$15,680
Cost of books	$1,250
Fees	$1,125

Financial Aid

% students receiving any aid	82
% students receiving grants	30
% students receiving loans	80
% aid that is merit-based	0
Average grant	$3,800
Average loan	$42,566
Average total aid package	$44,021
Average debt	$148,162

Northwestern University
Feinberg School of Medicine

Admissions Office, Morton 1-606, 303 East Chicago Ave, Chicago, IL 60611-3008 • Admission: 312-503-8206
Fax: 312-503-05507 • E-mail: MED-ADMISSIONS@NORTHWESTERN.EDU • Website: MED-ADMISSIONS.NORTHWESTERN.EDU

STUDENT BODY

Type	Private
Enrollment of parent institution	19,000
Enrollment of medical school	712
% male/female	60/40
% underrepresented minorities	2
% out-of-state	75
% international	18
# countries represented	25
Average age of entering class	24

FACULTY

Total faculty	2,016
% female faculty	47
% minority faculty	5
% part-time faculty	8
Student-faculty ratio	0.4:1

ADMISSIONS

# applied	6,910
% accepted	7
% enrolled	31

Average GPA and MCAT Scores

Overall GPA	3.8
MCAT Bio	12.0
MCAT Phys	11.7
MCAT Verbal	10.6
MCAT Essay	Q

Application Information

Regular application	10/15
Regular notification	12/15
Are transfers accepted?	Yes
Admissions may be deferred?	Yes
Admissions need-blind?	No
Application fee	$85

Academics

The FSM curriculum retains the best features of traditional medical education and incorporates innovative, interactive methods designed for the independent adult learner. Four main curricular elements weave through the four years of study which are divided into 3 phases. Science in Medicine, Clinical Medicine, Health and Society, and Professional Development each provide context for the other elements.

BASIC SCIENCES: During the first phase of the curriculum the material is organized into organ-based units. Each unit includes the study of normal and pathologic changes. The format includes 10-15 hours of lecture per week, and is complemented by problem-based learning sessions, team based learning, laboratories, and small-group discussions and tutorials.

CLINICAL TRAINING

Clinical Medicine starts in Phase 1, concurrent with the beginning of Science in Medicine. Focused Clinical Experiences and the Education Centered Medical Homes provide key early exposure. In phase 2 (clerkship year) students rotate through the traditional medical disciplines at the Northwestern Hospitals. The last year (Phase 3) is largely elective and includes time for completion of the Area of Scholarly Concentration project.

Students

We seek an incoming class which is racially and ethnically diverse, gender balanced, represents a variety of ages, and has geographically diverse origins. Our students hail from major research universities and liberal arts colleges.

STUDENT LIFE

Northwestern students spend less time in lecture than students in more traditional schools and have opportunities to perform community service, get involved in research and enjoy the cultural life of Chicago. The school is located in one of the most vibrant cities in the world. An excellent public transportation system makes Chicago's museums, shopping, parks, restaurants, theaters, and other attractions easily accessible. About 75% of our students live in central Chicago, within walking distance of the school and Northwestern Memorial Hospital; others live in a variety of neighborhoods throughout the city.

GRADUATES

Northwestern graduates are accepted to competitive residencies throughout the nation. Today there are more than 12,000 medical school alumni living in the United States and around the world. Northwestern alumni are particularly well represented in academic medicine.

Admissions

REQUIREMENTS

At minimum, one full year of Biology/lab, General Chemistry/lab, Organic Chemistry/lab, Physics/lab, and a semester of English are required. However, students accepted to Feinberg have usually taken additional science courses in preparation for the rigors of the medical school curriculum. The Medical College Aptitude Test (MCAT) with scores not more than three years old, exposure to clinical medicine and community service are required.

SUGGESTIONS

Feinberg students have strong academic records and clear motivation for a career in medicine. We look for well-rounded individuals and applicants who have studied the humanities and arts are welcome. Most of our successful applicants have been involved in research and have varied interest outside of academics.

PROCESS

All AMCAS applicants applying to Feinberg are sent a supplemental application. Of those returning the supplemental, about 10 percent are interviewed between September and February. An interview is required for acceptance and the medical school uses a combined interview approach (both individual and panel interview). The individual interview is conducted by a member of the dean's administration or admissions committee, and the panel is conducted by three members of the interview committee (usually two faculty and one senior student). During the panel interview special attention is paid to interpersonal and communication skills as manifested in the group problem solving activity. The interview day further includes a campus tour, lunch and a financial aid session. Applicants are accepted, declined, or placed on an alternate list.

Admissions Requirements (Required)

MCAT Scores, Essays, Science GPA, Extracurricular activities, Non-Science GPA, Exposure to medical profession, Recommendation, Interview

Admissions Requirements (Optional)

State Residency

COSTS AND AID

Tuition & Fees

Annual tuition	$48,399
Room & board	$16,620
Cost of books	$2,000
Fees	$309

Financial Aid

% students receiving any aid	70
% students receiving grants	52
% students receiving loans	61
% aid that is merit-based	8
Average grant	$19,028
Average loan	$47,223
Average total aid package	$55,010
Average debt	$143,027

THE OHIO STATE UNIVERSITY
COLLEGE OF MEDICINE

155 D MEILING HALL, 370 WEST 9TH AVENUE COLUMBUS, OH 43210 • **ADMISSION:** 614-292-7137
FAX: 614-247-79597 • **E-MAIL:** MEDICINE@OSU.EDU • **WEBSITE:** MEDICINE.OSU.EDU

Academics

Ohio State's Lead.Serve.Inspire (LSI) curriculum has been developed to prepare tomorrow's physicians to deliver the highest quality care to a diverse population of patients. Presented as a three-part, four year experience, the LSI curriculum fully integrates foundational and clinical science throughout the four-year period. The curriculum emphasizes critical thinking skills using a clinical analysis and problem solving framework. Students gain hands-on experience early in the program through a longitudinal, practice-based clinical service that offers opportunities to apply classroom knowledge to actual patient situations. A team-based environment emphasizing self-directed learning with multiple competency based assessments provides students with individualized learning opportunities, while producing standardized outcomes. The goal of the LSI curriculum is to ensure that all students are prepared to excel in their chosen post-graduate residency programs and from there to move on to their areas of specialization and physician practices.

BASIC SCIENCES: Lead Serve Inspire is the new medical curriculum that was implemented at The Ohio State University with the entering medical class of 2012. The Lead Serve Inspire curriculum is designed to integrate basic, behavioral, and clinicalscience, to develop independent and life long learning skills, and promote clinical reasoning in our students. The curriculum is divided into three parts, the first of which, Clinical Foundations, is designed to provide the foundational medical knowledge and skills necessary to prepare each student for success as they advance into more focused and advanced clinical training. Key features of the Clinical Foundations curriculum is the integration of content across disciplines, utilization of a variety of teaching and learning methods to meet individual student learning styles, and early exposure and participation in clinical activities. The learning objectives are organized in blocks of material focused on the normal and pathophysiology of organ systems. Blocks during the first year include Medical Practice and Patient Care, Bone and Muscle Disorders, Neurological Disorders, and Cardiopulmonary Disorders. Second year blocks include Gastrointestinal and Renal Disorders, Endocrine and Reproductive Disorders, Host Defense, and Clinical Foundations Review. Blocks are divided into content components that focus on a basic science principle and a related disease. As they progress through the curriculum, the student learns the underlying normal anatomy, physiology, and biology of each system, which is followed by the presentation of the pathology and clinical disease manifestations associated with each system. Various methods of content delivery are used in addition to the lecture format, including eLearning, readings, team based learning, small group sessions, laboratories, and case based correlations and discussion sessions. Lectures are recorded and available for review as podcasts providing greater opportunity for students with differing learning styles to be successful. During the first few weeks of the Medical Practice and Patient Care Block, students will also be trained in basic clinical skills. After demonstrating competency in these skills, students will actively participate in a clinical practice one afternoon every two weeks. Students will meet in longitudinal small groups each week to integrate their clinical experiences with additional behavioral and clinical skills training. Students will also empanel selected patients they encounter within their practices to further integrate their clinical experiences with the foundational science concepts and learning objectives of the Clinical Foundations curriculum. The lead Serve Inspire curriculum is designed to provide greater opportunities for medical students to excel as physician trainees.

CLINICAL TRAINING

Part 2 of the OSU COM curriculum will provide students with integrated clinical experiences to apply and practice clinical skills, critical analysis of patient information, diagnostic reasoning, and patient management. Students will encounter patients in both inpatient and outpatient settings, in the clinical areas traditionally experienced in medical school, in a manner that encourages more longitudinal activities and integration of areas of knowledge and skills. Three sixteen-week blocks will each begin with "ground school" to prepare students to succeed in the subsequent clinical areas, followed by combined clinical work in surgery and ob-gyn, pediatrics and family medicine/ambulatory care, and internal medicine, neurology and psychiatry. Short exploratory periods will occur within these longer blocks to permit students to experience specialty areas and fields such as anesthesiology and radiology during what represents the typical Med 3 year time frame. Part 3 of the curriculum (fourth year) will encourage students' further development in three tracks: advanced care of the acutely ill patient, including emergency care and acute hospital care; advanced clinical competencies in procedural skills and areas such as care of chronically ill patients, patient safety, quality improvement, global health and geriatrics; and coordinated advanced clinical track experiences in a field of the student's career choice. Successful completion of USMLE Step 2 CK and Step 2 CS are required for graduation.

Students

The class profile for the most recent entering class shows diversity of not only gender, race and ethnicity but of thought as shown by the undergraduate institutions and majors represented. The class profile details are at: http://medicine.osu.edu/students/admissions/Pages/ClassProfile.aspx

STUDENT LIFE

There are numerous medical student organizations and interest groups. Student Council is very active and is the voice of the medical students. Medical students serve on all major committees within the College of Medicine. Medical students have access to all of the resources and facilities of the University including the Recreation and Physical Activity Center which contains 25,000 square feet of fitness space. Campus and city bus transportation is free with the presentation of student ID. University graduate residence halls and family housing are available.

Admissions

REQUIREMENTS

One year each of: Biology with labs General Chemistry Organic Chemistry with labs Physics with lab One quarter or one semester each of: Biochemistry and any area of Anatomy are required. Courses in writing/speech, social sciences, humanities and diversity/ethics are recommended. To receive consideration for the current application cycle, applicants must submit the AMCAS application, Ohio State secondary application, MCAT scores, and reference letters. All applicants are required to take the MCAT within three years of their application. The last month to take the MCAT is September for the year prior to intended matriculation. Although the MCAT is offered in January, first-time takers' scores will be received too late for consideration for that year's entering class. Consideration will be given to applicants who have interview dates and elect to repeat the January test in an effort to improve previous scores.

SUGGESTIONS

The Admissions Committee evaluates candidates according to competitive standards. Applicants are judged on the basis of academic performance as well as personal qualities such as integrity, leadership, and interpersonal skills. Clinically related experiences, as well as physician shadowing, community service, leadership roles, and research positions are essential to exhibiting motivation for a career in medicine.

Admissions Requirements (Required)

MCAT Scores, Essays, Science GPA, Extracurricular activities, Non-Science GPA, Exposure to medical profession, Recommendation, Interview

Admissions Requirements (Optional)

State Residency

COSTS AND AID

Tuition & Fees

Annual tuition	$31,425
Room & board	$10,400
Cost of books	$3,314
Fees	$1,023

Financial Aid

% students receiving any aid	93
% students receiving grants	54
% students receiving loans	85
% aid that is merit-based	4
Average grant	$10,954
Average loan	$43,690
Average total aid package	$46,212
Average debt	$152,028

OREGON HEALTH & SCIENCE UNIVERSITY
SCHOOL OF MEDICINE

OFFICE OF ADMISSIONS, L102, 3181 SW SAM JACKSON PARK RD., PORTLAND, OR 97239-3098
ADMISSION: 503-494-2998 • FAX: 503-494-34007 • E-MAIL: TONERL@OHSU.EDU
WEBSITE: WWW.OHSU.EDU/XD/EDUCATION/SCHOOLS/SCHOOL-OF-MEDICINE/
ACADEMIC-PROGRAMS/MD-PROGRAM/ADMISSIONS

STUDENT BODY

Type	Public
Enrollment of parent institution	1,986
Enrollment of medical school	522
% male/female	45/55
% out-of-state	37
% international	18
Average age of entering class	26

FACULTY

Total faculty	1,737
% female faculty	47
% minority faculty	15
% part-time faculty	20
Student-faculty ratio	3.0:1

ADMISSIONS

# applied	4,622
% accepted	5
% enrolled	59

Average GPA and MCAT Scores

Overall GPA	3.7
MCAT Bio	11.0
MCAT Phys	10.5
MCAT Verbal	10.0
MCAT Essay	Q

Application Information

Regular application	10/15
Are transfers accepted?	Yes
Admissions may be deferred?	No
Admissions need-blind?	No
Application fee	$100

Academics

Although most students complete a four-year M.D. curriculum, others follow alternative courses of study, including joint-degree programs. The five-year M.D./M.P.H. Degree Program is offered by the School of Medicine's Department of Public Health and Preventive Medicine in conjunction with appropriate departments at Oregon State University and Portland State University. Generally, students indicate their interest in this program when they apply to the School of Medicine. First-year medical students may pursue an Epidemiological and Biostatistics track, which also serves as preparation for careers in public health. The M.D./Ph.D. joint-degree program is in the following fields: Biochemistry and Molecular Biology, Cancer Biology, Cell and Developmental Biology, Molecular and Medical Genetics, Molecular Microbiology and Immunology, Physiology and Pharmacology, Neuroscience, Behavioral Neuroscience, Medical Informatics and Clinical Epidemiology, and Biomedical Engineering. Grades are Honors, Near Honors, Satisfactory, Marginal, and Fail. Taking both steps of the USMLE is a requirement for graduation.

BASIC SCIENCES: Students spend two hours per day in lecture. An additional two hours each day are used for small-group sessions and/or laboratory activities. One afternoon each week is devoted to Principles of Clinical Medicine in which students work one-on-one with physicians and an additional afternoon studying issues related to public health, behavioral sciences, history taking and learning physical diagnosis skills. First-year courses are Gross Anatomy, Embryology and Imaging; Cell Structure and Function; Systems Process and Homeostasis; Biological Basis of Disease; and Principles of Clinical Medicine, which continues into the second year. The second year is organized around organ systems and physiological concepts, which include Blood, Circulation, Neuroscience and Behavior, Metabolism, and Human Growth & Development. The first two years are spent largely in the Basic Sciences and Education buildings, which have facilities for lectures, discussions, computer learning, and laboratories. The library contains over 150,000 volumes and 2,500 periodicals.

CLINICAL TRAINING
Required third-year rotations are Transition to Clerkship (1 week); Medicine (10 weeks); Rural and Community Health (5 weeks); Ob/Gyn (5 weeks); Pediatrics 1 (5 weeks); Psychiatry (5 weeks); Family Medicine (5 weeks); and Surgery (5 weeks). During the fourth year, students fulfill advanced clerkship requirements in Sub I, ICU/MICU, Surgery Subspecialty, Pediatrics II, and Neurology (4 weeks each) in addition to electives. The fourth year culminates in Transition to Residency, a week-long experience. Clinical training takes place at the University Hospital and Clinics and at affiliated institutions, which include Doernbecher Children's Hospital and Portland's Veterans Affairs Medical Center. The School of Medicine's research touches all realms of modern medical sciences. Some investigate the causes and treatments of learning disorders, addiction, heart disease, stroke, cancer, infertility, movement disorders, and emotional disorders. Others work at the molecular and cellular levels to unravel the most basic aspects of human health.

Students

The student body consists of ober 500 outstanding students with academic credentials exceeding national averages: 55% female, 45% male, and 68% Oregon residents. The average age of incoming students is 26. The incoming class size is 132.

STUDENT LIFE

Portland is an ideal location for students, offering the comforts of a medium-sized city and proximity to spectacular outdoor destinations. Close to campus are parks and other places to run, walk, or bike ride. A bit further are mountains for hiking and skiing. For an urban area, Portland is relatively affordable and safe. On-campus activities are also popular with medical students. The Student Center provides social, cultural, and recreational opportunities to students and members of the OHSU community. The Center for Diversity and Inclusion leads and supports university-wide initiatives to create an environment of respect and inclusion for all. The Global Heath Center promotes global health awareness through interprofessional education, service, advocacy, and research efforts among students, faculty, staff, and community partners. Numerous clubs and organizations bring students together around professional or extracurricular interests.

GRADUATES

Graduates are successful in securing residency positions at prestigious institutions all over the country. Graduates are successful in securing residency positions at prestigious institutions all over the country. About 85% of graduates obtain one of their top three choices for residency training and education. Roughly 45% enter primary care residencies. One-third of Oregon's physicians have received some or all of their education at OHSU.

Admissions

REQUIREMENTS

A Bachelor of Arts or Bachelor of Science degree, or its equivalent, from an accredited college or university is required prior to matriculation to medical school. One academic year of general biology to include one genetics course. One course each of general chemistry, organic chemistry and biochemistry. One academic year of general physics. One mathematics course (not including statistics). Two academic years of humanities and/or social sciences to include one course in English composition (or equivalent writing emphasis). An eligible MCAT is required. An eligible MCAT is one that is taken from one to three years prior to the year in which the applicant seeks matriculation to medical school. Applicants must have United States citizenship or resident alien status with a current green card indicating they are a permanent resident of the United States. (Resident aliens are encouraged to have at least one year of full-time course work at a college or university in the United States.) Applicants must meet the minimum academic and MCAT qualifiers set for that admissions cycle. The minimum qualifiers to receive further consideration in the process are: a cumulative total GPA, as reported by AMCAS, of 2.8 and a cumulative score of 24 on the most recent eligible MCAT. Minimum qualifiers are subject to change from one admissions cycle to the next.

SUGGESTIONS

Laboratories are recommended. A course in statistics is strongly recommended.

PROCESS

After the Admissions Office receives your application packet from AMCAS, the admissions staff will send a secondary application notice via email. It takes approximately 4-6 weeks from the time you certify and submit your application to AMCAS until we receive it. OHSU has an online secondary application that is made available to applicants through the Admissions Portal once we have received and processed your AMCAS application. Interviews are by invitation only and consist of seven multiple mini interview (MMI) stations and one one-on-one interview station.

Admissions Requirements (Required)

MCAT Scores, Essays, Science GPA, Extracurricular activities, Non-Science GPA, Exposure to medical profession, Recommendation, Interview

Admissions Requirements (Optional)

State Residency

COSTS AND AID

Tuition & Fees

Annual tuition (in-state out-of-state)	$37,045/$51,843
Room & board	$12,640
Cost of books	$7,276
Fees	$6,636

Financial Aid

% students receiving any aid	89
% students receiving grants	55
% students receiving loans	81
Average grant	$16,025
Average loan	$55,989
Average total aid package	$61,258
Average debt	$190,063

PENNSYLVANIA STATE UNIVERSITY
COLLEGE OF MEDICINE

OFFICE OF STUDENT AFFAIRS, P.O. BOX 850, HERSHEY, PA 17033 • ADMISSION: 717-531-8755
FAX: 717-531-62257 • E-MAIL: HMCSAFF@PSU.EDU • WEBSITE: WWW.HMC.PSU.EDU

STUDENT BODY

Type	Private
Enrollment of medical school	423
% male/female	56/44
% out-of-state	60
% international	28
Average age of entering class	23

FACULTY

Total faculty	155
% female faculty	18
% minority faculty	23

ADMISSIONS

# applied	6,615

Application Information

Regular application	11/15
Are transfers accepted?	Yes
Admissions may be deferred?	Yes
Admissions need-blind?	No
Application fee	$40

Academics

Penn State was one of the first medical schools in the country to institute departments of Humanities and Behavioral Science and to incorporate these perspectives into the basic science and clinical education programs. The College of Medicine was also among the first to develop a separate Family and Community Medicine department. A combined M.D./Ph.D. program is offered, allowing students to earn the doctorate degree in Biochemistry, Biomedical Engineering, Cell Biology, Genetics, Immunology, Microbiology, Molecular Biology, Pharmacology, and Physiology. There are also numerous opportunities to pursue discrete research projects as electives or during summers. Grading designations are Honors, High Pass, Pass, and Fail. Students must pass USMLE Step 1 after the pre-clinical years, and Step 2 in order to graduate.

BASIC SCIENCES: During the first and second years, students are in class or other scheduled sessions for approximately 23 hours per week. This schedule gives students the opportunity for independent and collaborative study. Clinical problems are used as a means of applying and correlating the basic science information that is presented in lectures or discussions. Labs and computer-assisted learning are also important parts of the curriculum. First-year courses are Structural Basis of Medical Practice; Cellular and Molecular Basis of Medical Practice; Biological Basis of Disease; and Physicians, Patients and Society, which touches on the psychological, social, ethical, legal, and humanistic aspects of medicine. Second-year courses are Pharmacology; Microbiology; Immunology; Psychiatry; Pathology; Introduction to Medicine III and IV; Physical Diagnosis; and Issues in Medical Practice. Instruction takes place in the Medical Sciences Building, which houses classrooms and laboratories. The Harrell Library is open 24 hours a day, and holds approximately 125,000 volumes and 2,000 periodicals in addition to modern computer and audiovisual resources.

CLINICAL TRAINING
Third-year required clerkships are Internal Medicine (8 weeks); Surgery (8 weeks); Pediatrics (6 weeks); Ob/Gyn (6 weeks); Psychiatry (4 weeks); Family and Community Medicine (4 weeks); selectives (8 weeks); and Primary Care (4 weeks). The fourth year is devoted to electives and selectives, which are chosen from clinical or research departments. An overseas elective program allows a number of fourth-year students to fulfill elective requirements at clinical sites in Asia, Africa, and Latin America. Generally, clinical training takes place at the University Hospital (463 beds), Children's Hospital, the Rehabilitation Center, and at other hospitals and clinics affiliated through an organized health network called Alliance Health. Additional facilities on campus are a Sports Medicine Center, the General Clinical Research Center, an Animal Research Center, and a Trauma Center.

Students

About 40 percent of students are Pennsylvania residents. Over 25 percent of students are underrepresented minorities, a tribute to the school's commitment to recruiting a diverse student body. The average age of incoming students is 23, with a wide age range. Class size is 110.

STUDENT LIFE

Educational facilities, clinical teaching sites, campus housing and recreational centers are within walking distance of one another. The College of Medicine is an attractive campus, occupying 550 acres. Hershey provides a comfortable, student-friendly community that is relatively safe. As a tourist destination, Hershey offers a variety of dining and entertainment possibilities. Medical students are involved in organizations such as honor societies, professional interest groups, local chapters of national organizations, and groups focused on community service or recreational pursuits. When in need of urban distractions, the state capital, Harrisburg, is 12 miles away, and both Philadelphia and Pittsburgh are easily accessible. On-campus housing options include one-, two-, and three-bedroom apartments.

GRADUATES

Graduates are successful at securing residencies nationwide. Penn State emphasizes primary care and encourages students to consider post-graduate training programs in primary care fields.

Admissions

REQUIREMENTS

Prerequisites are one year each of Biology, Physics, Chemistry, Organic Chemistry, and college-level Math. All science courses should have associated labs. One semester each of Social Sciences and Humanities is also required. The MCAT is required, and scores must be no more than two years old. For applicants who have taken the exam on multiple occasions, all sets of scores are considered.

SUGGESTIONS

Beyond requirements, course work in Calculus, Psychology, Statistics, Sociology, Genetics, and Anthropology are recommended. The April, rather than August, MCAT is strongly advised. Health care related experience is valued, as are interpersonal and communication skills. State residency is not a consideration in the application process.

PROCESS

All AMCAS applicants are sent secondary applications. About 10 percent of those returning secondaries are interviewed between September and March. Interviews consist of two or three sessions each with a faculty member. On interview day, candidates also tour the campus and have lunch with current medical students. About one-third of interviewees are accepted on a rolling basis. Another group is wait-listed. Wait-listed candidates are not encouraged to send supplementary material.

Admissions Requirements (Required)

MCAT Scores, Essays, Extracurricular activities, Exposure to medical profession

Admissions Requirements (Optional)

Science GPA, Non-Science GPA, Recommendation, Interview, State Residency

COSTS AND AID

Tuition & Fees

Annual tuition	$42,742
Room & board	$6,144
Cost of books	$1,205
Fees	$448
Financial Aid	
% students receiving any aid	91
% students receiving loans	83
Average grant	$10,248
Average loan	$23,500
Average debt	$98,061

PONCE SCHOOL OF MEDICINE

PONCE SCHOOL OF MEDICINE

PO BOX 7004, PONCE, PR 00732-7004 • **ADMISSION:** 787-840-2575 • **FAX:** 787-842-04617
E-MAIL: ADMISSIONS@PSM.EDU • **WEBSITE:** WWW.PSM.EDU

STUDENT BODY	
Type	Private

ADMISSIONS	
# applied	968
% accepted	15
% enrolled	45

Average GPA and MCAT Scores	
Overall GPA	3.3
MCAT Bio	7.8
MCAT Phys	7.0
MCAT Verbal	7.2
MCAT Essay	M

Application Information	
Regular application	12/15
Early application	6/1
Early notification	11/15
Are transfers accepted?	Yes
Admissions may be deferred?	No
Admissions need-blind?	Yes
Application fee	$100

Academics

The primary goal of the School of Medicine is to provide quality medical education to bilingual students, with an emphasis on primary care and family medicine. The curriculum includes a strong emphasis on basic sciences, enabling students to get the most out of their clinical training. Longitudinal programs in preventive medicine and medical ethics are integrated into the four-year curriculum.

BASIC SCIENCES: Basic sciences are taught during the first two years. Year one courses include: Gross Anatomy Imaging and Embryology, Cellular Biology and Histology, Neuroscience, Biochemistry, Microbiology and Immunology, Behavioral Science, Physiology, General Pathology, Bioethics, Human Genetics, and a year-long session devoted to clinical correlation. Second year courses are: Pathophysiology, Pathology, Pharmacology, Psychiatry, Introduction to Clinical Medicine, Infectious Diseases, Family and Community Medicine, and Bioethics. Instructional methods include computer-assisted learning, lectures, labs, and problem-based learning. Standardized patients are used for teaching and evaluation of basic clinical skills. During the first two years, students are in class or other scheduled sessions for about 30 hours per week. Students must pass Step I of the USMLE for promotion to year three.

CLINICAL TRAINING

The third year begins in July with two weeks of a course called Introduction to Hospital Life. Following this orientation, students begin required clerkships. These are: Internal Medicine (10 weeks), Surgery (10 weeks), Pediatrics (10 weeks), Ob/Gyn (5 weeks), Psychiatry (5 weeks), and Family Medicine (5 weeks). The third year also includes a Dean's Hour, which emphasizes Medical Humanities, Health Economics, Law, Bioethics, and Literature. In the fourth year, students participate in a required clerkship in Medicine (4 weeks), a Sub-internship (Medicine, Ob/Gyn, Pediatrics, or Family Medicine), a clerkship in Emergency Medicine (4 weeks), and a Primary Care Selective (4 weeks). Students are also required to complete 16 weeks of elective rotations, of which five weeks may be completed at sites other than Ponce. USMLE Step II must be passed prior to graduation.

Students

STUDENT LIFE

The relatively small class size of 60 students encourages communication among students and faculty. The School's location is an asset, offering a pleasant environment for living and studying.

Admissions

REQUIREMENTS

Required undergraduate course work includes eight semester credits in Biology, General Chemistry, Organized Chemistry, and Physics in addition to six credits in Advanced Math and Spanish. Twelve credits in both Behavioral Sciences and English are also required. Behavioral science includes Psychology, Sociology, Anthropology, Political Sciences, Economics, and Anthropology. Applicants must have a minimum overall grade point average of 2.7 and an average of 2.5 in science courses. The MCAT is required, and scores should be from within one year of application. Applicants should have at least the mean on all sections of the MCAT.

SUGGESTIONS

In evaluating applicants, the Admissions Committee considers academic achievements, MCAT scores, interview reports, letters of recommendation, and other supplementary information. Preference is given to residents of Puerto Rico.

PROCESS

Ponce takes part in the AMCAS application process. The deadline for submission to AMCAS is December 15. Secondary applications are sent to all qualified applicants, and interviews are conducted throughout the spring.

Admissions Requirements (Required)

MCAT Scores, Essays, Science GPA, Non-Science GPA, Recommendation, Interview

Admissions Requirements (Optional)

Extracurricular activities, Exposure to medical profession, State Residency

COSTS AND AID

Tuition & Fees

Annual tuition	$26,590
Fees	$2,625

Financial Aid

Average grant	$8,000
Average loan	$35,954
Average total aid package	$38,085
Average debt	$96,931

QUEEN'S UNIVERSITY
SCHOOL OF MEDICINE

68 BARRIE STREET, KINGSTON, ON K7L 3N6 • ADMISSION: 613-533-2542 • FAX: 613-533-61907
E-MAIL: JEB8@POST.QUEENSU.CA • WEBSITE: HTTP//MEDS.QUEENSU.CA

STUDENT BODY	
Type	Public
Enrollment of medical school	100
% male/female	52/48
% international	2

ADMISSIONS	
# applied	1,388
% accepted	13
% enrolled	57

Average GPA and MCAT Scores

Overall GPA	3.6
MCAT Bio	11.0
MCAT Phys	11.1
MCAT Verbal	10.8
MCAT Essay	P

Application Information

Regular application	10/1
Regular notification	5/31
Are transfers accepted?	No
Admissions may be deferred?	Yes
Admissions need-blind?	No
Application fee	$250

Academics

Most students follow a four-year curriculum leading to an MD degree. Masters and Doctoral degree programs are also offered in Biochemistry, Biostatistics, Environmental and Occupational Health, Epidemiology, General Community Health, Health-Care Systems, Pathology, and Preventive Medicine. Although there are no formally structured combined programs, superior students may be permitted the flexibility to work toward an M.Sc. or a Ph.D. concurrently with the M.D. Grading uses a Honours/Pass/Fail system.

BASIC SCIENCES: Most basic science instruction takes place during the first three years. First-year course starts with Phase I, Introduction to the Sciences Relevant to Medicine, an introduction to the fundamental language and concepts of medical science, and Communication/Clinical Skills. Phase IIA includes Dermatology/Musculoskeletal systems, Haematology and Oncology, Microbiology and Infectious Diseases, Allergy and Immunology, and Clinical Skills. Second year courses are Psychiatry/Neuroscience/Ophthalmology/ ENT, Genitourinary/Cardiovascular/Respirology, and Clinical Skills. In addition, eight weeks are left open for an elective. Third year courses are: Endocrine/Metabolism/Reproduction, Gastrointestinal, and Clinical Skills. In addition to problem-based learning, teaching methods include lectures, seminars, small group discussions, laboratory experience, and computer-based instruction. Basic science instruction takes place primarily at Botterell Hall, which also houses administrative offices and Bracken Library. The Clinical Learning center is an important educational facility within the Faculty of Health Sciences specifically designed for the teaching, learning, and evaluation of important clinical skills, and is used during both preclinical and clinical years. The Health Sciences library subscribes to approximately 844 serials and its total collection consists of 156,000 volumes. In the library is the Multimedia Learning Centre, which offers both video- and computer-assisted instruction.

CLINICAL TRAINING

Clerkships begin in January of the third year. They are: Medicine (12 weeks), Surgery (8 weeks), Psychiatry (6 weeks), Ob/Gyn (6 weeks), Pediatrics (6 weeks), Family Medicine (4 weeks), Geriatrics (2 weeks), and Emergency Medicine (2 weeks). Four weeks of selectives and 12 weeks of electives are also required. Clerkships takes place at a number of affiliated hospitals including Kingston General Hospital, Hotel Dieu Hospital, St. Mary's of the Lake Hospital, Kingston Psychiatric Hospital, and Ongwanada Hospital. The provision of healthcare services in Kingston is presently being restructured and will change over the next few years.

Students

Each class has 90 students, about 50 of whom are typically from the province of Ontario. The student body is approximately 50 percent women.

STUDENT LIFE

Medical students enjoy the recreational, cultural, and social activities of the greater university and the city of Kingston. On-campus attractions include museums, concert halls, cinema, and an observatory. Student services include a child care resource center, a foundation supporting women, comprehensive health services, an international center, a physical education center and a student center. The University provides accommodations in single and double occupancy rooms for approximately 300 graduate students. In addition, the Apartment and Housing office manages University-owned rentals in the area.

Admissions

REQUIREMENTS

In order to apply, students must have completed three years of full-time study at a university. In addition, one year each of Biological sciences, Physical sciences, and Humanities/Social Sciences are required. The MCAT is required. To be eligible for admission, applicants must be Canadian citizens, Canadian permanent residents, or children of Queen's University alumni.

SUGGESTIONS

The Admissions Committee looks for both academic abilities, such as commitment, achievement, critical thinking, and self-directed learning, and personal characteristics such as communication skills, creativity, and sensitivity. No preference is given to a particular undergraduate program of studies, and college students seeking admission are encouraged to pursue studies in their area of interest.

PROCESS

Applicants seeking further information about admission should contact the School of Medicine. Applications are made through: Ontario Medical Schools', Application Service, 70 Research Lane, Guelph, Ontario N1G 5E2. The deadline is October 15. The first admissions cutoff is based on the cumulative converted grade point average, and the second is made on the basis of MCAT scores. Those applicants who qualify are interviewed. Applicants are then ranked according to evaluation of letters of reference, autobiographic sketch, and interview results.

Admissions Requirements (Required)

MCAT Scores, Essays, Science GPA, Extracurricular activities, Non-Science GPA, Recommendation, Interview

COSTS AND AID

Tuition & Fees

Annual tuition	$13,500
Fees	$13,500

ROSALIND FRANKLIN UNIVERSITY OF MEDICINE & SCIENCE

CHICAGO MEDICAL SCHOOL

OFFICE OF ADMISSIONS, 3333 GREEN BAY ROAD NORTH CHICAGO, IL 60064 • ADMISSION: 847-578-3204
FAX: 847-775-65597 • E-MAIL: CMS.ADMISSIONS@ROSALINDFRANKLIN.EDU • WEBSITE: WWW.ROSALINDFRANKLIN.EDU

STUDENT BODY

Type	Private
Enrollment of parent institution	2,157
Enrollment of medical school	754
% male/female	52/48
% underrepresented minorities	5
% out-of-state	55
% international	5
# countries represented	36
Average age of entering class	25

ADMISSIONS

# applied	8,663
% accepted	5
% enrolled	40

Average GPA and MCAT Scores

Overall GPA	3.6
MCAT Bio	10.5
MCAT Phys	10.1
MCAT Verbal	9.4

Application Information

Regular application	11/1
Are transfers accepted?	Yes
Admissions may be deferred?	Yes
Admissions need-blind?	No
Application fee	$105

Academics

Founded in 1912, The Chicago Medical School has been dedicated to excellence in medical education for over a century. The Chicago Medical School has educated thousands of professionals with recognized innovation in health education, excellence in the creation of knowledge and scientific discovery focused on prediction and prevention of disease, outstanding clinical programs, and compassionate community service. Major hospital affiliates include Advocate Christ Medical Center, Advocate Condell Medical Center, Advocate Illinois Masonic, Advocate Lutheran General Hospital, John H. Stroger, Jr. Hospital of Cook County, Mount Sinai Hospital and Medical Center, and the Captain James A. Lovell Federal Health Care Center.

BASIC SCIENCES: The Chicago Medical School curriculum offers a strong grounding in the sciences basic to medicine along with assuring competency in skills necessary for the practice of medicine. The CMS curriculum features a unique interprofessional approach with interaction among a broad range of health professional students and practitioners. The curriculum is a mix of lectures, labs, small group discussions, team based learning, and opportunities for peer to peer learning. Topic integration across courses and a unique Interprofessional Teams course are the hallmark of the M1 curriculum. Our educational information system, Desire to Learn (D2L), provides 24-hour access to materials, electronic databases, and; medical textbooks are available through Access Medicine.

CLINICAL TRAINING

Students engage in their clinical experiences in a state-of-the-art Education and Evaluation Center, through high-fidelity simulation, and through participation with physician preceptors. The required junior clinical clerkships include Medicine, Ambulatory Care, Surgery, Family Medicine, Obstetrics/Gynecology, Psychiatry, MedCore, Pediatrics, Neurology, and Emergency Medicine. The senior requirements include four weeks in a Medicine or Pediatrics Subinternship, plus 32 weeks of approved electives (14 of which must be intramural). The elective period gives students an opportunity, through both intramural and extramural experiences, to explore and strengthen their personal career interests.

Students

Rosalind Franklin University of Medicine and Science is situated in the northern suburbs of Chicago, with easy access to downtown Chicago and the surrounding areas by car or public transportation. State-of-the-art facilities include a $10 million research wing expansion, the Morningstar Interprofessional Education Center, The Rothstein Warden Centennial Learning Center, a gross anatomy laboratory and classrooms fully-equipped for multimedia-enhanced learning, and the Education and Evaluation Center for physical examination skills training. Recreational facilities include a brand new fitness center, game room, and the brand-new Student Union (home to the University Bookstore, Union Cafe, and computer lab).

STUDENT LIFE

Most first and second-year students live in the vicinity of campus and drive to school. On-campus housing is available at Rosalind Franklin University. On-campus housing is available at Rosalind Franklin University. The University's three residential buildings offer one and two-bedroom apartments. Each on-campus apartment building includes study and lounge areas, shared laundry facilities on every floor and individual storage units. For information on student housing, please visit the following website: http://www.rosalindfranklin.edu/prospectivestudents/studenthousing.aspx Often, third and fourth-year students elect to live in Chicago, where they are closer to clinical training sites. Public transportation from downtown Chicago to campus facilitates such living arrangements. Chicago is one of the largest and most culturally rich cities in the country, providing a wealth of entertainment, museums, theater, restaurants, nightlife, indoor and outdoor athletic activities, and spectator sporting events. The city provides distraction for medical students when they need it. Students have a voice in school administrative affairs through the University Student Council and through participation on various boards and committees. The Chicago Medical School has chapters of most national medical student associations and has special interest clubs and organizations based on recreational activities, professional interests, and ethnic/social background. For information about Rosalind Franklin University's Student Life department, please visit the following website: http://www.rosalindfranklin.edu/campuslife.aspx

GRADUATES

The most popular specialties chosen by graduates of the Chicago Medical School include: Emergency Medicine, Internal Medicine, Anesthesiology, Pediatrics, and Diagnostic Radiology.

Admissions

REQUIREMENTS

One year of Biology, Chemistry, Organic Chemistry, and Physics, all with labs, are required. The MCAT is required and must be no more than three years old at time of matriculation. For multiple exams, the most recent set of scores are used. The September MCAT test is the last test accepted.

SUGGESTIONS

CMS looks for students who not only have strong grades and test scores, but also demonstrate a commitment to community service and experience in the medical field. A student's potential for the study and practice of medicine will be evaluated on the basis of academic achievement, MCAT results, appraisals by a preprofessional advisory committee or individual instructors, and a personal interview, if requested by the Student Admissions Committee. To fulfill the mission of The Chicago Medical School, admissions policies are designed to ensure that the selection process matriculates a class made up of individuals capable of meeting the needs of current and future patients. Applicants will be evaluated not only for educational potential, but with the aim of providing diverse educational experience for other members of the class. For information on selection factors, see: www.rosalindfranklin.edu/degreeprograms/allopathicmedicine/appneeds.aspx

PROCESS

In addition to the AMCAS, a secondary application is required. Interviews take place from September through April and consist of two sessions with faculty, administrators, and/or medical students. Notification of acceptance begins in October and is an ongoing process until the class is filled.

Admissions Requirements (Required)

MCAT Scores, Essays, Science GPA, Non-Science GPA, Exposure to medical profession, Recommendation, Interview

Admissions Requirements (Optional)

Extracurricular activities, State Residency

COSTS AND AID

Tuition & Fees

Annual tuition	$49,920
Room & board	$17,156
Cost of books	$2,656
Fees	$736

Financial Aid

% students receiving any aid	83
% students receiving grants	30
% students receiving loans	81
Average grant	$9,225
Average loan	$57,442
Average total aid package	$72,212
Average debt	$201,895

RUSH MEDICAL COLLEGE OF RUSH UNIVERSITY
RUSH MEDICAL COLLEGE

OFFICE OF ADMISSIONS, 600 SOUTH PAULINA ST., SUITE 524 CHICAGO, IL 60612 • ADMISSION: • FAX: 312-942-68407
E-MAIL: RMC_ADMISSIONS@RUSH.EDU • WEBSITE: WWW.RUSHU.RUSH.EDU

STUDENT BODY

Type	Private
Enrollment of parent institution	2,206
Enrollment of medical school	542
% male/female	50/50
% out-of-state	32
% international	31
# countries represented	15
Average age of entering class	24

FACULTY

Total faculty	883
% minority faculty	32
Student-faculty ratio	1.6:1

ADMISSIONS

# applied	4,648
% accepted	6
% enrolled	49

Average GPA and MCAT Scores

Overall GPA	3.6
MCAT Bio	10.8
MCAT Phys	10.1
MCAT Verbal	9.4
MCAT Essay	Q

Application Information

Regular application	11/1
Are transfers accepted?	No
Admissions may be deferred?	Yes
Admissions need-blind?	No
Application fee	$75

Academics

Rush provides a comprehensive background in the science of medicine and clinical practice through a four-year curriculum designed to provide educational flexibility. The faculty have created an environment that fosters a commitment to competent and compassionate patient care and to attitudes of inquiry and life-long learning.

BASIC SCIENCES: The first- and second-year curriculum provides students with foundations in both the basic sciences and the clinical skills required for patient care. Classes consist of lectures, laboratories, small group discussions, workshops and team-based and self-directed learning. The hallmark of the curriculum is the merging of traditional science disciplines with patient interaction and clinical skills development. The pre-clerkship curriculum is organized into organ-based blocks, each covering traditional basic science disciplines taught through the use of case studies.

CLINICAL TRAINING

The first- and second-year curriculum provides students with foundations in both the basic sciences and the clinical skills required for patient care. The third- and fourth-year curriculum provides students with training in patient care, diagnosis, and treatment in a variety of clinical settings. The M3 year is comprised of both required core clerkships and elective clerkships through which students have the opportunity to begin exploring areas of interest. Core clerkships are offered at Rush University Medical Center or at The John H. Stroger, Jr. Hospital of Cook County (formerly Cook County Hospital); ambulatory weeks take place throughout the greater Chicago area. In the M4 year, students complete their Subinternship and the Emergency Medicine Core Clerkship, and further explore areas of interest via elective clerkships.

Students

Rush Medical College is located on the near west side of Chicago; the John H. Stroger, Jr. Hospital of Cook County, a major teaching affiliate, is two blocks away. The community is thriving and culturally diverse, with easy access by public transportation. January 2012 marked the opening of a new, state-of-the art hospital at Rush University Medical Center. Called "The Tower," the building reorients the facilities and care around patients and their families and is Chicago's first full-service, "green" hospital. The Tower has 304 individual adult and critical care beds, giving Rush 664 total beds across the existing and new facilities. Housed on the ground floor is the emergency room, designed to provide an unprecedented level of readiness for large-scale health emergencies from a mass outbreak of an infectious disease, a bioterrorist attack, or an accident that spills hazardous materials.

STUDENT LIFE

Center Court Gardens, located on Harrison Street across from the Marriott Chicago Downtown at the Medical District, consists of apartment-style living, with over 280 units available as studios, one-bedrooms and two-bedrooms. All apartments are carpeted, have individually controlled heating and air conditioning, modern appliances, and bathtubs with showers. Basic cable and internet are included in the rent, but utilities and heating are not. One parking space is available per apartment. Additional information may be obtained from the Office of Student Life.

GRADUATES

In 2013, Rush students matched in 19 distinct specialties at institutions throughout the country.

Admissions

REQUIREMENTS

Prerequisites are eight semester hours each of inorganic chemistry, organic chemistry, biology, and physics. The MCAT is required. For the entering class of 2014, scores must be dated January 2011 or later. Only U.S. citizens and Permanent Residents are considered for admission.

SUGGESTIONS

The Committee on Admissions considers both academic and non-academic qualifications of applicants in making decisions. The Committee looks for objective evidence that the applicant will be able to handle the academic demands of the curriculum. In addition, the Committee places strong emphasis on the applicant's humanistic concerns, unique experiences and demonstrated motivation for a career in medicine, including healthcare experience, academic achievement, letters of recommendation, MCAT performance, healthcare experience and interviews are considered in the final evaluation of all applicants.

PROCESS

All AMCAS applicants are invited to complete a Supplemental Application. Approximately 425 applicants will be interviewed on campus between September and March. The interview day consists of two 30-minute interviews, tours of the clinical and academic facilities, and the opportunity to meet with current students. Each year, 128 students matriculate.

Admissions Requirements (Required)

MCAT Scores, Essays, Science GPA, Extracurricular activities, Non-Science GPA, Exposure to medical profession, Recommendation, Interview, State Residency

COSTS AND AID

Tuition & Fees

Annual tuition	$46,272
Room & board (on-campus off-campus)	$13,170/$11,430
Cost of books	$2,063
Fees	$0

Financial Aid

% students receiving any aid	85
% students receiving grants	60
% students receiving loans	84
% aid that is merit-based	0
Average grant	$8,114
Average loan	$55,997
Average total aid package	$64,522
Average debt	$201,720

RUTGERS

RUTGERS NEW JERSEY MEDICAL SCHOOL

OFFICE OF ADMISSIONS, 185 SOUTH ORANGE AVENUE, MEDICAL SCIENCE BUILDING, RM. C-653 NEWARK, NJ 07103
ADMISSION: 973-972-4631 • FAX: 973-972-79867
E-MAIL: NJMSADMISS@NJMS.RUTGERS.EDU • WEBSITE: NJMS.RUTGERS.EDU

STUDENT BODY

Type	Public
Enrollment of medical school	695
% male/female	51/49
% out-of-state	10
% international	32

ADMISSIONS

# applied	4,331
% accepted	4
% enrolled	100

Average GPA and MCAT Scores

Overall GPA	3.7
MCAT Bio	11.1
MCAT Phys	10.0
MCAT Verbal	1102.0
MCAT Essay	P

Application Information

Regular application	12/1
Regular notification	10/15
Early application	8/1
Early notification	10/1
Are transfers accepted?	Yes
Admissions may be deferred?	Yes
Admissions need-blind?	No
Application fee	$95

Academics

All applicants are processed and reviewed. The Minimum course requirements are eight semester hours of Biology, Physics, Chemistry and Organic Chemistry, all with associated labs and six semester hours of English, biochemistry and genetics are recommended. The MCAT is required. Just over 15 percent of applicants are interviewed. Wait list candidates may send supplementary information to update their files.

BASIC SCIENCES: During the first two years, small group sessions and tutorials account for about a substantial part of the curriculum, with the remainder of class time used for lectures and labs. Students are paired with physicians in the community, working with them one afternoon each week as part of primary care preceptorships. Courses demand about 27 hours per week, in addition to individual study time. First-year courses are Biochemistry and Molecular Biology; Cell and Tissue Biology; Genetics; Gross and Developmental Anatomy; Neuroscience; Physiology; Psychiatry; Public Health; The Art of Medicine; Problem-Based Learning; and Clinical Skills, which focuses on the physical examination. During the second year, topics are coordinated among courses and are organized around organ systems. Courses are Clinical Preventive Medicine and Nutrition; Immunology; Microbiology; Pathology; Pharmacology; Introduction to Clinical Sciences; and Psychiatry and the Clinical Interview. The Medical Sciences Building, where basic sciences are taught, is connected to the University Hospital and the George F. Smith Library, the latter of which houses 70,000 volumes and over 2,000 periodicals. The proximity of clinical facilities to classrooms and labs encourages first- and second-year students' involvement in clinical activities. The Office of Student Affairs provides services ranging from personal counseling to guidance on elective and residency selection.

CLINICAL TRAINING

Required third-year clerkships are Internal Medicine (12 weeks); General Surgery (8 weeks); Pediatrics (8 weeks); Ob/Gyn (8 weeks); Psychiatry (6 weeks); and Family Medicine (6 weeks). During the fourth year, 16 weeks of electives are required in addition to Neurology (4 weeks); Emergency Medicine (4 weeks); Substance Abuse (2 weeks); Physical Medicine and Rehabilitation (2 weeks); Ophthalmology, Orthopedics, Otolaryngology, Urology (1 week each); and an acting internship in Medicine, Pediatrics, Family Medicine, Obstetrics, or Surgery (4 weeks). Much of the clinical training takes place at the contiguous 518-bed University Hospital, which serves the needs of the immediate community and, with its specialized care units, attracts patients from around the state. Other affiliated teaching hospitals are Barnabus Healthcare System, Hackensack University Hospital, Morristown Memorial Hospital, Veterans Affairs Health Care System, East Orange, and Kessler Institute for Rehabilitation.

Students

90 percent of the NJMS entering students are New Jersey residents. Underrepresented Minorities account for about 20 percent of the student body. The average age of students entering the class of 2013 was 26, ranging from 19-41 and a Matriculated class size of 170. George F. Smith Library (www3.umdnj.edu/stlibweb) provides access to more that 40-online databases, 185 electronic books, and more that 2,000 online journals. The online catalog enables users to identify materials in the print, media, and electronic collections. Students, faculty and staff may access these resources from on campus computers or

remotely, via the university library's microcomputer lab also provide access to the desktop applications (Microsoft Office Suite), educational software, and tutorials. Scanning and slide production equipment is also available in the microcomputer lab. Staff support and user training is available for all programs.

STUDENT LIFE

Students are involved in intramural sports and organized student events. Each entering student is assigned to a peer group of first- and second-year students. There is a HOUSE SYSTEM which combines students from all four years. Students initiate and develop service activities such as: AMA (American Medical Assoc.), AMSA (American Medical Students Assoc.), AMWA (American Medical Women's Assoc.), BLHO (Boricua Latino Health Organization), Center for Humanism and Medicine, Community 2000, which conducts clinical screening and health education with local churches, Early Start Mentoring Program, Family Medicine Interest Group, New Moms, Peer Support, Project Pediatrics (Border Babies), Students Health Advocates for Resources and Education (S.H.A.R.E.), Students are actively involved in community-service projects through the SHARE center. Student Family Health Care Center (SFHCC) (Clinic), SNMA (Student National Assoc.), STATS (Students Teaching AIDS to Students), Student Council, Unite for Site. NJMS is located in University Heights. Newark offers many artistic and creative activities including the performing arts, jazz clubs, and diverse neighborhoods. It is home to the Newark Bears, the NJ Symphony Orchestra, the NJ State Opera, NJ Performing Arts Center, the Newark Museum, the Ballantine House, Newark Symphony Hall, the Newark Library, the Cathedral Basilica of the Sacred Heart and the Garden State Ballet and several institutions of Higher Education. New York City is an easy train ride and serves as a convenient distraction for medical students.

GRADUATES

Each year, graduates are successful in obtaining residencies at prestigious institutions such as Massachusetts General, New York Presbyterian (Cornell and Columbia campuses), the Children's Hospital in Washington, DC, New Haven Hospital at Yale. The alumni association is very enthusiastic, and among its activities is the provision of scholarships and research stipends to medical students.

Admissions

REQUIREMENTS

The minimum course requirements are 8-semester hours of biology; 8- semester hours of physics, 16- semester hours chemistry (general or inorganic chemistry and organic chemistry), all with associated labs; and 6-semester hours of English. Although math is not required it is strongly recommended. The MCAT is required; we do accept scores from any year. There is no minimum GPA or MCAT requirement but intense competition tends to favor those with stronger credentials, as the average GPA of our accepted applicants is 3.6 with an average MCAT of 32.4. Approximately 15 percent of the 4,047 applicants are interviewed with interviews taking place between August and April. About one-third of interviewees are accepted. Wait-listed candidates may send supplementary information to update their files. Applicants are selected on the basis of academic excellence, leadership qualities, demonstrated compassion for others and broad extracurricular experiences. The Admissions Committee considers related factors such as passion, motivation, perseverance, special aptitudes and stamina (personal statement, letters of recommendation and the interview are also very important factors in evaluation). NJMS encourages non-residents to apply but New Jersey residents will be given some preference.

SUGGESTIONS

Research or experience in a health care setting is useful. Personal traits, such as compassion, dedication, and interpersonal skills, are very important.

RUTGERS
RUTGERS ROBERT WOOD JOHNSON MEDICAL SCHOOL

OFFICE OF ADMISSIONS, 675 HOES LANE, PISCATAWAY, NJ 08854 • ADMISSION: 732-235-4576 • FAX: 732-235-50787
E-MAIL: RWJAPADM@UMDNJ.EDU • WEBSITE: RWJMS.UMDNJ.EDU

STUDENT BODY

Type	Public
Enrollment of medical school	642
% male/female	47/53
% out-of-state	3
% international	16
Average age of entering class	23

FACULTY

Total faculty	850
% female faculty	35
% minority faculty	23

ADMISSIONS

# applied	3,170
% accepted	11
% enrolled	46

Average GPA and MCAT Scores

Overall GPA	3.6
MCAT Bio	10.5
MCAT Phys	10.4
MCAT Verbal	9.7
MCAT Essay	P

Application Information

Regular application	12/1
Early application	8/1
Early notification	10/1
Are transfers accepted?	Yes
Admissions may be deferred?	Yes
Admissions need-blind?	No
Application fee	$75

Academics

Students are encouraged to pursue a variety of educational opportunities. In addition to the traditional four-year medical school curriculum, students may enroll in one of the dual degree options including MD/PhD, MD/JD, MD/MPH, MD/MBA, MS/MS Biomedical Informatics, and MD/MS Jurisprudence. A MS in Clinical and Translational Research planned for 2007. The flexible curriculum allows the rearranging of certain courses to enable students to pursue the dual degrees, relevant projects, personal interests, research or employment. Student scholars may take an additional year to pursue the basic science or clinical research or off-campus community health projects. Students who complete a thesis graduate with Distinction in Research. A new distinction in service to the community program has been established. The grading policy uses Honors/High Pass/Pass/Low Pass/Fail. Both Steps of the USMLE are required for graduation. Research facilities: Center for Advanced Biotechnology and Medicine, Child Health Institute, The Cancer Institute of New Jersey, Environmental and Occupational Health Science Institute, Stem Cell Institute, and Cardiovascular Institute.

BASIC SCIENCES: Curricular changes in the first two years have been implemented towards a two-fold mission: better preparation of clinicians as lifelong learners and a shift toward self-directed learning. The changes include more small group learning, a new course in patient centered mediine structured as small clinic groups facilitated by a mentor, problem-based approaches, a reduction in lecture time in addition to a systems based approach in the second year. Clinical correlation is emphasized in all first year disciplines. First year courses: Cellular and Genetic Mechanisms and Histology, Gross and Developmental Anatomy, Neuroscience, Epidemiology and Biostatistics, Biological Chemistry, Principles of Environmental and Community Medicine, Patient Centered Medicine, Medical Physiology, Medical Microbiology and Immunology, and Basic Life Support I. Second year courses: Clinical Pathophysiology, Behavorial Science and Psychiatry, Human Sexuality, Pathology and Laboratory Medicine, Patient Centered Medicine, Pharmacology, Clinical Prevention and Environmental Medicine, Biochemical Basis of Nutrition, Basic Life Support II, and Universal Precautions/Venipuncture. A vast array of non-credit preclinical electives enriches the experience during the first and second years. Courses inlcude: Issues in Women's Health, Community and Child Health, Humanities in Medicine, Business in Medicine Elective, Emergency Room Elective, Geriatric Issues, Alternative and Complementary Medicine, to name a few. Renovations at the Medical Science Complex bring 26-state of the art multipurpose classrooms and anatomy laboratories for the educational programs.

CLINICAL TRAINING

Most clinical training takes place at the principal teaching hospitals, Robert Wood Johnson University Hospital on the New Brunswick Campus and Cooper Hospital University Medical Center on the Camden Campus. A Clinical Skills Center with a standardized patient program is used to teach and assess the clinical skills of first, second, third and fourth year medical students. During the third year of medical school students rotate through clerkships in Medicine, Surgery, Pediatrics, Family Medicine, Psychiatry, Neurology, and Obstetrics/Gynecology. Additionally there is a significant amount of elective work during the third year. During the fourth year students are required to take rotations in emergency medicine and critical care. A longitudinal care experience runs through the third and fourth years.

Students

Approximately 80 percent of the students apply as New Jersey residents. There is great diversity among the student body, Fifty-one percent of students self-describe as minorities with 14 percent from under-represented groups. Typically between 10-20 percent of the student body took off some time between undergraduate studies and medical school. The class size is 156. One third of the class completes their clinical training on the Camden Campus.

STUDENT LIFE

New Brunswick offers the many amenities of a university city. Princeton and New York City are short train rides away. Students who complete clinical training on the Camden Campus enjoy the proximity of Philadelphia. The medical school does not have on-campus housing, however the school helps students secure accomodations in the area. Medical students have access to Rutgers University athletic facilities which include golf, swimming pools, gyms, squash, racquetball, and volleyball courts. Rutgers also offers social, cultural and recreational activities for medical students. There are many student organizations and interest groups, including chapters of the major national medical student associations. Many students participate in volunteer organizations including the student run HIPHOP (Homeless and Indigent Persons Health Outreach Project) and UIP (Urban Health Initiatives). Honor societies include AOA and the Humanism in Medicine Honor Society.

GRADUATES

Graduates have done particularly well in securing outstanding training positions throughout the country as well as within our own training programs. About one half of the class chooses a internal medicine, pediatrics or family medicine, but all specialties are represented.

Admissions

REQUIREMENTS

Two semesters of Biology, General Chemistry, Organic Chemistry, and Physics, with laboratory, two semesters of English or writing intensive courses, and one semester of college-level mathematics are required. The MCAT is required and must be no more than four years old. For applicants who have taken the exam more than once, all scores are considered, but the most recent score is given the most weight.

SUGGESTIONS

Coursework in the Behavioral Sciences and Humanities is recommended. Medically related experiences, research, and community service are all valued by the Admissions Committee.

PROCESS

As a state institution, preference is given to in-state residents, however the importance of geographic diversity is recognized and out-of-state residents are encouraged to apply. A new process allows accepted out-of-state residents to become in-state residents and hence be eligible for in-state tuition. Approximately one half of New Jersey applicants and five percent of out-of-state applicants are interviewed on one of the three campuses: Piscataway, New Brunswick, or Camden. Generally students are interviewed by one faculty member. Some applicants also are interviewed by a student member of the Admissions Committee. All applicants have the opportunity to meet and tour with a current student. About one-third of those interviewed are accepted. Acceptances are offered on a rolling basis. Several alternative means of acceptance exist. There is a combined BA/MD program with Rutgers University. There is also an Accelerated Acceptance program for post-baccalaureate students completing post-baccalaureate studies at a number of institutions including University of Pennsylvania, Columbia, Johns Hopkins, Rutgers, Drexel, NYU and Bryn Mawr, and LaSalle.

Admissions Requirements (Required)
MCAT Scores, Essays, Science GPA, Extracurricular activities, Non-Science GPA, Exposure to medical profession, Recommendation, Interview

Admissions Requirements (Optional)
State Residency

COSTS AND AID

Tuition & Fees

Annual tuition (in-state out-of-state)	$22,246/$34,811
Room & board	$10,026
Cost of books	$1,768
Fees	$3,112

Financial Aid

% students receiving any aid	78
% students receiving grants	24
% students receiving loans	80
Average grant	$5,000
Average loan	$25,000
Average total aid package	$30,000
Average debt	$102,000

SAINT LOUIS UNIVERSITY

SAINT LOUIS UNIVERSITY SCHOOL OF MEDICINE

COMMITTEE ON ADMISSIONS, 1402 S. GRAND BLVD., C130 ST. LOUIS, MO 63104 • ADMISSION: 314-977-9875
FAX: 314-977-98257 • E-MAIL: SLUMD@SLU.EDU • WEBSITE: MEDSCHOOL.SLU.EDU

STUDENT BODY

Type	Private
Enrollment of parent institution	12,622
Enrollment of medical school	709
% male/female	54/46
% underrepresented minorities	4
% out-of-state	74
% international	6

FACULTY

Total faculty	720
% female faculty	35
% minority faculty	6
% part-time faculty	12

ADMISSIONS

# applied	6,635
% accepted	8
% enrolled	34

Average GPA and MCAT Scores

Overall GPA	3.8
MCAT Bio	11.1
MCAT Phys	10.9
MCAT Verbal	10.3

Application Information

Regular application	12/15
Regular notification	10/15
Early application	8/1
Early notification	10/1
Are transfers accepted?	Yes
Admissions may be deferred?	Yes
Admissions need-blind?	No
Application fee	$100

Academics

The medical curriculum is continually evolving to respond to the rapid changes in the health care field and to reflect national trends in medical education. Current students enjoy a program of study that uses a block schedule and human organ systems based learning and emphasizes small-group and independent study. SLU offers several options for students interested in research. Qualified students may enter an M.D./Ph.D. program, allowing them to complete both degrees within 6-7 years. The doctorate is offered in Anatomy, Health Care Ethics, Biochemistry, Cell Biology, Genetics, Immunology, Microbiology, Molecular Biology, Neuroscience, Pathology, Pharmacology, and Physiology. Students interested in summer or elective research experiences may graduate in four years, earning an M.D. with distinction in research. The first two years of the M.D. curriculum are pass/fail. The final two years are Honors/Near Honors/Pass/Fail. Passing the USMLE Step 1 is a requirement for promotion to year three, and passing Step 2 CK and taking Step 2 CS is a requirement for graduation.

BASIC SCIENCES: Year 1 consists of Cell and Molecular Biology, Epidemiology and Biostatistics, Clinical Anatomy, Microbes and Hosts Responses, Pharmacology and Pathology. Year 1 also includes Applied Clinical Skills 1 that focuses on communication skills and physical diagnosis. Year 2 uses an organ-based approach that also incorporates Applied Clinical Skills 2 and Bedside Diagnosis. An important resource for students is the Learning Resources Center, which houses the Health Sciences Center Library and the Simulation lab. The new Education Union houses the Clinical Skills Center, where diagnostic and treatment skills are taught.

CLINICAL TRAINING

Year 3 incorporates the core clerkships including Family Medicine and the opportunity for some students to take an elective. During Year 4 students are able to design programs to fit their individual career goals. Required coursework includes 3 weeks of subinternship, 3 weeks of surgical subspecialty, 3 weeks of required capstone and 27 weeks of electives. Training is conducted at the St. Louis University Hospital, a 365-bed tertiary care facility. It is also a Level I trauma center. Other affiliated institutions include Cardinal Glennon Children's Medical Center, Anheuser-Busch Eye Institute, St. Mary's Health Center, and Saint Louis University Cancer Center. A portion of electives may be taken at other academic and clinical institutions.

Students

Students come from all regions of the country. About 8 percent of the entering class are underrepresented minorities and about 40 percent are nontraditional, having pursued other careers or interests between college and medical school.

STUDENT LIFE

Since 1994, the students and physicians of the School of Medicine have been committed to providing free primary health care services in an academic environment. Currently we offer three different clinic sessions to meet our patients' needs: Regular Clinic, Pediatric Clinic, and Well Woman Clinic.

GRADUATES

About 40 percent of graduates enter primary care residencies. Our students are competitive applicants for specialty and surgical fields as well.

Admissions

REQUIREMENTS

8 hrs. Biology, 8 hrs. Inorganic Chemistry, 8 hrs. Organic Chemistry, 8 hrs. Physics-a lab is required for all science courses. 6 hrs. English and 12 hrs. Humanities and Behavioral Sciences.

SUGGESTIONS

The Committee recommends applicants have shadowing and volunteer experience.

PROCESS

All AMCAS applicants receive secondary applications. Of the approximately 6,000 applicants who return secondaries, about 18 percent are interviewed on a rolling basis. Interviews are one hour in length and are conducted by a faculty member. The remainder of the interview day includes a tour of the campus, group informational sessions, and lunch with current students. Applicants are notified of committee decisions in 6 to 8 weeks of the interview and are either accepted, rejected, or put into a hold category. For wait-listed applicants, additional grades or MCAT scores are useful supplementary information.

Admissions Requirements (Required)

MCAT Scores, Essays, Science GPA, Non-Science GPA, Recommendation, Interview

Admissions Requirements (Optional)

Extracurricular activities, Exposure to medical profession, State Residency

COSTS AND AID

Tuition & Fees

Annual tuition	$48,390
Room & board	$10,380
Cost of books	$980
Fees	$690

Financial Aid

% students receiving any aid	83
% students receiving grants	74
% students receiving loans	76
% aid that is merit-based	0
Average grant	$9,375
Average loan	$51,422
Average total aid package	$54,169
Average debt	$187,266

SOUTHERN ILLINOIS UNIVERSITY
SCHOOL OF MEDICINE

PO Box 19624, SPRINGFIELD, IL 62794-9624 • **ADMISSION:** 217-545-6013 • **FAX:** 217-545-55387
E-MAIL: ADMISSIONS@SIUMED.EDU • **WEBSITE:** WWW.SIUMED.EDU

STUDENT BODY

Type	Public
Enrollment of parent institution	21,441
Enrollment of medical school	289
% male/female	47/53
% international	14
Average age of entering class	23

FACULTY

Total faculty	336
% female faculty	37
% minority faculty	19
% part-time faculty	6
Student-faculty ratio	1.0:1

ADMISSIONS

# applied	1,184
% accepted	13
% enrolled	49

Average GPA and MCAT Scores

Overall GPA	3.6
MCAT Bio	10.1
MCAT Phys	9.4
MCAT Verbal	9.6
MCAT Essay	O

Application Information

Regular application	11/15
Regular notification	10/15
Are transfers accepted?	Yes
Admissions may be deferred?	Yes
Admissions need-blind?	No
Application fee	$50

Academics

SIU offers a case-based, small group-oriented curriculum with an abundance of patient contact and early clinical exposure. In cooperation with the SIU School of Law, a joint M.D./J.D. degree program is also offered. The school also offers a masters of science in physician assistant studies and a MD/MPH concurrent degree in medicine and public health. Medical students are evaluated on Pass/Fail and with honors system. The USMLE Step 1 must be passed as a graduation requirement.

BASIC SCIENCES: The instructional format emphasizes small-group instruction, self-directed study, and a case-based approach, but also incorporates lectures and an organ system organizational scheme. Topics covered in the first year are cardiovascular, respiratory, renal, endocrine, reproductive, gastrointestinal, and sensorimotor systems and behavior. In Carbondale, basic science instruction takes place in Lindegren Hall. Early clinical experiences are offered at Memorial Hospital in Carbondale (151 beds), the Carbondale Clinic, offices of local physicians, and at the VA Hospital (171 beds). In Springfield, the Medical Instructional Facility contains lecture halls, classrooms, labs, and a teaching museum. A four-year doctoring curriculum (physicians conduct and attitude, clinical skills development, and medical humanities issues) begins immediately. Both simulated and real patients are used. Topics covered in the second year include circulation, infection, and host diseases, neoplasia, population health and preventive medicine, neuromuscular, and medicine and behavior. Computer assisted instruction is used as a learning aid, and computers are available in the Student Computer Lab and at other sites. The Morris Library at Carbondale houses more than 100,000 volumes, while the Medical Instruction Facility in Springfield contains 113,000.

CLINICAL TRAINING

Extensive clinical activities are the hallmark of our education throughout all four years. From the first week of school, supervised students engage in patient care. Third-year required multidisciplinary rotations are Internal Medicine, Surgery, Family and Community Medicine, Psychiatry, Obstetrics, Gynecology, and Pediatrics. Four weeks of electives, which may include emergency medicine, radiology, anesthesiology, are allowed in the third year. The doctoring curriculum continues during this year. At the conclusion of the third year, students must pass an examination that evaluates their skills in assessing and managing patient problems. During the fourth year, students complete one additional required clerkship: Neurology (4 weeks). Thirty-one weeks are reserved for elective studies. Clinical training sites include Memorial Medical Center (580 beds), St. John's Hospital and Pavilion (715 beds), and the clinics and offices of faculty and community physicians. Electives may be taken off campus.

Students

All regular M.D. students are Illinois residents. The average age of incoming students is 24. Underrepresented minorities account for 14 percent of the student body. Class size is 72.

STUDENT LIFE

On-campus recreational facilities at Carbondale include a complete fitness room, swimming pools, racquetball courts, and a student center. Intramural sports and inter-collegiate sporting events are popular activities. The area features a state park and the Shawnee National Fores for hiking, biking, camping, canoeing, and swimming. Springfield is a family-friendly community that offers numerous recreational activities including parks, golf courses, bike trails, a water park, great shopping and numerous cultural and historical sites. Medical students enjoy membership at a local fitness center. Lake Springfield offers fishing, swimming, boating, and sailing. All students live off campus in both Carbondale and Springfield. St. Louis is a two-hour drive from both communities.

GRADUATES

Among the 2013 graduating class, the most prevalent fields for post-graduate training were family medicine (13%), internal medicine (12%), and pediatrics (12%). Students generally score around the national mean on the USMLE Part 1, and above the mean on Part 2, making them well-positioned for securing residency positions.

Admissions

REQUIREMENTS

In order to do well on the MCAT, students should have taken at least one year each of Biology, Chemistry, Organic Chemistry, Physics, English, and Math, the last of which should have included some Statistics. The MCAT is required and scores must be no more than two years old. For applicants who have taken the exam on multiple occasions, the most recent set of scores is considered.

SUGGESTIONS

As a state school, preference is given to applicants from central and southern Illinois who are interested in practicing in the region. Applicants are expected to have a good foundation in the natural sciences, social sciences, and humanities in addition to sound English skills. The Admissions Committee looks beyond scholastic achievement for evidence of responsibility, integrity, compassion, motivation, interest in medicine, community service, and sound interpersonal skills. The Medical Education Preparatory Program (MEDPREP) is a nondegree post-baccalaureate program that assists disadvantaged students with meeting the requirements for medical schools throughout the country.

PROCESS

About 1/4 of applicants are interviewed. Interviews are conducted between August and March, and consist of two sessions with individual faculty and/or administrators. About 30 percent of interviewed candidates are accepted on a batch basis. Others are rejected or wait-listed. Wait-listed candidates may send supplemental material to update their files.

Admissions Requirements (Required)

MCAT Scores, Essays, Science GPA, Non-Science GPA, Recommendation, Interview, State Residency

Admissions Requirements (Optional)

Extracurricular activities, Exposure to medical profession

COSTS AND AID

Tuition & Fees

Annual tuition (in-state out-of-state)	$20,144/$54,936
Room & board	$6,956
Cost of books	$5,650
Fees (in-state out-of-state)	$2,140/$1,673

Financial Aid

% students receiving any aid	93
% students receiving grants	36
% students receiving loans	88
% aid that is merit-based	0
Average grant	$13,681
Average loan	$29,338
Average total aid package	$36,065
Average debt	$28,736

ST. GEORGE'S UNIVERSITY
ST. GEORGE'S UNIVERSITY SCHOOL OF MEDICINE

UNIVERSITE CENTRE, GRENADA, WEST INDIES, ONE EAST MAIN STREET BAY SHORE, NY 0 • **ADMISSION:** 800-899-6337
FAX: 631-665-55907 • **E-MAIL:** SGUINFO@SGU.EDU • **WEBSITE:** WWW.SGU.EDU

STUDENT BODY

Type	Private
Enrollment of medical school	4,110
% male/female	55/45
% underrepresented minorities	34
# countries represented	90
Average age of entering class	26

FACULTY

Total faculty	2,082
% part-time faculty	24

ADMISSIONS

# applied	2,082

Average GPA and MCAT Scores

Overall GPA	3.4
MCAT Bio	10.0
MCAT Phys	9.0
MCAT Verbal	8.0

Application Information

Admissions need-blind?	No
Application fee	$75

Academics

Founded as an independent School of Medicine over 32 years ago, St. George's University (SGU) has evolved into a top center of international education. The University offers advanced degrees in its Schools of Medicine and Veterinary Medicine, as well as independent and dual graduate degrees in exciting areas of science, public health, and business. Undergraduate degree programs are available in the life sciences, business, management information systems, information technology, medical sciences, psychology, nursing, and liberal studies through St. George's University School of Arts and Sciences. Over 8,000 physicians have graduated from the St. George's University School of Medicine and are practicing medicine in over 35 countries and every state in the United States. They practice in virtually every specialty and subspecialty, and in positions in academic medicine, as well as public health and institutional practice. Their scores on standardized tests over the years attest to the academic excellence of the SGUSOM curriculum. According to a study recently released in the journal, Academic Medicine, Grenada was ranked #1 in USMLE Step One and Step Two/CK in the Caribbean for the highest first time pass rate among all countries with medical schools in the Caribbean over the past 15 years. Grenada-with St. George's University School of Medicine as the only medical school in Grenada-had an 84.4% pass rate in Step One, outperforming the other counties that had an average pass rate of 49.9% during the same 15 year time period. State Education Departments across the United States and various Government Councils around the world have conducted site visits and extensive evaluations of the St. George's University Doctor of Medicine program, and St. George's University has received a favorable review each time, meeting or exceeding all standards.

BASIC SCIENCES: Students in the four-year Doctor of Medicine degree program may spend the first two years on the True Blue campus in Grenada studying the Basic Medical Sciences. The Keith B. Taylor Global Scholars Program (KBTGSP) allows students who are accepted to the St. George's University Doctor of Medicine degree program to spend their first year of Basic Medical Sciences on the campus of Northumbria University in Newcastle, England. This unique partnership gives a select group of students the opportunity to study in the United Kingdom, Grenada, and the United States. In the final two years, students complete their clinical training in one of the affiliated centers in the United States or the United Kingdom.

CLINICAL TRAINING
St. George's offers a highly integrated system of affiliated hospitals and Clinical Centers in the United States, all of whose core rotations have ACGME-approved residency training programs running concurrently. Our program in the United Kingdom is similar to that in the United States, providing students with clinical opportunities at over 60 affiliated hospitals in the United States and the United Kingdom. Although clinical training may be completed in one country, students may combine clinical experiences in the United States and the United Kingdom for a more international experience.

Students

SGU's $250 million+, technologically advanced campus is set on the beautiful, safe island of Grenada. Over 50 state-of-the-art buildings create the perfect environment in which to learn, play and make lifelong networks of colleagues and friends. The brand new administrative, residential, academic, and scientific buildings include a 45,000 square-ft. fully electronic library; gross anatomy laboratory; microbiology, pathology, and histology laboratories with extensive microscopic and gross preparations collections and an up-to-date array of audiovisual and computerized materials in all subjects. The student center is home to two restaurants, a fully equipped weight room and exercise facilities. After classes and on weekends students can also be found on the new sports fields and basketball courts, participating in many sporting activities and team sports. To accommodate our growing population we have expanded our on-campus housing to include a wide variety of comfortable, attractive and convenient living arrangements. In addition, there are numerous choices for living off-campus which can be accessed by the University bus system. From the first contact with the University, the welfare of each student is carefully considered and safeguarded. Our financial counselors stay closely involved with students through the course of their study and beyond, to ensure their financial health; the Dean of Students Office monitors and supports students in academic progress as well as non-academic activities and concerns, and Department of Educational Services provides coursework tutorials, workshops in study, test-taking, and time-management skills. Additionally, our Counseling Service offers both formal clinical and peer counseling services. Throughout clinicals and after graduation the Office of Career Guidance advises students and graduates in specialty selection, residency application processes, and CV development. The University also supports programs and opportunities for spouses and dependents through our Significant Others Organization which sponsors a regular series of events and gatherings, developing a close camaraderie among club members.

STUDENT LIFE

Students attend their basic science years on the True Blue campus in Grenada. The inhabitants of Grenada are English speaking, and all course work is delivered in English. Students have options of taking clinical rotations in the United States and/or in the United Kingdom. The community at St. George's University gathers there from all four corners of the world—it is extremely diverse. Over 90 nations are represented in the student population and over 50 student organizations are organized around various interests—cultural, religious, avocational, community service, etc.—fostering a sense of belonging as well as collegiality. Students participate in many types of sporting activities and team sports such as basketball, tennis, flag football, soccer, cricket, badminton, volleyball, street hockey, ultimate frisbee, lacrosse, and softball to name a few. Water sports include sailing, boating, swimming, snorkeling and scuba diving. Aerobics, fitness, and martial arts classes are held regularly. In addition to on-campus activities, students have access to markets, shops, banks, and the movie theatre. Local buses will deliver you to hiking trails in the rain forest, or to the seashore for boating, scuba diving, snorkeling, and other outdoor activities.

Admissions Requirements (Required)

MCAT Scores, Essays, Science GPA, Extracurricular activities, Non-Science GPA, Recommendation, Interview

Admissions Requirements (Optional)

Exposure to medical profession, State Residency

COSTS AND AID

Tuition & Fees

Annual tuition $40,664

STANFORD UNIVERSITY

STANFORD UNIVERSITY SCHOOL OF MEDICINE

OFFICE OF MD ADMISSIONS, 1265 WELCH RD., MSOB XC301, STANFORD, CA 94305-5404 • ADMISSION: 650-723-6861
FAX: 650-725-78557 • E-MAIL: MDADMISSIONS@STANFORD.EDU • WEBSITE: WWW.MED.STANFORD.EDU

STUDENT BODY

Type	Private
Enrollment of parent institution	15,877
Enrollment of medical school	468
% male/female	52/48
% underrepresented minorities	3
% out-of-state	58
% international	59
Average age of entering class	24

FACULTY

Total faculty	897
% female faculty	29
% minority faculty	6
% part-time faculty	1
Student-faculty ratio	0.5:1

ADMISSIONS

# applied	7,341
% accepted	3
% enrolled	52

Average GPA and MCAT Scores

Overall GPA	3.8
MCAT Bio	12.4
MCAT Phys	12.5
MCAT Verbal	11.6
MCAT Essay	Q

Application Information

Regular application	10/15
Are transfers accepted?	No
Admissions may be deferred?	Yes
Admissions need-blind?	No
Application fee	$85

Academics

Generally, about 60 percent of Stanford students receive their M.D. in five rather than four years, which allows for individual research and elective study. Stanford supports a range of opportunities for candidates to pursue an advanced degree in addition to the M.D., including Ph.D. degrees in Bioengineering, Biomedical Informatics, or one of the 13 Biosciences home departments. MD-MS degree opportunities include Health Services Research, Epidemiology, Medical Informatics, and Biomechanical Engineering. MD-MA Degrees include: Education, IPER: Interdisciplinary Program in Environment and Resources, and Public Policy. There are opportunities to obtain an MBA or JD degree. A collaboration with UC Berkeley allows Stanford MD students to pursue and obtain a Master of Public Health. Approximately eight to ten Medical Scientist Training Program (MSTP) students begin that program each year. In addition to formal degree programs, students may take electives in non-medical departments. Through the Medical Student Scholars Program and other programs, students enjoy a range of research opportunities, most of which are remunerated.

BASIC SCIENCES: The Stanford curriculum melds a strong introduction to basic science and clinical experience with in-depth study and independent research through the Scholarly Concentrations. In the first five quarters, in-depth instruction in basic science and the pathophysiology of disease runs in parallel with clinical skills instruction and the introduction to patient care in the Practice of Medicine course sequence. Clinical skills instruction is led by 16 faculty who provide longitudinal mentorship. The Practice of Medicine sequence is held on two afternoons per week using a combination of small and large group instructional formats. Topic areas include clinical skills (history-taking and physical examination), medical ethics, biostatistics and epidemiology, health care systems, clinical psychiatry, and other aspects of the practice of medicine in society. In Quarters One and Two, the Foundations of Medicine courses include anatomy (taught through a traditional cadaver lab), molecular biology, cells to tissues, applied biochemistry, genetics, development and disease mechanisms, immunology, and overview of the nervous system. Wednesdays remain unscheduled throughout the first six quarters so that students may engage in electives and course work for their Scholarly Concentration. Quarter Three initiates the integrated Human Health and Disease course sequence using a modular organ system based approach with instruction in physiology, infectious disease, histology, pathology, and pharmacology. Instruction in the Practice of Medicine continues at the same time over the first five quarters, culminating in Quarter 6 with a four-week intensive course that prepares students for clinical clerkships. In conjunction with their MD studies, students also participate in course work and complete a project in a Scholarly Concentration. The Stanford curriculum is structured to encourage students to engage in individual or group study, elective course work, research, and other opportunities for professional growth, with many students electing to extend their studies for an additional year. Grading for pre-clerkship courses, elective clerkships and sub-internships is Pass/Fail; students demonstrating exceptional performance in required clerkships may receive Pass with Distinction in the domains of professionalism/interpersonal communication, patient care, and knowledge. Step 1 of the USMLE must be passed no later than February 1st of the first clinical year, with two months available for study between Quarter Six and the beginning of clinical clerkships. Step 2 must be passed prior to graduation.

CLINICAL TRAINING

Patient contact begins in the fall quarter of the first year, and there are opportunities for clinical experiences during the first two years. Third- and fourth-year clerkships take place at the major affiliated teaching hospitals, which include Stanford Hospital, the Lucile Salter Packard Children's Hospital, Santa Clara Valley Medical Center, the Palo Alto VA Hospital, and Kaiser Permanente in Santa Clara. These facilities serve both rural and urban populations with diverse needs. Students complete 15 and a half months of clinical clerkships, including 12 and a half months of required core clerkships in General Medicine, General Surgery, Pediatrics, Ob/Gyn, Psychiatry, Family Medicine, Ambulatory Internal Medicine, Neurology, and Critical Care. Two months are spent training in areas related to required clerkships through "selectives," in which students choose from Fundamentals of Clinical Care and Sub-internship options. The final month is designated as elective clerkship.

Students

Stanford students benefit from an academic environment that fosters collaboration among students and mentorship by faculty through the E4C (Educators for Care) Program. Special efforts are made to recruit diverse students from underrepresented minority backgrounds and socioeconomically disadvantaged life experiences. Student organizations enrich the intellectual, social and cultural vibrancy of the school. With 90 to 100 students per class, Stanford is relatively small.

STUDENT LIFE

The campus and the surrounding area offer excellent sports and other outdoor activities. San Francisco is 35 minutes to the north, San Jose is 20 minutes south, and Oakland is 45 minutes northeast. All are accessible by public transportation—train and subway. Numerous on-campus housing options exist, including family housing, apartments, dormitories, and co-ops.

GRADUATES

Stanford itself offers excellent residency programs, and many graduates opt for post-graduate training at Stanford. Perhaps as a result of the teaching and research experience students gain while in school, many go on into academic medicine. Increasingly, graduates are entering primary care fields.

Admissions

REQUIREMENTS

Biology with lab (1 year); Chemistry/Organic Chemistry with labs (2 years); and Physics with lab (1 year). Applicants must have received an undergraduate degree from an accredited college or university by the time of matriculation. The institution must have been accredited at the time of Stanford's application deadline.

SUGGESTIONS

Biochemistry, Calculus, and Behavioral Sciences are recommended, as is knowledge of a second language. No preference is given to California residents or to Stanford undergraduates. Successful applicants generally have significant medical, health-related, research, or community service experience.

PROCESS

Secondary applications are sent out on a rolling basis. Stanford implements the Multiple Mini-Interview (MMI) process to evaluate candidates. Of interviewed candidates, about one third are accepted, with responses given within four to six weeks of the interview. During the past few years, from 0–15 applicants were eventually accepted off of the wait-list.

Admissions Requirements (Required)

MCAT Scores, Essays, Science GPA, Extracurricular activities, Non-Science GPA, Exposure to medical profession, Recommendation, Interview

Admissions Requirements (Optional)

State Residency

COSTS AND AID

Tuition & Fees

Annual tuition	$48,999
Room & board (on-campus off-campus)	$20,520/$19,650
Cost of books	$1,500
Fees	$596

Financial Aid

% students receiving any aid	78
% students receiving grants	66
% students receiving loans	62
% aid that is merit-based	17
Average grant	$39,469
Average loan	$27,491
Average total aid package	$54,381
Average debt	$96,385

STATE UNIVERSITY OF NEW YORK DOWNSTATE MEDICAL CENTER
SUNY DOWNSTATE MEDICAL CENTER

OFFICE OF ADMISSIONS, 450 CLARKSON AVENUE, BOX 60M, BROOKLYN, NY 11203 • ADMISSION: 718-270-2446
FAX: 718-270-47757 • WEBSITE: WWW.DOWNSTATE.EDU

STUDENT BODY

Type	Public
Enrollment of medical school	757
% male/female	56/44
% out-of-state	4
% international	15
Average age of entering class	23

ADMISSIONS

# applied	3,505

Application Information

Regular application	12/15
Are transfers accepted?	No
Admissions may be deferred?	Yes
Admissions need-blind?	No
Application fee	$65

Academics

The curriculum emphasizes the development of clinical reasoning and problem-solving skills, it integrates basic and clinical sciences, and exposes students from the first year to patient care. Each student spends one afternoon biweekly in a physician's private office or clinic; the practicing physician serves as the student's clinical mentor for the entire year. Students are also encouraged to participate in research. Opportunities are available throughout the 4 years of medical school. Those who make a significant research contribution are eligible to graduate with Distinction in Research. A M.D./Ph.D. program is open in one of two modern biomedical science areas, Neuroscience or Molecular and Cell Biology. Medical students are evaluated with an Honors/High Pass/Pass/Fail system. Students must pass Step 1 of the USMLE in order to be promoted to year three. Students are encouraged to take Step 2 prior to graduation, but it is not a requirement.

BASIC SCIENCES: Basic science courses have been integrated into "topics" or blocks. Each block is taught using a combination of traditional lectures, case-based, small-group sessions, laboratories, conferences, and a weekly clinical experience. First year topics are Genes to Cells, Skin and Connective Tissue, Musculoskeletal System, Blood/Hematopoiesis/ Lymphoid, Cardiovascular System, Respiratory System, Gastrointestinal System/ Intermediary Metabolism, Renal/Urinary System, Endocrine and Reproduction Systems, Head and Neck, and Neuroscience. The current second-year curriculum includes courses in Pathology, Pathophysiology, Pharmacology, Microbiology and Immunology, Preventive Medicine, Preparation for Clinical Medicine, Psychopathology, and Nutrition. With the exception of the last two, each course runs throughout the full academic year, with each discipline presenting material related to specific organ systems. The Office of Academic Development promotes students' academic success through seminars, workshops, and individual tutoring. The Health Science Education Building holds two floors of study carrels, which serve as "home base" to students during the first two years. In the same building is the Medical Research Library, one of the largest medical school libraries in the country, and a 500 seat auditorium. A Learning Resource Center has 90 computer work stations loaded with an array of medical applications.

CLINICAL TRAINING
The current clerkships are Medicine (10 weeks); Surgery (8 weeks); Anesthesia (2 weeks); Pediatrics (6 weeks); Ob/Gyn (6 weeks); Psychiatry (6 weeks); and Neurology (4 weeks). Primary care; a Subinternship (4 weeks), and at least 20 weeks of electives. Training takes place at a number of major affiliates, University Hospital, and Kings County Hospital. Electives can be completed at those institutions or at extramural hospitals or medical centers.

Students

This year's first-year class is 185 students from more than 60 individual colleges. About 93 percent are New York State residents. Approximately 13 percent of students are underrepresented minorities. The age range of the 2001 entering class is 20–35, with a median of 22.

STUDENT LIFE

All entering students are assigned a clinical faculty mentor who provides guidance and support throughout the first year. The focal point for recreational, social, and cultural activities on campus is the Student Center, which has lounges, a piano room, an athletic center, a swimming pool, squash courts, and a spa. Student organizations focus on professional, ethnic, service related, social, and recreational interests, and also provide support for groups of students. For example, the Daniel Hale Williams Society, named for a prominent black physician, is a voice for minority students on campus and also brings students together to participate in educational, social, and service-related goals. Brooklyn is a culturally rich, active community that provides an exciting extracurricular life for medical students. Manhattan is easily accessible on the subway. On-campus housing options are single or shared studios, or dormitory rooms. Students who live off campus often reside in the nearby neighborhood of Park Slope.

GRADUATES

SUNY Brooklyn graduates perform above the national average in terms of securing residency positions at top institutions nationwide. Alumni hold faculty positions at universities such as Harvard, Case Western, Stanford, Yale, Hopkins, Columbia, Cornell, and the University of Pennsylvania, among other prestigious institutions. 40 percent of 2002 graduating students entered residency programs in primary care. More than 69 percent of graduates chose to stay within New York State.

Admissions

REQUIREMENTS

Fifteen positions in each class are reserved for students in a B.A./M.D. program organized with Brooklyn College. Five positions are reserved for early assurance applicants from Queens College and the College of Staten Island. New York residents are given strong preference for the remaining spots. Prerequisites are eight semester credits each of Biology, Chemistry, Organic Chemistry, and Physics, all with associated labs. Six semester hours of English are also required. The MCAT is required and scores must be from within three years of the date of anticipated enrollment. Component scores for each MCAT series are looked at individually.

SUGGESTIONS

In addition to required courses, one year each of college-level Math, Biochemistry, and another advanced science are recommended. Medically related experience and demonstrated commitment to social service and community outreach activities are important factors in admission.

PROCESS

All AMCAS applicants are sent secondary applications. About 20 percent of those returning secondaries are interviewed between September and April. Interviews consist of one one-hour session with a faculty member. On interview day, candidates also have a group orientation session, lunch with current students, and a campus tour. Of interviewed candidates, about 40 percent are accepted on a rolling basis. Wait-listed candidates are not encouraged to send supplementary information.

Admissions Requirements (Required)

MCAT Scores, Science GPA, Extracurricular activities, Non-Science GPA, Exposure to medical profession, Recommendation, Interview

Admissions Requirements (Optional)

Essays, State Residency

COSTS AND AID

Tuition & Fees

Annual tuition (in-state out-of-state) $18,800/$33,500
Fees $450

Financial Aid

Average debt $59,906

State University of New York Upstate Medical University
College of Medicine

OFFICE OF STUDENT ADMISSIONS, 766 IRVING AVENUE, SYRACUSE, NY 13210 • ADMISSION: 315-464-4570
FAX: 315-464-88677 • E-MAIL: ADMISS@UPSTATE.EDU • WEBSITE: WWW.UPSTATE.EDU

STUDENT BODY

Type	Public
Enrollment of parent institution	1,245
Enrollment of medical school	643
% male/female	53/47
% underrepresented minorities	1
% out-of-state	26
% international	36
# countries represented	5
Average age of entering class	24

FACULTY

Total faculty	693
% female faculty	28
% minority faculty	22
% part-time faculty	32
Student-faculty ratio	1.0:1

ADMISSIONS

# applied	4,945
% accepted	8
% enrolled	43

Average GPA and MCAT Scores

Overall GPA	3.6
MCAT Bio	10.5
MCAT Phys	10.0
MCAT Verbal	9.6
MCAT Essay	P

Application Information

Regular application	12/1
Regular notification	5/1
Early application	8/1
Early notification	10/1
Are transfers accepted?	Yes
Admissions may be deferred?	Yes
Admissions need-blind?	No
Application fee	$100

Academics

The College of Medicine curriculum integrates the basic and clinical sciences—with basic science courses teaching the clinical implications of the material—and provides clinical experience starting in the first semester. All courses are aligned by organ systems. For example, in the first year, students learn the structure and function of the brain in February, the heart in March and the lungs in April. Similarly, the second year aligns the pharmacology, microbiology and pathology of each organ system. The curriculum also addresses the humanistic aspects of medicine, including its ethical, legal and social implications. Throughout their four years at Upstate, students acquire the knowledge, skills and attitudes necessary to become competent, caring physicians. All College of Medicine students spend their first two years on the Upstate campus in Syracuse. At the start of the third year, one-quarter of the class moves to the Binghamton Clinical Campus. The rest of the class remains in Syracuse, and completes clinical education at University Hospital and its clinical affiliates. Students learn the same skills at both campuses, but the ambiance is different. Much of the clinical training in Syracuse takes place in a tertiary care setting, the special focus of a university hospital. In Binghamton, most of the training occurs in a community-based setting that is more akin to the environment in which most physicians will practice later on. Applicants indicate their campus preference within two weeks of the admissions interview, and are assigned to a clinical campus upon acceptance to the College of Medicine.

Students

80 percent of students are New York residents, applications from non NY state residents are welcome. About 12 percent of students are underrepresented minorities, and about 15 percent took some significant time off between college and medical school. Class size is 160.

STUDENT LIFE

A large part of college life takes place outside the classroom, and Upstate is no exception. We offer 45 student clubs and organizations including ballroom dancing and student government, special events and athletic programs. The Campus Activities Governing Board schedules social, cultural and recreational programs for students including first-run movies on weekends, a guest lecture series, comedy hours, weekend getaways and discount tickets to local sports and cultural events. The Campus Activities Building (CAB), located next door to our residence hall, has a computer lounge, snack bar, bookstore, TV lounge, pool, sauna, gym, squash and racquetball courts, treadmills, step machines, Nautilus, tennis courts, billiards, ping pong and more. Our intramural sports program runs men's, women's and/or co-ed leagues in basketball, volleyball, softball, football, racquetball and soccer. Syracuse is a medium-sized city surrounded by countryside. It is a one-hour drive to Lake Ontario's beaches, and four hours to New York City. The Binghamton campus is conveniently situated about three hours from New York City, Philadelphia, and Buffalo. Modern residence halls at the Syracuse campus provide dormitory rooms, studios, and one-bedroom apartments for single and married students. Off campus housing is readily available for students choosing to attend the Binghampton campus during their last two years of study.

210 • THE BEST 167 MEDICAL SCHOOLS

GRADUATES

Graduates are successful in securing residencies in all fields.

Admissions

REQUIREMENTS

Prerequisites are General Chemistry (6–8 semester hours); Organic Chemistry (6–8 hours); General Biology (6–8 hours); General Physics (6–8 hours); and English (6 hours, at least 3 of which must be composition).

SUGGESTIONS

Academic work in the Humanities and Social Sciences is considered equally as important as science course work.

PROCESS

All applicants are sent secondary applications. Of those returning secondaries, about 20 percent are invited to interview between September and March. Interviews consist of two sessions each with faculty members, administrators, students or alumni. About 20 percent of interviewed candidates are accepted on a rolling basis, while others are may be admitted later in the year.

Admissions Requirements (Required)

MCAT Scores, Essays, Science GPA, Extracurricular activities, Non-Science GPA, Exposure to medical profession, Recommendation, Interview

Admissions Requirements (Optional)

State Residency

COSTS AND AID

Tuition & Fees

Annual tuition (in-state out-of-state)	$24,850/$48,770
Room & board	$17,727
Cost of books	$2,476
Fees	$1,340

Financial Aid

% students receiving any aid	87
% students receiving grants	30
% students receiving loans	82
% aid that is merit-based	13
Average grant	$9,653
Average loan	$39,760
Average total aid package	$39,332
Average debt	$123,078

STATE UNIVERISTY OF NEW YORK—UNIVERSITY AT BUFFALO
SCHOOL OF MEDICINE AND BIOMEDICAL SCIENCES

131 BEB, BUFFALO, NY 14214-3013 • ADMISSION: 716-829-3466 • FAX: 716-829-38497
E-MAIL: JJROSSO@BUFFALO.EDU • WEBSITE: MEDICINE.BUFFALO.EDU

STUDENT BODY

Type	Public
Enrollment of medical school	575
% male/female	48/52
% out-of-state	16
% international	7
Average age of entering class	23

ADMISSIONS

# applied	3,824
% accepted	10
% enrolled	36

Average GPA and MCAT Scores

Overall GPA	3.7
MCAT Bio	10.4
MCAT Phys	10.1
MCAT Verbal	10.2
MCAT Essay	P

Application Information

Regular application	11/15
Regular notification	10/15
Early application	8/1
Early notification	10/1
Are transfers accepted?	No
Admissions may be deferred?	Yes
Admissions need-blind?	No
Application fee	$65

Academics

In addition to the M.D., the School of Medicine and Biomedical Sciences awards the Ph.D., M.A., M.S., and the combined M.D./Ph.D. There are four M.S.T.P.-sponsored M.D./Ph.D. positions available each year. Departments awarding graduate degrees include: Anatomy, Biochemistry, Biophysics, Cell Biology, Genetics, Immunology, Microbiology, Molecular Biology, Neuroscience, Pathology, Pharmacology, and Physiology. A new joint-degree program, leading to the M.D./M.B.A. began in 1997. Evaluation of medical students uses Honors/Pass/Fail. Passing the USMLE Step 1 is required before matriculants can enter third year.

BASIC SCIENCES: Basic sciences are taught through a combination of lectures, labs, small group sessions, problem-based learning and clinical experiences. On average, students are in class or scheduled sessions for about 20 hours per week. First-year courses are: Gross Anatomy; Biochemistry; Human Behavior; Histology; Embryology; Physiology; Neuroscience, Medical Genetics; Scientific Basis of Medicine; Social and Preventive Medicine; and Clinical Practice of Medicine, which provides early patient-contact experiences. Second-year courses are: Hematology; Pathology; Microbiology; Pharmacology; Scientific Basis of Medicine; Social and Preventive Medicine; Genetics; Human Behavior; and the continuation of Clinical Practice of Medicine. Summer externships, which allow up to 60 first- and second-year medical students to shadow primary care physicians are available with stipends. Stipends are also available on a limited basis for summer research projects. The Health Sciences Library features a Media Resources Center with approximately 2,000 multimedia items, a History of Medicine Collection with 12,000 volumes, and a comprehensive general medicine/scientific book and journal collection.

CLINICAL TRAINING

Third-year required rotations are: Internal Medicine (8 weeks); Surgery (8 weeks); Ob/Gyn (7 weeks); Pediatrics (7 weeks); Psychiatry (7 weeks); and Family Medicine (7 weeks). The Family Medicine Clerkship includes six sessions in a community-based family physician's office, two sessions in a problem-based learning format, one session focusing on a community project, and one session devoted to independent learning. During the third year, students also choose a week-long seminar from diverse selective offerings. Fourth-year requirements are four weeks each of Neurology, Medicine, and Surgery, and four weeks of an ambulatory experience. Four-year electives are also available. Training takes place at: The Buffalo General Hospital; Children's Hospital of Buffalo; Erie County Medical Center; Mercy Hospital; Millard Fillmore Health System; Sisters of Charity Hospital; Roswell Park Cancer Institute; and the Buffalo VA Medical Center. The Community Academic Practice Program identifies community-based sites for clinical training. With faculty approval, up to 16 weeks of electives may be taken at other academic institutions.

Students

Approximately 30-35 students in each class are Out of State residents. About 20 percent of entering students are over 25 years old. Approximately 5 percent of students are underrepresented minorities. Class size is 140.

STUDENT LIFE

The first year begins with a relaxed orientation week that allows students to get acquainted with each other and their new surroundings. Several student centers serve as focal points for student life on campus. The Student Union houses more than 75 clubs and organizations in addition to recreational facilities, dining areas, and a theater. The Oasis Recreation Center features pool tables, music, and a TV room. The Harriman Student Activities Center is an alternate student union, and the Creative Craft Center provides ongoing craft programs and courses. The Living Well Center (LWC) is dedicated to improving students' overall health and wellness. It offers a range of services to students, including counseling, health education, fitness assessments, seminars on personal health issues, relaxation services such as massage, and special events with outside speakers. For medical students, the LWC also provides opportunities for volunteer work in areas related to preventive medicine. Buffalo is an affordable and student-friendly community. Residence Halls and graduate student apartments are available close to campus.

GRADUATES

Among graduates in a recent class, the most prevalent specialty fields were: Internal Medicine (28%); Pediatrics (25%); Family Practice (15%); Ob/Gyn (10%); Surgery (11%); and Emergency Medicine (5%). Approximately half of graduates entered residency programs in New York State.

Admissions

REQUIREMENTS

Prerequisites are Biology (two semesters); Chemistry (four semesters, including two of Organic Chemistry); Physics (two semesters); and English (two semesters). The MCAT is required, and must be from after 2007. For applicants who have taken the exam on multiple occasions, the best set of scores is generally considered. Thus, there is no advantage in withholding scores.

SUGGESTIONS

In addition to science requirements, two years of course work in Social Sciences and one year in the Humanities are advised. For applicants who have taken time off after college, some recent course work is recommended. Medically related experience is important.

PROCESS

All applicants are sent secondary applications. Between 600 and 700 applicants are interviewed from August through April. These candidates are selected from a pool of about 4,300, meaning that about 15 percent of applicants make it to the interview stage. Interviews consist of two sessions each with a faculty member or medical student. On interview day, there are also group informational sessions, a campus tour, and the opportunity to have lunch with current medical students. The first acceptance letters are mailed in October, with subsequent batches of letters sent at 4-6-week intervals throughout the year. Approximately 20 percent of interviewees are accepted initially. Others are rejected or placed on a wait-list. Supplementary material from wait-listed candidates is not encouraged. Usually 60 percent of interviewees are eventually offered an acceptance before orientation begins.

Admissions Requirements (Required)
MCAT Scores, Essays, Science GPA, Recommendation, Interview

Admissions Requirements (Optional)
Extracurricular activities, Non-Science GPA, Exposure to medical profession, State Residency

COSTS AND AID

Tuition & Fees

Annual tuition (in-state out-of-state)	$27,000/$55,000
Room & board	$8,000
Cost of books	$4,000
Fees	$1,300

Financial Aid

% students receiving any aid	85
Average grant	$2,000
Average loan	$40,000

STONY BROOK UNIVERSITY

STONY BROOK UNIVERSITY, SCHOOL OF MEDICINE

COMMITTEE ON ADMISSIONS, LEVEL 4, ROOM 147, HEALTH SCIENCES, STONY BROOK, NY 11794
ADMISSION: 631-444-2113 • FAX: 631-444-60327 • E-MAIL: SOMADMISSIONS@STONYBROOKMEDICINE.EDU
WEBSITE: HTTP://MEDICINE.STONYBROOKMEDICINE.EDU

STUDENT BODY	
Type	Public
Enrollment of parent institution	27,000
Enrollment of medical school	506
% male/female	55/45
% out-of-state	5
% international	13
Average age of entering class	24

FACULTY	
Total faculty	808
% part-time faculty	13

ADMISSIONS	
# applied	5,196
% accepted	7
% enrolled	36

Average GPA and MCAT Scores	
Overall GPA	3.7
MCAT Bio	11.0
MCAT Phys	11.0
MCAT Verbal	10.0
MCAT Essay	P

Application Information	
Regular application	12/1
Regular notification	10/15
Early application	8/1
Early notification	10/1
Are transfers accepted?	Yes
Admissions may be deferred?	Yes
Admissions need-blind?	No
Application fee	$100

Academics

Most students earn the M.D. degree in four years. Students who engage in relevant projects or course work may be eligible for The Scholarly Concentrations Program, which is a four-year track opportunity for medical students to engage in and attain recognition for scholarly pursuits in related areas of medicine. A combined M.D./ Ph.D. program is offered as part of the M.S.T.P. The doctorate degree may be earned in Anatomy, Biochemistry, Biomedical Engineering, Cell Biology, Genetics, Immunology, Microbiology, Molecular Biology, Neuroscience, Pathology, Pharmacology, and Physiology. Medical students are evaluated with Honors/Pass/Fail and must take both steps of the USMLE in order to graduate. There is also a combined MD/MPH and MD/ MBA track.

CLINICAL TRAINING

Stony Brook School of Medicine curriculum will provide the opportunity for extensive and integrated training in the basic medical sciences and clinical disciplines of medicine. The curriculum includes three phases. Phase one begins with an orientation and transition course and then a six month course which covers the basic building blocks of medicine: anatomy with an introduction to radiology and orthopaedics, biochemistry, genetics, cell biology, cellular physiology, basic principles of pharmacology and pathogens and host defense mechanisms. The next twelve months of phase one are spent learning an organ systems-based approach to pathophysiology and therapeutics. Themes in medical education are also spread throughout this phase. They include such topics as medical ethics, health maintenance and prevention, patient safety and an introduction to clinical medicine. Phase one provides time for a summer vacation and/ or research/global health studies. It also provides structured time to prepare for USMLE Step 1. Phase two spans one year and includes the core clerkships: internal medicine, primary care medicine, pediatrics, obstetrics and gynecology, surgery, emergency medicine, anesthesiology, neurology, psychiatry and radiology. Phase three represents the transition to residency. This phase includes a subinternship requirement, an advanced clinical experience, a transition to residency course and electives. This phase is to create a well-rounded medical student who is also specifically prepared for the rigors of their specialty choice. Throughout phases two and three, are translational pillars which are designed to integrate basic medical sciences with the clinical phases.

Students

Typically, approximately 75 percent of students are New York residents. About 16–17 percent are underrepresented minorities. Class size is 124.

STUDENT LIFE

Stony Brook is located on the North Shore of Long Island, just over an hour's train ride from Manhattan. Students enjoy both the comfort of their school's suburban location and its proximity to NYC. The campus offers a vast sports complex,recreation center and the immediate area offers bike trails, beaches, and parks. The Stony Brook Student Activities Bldg. is the campus center for hundreds of activities. On-campus child care is available to students. University-owned housing includes residence halls and several apartment complexes with units of all sizes. Most students own cars, which are particularly important during the clinical years.

GRADUATES

Close to 40% of the graduating Class of 2013 entered primary care specialities (family practice, general pediatrics, general internal medicine and ob/gyn).

Admissions

REQUIREMENTS

Academic prerequisites commencing with the 2015 entering class are: Biology—2 semesters with lab, one of which should include a course in cell biology or genetics; Chemistry—minimum of 4 semesters including coursework in general and organic chemistry with lab and a course in biochemistry; English/Writing—1 semester; Physics—1 semester with lab; Social Science/Humanities—1 semester of either psychology, sociology, logic or ethics, or anthropology; Statistics—1 semester Advanced Placement (AP) credit will be considered for a course in which the applicant achieved a score of 4 or 5. AP credit not to exceed one course in a specific discipline. Applicants may be invited for an interview prior to fulfilling all the requirements. These requirements must be satisfactorily completed in full prior to matriculation into the School of Medicine. Applicants offered an acceptance who lack any of these requirements will be required to complete the course(s) with a grade of C or better prior to matriculation. The MCAT is required, and scores must be no more than 5 years old. For applicants who have taken the exam more than once, the best scores are considered.

SUGGESTIONS

Applicants who have taken significant time off after college should have some recent course work. For all applicants, some medically related experience is important, and patient contact is particularly valued.

PROCESS

All AMCAS applicants receive secondary applications. About 13 percent are interviewed between September and March. Two interviews are conducted with members of the Admissions Committee in addition to a group orientation session, tour, and the opportunity to meet with current medical students. About 50 percent of interviewed candidates are accepted, with notification occurring on a rolling basis. An alternate admissions path is through the Bachelors/Medical Scholars for Medicine Program, which admits a limited number of high school students into an eight-year combined program at the University. In addition, seven post-bacc programs, including Bryn Mawr, Johns Hopkins, Stony Brook, NYU, Queens, Hunter, and Columbia have admission arrangements with Stony Brook through a linkage program.

Admissions Requirements (Required)

MCAT Scores, Essays, Science GPA, Extracurricular activities, Non-Science GPA, Exposure to medical profession, Recommendation, Interview

Admissions Requirements (Optional)

State Residency

COSTS AND AID

Tuition & Fees

Annual tuition (in-state out-of-state)	$32,190/$57,380
Room & board	$11,413
Fees	2,670

Financial Aid

% students receiving any aid	83
% students receiving grants	25
% students receiving loans	67
% aid that is merit-based	83
Average debt	$148,35

TEMPLE UNIVERSITY

TEMPLE UNIVERSITY SCHOOL OF MEDICINE

3500 NORTH BROAD STREET, MERB, SUITE 124 PHILADELPHIA, PA 19140 • ADMISSION: 215-707-3656
FAX: 215-707-69327 • E-MAIL: MEDADMISSIONS@TEMPLE.EDU • WEBSITE: WWW.TEMPLE.EDU / MEDICINE

Academics

The academic program has options that appeal to all students, be they interested in research and/or intensive clinical training. Summer research projects in both basic and clinical sciences are encouraged and are often funded. Qualified students may pursue an MPH, MBA or PhD concurrently with an MD. PhD degrees may be obtained in Biomedical Sciences with a concentration in one of the following areas: Cancer Biology and Genetics, Infectious Diseases and Immunity, Molecular and Cellular Biosciences, Neuroscience, or Organ Systems and Translational Medicine. Temple's system of student evaluation uses Honors/Pass/Fail in the first two years and Honors/High Pass/Pass/Fail in the third and fourth year. A grade of Pass or higher is required for promotion, and passing both steps of the USMLE and an internally-administered Objective Structured Clinical Examination are graduation requirements.

BASIC SCIENCES: During the first two years, students are assigned to basic science faculty advisors who are available to discuss academic matters as well as personal issues. Students are in class for about 25 hours per week, with about half of scheduled sessions utilizing a lecture format. Other instructional methods include small-group discussions, labs, patient simulators and interactive clinical training. All formal classes are held in the morning, with afternoon hours used for workshops and the Doctoring course. The curriculum was modified in August 2006 to a hybrid organ-based curriculum. First-year blocks cover Human Gross Anatomy, Elements of Bioscience, Biological Systems 1 (Cardiovascular, Pulmonary, Gastrointestinal and Urinary), Biological Systems 2 (Integument, Musculoskeletal, Endocrine and Reproductive), Biological Systems 3 (Neuroscience), and Introduction to Principles of Immunology, Pathology, and Pharmacology. Doctoring 1 and a choice of electives runs throughout the year. Second-year blocks cover Microbiology of Infectious Diseases, Diseases of the Cardiovascular and Respiratory Systems, Diseases of the Endocrine, Reproductive and Renal Systems, Diseases of the Nervous System, and Diseases of the Gastrointestinal System, Hematology/Oncology, and Musculoskeletal System. Doctoring 2 and a choice of electives run concurrently. Students are evaluated based on a series of internal exams, National Board-style exams and standardized patient exams.

CLINICAL TRAINING

Students are introduced to clinic medicine in the first two years, in our Doctoring course, in which students learn to take a medical history, perform a physical examination, and receive training in medical ethics and professionalism. Clinical skills are learned through use of patient simulators, standardized patients and real patient encounters. In the third year, students are assigned to a clinical faculty advisor who assists with decisions about clinical electives and post-graduate training. Third-year required rotations are Internal Medicine (8 weeks); Surgery (8 weeks); Ob/Gyn (6 weeks); Pediatrics (6 weeks); Family Medicine (6 weeks); Psychiatry (6 weeks); Neurology (4 weeks); and an Elective (4 weeks). During the fourth year, 20 weeks of electives are required, in addition to clerkships in Emergency Medicine (4 weeks), Radiology (4 weeks), and a subinternship in medicine (4 weeks). Students may choose from 2 of the following 3 for additional clerkships in critical care, a surgical subspecialty, or an additional subinternship in Internal Medicine, Pediatrics, Surgery, Family Medicine, Obstetrics-Gynecology or Psychiatry. Training takes place at the Temple University Hospital, Temple Episcopal Hospital, St. Christopher's Hospital for Children, and affiliated hospitals including Abington

Memorial Hospital and Fox Chase Cancer Center. Clinical Campus students complete the third and fourth year of medical training at Crozer-Chester Medical Center in Upland, Geisinger Medical Center in Danville or West Penn Allegheny Health System in Pittsburgh. A regional campus has been established at St. Luke's Hospital in Bethlehem which has students completing the first year of medical school at Temple in Philadelphia and the second, third and fourth years at St. Luke's in Bethlehem.

Students

Approximately 50 percent of students are Pennsylvania residents. About 15 percent of students are underrepresented in medicine. In particular, Temple has a strong contingent of African American and Latino students. Class size is 210. The Ginsburg Health Sciences Library supports education, patient care, and research at Temple, providing access to a variety of online and print materials and offering extensive space for individual study, collaborative learning, and information instruction. An 11 story, 480,000 square foot academic and research building opened in 2009.

STUDENT LIFE

Temple students benefit from rich extracurricular offerings both on and off campus. Both Temple Medical School and the main Temple campus have comprehensive athletic and recreational facilities. Medical students are active in school governance, and are members of the Curriculum, Financial Affairs, and Admissions Committees. A special support program is designed primarily for groups underrepresented in medicine, but is open to all students. There are numerous student organizations that range from community outreach to political advocacy to specialty interest groups. Philadelphia is a historically and culturally rich city. It is also a very student-friendly city, where medical students in particular abound. Students live off campus in a variety of neighborhoods within and close to Philadelphia.

GRADUATES

About forty percent of Temple's graduates enter residency programs in Pennsylvania. Among students graduating in 2013, the most prevalent of the 26 specialties chosen were Internal Medicine (21%); Emergency Medicine (14%); Family Medicine (10%); Pediatrics (7%); Anesthesiology (7%)Radiology (7%); Surgery (5%); and Neurology (4%).

Admissions

REQUIREMENTS

1 year each (with lab) of biology, chemistry, organic chemistry, and physics are required as well as 6 semester hours of humanities. The MCAT is required, and scores must be no more than three years old.

SUGGESTIONS

As a state-related school, Temple strongly considers Pennsylvania residents, although a significant number of out-of-state applicants are admitted. For applicants who have been out of school for a period of time, recent course work is important. The spring, rather than August/September, MCAT is advised. Medically-related and community-service activities are valued, and the Admissions Committee is serious about selecting students who will make supportive class members and caring physicians.

PROCESS

All "complete" applications are reviewed by a member of the Admissions Committee. There is no absolute cutoff for MCAT scores and GPAs. All applicants are sent secondary application material, and about 20 percent of those completing their application are invited to interview. Interviews take place between September and April and applicants will meet with a faculty member as well as a medical student. Applicants also meet with the Admissions Director, a representative of the Office of Student Financial Services, and take the campus tour and have lunch with second year medical students. About one-third of interviewees are accepted, with notification occurring on a rolling basis.

Admissions Requirements (Required)

MCAT Scores, Essays, Science GPA, Extracurricular activities, Non-Science GPA, Exposure to medical profession, Recommendation, Interview

Admissions Requirements (Optional)

State Residency

COSTS AND AID

Tuition & Fees

Annual tuition (in-state out-of-state)	$43,654/$53,468
Room & board	$13,180/$0
Cost of books	$1,700
Fees	$750

Financial Aid

% students receiving any aid	94
% students receiving grants	44
% students receiving loans	88
% aid that is merit-based	25
Average grant	$9,547
Average loan	$56,831
Average total aid package	$57,932
Average debt	$208,122

Texas A&M Health Science Center

Texas A&M Health Science Center College of Medicine

3050 Health Professions Education Bldg, 8447 State Highway 47 Bryan, TX 77807
Admission: 979-436-0237 • Fax: 409-436-00977 • E-mail: ADMISSIONS@MEDICINE.TAMHSC.EDU
Website: WWW.MEDICINE.TAMHSC.EDU

STUDENT BODY

Type	Public
Enrollment of parent institution	2,122
Enrollment of medical school	633
% male/female	54/46
% out-of-state	6
% international	45
Average age of entering class	24

FACULTY

Total faculty	1,876
% female faculty	30
% minority faculty	26
% part-time faculty	9
Student-faculty ratio	1.0:1

ADMISSIONS

# applied	2,635
% accepted	20
% enrolled	38

Average GPA and MCAT Scores

Overall GPA	3.6
MCAT Bio	10.2
MCAT Phys	9.6
MCAT Verbal	9.2
MCAT Essay	Q

Application Information

Regular application	10/1
Regular notification	11/15
Early application	5/1
Early notification	10/15
Are transfers accepted?	Yes
Admissions may be deferred?	Yes
Admissions need-blind?	Yes
Application fee	$75

Academics

Students may pursue a joint MD/PhD in conjunction with graduate departments of the Health Science Center in the following fields: Biochemistry and Structural Biology, Bioengineering and Biomedical Imaging, Cell and Developmental Biology, Genetics and Genomics, Immunology, Microbiology and Infectious Diseases, Molecular Biology, Neuroscience, Physiology and Biophysics, and Space Life Sciences. MD Plus is a new pathway for students who are interested in pursuing a Master of Science or a Master of Public Health at the Bryan, Houston, or Temple campuses. The MD Plus program of study typically begins in the summer semester one year prior to beginning medical school at the College of Medicine. Students are considered only after acceptance to the College of Medicine.

BASIC SCIENCES: The focus of the medical curriculum is an enhanced level of integration of material that is taught to students in the first two years. Students in the curriculum do not take separate courses in the traditional basic science disciplines of gross anatomy, biochemistry, genetics, physiology, histology, microbiology, immunology, pharmacology, pathology and neuroscience. Rather, this material is appropriately organized into integrated blocks of instruction of three to 10 weeks in duration depending on the theme of the block. Grades are issued for the individual blocks and not the separate disciplines taught within the blocks. Students are required to take and pass National Board of Medical Examiners (NBME) Customized Comprehensive Exams at various points in the program that include questions in all medical science disciplines taught in the structured phases of the curriculum. A second critical focus of the curriculum is a revised approach to how students are taught clinical skills particularly in the first year. Students learn physical diagnosis techniques earlier in the first year than in previous iterations of the curriculum. The organization of the curriculum during the first two years consists of two phases as follows: Phase I begins when students start the first year of medical school and continues through the end of December (6 months). Phase I emphasizes the basic structure of the human body and basic principles of other medical science disciplines including gross anatomy, histology, biochemistry, genetics, pharmacology and cell-physiology. Additionally, courses are taught in medical humanities and ethics; clinical skills, including patient history and doctor-patient communication skills. Phase II begins in early January of the following calendar year, continues through the entire second year and concludes the following spring (18 months) with a summer break after the first two blocks of Phase II are completed. Phase II covers normal function and disease-related aspects of the specific organ systems including the treatment of these diseases, specifically organ-based physiology, organ system/disease-related topics in biochemistry and genetics, pathology, microbiology, immunology, pharmacology and medicine. The Office of Student Affairs in conjunction with the Academic Enhancement Program coordinates tutoring activities for students facing academic difficulty. Tutoring is also available from professors and qualified upperclassmen, and academic consultation and counseling are provided by an educational specialist in the Office of Academic Support Services. During the third and fourth years, students select a faculty advisor with whom they can meet and discuss choices of electives, residency training and career opportunities. Study facilities include academic and clinical libraries at all campus communities, Learning Resources, a student-centered hub that provides study space and curriculum materials in 24-hour facilities on the Temple and Bryan-College Station campuses. Students have access to computers, HSC Wi-Fi, rquired and recommended curriculum materials, as well as other electronic and print educational resources. Media, Blackboard and other staff specialists will answer questions and provide assistance in using equipment and resources. Evaluation of performance during years one and two uses an A-F scale. Passing the USMLE Step 1 is required for promotion to year three. The passing rate for Texas A&M Medical Students exceeds the national average.

CLINICAL TRAINING

Patient contact begins in year one. Students learn physical diagnosis techniques and clinical skills including patient history taking and doctor-patient communication skills. In addition to covering normal function and disease-related aspects of the specific organ systems, including the treatment of disease in year two, students participte regularly in the preceptorship for Primary Care program. Early informal patient contact is also possible for those who engage in certain community service or volunteer activities. Year three begins with a week-long orientation, followed by required rotations: Ob/Gyn (6 weeks); Pediatrics (6 weeks); Family Medicine (6 weeks); Psychiatry (6 weeks); Internal Medicine (12 weeks); and Surgery (12 weeks). Year four consists of 24 weeks of electives plus five required clerkships: Acting Intership (4 weeks); Emergency Medicine (4 weeks); Intensive Care (4 weeks); Alcohol and Drug Dependence (2 weeks); and Professionalism (2 weeks). Training takes place at several patient care venues, including Austin, Bryan-College Station, Corpus Christi, Dallas, Houston, Round Rock and Temple. Libraries are available for third- and fourth-year students at all of our campus communities. During year three, students are evaluated by using an A-F scale. During year four, most rotations are evaluated with Pass/Fail. Passing the USMLE Step 2 is required for graduation. The curriculum allows for a highly personalized medical education from the onset. Students interact one-on-one with basic science teaching faculty, physicians and patients early in the first and second phases of instruction and, therefore, use these close interactions to build the skills and confidence necessary for the applied and advanced core principles of medicine in the later phases of training. Another important dimension of clinical training is clinical simulation. Clinical simulation provides students with immediat feedback, repetitive practice, curriculum integration, adapted learning, individualized learning, reflective learning and the opportunity to learn from mistakes without risk. SIM facilities are available at all campus communities.

Students

Ninety to ninety-five percent of students are from Texas. About 24 percent percent of students are underrepresented minorities, most of whom are Hispanic and Black/African American. About 77 percent of new entrants have majors in the biomedical sciences.

STUDENT LIFE

Central to the extraordinary educational experience, COM students enjoy individual attention and a family-like atmosphere. This intimacy generates comraderie and loyalty evident in all phases of student life—academic, professional, recreational, and community service. Community service has always been a priority for students at the COM. Each class chooses to support different human service organizations throughout the year, thereby focusing their energy and enthusiasm on a variety of cases withing the community, the state and beyond. These organizations allow students to grow through leadership, teamwork, and participation. Within the COM are many opportunities for students to express themselves and to demonstrate a variety of talents and interests far beyond classrooms and laboratories. This added dimension to a challenging academic regimen plays a vital role in the development of well rounded individuals and physicians.

GRADUATES

Of those who graduated recently, the following residencies were the most popular: Family Practice; Internal Medicine; Pediatrics; and General Surgery. Half of the graduates enter residency training programs at University-affiliated hospitals aross the state and country.

Admissions

REQUIREMENTS

The College of Medicine considers for enrollment individuals who have completed at least 90 credit hours of undergraduate course work. By state mandate, enrollment of out-of-state residents may not exceed 10 percent.

Admissions Requirements (Required)

MCAT Scores, Essays, Science GPA, Non-Science GPA, Recommendation, Interview, State Residency

Admissions Requirements (Optional)

Extracurricular activities, Exposure to medical profession

COSTS AND AID

Tuition & Fees

Annual tuition (in-state out-of-state)	$12,350/$25,450
Room & board	$13,085
Cost of books	$12,197
Fees	$2,687

Financial Aid

% students receiving any aid	88
% students receiving grants	49
% students receiving loans	83
% aid that is merit-based	5
Average grant	$3,818
Average loan	$29,375
Average total aid package	$29,648
Average debt	$104,390

TEXAS TECH UNIVERSITY

TEXAS TECH UNIVERSITY HEALTH SCIENCES CENTER SCHOOL OF MEDICINE

3601 4TH STREET, MS 6216 LUBBOCK, TX 79430 • ADMISSION: 806-743-2297 • FAX: 806-743-27257
E-MAIL: SOMADM@TTUHSC.EDU • WEBSITE: WWW.TTUHSC.EDU / SOM / ADMISSIONS

STUDENT BODY

Type	Public
Enrollment of parent institution	571
Enrollment of medical school	579
% male/female	55/45
% underrepresented minorities	4
% out-of-state	11
% international	57
# countries represented	12
Average age of entering class	23

FACULTY

Total faculty	388
% female faculty	37
% minority faculty	32
% part-time faculty	35

ADMISSIONS

# applied	3,364
% accepted	4
% enrolled	100

Average GPA and MCAT Scores

Overall GPA	3.7
MCAT Bio	10.8
MCAT Phys	10.4
MCAT Verbal	9.8
MCAT Essay	0

Application Information

Regular application	10/1
Regular notification	2/1
Early application	8/1
Early notification	10/1
Are transfers accepted?	Yes
Admissions may be deferred?	Yes
Admissions need-blind?	No
Application fee	$50

Academics

Most students complete a four-year curriculum designed to prepare physicians with a broad base of medical knowledge and sound analytic and problem-solving skills. It is organized in two stages—basic science and clinical training. Some students devote an additional year to research and earn the M.D. degree in five years. Others are involved in summer research projects. Qualified students interested in Biomedical research or academic medicine can earn a Ph.D. along with the M.D. degree. To address the needs of a rapidly changing health care system, students can participate in an M.D./M.B.A. joint-degree program in which both degrees are earned in four years. Medical students are graded on a categorical system and pass for promotion and graduation.

BASIC SCIENCES: First-year courses are Clinicall Oriented Anatomy; History of Cells and Tissues; Structure of Major Organ Systems; Host Defense and Early Clinical Experience I. Second-year courses are General Principles & Integrated; Multisystem Disorders and Cancer; System Disorders I; Systems Disorders II and Life Span Issues; Basic Medical Spanish, and Early Clinical Experience II. During the first and second years, instruction primarily uses block system format. However, some concepts are addressed in small-group sessions. Students are in classes or other scheduled sessions for about 20 hours per week. All instruction takes place in the new academic classroom facility with wireless technology on the Lubbock campus.

CLINICAL TRAINING

Third-year required rotations are Internal Medicine (8 weeks); Surgery (8 weeks); Pediatrics (8 weeks); Family Medicine (8 weeks); Ob/Gyn (8 weeks); and Psychiatry (8 weeks). Fourth-year requirements are Neurology (4 weeks); Selectives (8 weeks); a Subinternship (16 weeks); and 20 weeks of electives. After successful completion of years one and two, approximately one-third of fist year students go on to Amarillo, Permian-Basin or Lubbock for clinical training. Amarillo, Permian-Basin (Odessa) and Lubbock all serve both urban and rural populations. Multiple clinical affiliations of each site provide a wealth of training opportunities for students. In Lubbock, students benefit from recreational and cultural opportunities available on the Texas Tech University campus of the main University. The primary teaching hospital is University Medical Center and Covanant Healthcare. Amarillo provides exposure to medicine primarily from a private hospital perspective. Teaching hospitals include Northwest Texas Health Care System, Baptist-St. Anthony Health Care System, and Veterans Administration Hospital.

Students

The 2011 entering class had the following characteristics: 90% Texas residents; 10% are non-residents; 12% underrepresented minorities; 85% science majors. Class size is 150.

STUDENT LIFE

During their first two years, students benefit from the resources of the Health Sciences Center and from being adjacent to Texas Tech University, a major undergraduate institution. Medical students are supportive of one another, as demonstrated by a student-initiated, peer-tutoring program. First-and second-year students are often involved in community service projects, which provide early clinical exposure. Student life during the third and fourth years varies according to location.

GRADUATES

Approximately 21 percent of graduates enter Texas Tech residency programs, which operate on all three campuses. Others are successful in obtaining positions throughout Texas and at institutions acrpss the entire country. Graduates are highly competitive and match with one of their top three residency choices.

Admissions

REQUIREMENTS

Requirements are Biology (12 semester hours); Biology lab (2 semester hours); General Chemistry with lab (8 semester hours); Organic Chemistry with lab (8 semester hours); Physics with lab (8 semester hours); English (6 semester hours), Biochemistry (3 semester hours) and Statitics (3 semester hours). All prerequisite courses require a grade of C or better. The MCAT is required, and should be taken within the past five years. For applicants who have taken the exam more than once, the best set of scores is weighed most heavily, but all scores must be reported. Texas residents and residents of neighboring counties in New Mexico and Oklahoma, which comprise the service areas of the school, are given preference in admission. Only nonresident applicants with GPAs of 3.60 or higher, and MCAT scores of 30 or higher will be considered for admission.

SUGGESTIONS

In addition to high intellectual ability and a record of strong academic achievement, the committee looks for qualities and traits, such as compassion, motivation, communication skills, maturity, and personal integrity.

PROCESS

Texas Tech participates in AMCAS application for the MD/PHD and JD/MD programs. Texas Tech participates with eight other state-supported medical schools in the Texas Medical and Dental Schools Application Service (TMDSAS). A single application is sent to TMDSAS for processing and then is forwarded to any or all of the participating schools as requested by the applicant. A secondary application is also required by Texas Tech. Both applications will be available via the internet. Texas Medical and Dental Schools Application Service, 702 Colorado Street, Suite 6400, Austin, TX 78701 receives all applications for all medical schools. Applicants are interviewed between August and December. Interviews consist of two sessions, each with an admissions clinical or basic science committee member. On interview day, applicants tour the campus, attend orientation, meet current students in person and in a panel format session. Early notification offers begin on October 15th with the dual-degree programs. It continues with a pre-match rolling-admissions basis from November 15th through December 30th. The Match process for any open seats is conducted on February 1st. Offers are made until the class is filled on a rolling admissions basis.

Admissions Requirements (Required)

MCAT Scores, Essays, Science GPA, Extracurricular activities, Non-Science GPA, Exposure to medical profession, Recommendation, Interview

Admissions Requirements (Optional)

State Residency

COSTS AND AID

Tuition & Fees

Annual tuition	$27,150
Cost of books	$1,271
Fees	$2,132

Financial Aid

% students receiving any aid	85
Average grant	$1,600
Average loan	$20,084
Average total aid package	$35,000
Average debt	$100,00

THOMAS JEFFERSON UNIVERSITY

JEFFERSON MEDICAL COLLEGE

1015 WALNUT STREET, ROOM 110, PHILADELPHIA, PA 19107 • ADMISSION: 215-955-6983 • FAX: 215-955-51517
E-MAIL: JMC.ADMISSIONS@JEFFERSON.EDU • WEBSITE: WWW.JEFFERSON.EDU/JMC

STUDENT BODY

Type	Private
Enrollment of parent institution	3,730
Enrollment of medical school	1,053
% male/female	49/51
% underrepresented minorities	5
% out-of-state	52
% international	35
# countries represented	37
Average age of entering class	23

FACULTY

Total faculty	2,672
% female faculty	29
% minority faculty	6
Student-faculty ratio	2.5:1

ADMISSIONS

# applied	10,018
% accepted	5
% enrolled	55

Average GPA and MCAT Scores

Overall GPA	3.7
MCAT Bio	11.1
MCAT Phys	10.8
MCAT Verbal	10.1
MCAT Essay	Q

Application Information

Regular application	11/15
Early application	6/1
Early notification	10/1
Are transfers accepted?	Yes
Admissions may be deferred?	Yes
Admissions need-blind?	No
Application fee	$80

Academics

Along with basic science and clinical training, Jefferson's curriculum emphasizes the social and public health issues related to medicine. Students with solid science backgrounds may pursue an MD and a PhD in one of the departments of the College of Graduate Studies. These include: Biochemistry & Molecular Biology, Genetics, Immunology & Microbial Pathologies, joint PhD programs, Molecular Cell Biology, Molecular Pharmacology & Structural Biology, Neuroscience, Physiology, and Tissue Engineering & Regenerative Medicine. A joint MD/MBA degree is offered in conjunction with Widener University in Chester, Pennsylvania, as is a combined MD/Masters in Hospital Administration. A five-year program is available in which Jefferson students have the opportunity to earn an MPH at the Jefferson School of Public and Population Health while earning their MD degree at Jefferson Medical College. This program is offered to students with special interests such as community health and in recognition of the increasing importance of population medicine. Pennsylvania State University and Jefferson Medical College allow students to pursue a combined B.S./MD program, which grants both degrees in a six- or seven-year period. In 2012, Thomas Jefferson University started its own post-bacc program, through which highly qualified students may be admitted to Jefferson prior to completion of their premedical requirements.

BASIC SCIENCES: We believe that the first year of medical school sets the stage for at least the first four years of medical education, if not for ones entire professional career. During this year, Jefferson students focus on the structure and function of the human organisim in its physical and psychosocial context. Course work in the basic sciences of human gross anatomy, cell biology, and microscopic anatomy, biochemistry, genetics, neuroscience, and physiology provides first-year sturdents with a strong basic science grounding. Practice related topics such as medical informatcs, evidence-based medicine, health policy and ethics are also introduced during the first year. Clinical coursework focuses on the patient-doctor relationship, medical interviewing, and history-taking, the human developmental trajectory, and behavioral science principles. This curricula provides students with both a behavioral science foundation and a clinical framework; it establishes an educational bridge between lay perspectives and the realities of medical practice. In addition to increasing emphasis on the study of "bedside" skills, the curriculum shifts in the second year to the study of pathophysiology and disease. After an introductory block of general pathology and general pharmacology, the subjects of immunology, microbiology, and systems-based pharmacology, pathology, physical diagnosis, and clinical medicine are presented as an interdisciplinary curriculum. The curriculum includes small group sessions focusing on the problem-solving evidence-based medicine and service based learning. Grades are Honors/Pass/Fail. Pre-clinical studies take place in the central Medical College building complex, which includes administrative offices, labs, lecture halls, common areas, and recreational facilities. The Scott Library includes 200,000 print volumes, a Learning Resources Center and computer labs in addition to videos, slides, and supplemental learning materials. MEDLINE and other electronic data systems are available, as well as more than 500 electronic journals and books. The Dorrance H. Hamilton Building opened in 2007 and includes three floors of clinical simulation.

CLINICAL TRAINING

Patient contact officially begins in Year One, with Medical Practice in the 21st century. There are also ongoing opportunities for medical students interested in volunteer clinical experience or clinical research through summer programs and part-time jobs. Formally, the clinical portion of the curriculum begins in year three with required rotations. These are: Family Medicine (6 weeks); Surgery (6 weeks general, 6 weeks surgical subspecialties); Pediatrics (6 weeks); Psychiatry and Human Behavior (6 weeks); and Ob/Gyn (6 weeks). Phase II of clinical rotations are selectives in which students choose specialties within broadly defined categories. Sixteen weeks are also designated as purely elective. Training sites include: Albert Einstein Medical Center; Abingotn Hospital; Aria Health System; Bryn Mawr Hospital; Bryn Mawr Rehabilitation Hospital; Christiana Care Medical Center; Chester-Crozier Medical Center; DuPont Hospital for Children; York Hospital and Latrobe Hospital providing rural exposure; Lankenau Hospital; Magee Rehabilitation Hospital; Reading Hospital; Underwood Hospital; Virtua Health System; and Wills Eye Hospital. The patients come from several states and represent extremely diverse populations.

Students

Approximately half the states are represented by the students within a class, mostly those of the eastern part of the country. About 38 percent of the students are Pennsylvania state residents. Applicants underrepresented in medicine make up about nine percent of the first year class. Class size is 260. Approximately 20 percent of each class is over 25 years of age upon matriculation. In recent years, about 5 percent of matriculants have held advanced degrees.

STUDENT LIFE

Numerous professional, athletic, and cultural student organizations exist on campus. Beyond campus, the city of Philadelphia provides ample recreational and cultural possibilities and New York is just over an hour away. On-campus housing options include residence halls and apartments of all sizes; housing is guaranteed to first-year students. With Jefferson's central and urban location, a car is unnecessary in the first two years.

GRADUATES

Approximately 75 percent of Jefferson graduates enter residency programs at University-affiliated hospitals around the nation. Jefferson graduates do very well in the residency-matching program, both in primary care and in more specialized fields.

Admissions

REQUIREMENTS

Required course work is one year of: Biology with lab; Chemistry with lab; Organic Chemistry with lab; and Physics with lab.

SUGGESTIONS

Applicants should demonstrate problem-solving capability, success in a range of subjects, and some in-depth knowledge of one or a few subjects. Strong writing skills are also valued. Experience in a medical or research environment is important. Delaware residents are given preference, as are applicants from programs that have special arrangements with Jefferson. Applicants are advised to submit all materials in a timely fashion.

PROCESS

On receipt of the verified AMCAS application, Jefferson will send, via email, notification of receipt. Also included will be instructions for completing the Jefferson Medical College online secondary application with online payment capability. The Committee on Admissions will begin reviewing the application when all supplementary materials have been received including: 1) the Jefferson Medical College Secondary Application Form, 2) the nonrefundable $80 application fee, 3) MCAT scores, and 4) the required letters of recommendation. Interviews are conducted from September through April, and approximately 10 percent of the applicant pool is interviewed. Interviews are 30-45 minutes in length and are conducted by a member of the faculty or administration. Admissions are rolling. Approximately 50 percent of those who interview are accepted. Others are either rejected or wait-listed. When places become available, later in the cycle, wait-listed applicants will be notified and offered positions. Indicating interest in Jefferson may help the prospects of wait-listed candidates.

Admissions Requirements (Required)

MCAT Scores, Essays, Science GPA, Extracurricular activities, Non-Science GPA, Exposure to medical profession, Recommendation, Interview

Admissions Requirements (Optional)

State Residency

COSTS AND AID

Tuition & Fees

Annual tuition	$51,240
Room & board	$17,050
Cost of books	$8,389
Fees	$715

Financial Aid

% students receiving any aid	72
% students receiving grants	66
% students receiving loans	88
% aid that is merit-based	26
Average grant	$9,141
Average loan	$52,100
Average total aid package	$57,208
Average debt	$178,726

TUFTS UNIVERSITY
SCHOOL OF MEDICINE

OFFICE OF ADMISSIONS, 136 HARRISON AVENUE, STEARNS 1, BOSTON, MA 02111 • ADMISSION: 617-636-6571
E-MAIL: SGP@COR.CDM.NEMC. • WEBSITE: WWW.TUFTS.EDU/MED

STUDENT BODY

Type	Private
Enrollment of medical school	695
% male/female	52/48
% out-of-state	66
% international	11
# countries represented	45

ADMISSIONS

# applied	8,207
% accepted	6
% enrolled	35

Average GPA and MCAT Scores

Overall GPA	3.5
MCAT Bio	10.5
MCAT Phys	10.3
MCAT Verbal	9.9

Application Information

Regular application	11/1
Regular notification	10/15
Early application	8/1
Early notification	10/1
Are transfers accepted?	Yes
Admissions need-blind?	Yes
Application fee	$95

Academics

The majority of students follow a four-year curriculum leading to the M.D. degree. Students with an interest in public health have the opportunity to earn an M.P.H. along with their M.D. This combined M.D./M.P.H. program may be completed in four years. Other combined-degree programs include the four year M.D./M.B.A. in Health Management in partnership with Brandeis University and Northeastern University, the M.D./Ph.D. in conjunction with the Sackler School of Graduate Biomedical Sciences, and the B.S. in Engineering and combined M.S./M.D. in Engineering degree program, a collaborative effort of the Tufts College of Engineering and the Tufts University School of Medicine. The doctorate may be earned in the following fields: Anatomy, Biochemistry, Biophysics, Cell Biology, Genetics, Immunology, Microbiology, Molecular Biology, Neuroscience, Pathology, Pharmacology, and Physiology. Each year, four funded M.D./Ph.D. positions are available. A primary care preceptorship program allows students with a particular interest in primary care to experience early patient contact.

BASIC SCIENCES: In addition to required courses, first and second-year students choose among pre-clinical selectives. These are graded as Pass/Fail and allow students to explore their interests early on in the program. A new Principles and Practice of Medicine Program (PPM) was developed to enhance the first- and second-year curriculum. PPM integrates basic science topics with interdisciplinary subjects such as Information Management, Computer Literacy, Negotiation/Team Building Skills, Health Care Economics, and Ethics. PPM also introduces important clinical techniques such as the patient interview, examination, and physical diagnosis. First-year courses are the following: Gross Anatomy; Histology; Biochemistry; Genetics; Epidemiology Biostatistics; Molecular Biology; Physiology; Cell Biology; Immunology; Hematology; Problem-Based Learning; Pre-clinical Selectives; and PPM. Second-year courses are the following: Pathology; Pathophysiology/Infectious Disease; Neuroscience; Psychopathology; Pharmacology; Microbiology; Problem-Based Learning; Addiction Medicine; Pre-clinical Selectives; and PPM, which focuses on clinical skills and serves as an important transition to third-year clerkships. During the first and second years, instruction involves lectures, labs, and small-group sessions. As an important learning aid, Tufts Health Sciences Library developed the Health Sciences Database. It contains the full text of many syllabi, lecture slides, reserve slide collections, lecture recordings, and other multimedia and resource materials.

CLINICAL TRAINING

Third-year required clerkships are the following: Medicine (12 weeks); Surgery (12 weeks); Ob/Gyn (6 weeks); Pediatrics (6 weeks); and Psychiatry (6 weeks). About four weeks are available for elective study during the third year. Fourth-year requirements are a 4-week primary care clerkship and a 4-week Neurology elective. At least 32 weeks of electives are also required, 20 of which must be completed at Tufts facilities. Twelve weeks of electives may be taken at other academic and clinical institutions. Some students fulfill a portion of elective requirements overseas.

Students

In last year's entering class, about 28 percent of students were Massachusetts residents, and about 14 percent of students went to Tufts as undergraduates. Another 28 percent of students were California residents, and 10 percent were New York residents. Approximately 30 percent of students were at least 23 years old, and 15 percent were 25 or older. Women accounted for 41 percent of the class, and underrepresented minorities accounted for about 11 percent.

STUDENT LIFE

Medical students at Tufts are generally cohesive and supportive of one another. Some students are involved in clubs or in local chapters of national medical student organizations. Off campus, students enjoy the offerings of Boston, a city filled with students, bookstores, coffee shops, restaurants, parks, and cultural activities. Residence facilities are available on a limited basis in Posner Hall, located close to the Medical School campus. Students who live off campus generally share apartments in neighborhoods that are convenient to the School.

GRADUATES

Graduates are successful in securing residency positions at institutions in all regions of the country. Tufts prepares graduates for careers in both primary care and specialty areas.

Admissions

REQUIREMENTS

Requirements are 8 semester credits of Biology, Chemistry, Organic Chemistry, and Physics all with associated labs. Applicants must possess the ability to speak and write English correctly. The MCAT is required, and scores should be from within the past three years. For applicants who have taken the exam on multiple occasions, the best scores are used.

SUGGESTIONS

In addition to prerequisite courses, recommended course work includes Calculus, Statistics, Computer Science, English, and Biochemistry. The selection of candidates for admissions is based not only on performance in the required pre-medical courses, but also on the applicant's entire academic record and extracurricular experiences.

PROCESS

All AMCAS applicants are sent secondary applications. Of those returning completed applications, about 12 percent are invited to interview between November and March. Interviews consist of two sessions, each with a faculty member, school administrator, or senior medical student. On interview day, applicants also attend informational sessions and a reception with current medical students. Approximately half of interviewed candidates are accepted. Notification occurs on a rolling basis and is completed by May. Wait-listed candidates are generally not encouraged to send additional information.

Admissions Requirements (Required)

MCAT Scores, Science GPA, Extracurricular activities, Non-Science GPA, Exposure to medical profession, Recommendation, Interview, State Residency

Admissions Requirements (Optional)

Essays

COSTS AND AID

Tuition & Fees

Annual tuition	$44,735
Room & board	$9,864
Cost of books	$1,500
Fees	$575

Financial Aid

% students receiving any aid	75
Average grant	$6,867
Average loan	$24,383
Average total aid package	$31,271

TULANE UNIVERSITY

TULANE UNIVERSITY SCHOOL OF MEDICINE

OFFICE OF ADMISSIONS, 1430 TULANE AVENUE, SL67, NEW ORLEANS, LA 70112 • ADMISSION: 504-988-5187
FAX: 504-988-64627 • E-MAIL: MEDSCH@TMCPOP.TMC.TULANE.EDU • WEBSITE: WWW.MCL.TULANE.EDU

STUDENT BODY

Type	Private
Enrollment of parent institution	12,590
Enrollment of medical school	747
% male/female	58/42
% underrepresented minorities	22
% out-of-state	82
% international	10
# countries represented	9
Average age of entering class	25

FACULTY

Total faculty	1,501
% female faculty	37
% minority faculty	12
% part-time faculty	70
Student-faculty ratio	2.0:1

ADMISSIONS

# applied	6,671
% accepted	7
% enrolled	43

Average GPA and MCAT Scores

Overall GPA	3.5
MCAT Bio	11.0
MCAT Phys	11.0
MCAT Verbal	10.0
MCAT Essay	P

Application Information

Regular application	1/15
Regular notification	10/15
Early application	9/1
Early notification	10/1
Are transfers accepted?	No
Admissions may be deferred?	Yes
Admissions need-blind?	No
Application fee	$100

Academics

The School of Medicine is one part of the Tulane University Health Sciences Center. In addition to the School of Medicine, the Health Sciences Center includes the School of Public Health and Tropical Medicine and the Primate Research Center. The following programs and centers of excellence are located within the Health Sciences Center: Center for Gene Therapy, the Center for Infectious Diseases, the Hayward Genetics Center, Hypertension and Renal Center, the Center for Bioenvironmental Research at Tulane and Xavier University, DePaul-Tulane Behavioral Health Center, Tulane Cancer Center, the Tulane Center for Abdominal Transplant, the Tulane Institute of Sports Medicine, the Tulane-Xavier National Women's Center, and Tulane Cardiovascular Center of Excellence.

BASIC SCIENCES: First-year courses include anatomy, histology, neuroscience, physiology and biochemistry, taught in an integrated fashion. Multi-media lectures, problem-based learning sessions, small group discussions, laboratories and clinical correlations are all employed by these first year courses. An emphasis is placed upon the clinical application of the basic science material. The second year takes a systems-oriented approach that integrates pharmacology, pathology, microbiology, immunology, pathophysiology, and physical diagnosis. During the second semester of the first year and throughout the entire second year, students choose from an extensive offering of both basic and clinical science electives, including many research opportunities. Each year, many students will use some of their elective time to take courses in the School of Public Health and Tropical Medicine; approximately 40 to 45 students each year graduate with the MD and the MPH degrees, having earned both degrees over a four year period. Combined degree programs are also available for students wishing to obtain MBA, MS, or JD degrees. Basic science instruction takes place in both the Medical School Building and a newly renovated facility located two blocks away, which are both central to both the research and clinical facilities. Computers are used as learning aids and research tools; a Computing Center serves the needs of the campus. The Rudolph Matas Library houses 130,000 volumes and receives 1,200 periodicals. The grading scale is Pass/Fail for the first two years and Honors/High Pass/Pass/Conditional/Fail for the clinical years. Students are required to pass USMLE Step 1 prior to entering the fourth year and are required to pass both USMLE Step 2 CK and 2CS in order to graduate.

CLINICAL TRAINING
During the first two years, clinical training is integrated with the basic science curriculum, with patient contact beginning immediately in year one through the Foundations in Medicine program. During these two years, students work with actual patients in hospitals near the school (the Tulane University Hospital, University Hospital, and Ochsner Medical Center), with patient simulators, and with surrogate, or standardized, patients. Students are also required to participate in community service activities which often involves direct patient care. Formal clinical training begins with the third and fourth years which are constructed as a 20-month clinical continuum, with students choosing the order of rotations depending on their own personal career goals. Required rotations include: Internal Medicine, Obstetrics and Gynecology, Pediatrics, Psychiatry, Neurology, Family Medicine, and Surgery. Students are also required to do a four-week Ambulatory Internal Medicine clerkship focusing on the undifferentiated patient, and a 2 week Outpatient Surgery rotation. Additionally, students complete a four-week subinternship in ward management, in addition to two weeks of Radiology, and Emergency

Medicine. Clinical students also have five elective months, which may include rotations taking place in locations either domestically or internationally. Established international rotations are available in Africa, South and Central America, and Asia. A formal exchange program exists with organizations in Sweden, Germany, and Japan.

Students

Students of the class of 2012 entering class represented 33 states and 3 countries. Of a class of 188 students, 24 came from the State of Louisiana, 30 from California, 14 from New York, and 10 from Massachusetts.. They received their undergraduate training at 77 different colleges and/or universities, with 26 earning the bachelor's degree from Tulane University. The average age of the class was 24, with a range of 21 to 39. About 14 percent of the class is from an underrepresented minority population.

STUDENT LIFE

Students are very much involved in life both on- and off-campus. Medical school extracurricular groups dedicated to student social life include MedArt, Music & Medicine, the Tulane Chorale, and Students Against Right Brain Atrophy. Organizations based upon academics, specialty interests, religion, hobbies, ethnicity and athletics bring medical students together around shared interests. An expansive support program is available for students experiencing problems, be those of an academic or personal nature. The medical school is within walking distance of the world famous French Quarter and Superdome, and New Orleans has many parks and areas suitable for fishing, biking, running, tennis and other outdoor activities, which are possible year-round. Of course the New Orleans cuisine and music scene is unparalleled in the United States. A housing facility, located adjacent to the Tulane University Health Sciences Center, makes over 250 apartments available to medical students, although most students choose to live off-campus, where houses and apartments are affordable and attractive. At the uptown, or university campus a large athletic facility, which includes an indoor track, two swimming pools, basketball and handball courts, and a very large selection of exercise equipment, is available for medical student use.

GRADUATES

Of the 2013 graduating class, the most popular residencies were Internal Medicine, Surgery, Pediatrics, Family Practice and Psychiatry. Approximately 35 percent of the class entered specialties considered to be primary care. Graduates from the class of 2012 will be pursuing residency training in 30 different states, with 36 staying in the State of Louisiana. Other popular states for residency training were Texas, California, Washington, Pennsylvania, Massachusetts, and Maryland.

Admissions

REQUIREMENTS

All students must have completed the following prerequisites prior to matriculation: English (six semester hours); general chemistry (six semester hours); organic chemistry (six semester hours); physics (six semester hours); and biology (six semester hours). While an undergraduate degree is not required, it is preferred. All required sciences courses must include a laboratory. The MCAT is required and should be no more than three years old; if the MCAT is taken more than once, the best set of scores is considered.

SUGGESTIONS

It is strongly required that applicants take the MCAT prior to September 1st in the year in which they intend to apply to medical school. Tulane's admission policy has no preference for any particular major; about one-third of the student body majored in a discipline other than science. While volunteer work in a hospital is useful, Tulane is more interested in seeing that applicants have an established history of providing service to a community, be it the college campus, church, or hometown, rather than a one-time exposure to a clinical environment. Activities that demonstrate strong interpersonal skills and/or evidence of self-discipline are valued, as are leadership positions.

Admissions Requirements (Required)

MCAT Scores, Essays, Science GPA, Extracurricular activities, Non-Science GPA, Exposure to medical profession, Recommendation, Interview

Admissions Requirements (Optional)

State Residency

COSTS AND AID

Tuition & Fees

Annual tuition	$50,600
Room & board	$14,100
Cost of books	$1,500
Fees	$3,655

Financial Aid

% students receiving any aid	79
% students receiving grants	30
% students receiving loans	71
% aid that is merit-based	6
Average grant	$14,086
Average loan	$60,670
Average total aid package	$68,747
Average debt	$216,83

UNIFORMED SERVICES UNIVERSITY OF THE HEALTH SCIENCES
F. EDWARD HEBERT SCHOOL OF MEDICINE

4301 JONES BRIDGE ROAD, ROOM A1041 BETHESDA, MD 20814 • ADMISSION: 301-295-3101
FAX: 301-295-35457 • E-MAIL: ADMISSIONS@USUHS.EDU • WEBSITE: WWW.USUHS.EDU

STUDENT BODY

Type	Public
Enrollment of medical school	691
% male/female	68/32
% out-of-state	91
% international	4
Average age of entering class	24

FACULTY

Total faculty	3,556
% female faculty	22
% minority faculty	9
% part-time faculty	1
Student-faculty ratio	6.0:1

ADMISSIONS

# applied	2,778
% accepted	11
% enrolled	56

Average GPA and MCAT Scores

Overall GPA	3.6
MCAT Bio	10.7
MCAT Phys	10.6
MCAT Verbal	10.0
MCAT Essay	P

Application Information

Regular application	11/15
Early application	6/1
Are transfers accepted?	No
Admissions may be deferred?	Yes
Admissions need-blind?	No
Application fee	$0

Academics

USU offers an extraordinary learning experience that blends science with a commitment to service. Although the quality of the core medical education remains consistent with other notable medical academic institutions, USU's School of Medicine curriculum contains an additional 500 hours of unique military content for medical students. This includes lecture and labs within the regular academic schedule as well as blocks of dedicated military medical training both on and off campus. The University's educational and research programs derive unparalleled benefits from its faculty members who deploy around the world to provide care for those in combat and in the wake of disasters as well as on humanitarian and research missions. This military unique curriculum is designed to give students a foundation and begin the development of skills and confidence necessary to provide quality medical care in austere and challenging environments. Educational resources abound at USU- from the alumni serving as mentors and role models, to the brick and mortar that house the centers of excellence. USU's unique educational resources provide a military medical education second to none. By the time they graduate, USU medical students receive more simulation practice than they would at most medical schools in the nation. During their four years at the University, students participate in approximately 40 different simulations in preparation for their careers as military medical officers. Much of this training occurs in our 30,000 square foot simulation center where we will soon debut our 8,000-square-foot, full-scale, immersive virtual-reality theater that will allow teams of students to participate in simulated mass casualty drills, biochemical attacks and other medical training scenarios. This unmatched facility, the National Capital Area Medical Simulation Center, is an integral part of USU's mission to provide state-of-the-art technology to conduct clinical and surgical skills training. The facility offers students some of the most advanced medical simulation technology available in the world. Going beyond the classroom, the training and simulations conducted at the center are critical components of the Washington, D.C. region's readiness and ability to respond to man-made or natural disasters.

BASIC SCIENCES: The F. Edward Hébert School of Medicine recently implemented a completely revised curriculum focusing on the theme "Molecules to Military Medicine." The new curriculum incorporates four key conceptual pillars: The integration of basic & clinical sciences throughout all four years, early patient contact, adaptability to unique learning styles, and the use of advanced educational technologies to promote student learning and development. Included in this transformation was a shift from a discipline or course based curriculum, to an integrated, organ-system based approach, which allows for medical science to be learned and applied in a clinical context. Moreover, students will start learning how to work with patients in a clinical setting, within their first few weeks of class. At the same time, they will study and master those aspects of the basic sciences that represent the foundation of all medical education. Coursework is graded on a Honors/Pass/Fail basis. Both steps of the USMLE must be taken and passed in order to graduate. The overall curriculum is divided into three major segments: the pre-clerkship, core clerkship and post-clerkship periods, all of which incorporate specialized instruction and training related to the unique aspects of military medicine. Of note is that the new curriculum includes an even greater amount of time for senior electives and/or advanced research opportunities.

CLINICAL TRAINING

Students engage in a total of 48 weeks of required clinical clerkships, which are accomplished in three sixteen-week blocks. The blocks may be completed in any order, but include a pairing of two clinical clerkships, each of which incorporate the integration of key clinical and basic science themes. Leave periods are provided after the first block, in early May, and after completion of the two other blocks in December. The basic science themes build on many of the fundamental anatomic, physiologic and pathologic concepts that were introduced in the pre-clerkship modules. Clinical threads will focus on topics of medical professionalism, ethics, patient safety, quality improvement, the skills necessary to practice life-long learning, and on evidence-based medicine. Block 1: Inpatient Medicine; Outpatient Medicine; Psychiatry. Block 2: Family Medicine; Pediatrics; Selective Rotation. Block 3: General Surgery; Surgical Specialties; Obstetrics and Gynecology The major objectives of the post-clerkship period are to prepare students for graduate medical education (residency training), and to foster advanced clinical decision making skills as students move from being able to Report medical information, to being able to Interpret information, in the interest of Managing and Educating patients in accordance with the "RIME" model of medical education. The first four-weeks of the post-clerkship phase of the USU curriculum will be used to help students prepare for successful completion of Step 1 of the USMLE exam. Students will then have an eight-week period of advanced curricular instruction entitled "Bench to Bedside and Beyond" (B3). B3 is an opportunity for students to further integrate basic science and clinical concepts in an advanced context. Emphasizing case-based examples, B3 will also incorporate topics such as patient safety, team-based care delivery patient-centered medical home), professionalism and evidence-based clinical decision making.

Students

For the 2012 First-Year Class, 68 percent had no prior military experience. Others have backgrounds in service academies, ROTC activities, as active and prior duty officers and enlisted service members, and as Reservists. Students are from all over the country, and represent a large number of undergraduate institutions. The most prevalent undergraduate majors were Biology (38%); Biochemistry (7%); and Chemistry (7%). About 6 percent of students are underrepresented minorities. The average age of entering students is 24. Class size is 171.

STUDENT LIFE

USUHS student groups include chapters of national organizations in addition to organizations focused on professional or service-oriented goals. These organizations are devoted to activities such as journalism, providing support to women medical students or spouses of medical students, and recreational pursuits. The school sponsors intramural athletic programs for men and women, and offers comprehensive athletic facilities. Nearby military posts and bases provide recreational and social activities for students and their families. Washington, D.C., with its museums, sites, parks, events, and diverse population, is an important resource and enriches the lives of medical students. All students live off campus, most in the immediate vicinity of the school or in Metro-accessible areas.

GRADUATES

Graduates must select residency programs at military hospitals, and often enter programs at the hospitals where they performed clerkships. Residencies vary in length, depending on the medical specialty. The residency period does not fulfill the seven-year commitment involved in attending USUHS. The military branch in which a graduate will serve is determined when he or she enters the School of Medicine and reflects both the student's preference and the needs of the organization.

Admissions

REQUIREMENTS

Applicants must be citizens of the United States; be at least 18 years old at the matriculation (but no older than 36 as of June 30) in the year of admission (age waivers will be considered); meet military regulations related to physical health; possess a baccalaureate degree by June 1 in the year of admission; and fulfill academic prerequisites. AP credit will be considered for courses. Applicants should consult our website at www.usuhs.edu/admissions.html for further details.

Admissions Requirements (Required)

MCAT Scores, Essays, Science GPA, Non-Science GPA, Exposure to medical profession, Recommendation, Interview

Admissions Requirements (Optional)

Extracurricular activities, State Residency

COSTS AND AID

Tuition & Fees

Annual tuition	$0
Cost of books	$0
Fees	$0

Financial Aid

% students receiving any aid	100
% aid that is merit-based	0
Average grant	$0
Average loan	$0
Average debt	$0

Universidad Central de Caribe

Universidad Central del Caribe

Universidad Central del Caribe, Call Box 60-327 Bayamon, PR 00960-6032
ADMISSION: (787) 798-3001 ext. 2403 • FAX: 787-269-75507 • E-MAIL: ICORDERO@UCCARIBE.EDU
WEBSITE: WWW.UCCARIBE.EDU

STUDENT BODY

Type	Private
Enrollment of medical school	240
% male/female	49/51
% international	5
Average age of entering class	22

FACULTY

Total faculty	332
% female faculty	52
% minority faculty	12
% part-time faculty	31
Student-faculty ratio	1.0:1

ADMISSIONS

# applied	726
% accepted	17
% enrolled	50

Average GPA and MCAT Scores

Overall GPA	3.3
MCAT Bio	7.2
MCAT Phys	6.3
MCAT Verbal	6.4
MCAT Essay	L

Application Information

Regular application	12/15
Regular notification	2/15
Are transfers accepted?	Yes
Admissions may be deferred?	No
Admissions need-blind?	No
Application fee	$50

Academics

The mission of the SOM is to develop competent physicians with an outstanding preparation within a humanistic and holistic framework. A guiding principle of our mission is to ensure that our gradutes possess a strong sense of professionalism and commitment to social duties and service to Puerto Rico, and Hispanic communities throughout the US mainland. The curriculum emphasizes techniques and values related to the provision of primary medical care. The first two years primarily teach basic medical sciences with a strong introduction to the clinical sciences through a longitudinal primary care preceptorship, human behavior, and clinical skills. The second two years are devoted to clinical rotations and to continuing interdisciplinary instruction.

BASIC SCIENCES: Basic sciences are taught primarily through lectures. Labs and small group sessions are also utilized. First year courses consist of Human Gross Anatomy, Histology, LPCP I, Physiology, Neurosciences, Behavioral Sciences, Bioethics and Humanities in Medicine I, Problem Base Learning I, and Introduction to Clinical Skills. Second year courses are: Microbiology and Immunology, Psychopathology, Pharmacology, Pathology, Pathophysiology, Clinical Skills, LPCP II, Bioethics and Humanities in Medicine II, and Problem Based Learning II. Most instruction during the first two years takes place in the new Biomedical Sciences building, which also houses laboratories and research facilities.

CLINICAL TRAINING

Clinical clerkships begin in the third year. These are comprised of Radiology (1 week), Internal Medicine (10 weeks), Family Medicine (6 weeks), Surgery (6 weeks), Pediatrics (6 weeks), Psychiatry (6 weeks), and Ob/Gyn (6 weeks). Major teaching hospitals are the Dr. Ramon Ruiz Arnau University Hospital, San Pablo Hospital, First Hospital Panamericano, San Jorge children's Hospital, and San Juan Veterans Administration Hospital.

Students

Around 50 percent of students are women. Virtually all students are from underrepresented minority groups.

STUDENT LIFE

To help students acclimate to medical school, an orientation is given to the entering first-year class. This also serves as an opportunity for students to interact with each other and with faculty members and administrators. Students are encouraged to develop an interest in culture and the arts. With this in mind, the Dean of Student Affairs sponsors an extracurricular activities program for medical students. Counseling services are aimed at helping students take advantage of the extensive educational opportunities at the Medical School. A comprehensive health plan is offered to all medical students. Housing facilities are available through individual arrangements in areas adjacent to the Medical School and the University Hospital.

GRADUATES

The Medical School has graduated about 1,750 physicians who serve the Commonwealth of Puerto Rico, and Hispanic communities in the United States.

Admissions

REQUIREMENTS

Applicants must demonstrate proficiency in both Spanish and English. This is essential, as lectures are conducted in the language preferred by the respective professor, most often Spanish. In addition, Spanish is necessary for most clinical work. Applicants must complete a minimum of 90 credits at an institution of higher education. A baccalaureate degree is highly recommended. Required premedical course are: General Biology (8 credit hours), General Chemistry (8 hours), Organic Chemistry (8 hours), Physics (8 hours), college-level Math (6 hours), English (12 hours), Spanish (6 hours), and Behavioral Sciences and Social Sciences (12 hours). The MCAT is required. Officials exam results from within the past two years must be submitted to the School of Medicine.

PROCESS

The Universidad Central del Caribe School of Medicine participates in the American Medical College Application Service (AMCAS). All applicants must file an AMCAS application. In addition, applicants should contact the School of Medicine for additional application materials and a processing fee, photographs, an essay, and a certificate of Certificate of Police Record. After applications, MCAT scores, and transcripts are given an initial review, applicants who are under consideration will be invited for personal interviews with members of the Faculty.

Admissions Requirements (Required)

MCAT Scores, Essays, Science GPA, Non-Science GPA, Recommendation, Interview

Admissions Requirements (Optional)

Extracurricular activities, Exposure to medical profession, State Residency

COSTS AND AID

Tuition & Fees

Annual tuition	$27,000
Room & board	$6,000
Cost of books	$15,000
Fees (in-state out-of-state)	$4,890

Financial Aid

% students receiving any aid	94
% students receiving grants	54
% students receiving loans	94
% aid that is merit-based	92
Average grant	$38,500
Average loan	$38,500
Average total aid package	$38,500
Average debt	$132,000

UNIVERSITE LAVAL
FACULTÉ DE MÉDECINE

PAVILLON VANDRY U.LAVAL, LOCAL 2222 QUÉBEC, QC G1V 0A6 • **ADMISSION:** 418-656-2131 2492
FAX: 418-656-24657 • **E-MAIL:** SANDRINE.CHARETTE-MARTINEAU@FMED.ULAVAL.CA
WEBSITE: WWW.FMED.ULAVAL.CA

STUDENT BODY	
Type	Public

FACULTY	
Total faculty	235
% female faculty	75
% minority faculty	5
Student-faculty ratio	4.0:1

ADMISSIONS	
# applied	2,145
% accepted	11

Application Information	
Regular application	3/1
Regular notification	5/15
Are transfers accepted?	No
Admissions may be deferred?	No
Admissions need-blind?	No
Application fee	$75

Academics

Laval offers a four-year curriculum leading to the M.D. degree. In addition, academic programs are available in a number of health and medical science fields including Molecular Biology, Community Health, Epidemiology, Occupational Health and Safety, and Physiology. Research is an important part of the academic experience at Laval, and students are encouraged to pursue research during summers and throughout the academic year.

BASIC SCIENCES: The first two years involve basic science instruction and opportunities for addressing clinical problems. The first year includes courses in Biochemistry, Physiology, Pharmacology, Microbiology-Immunology, Histology-Pathology, and Introduction to Problems. During the second part of the first year, instruction is organized around anatomical systems and medical concepts. These are Cardiovascular System, Respiratory System, Uro-nephrology, Microbiology/Infectious Disease, and Physiological/Sociological. Introduction to Problems continues during the second semester. Students also study Endocrinology, Ob/Gyn, and Growth/Development during their first year. Year two subjects are Nervous System, Locomotor System, Medical Ethics, Problem Discussion, The Art of Interviewing, ENT, Ophthalmology, Hematology, Gastroenterology, Psychopathology, Preventive Medicine, and Skin. Laval's library system is an important academic resource for students, holding millions of volumes and periodicals.

CLINICAL TRAINING

Years three and four are devoted to clinical rotations. Required clerkships are Introduction to Clinical Medicine (5 weeks), Medicine (8 weeks), Surgery (8 weeks), Pediatrics (8 weeks), Psychiatry (8 weeks), Ob/Gyn (8 weeks), Preventive Medicine (4 weeks), Geriatrics/Rehabilitation Medicine (4 weeks), Family Practice (4 weeks), and Emergency Medicine (4 weeks). In addition, up to 20 weeks are open for various clinical and basic science electives. Training takes place at a number of affiliated hospitals including Centre Hospitalier de l'Universite Laval, IUCPQ, Hôpital de l'Enfant-Jesus, Hôtel-Dieu de Levis, Hôtel-Dieu de Quebec, Hôpital du Saint-Sacrement and Hôpital Saint-Francois d'Assise.

Students

For more information about campus life, see the web site: http://www2.ulaval.ca/la-vie-universitaire/vie-etudiante.html

STUDENT LIFE

Laval University supports medical students both inside and outside the classroom. The services offered include orientation and counseling services, religious organizations, career placement services, social and athletic organizations, childcare, and attractive, low-cost student housing. The Laval campus is situated in an urban environment.

GRADUATES

For more information about graduates of Laval University, see the web site: http://www.adul.ulaval.ca/

Admissions

REQUIREMENTS

DEC sciences, humanities and arts; or DEC in the natural sciences and have passed the following courses: Biology 401; Chemistry 202, or Other DEC; Mathematics NYA, NYB, Mathematics 103-77, 203-77, or Mathematics 103-RE, RE-203; Physics NYA, NYB, NYC (or 101, 201, 301); Chemistry NYA, NYB (or 101, 201) and 202; NYA Biology (or 301) and 401; or International Baccalaureate science option of nature: the candidate is exempt from NYC Physics course (or 301); or Diploma in Health Sciences in New Brunswick; or Pre-university degree totaling 13 years of education (pre-university diploma or total of 12 years of schooling and one year of university studies) and satisfactory training in science (mathematics, physics, chemistry, biology). For more information, see the web site: http://www2.ulaval.ca/les-etudes/programmes/repertoire/details/doctor-at-en-medecine-md.html#description-officielle&conditions-admission

SUGGESTIONS

Priority is given to residents of the province of Quebec. Candidates are evaluated on the basis of academic achievement, interpersonal skills, experience, and personal characteristics.

PROCESS

Applications are coordinated in part by the organization of Quebec Colleges and Universities. For entrance in the Fall, the application deadline is March 1 for the college student ans and is February 1 for the university students. An application for admission must be submitted online at the following address: http://www2.ulaval.ca/admission/deposez-votre-demande-dadmission.html. The selection criteria are academic record (60%) and MMI (40%). Some particular features are require for some applicant category. For detailed criteria by applicant category, refer to the following site: http://www.fmed.ulaval.ca/site_fac/formation/1er-cycle/medecine/admission/. Generally, about 10 to 15 percent of applicants are admitted in a given year.

Admissions Requirements (Required)

Science GPA, Non-Science GPA, Interview, State Residency

Admissions Requirements (Optional)

Essays, Extracurricular activities

COSTS AND AID

Tuition & Fees

Annual tuition (in-state out-of-state)	$2,021/$8,416
Room & board	$7
Cost of books	$800
Fees (in-state out-of-state)	$287/$200

University of Alabama at Birmingham

University of Alabama School of Medicine

Medical Student Services, VH 100 , 1720 2nd Avenue South, Birmingham, AL 35294-0019
Admission: 205-934-2433 • Fax: 205-934-87407 • E-mail: MEDSCHOOL@UAB.EDU
Website: WWW.UAB.EDU / MEDICINE / HOME

STUDENT BODY

Type	Public
Enrollment of parent institution	18,568
Enrollment of medical school	759
% male/female	57/43
% out-of-state	9
% international	24
# countries represented	87
Average age of entering class	24

FACULTY

Total faculty	1,286
Student-faculty ratio	0.6:1

ADMISSIONS

# applied	2,866
% accepted	9
% enrolled	69

Average GPA and MCAT Scores

Overall GPA	3.7
MCAT Bio	10.3
MCAT Phys	9.9
MCAT Verbal	9.8
MCAT Essay	Q

Application Information

Regular application	11/1
Early application	8/1
Early notification	10/1
Are transfers accepted?	Yes
Admissions may be deferred?	Yes
Admissions need-blind?	No
Application fee	$80

Academics

The School of Medicine provides an integrated curriculum that focuses on teaching the basic sciences and is organized around organ systems rather than the traditional sciences disciplines. The objective of our curriculum is for students to learn basic sciences in a more clinically relevant context, teaching them to think comprehensively about organ function and diseases rather than simply memorize mountains of facts. Students receive instruction in clinical skills from the very first day of medical school. In addition to basic science and clinical clerkships, students engage in a Scholarly Activity and have their choice from numerous fourth-year electives. A joint MD/PhD program and an MD/MPH program are also offered.

BASIC SCIENCES: Basic science principles are taught in clinical context and incorporate active, case-based learning. Unlike traditional medical curricula, there are no individual basic science courses (Gross Anatomy, Biochemistry, Physiology, etc.). Concepts from these courses are still taught, but in an integrated clinical context. Consequently, students learn to think like a doctor from the beginning. Each module includes concepts from Anatomy, Histology, Genetics, Physiology, Nutrition, Correlative Pathology, Pharmacology, Microbiology, and Immunology, including Ethics, Geriatrics, and Evidence-Based Medicine components, where applicable. Gross anatomy is taught in conjunction with the organ-based modules. All courses in the first two years are taught on the Birmingham campus.

CLINICAL TRAINING

Clinical training begins on the first day of medical school. In addition to the introductory clinical course work of the first two years, some students are involved in community-based programs which provide patient exposure to public health issues, such as the student-led Equal Access Birmingham free medical clinic for the medically underserved. In the final two years of the curriculum students complete required clerkships in Medicine, Surgery, Pediatrics, Psychiatry, Family Medicine, Obstetrics and Gynecology, and Neurology. After a campus preference and assignment process, students take these core clinical clerkships and electives at either the main campus in Birmingham or at one of the three branch campuses in Huntsville, Montgomery, and Tuscaloosa. Each campus is affiliated with several teaching hospitals, and rotations take students to a variety of learning environments. In addiiton to Pass/Fail grading, students may be given a grade of Honors in clerkships.

Students

The school seeks a diverse student body to reflect the diverse health care needs of the state of Alabama. Special programs to promote both clinical and basic science research and to address unmet health care needs of the State of Alabama are available.

STUDENT LIFE

Students are involved in a wide range of recreational and volunteer activities. Some are active in student organizations, including national medical groups. The Student Government Association consists of elected members of each class. Most students live off campus, where housing is ample and relatively affordable.

GRADUATES

Primary care residencies are popular among graduates. Graduates are competitive for residencies nationwide, with a significant number entering residency programs in Alabama, at University-affiliated hospitals, or at other locations in the state.

Admissions

REQUIREMENTS

Undergraduate requirements are Biology or Zoology (8 semester hours); Chemistry with lab (8 semester hours); Organic Chemistry with lab (8 semester hours); Physics with lab (8 semester hours); Math (6 semester hours); and English (6 semester hours). A minimum total MCAT score of 24, not more than two years old at the time of application, is required. An AMCAS application is required.

SUGGESTIONS

The Admissions Committee values experience with patient care and exposure to health care environments. The University of Alabama School of Medicine welcomes nontraditional applicants. Alabama residents are given significant preference in the admissions process.

PROCESS

All verified AMCAS applicants who are US Citizens or Permanent Residents receive an invitation to complete the secondary application. Notification begins in October, and the class is filled by April 1. Interviews are held beginning mid-September through March.

Admissions Requirements (Required)

MCAT Scores, Essays, Science GPA, Extracurricular activities, Non-Science GPA, Exposure to medical profession, Recommendation, Interview

Admissions Requirements (Optional)

State Residency

COSTS AND AID

Tuition & Fees

Annual tuition (in-state out-of-state)	$24,510/$58,590
Room & board	$12,116
Cost of books	$1,713
Fees	$1,445

Financial Aid

% students receiving any aid	79
% students receiving grants	39
% students receiving loans	66
% aid that is merit-based	15
Average grant	$12,241
Average loan	$40,453
Average total aid package	$40,564
Average debt	$125,760

UNIVERSITY OF ALBERTA
FACULTY OF MEDICINE AND DENTISTRY

2-45 MEDICAL SCIENCES BUILDING, EDMONTON, AB T6G 2H7 • ADMISSION: 780-492-6350 • FAX: 780-492-95317
E-MAIL: ADMISSION@MED.UALBERTA.CA • WEBSITE: WWW.MED.UALBERTA.CA

STUDENT BODY	
Type	Public

ADMISSIONS	
# applied	1,095

Average GPA and MCAT Scores	
MCAT Bio	10.8
MCAT Phys	11.3
MCAT Verbal	9.7

Application Information	
Regular application	1/31
Admissions may be deferred?	Yes
Admissions need-blind?	No
Application fee	$60

Academics

Alberta's curriculum reflects the school's emphasis on clinical care and research. The preclinical curriculum has been revised and is largely centered on organ systems. It is multidisciplinary, including both biological and social science perspectives. Although basic sciences are the focus of study during the first two years, courses are taught with clinical applications in mind. The second two years integrate classroom and hospital-based instruction. While most medical students earn an MD degree in four years, qualified students may pursue joint degrees such as the MD/PhD or MD/MPH in a longer period of study.

BASIC SCIENCES: Basic sciences are taught in a variety of forums, including lectures, small-group discussions, laboratories, problem-based learning, independent study, and computer-based instruction. The academic period begins in August, covers thirty-five weeks, and includes courses in introduction to medicine; immunity, infection and inflammation; practice of medicine (part I); cardiology, renal, and pulmonary; and endocrine and metabolism. On average, students are in class or other scheduled sessions for about twenty-five hours per week. The second academic period also begins in August and includes gastroenterology, reproduction and urology, musculoskeletal, neurosciences, oncology, and practice of medicine (part II) in addition to a systems-based curriculum. Systems studied are cardiovascular, endocrinology, gastrointestinal, hematology, medical ethics, nephrology, ophthalmology, pediatrics, pulmonary, surgery, and urology. Basic science instruction takes place mainly at the medical sciences building and uses the resources of the John W. Scott Health Sciences Library. Medical students may use all university libraries and computer facilities. All enrolled students have access to free online service.

CLINICAL TRAINING

The third and fourth academic periods primarily teach clinical skills and consist of classroom instruction, required rotations, electives, and selectives. Required clerkships are anesthesia (two weeks), geriatrics (two weeks), medicine (ten weeks), obstetrics/gynecology (eight weeks), pediatrics (eight weeks), psychiatry (eight weeks), radiology (two weeks), rural family medicine (four weeks), and surgery (ten weeks). Selectives include two weeks in internal medicine and two weeks in surgery. Training takes place at University of Alberta hospitals, the Royal Alexandra Hospital, Edmonton General Hospital, Misericordia Hospital, Alberta Hospital, Glenrose Hospital, Cross Cancer Institute, and Grey Nuns Hospital. A certain number of electives may be taken at non-affiliated institutions.

Students

Among 102 students in the 1998 entering class, 42 percent are female. About 15 percent are from outside of Alberta. A total of eighty-one students completed at least four years of university.

STUDENT LIFE

Campus housing is available, although most students opt to live off campus in the surrounding area. The students' union provides a registry informing students of available housing. Medical students participate in clubs, events, and recreational activities geared toward medical students and the student body in general. Counseling and other support services are available to students, as are groups focused on special interests and minority groups. Edmonton is a midsize city, offering plenty of restaurants, shops, parks, theaters, sporting events, and outdoor activities. Although public transportation is available, most medical students own cars.

GRADUATES

Graduates enter both clinical medicine and research-oriented careers.

Admissions

REQUIREMENTS

Only Canadian applications are accepted. All applicants should have completed at least sixty units of university course work (approximately two years of full-time studies). Requirements are six units each of general chemistry, organic chemistry, biology, physics, and English, along with three units each of statistics and biochemistry. The MCAT is required and scores are valid for three years after the exam is taken. In addition to an application form, an autobiographical essay and two letters of reference are required.

SUGGESTIONS

Residency is an important consideration in admissions decisions. For admissions purposes, a resident of Alberta is defined as a Canadian Citizen or Permanent Resident who has lived in the Province of Alberta or Yukon or Northwest Territories for at least one continuous year immediately prior to the date of intended matriculation. At least 85 percent of available positions in an entering class are reserved for Alberta residents. The remaining 15 percent are available to other Canadians. Typically, successful applicants have completed four years of university with a grade point average of 7.0 on the University of Alberta's nine point grading system. An MCAT score of less than 7 in any category is not accepted.

PROCESS

Requests for applications should be directed to the address above. Applications are accepted between July 1 and November 1 in the year preceding anticipated matriculation. The essay and reference letters must be received by January 15, and transcripts must be submitted by January 31. Interviews are conducted between February and March, and admissions decisions are made between May and July. For the 1998 entering class, 1,011 students applied for 102 positions. Applicants who feel that they may merit special consideration (because of studies in a nontraditional area or unusual pattern) should write to the Admissions Officer outlining their situation and goals. All native (Aboriginal) students who are interested in medical studies are encouraged to contact Coordinator, Native Health Care Careers Program in care of the address above.

Admissions Requirements (Required)

Interview

COSTS AND AID

Tuition & Fees

Annual tuition	$6,066
Cost of books	$900
Fees	$6,000

UNIVERSITY OF ARIZONA
COLLEGE OF MEDICINE

ADMISSIONS OFFICE, ROOM 2209, P.O. BOX 245075, TUCSON, AZ 85724 • ADMISSION: 520-626-6214
FAX: 520-626-48847 • E-MAIL: • WEBSITE: WWW.AHSC.ARIZONA.EDU/PRE-MED

STUDENT BODY

Type	Public
Enrollment of medical school	406
% male/female	52/48
% international	15

ADMISSIONS

# applied	608
% accepted	8

Application Information

Regular application	11/1
Are transfers accepted?	No
Admissions may be deferred?	Yes
Admissions need-blind?	Yes
Application fee	$0

Academics

Students may apply to joint Ph.D./M.D. programs in the following: Anatomy, Biochemistry, Cell Biology, Genetics, Immunology, Microbiology, Molecular Biology, Neuroscience, Pharmacology, and Physiology. Combined studies in other fields are possible as well, including a collaborative program of Arizona State University, Northern Arizona University, and the College of Medicine at the University of Arizona. This program focuses on the health needs of underserved communities and leads to a Master's in Public Health along with the M.D. Through this and other venues, medical students at the University of Arizona take advantage of the resources of the academic and medical institutions throughout the state.

BASIC SCIENCES: The basic sciences are taught in the Basic Science Building of the Tucson campus. Traditional lectures with labs are the primary mode of instruction, occupying about 24 hours per week. Alternative teaching methods, including small-group and case-based learning, account for the remaining six hours per week of structured classroom time. First-year courses are Anatomy; Histology and Cell Biology; Physiology; Neuroscience; Biochemistry; Medical and Molecular Genetics; Preparation for Clinical Medicine; and Social and Behavioral Science. During year two, students take Microbiology; Pathology; Pharmacology; Preparation for Clinical Medicine; and Social and Behavioral Science. In the course Preparation for Clinical Medicine, students focus on clinical problem-solving and learn patient evaluation skills. This course links basic science principles with clinical applications. Computers, located in the Learning Resource Center, supplement lectures and are an important component of the basic science education. The Arizona Health Science Library houses nearly 200,000 volumes, operates extensive online database and informational services, and is connected electronically to the library system of the greater university. To accommodate the study schedules of all students, the library is open 24 hours a day. Students are evaluated with an Honors/Pass/Fail scale. The USMLE Step 1 is required upon completion of basic science course work.

CLINICAL TRAINING

Patient contact begins during year one in Preparation for Clinical Medicine. Throughout the four years, there are opportunities for clinical exposure through volunteer and outreach programs. In addition, clinical research is often community based and gives medical students a chance to help others while they learn. The Commitment to Underserved People (CUP) is a program through which many medical students volunteer. In CUP, students are involved in health education for, and supervised treatment of, people in underserved communities. The formal clinical curriculum begins in year three, when students rotate through the following clerkships: Medicine (12 weeks); Pediatrics (6 weeks); Family Medicine (6 weeks); Ob/Gyn (6 weeks); Psychiatry (6 weeks); Surgery (6 weeks); Specialty Surgery (3 weeks); and Neurology (3 weeks). Year four is composed of electives, many of which can be taken at alternate locations throughout the state. Clinical facilities in Tucson are the University Medical Center, the University Outpatient Clinic, the Children's Research Center, and the Arizona Cancer Center. The hospitals serve managed care participants, and the medical school seeks to respond to the ongoing changes in the economics of health care, as seen in the public health/health policy components of medical school training. Evaluation of clinical performance is Honors/Pass/Fail. Passing the USMLE Step 2 is a requirement for graduation.

Students

Students are either Arizona residents, or are from western states that do not have their own medical schools. Generally, about 15 percent of the student body are underrepresented minorities, most of whom are of Mexican American descent. Older students comprise about one-third of each class. A wide range of undergraduate institutions and majors are represented in a typical class. Class size is 100.

STUDENT LIFE

With access to both the campus community of over 36,000 students, and a medium-sized urban community, students have active social lives. Recreational facilities are extensive at the University. The Medical School's emphasis on community involvement promotes extracurricular activities that are medically related. Student clubs also provide mechanisms for support and social interaction. The Chicano/Latino Club is linked to similar organizations at California universities, providing a larger network for those involved. On-campus housing options include apartments and dorms. Most students, however, opt to live off campus.

GRADUATES

At least 60 percent of graduates enter primary care fields, which include Family Medicine, Ob/Gyn, Internal Medicine, and Pediatrics. About 50 percent of graduates enter residency programs within the state.

Admissions

REQUIREMENTS

Applicants should have completed one year of each of the following subjects: Biology, Physics, Chemistry, Organic Chemistry, and English. In addition, at least 30 hours of upper-division course work as part of the undergraduate record is required. For older applicants, recent science course work is necessary. The MCAT is required, and only the best scores are considered, suggesting that applicants should not withhold scores. Together, the MCAT and college record are used for initial screening.

SUGGESTIONS

Hands-on clinical experience is important, as are other activities that demonstrate an applicant's commitment to community service. The Admissions Committee is interested in applicants whose undergraduate records include significant course work in the Humanities and Social Sciences. Applicants are advised to take the April rather than August MCAT.

PROCESS

All AMCAS applicants receive secondary applications, and virtually all who meet residency requirements are interviewed. Interviews are conducted from September through March and consist of three short meetings with faculty members and one longer session with a practicing clinician from the area. About one quarter of those who interview are accepted, with notifications occurring on a rolling basis. A ranked wait list is established, but those who find themselves on this list are not encouraged to send additional information.

Admissions Requirements (Required)

MCAT Scores, Science GPA, Extracurricular activities, Non-Science GPA, Exposure to medical profession, Recommendation, Interview, State Residency

Admissions Requirements (Optional)

Essays

COSTS AND AID

Tuition & Fees

Annual tuition	$15,786
Fees	$170

Financial Aid

% students receiving any aid	87

UNIVERSITY OF ARKANSAS COLLEGE OF MEDICINE

COLLEGE OF MEDICINE

4301 WEST MARKHAM STREET, SLOT 551, LITTLE ROCK, AR 72205-7199 • ADMISSION: 501-686-5354
FAX: 501-686-58737 • E-MAIL: SOUTHTOMG@UAMS.EDU • WEBSITE: WWW.UAMS.EDU

STUDENT BODY

Type	Public
Enrollment of medical school	576
% male/female	56/44
% out-of-state	1
% international	10
Average age of entering class	24

ADMISSIONS

# applied	675
% accepted	25
% enrolled	82

Average GPA and MCAT Scores

Overall GPA	3.6
MCAT Bio	9.0
MCAT Phys	9.0
MCAT Verbal	9.0
MCAT Essay	O

Application Information

Regular application	11/1
Regular notification	2/15
Early application	6/1
Early notification	12/15
Are transfers accepted?	Yes
Admissions may be deferred?	Yes
Admissions need-blind?	No
Application fee	$100

Academics

The College of Medicine, along with the schools of Nursing, Pharmacy, Public Health, Health Related Professions, and Graduate Studies, comprise the University of Arkansas for Medical Sciences, one of six campuses of the University of Arkansas system. Most students complete the M.D. curriculum in four years, but a few students each year take part in joint M.D./Ph.D. or M.D./MPH, and MD/MBA programs. Joint degrees can be pursued in the following fields: Anatomy, Biochemistry, Immunology, Microbiology, Neuroscience, Pharmacology, and Physiology.

BASIC SCIENCES: Throughout year one, students learn skills related to patient care in Introduction to Clinical Medicine. Fall semester courses are Cell Biology, Genetics, Gross Anatomy, and Microscopic Anatomy. Spring semester courses are Biochemistry, Neuroscience, and Physiology. In the fall semester of year two, students take Behavioral Sciences, Medical Ethics, Microbiology, and Pathophysiology I. In the spring, classes are Introduction to Clinical Medicine II, Pathophysiology II, and Pharmacology. Scheduled class time accounts for about 20 hours per week, most of which is devoted to lecture and lab. Alternately, for perhaps two hours per week, small groups are used as the instructional format. Grading uses an A–F scale. Passing the USMLE Step 1 is a requirement for promotion to year three, and USMLE 2 for graduation. Basic-science teaching facilities, including libraries and labs, are part of the medical complex, which includes the main hospitals as well as residence halls.

CLINICAL TRAINING

Patient contact begins in year one, in Introduction to Clinical Medicine. The third year consists of required clerkships in the following: Internal Medicine (12 weeks); Surgery (8 weeks); Ob/Gyn (6 weeks); Psychiatry (6 weeks); Pediatrics (8 weeks); Specialties (4 weeks); Geriatrics (unspecified); and Family Medicine (4 weeks). During year four, students choose among Primary Care Selectives (8 weeks) and Specialties Clerkships (4 weeks). The remainder of the year is designated as elective study, some of which may be taken off campus, out of state, or overseas. Training takes place primarily at the University Hospital (400 beds), located in the Medical Center complex. Other training sites are the Arkansas Children's Hospital (the 6th largest children's hospital in the country) and two VA hospitals (500 and 2000 beds). In addition, outreach-training sites in small communities around the state provide exposure to rural medicine. The primary care clerkships involve rotations to these sites, located in El Dorado, Fayetteville, Fort Smith, Jonesboro, Pine Bluff, and Texarkana. Specialized research institutes in Little Rock include The Child Study Center, The Ambulatory Care Center, The Arkansas Cancer Research Center, and the Jones Eye Institute. Evaluation of clinical progress in required clerkships uses an A-F scale, and electives are graded as Pass/Fail. Students must pass the USMLE Step 2 as a requirement for graduation.

Students

Virtually all students are Arkansas residents. About 70 percent of students earned undergraduate degrees in Arkansas. Approximately 79 percent of incoming students in a recent class had undergraduate majors in science disciplines. Classes include a significant number of older students, including some who were older than 50 years old at the time of admission. Class size is 150.

STUDENT LIFE

Little Rock is a small but lively city, with indoor and outdoor recreational activities. Students take part in volunteer and community activities. Many single first- and second-year students live on campus in residence halls. Most upperclass students and married students live off campus.

GRADUATES

Many graduates enter post-graduate programs in Arkansas. Programs in about 20 specialty areas are offered at university-affiliated hospitals in Little Rock. In addition, a number of family practice residencies are available at rural locations around the state. At least half of the graduates of the School of Medicine enter primary care fields.

Admissions

REQUIREMENTS

Within each class, 70 percent of students must be equally divided from among the four congressional districts in the state. The College of Medicine is allowed to admit a few out-of-state applicants each year, but only if they do not displace Arkansas residents with equal qualifications. Out-of-state applicants should be highly qualified and have close ties to Arkansas. Students must have successfully completed the following courses prior to matriculation: Biology (one year); Chemistry (one year); Organic Chemistry (one year); Physics (one year); English (one year); and Math (one year) or through Calculus I. The MCAT is required, and scores must be no more than 3 years old. Scores from all sections of the MCAT, including the writing sample, are considered.

SUGGESTIONS

Other courses deemed helpful are Biochemistry, Zoology, Botany, Embryology, Genetics, Histology, Calculus, Physical Chemistry, Statistics, Sociology, Speech, Anthropology, Psychology, Human Ecology, Composition, Literature, History, and Logic. For students who graduated from college several years ago, some recent course work is useful. All medically related extracurricular activities are valued.

PROCESS

All AMCAS applicants are asked to submit secondary applications. All Arkansas residents, and highly qualified out-of-state residents are interviewed, with interviews taking place between October and January. Team interviews consist of a one-hour session with faculty. All applicants are notified by February 15. A ranked wait list is established, and about 25 students from the list are usually admitted. Wait-listed candidates who commit to practicing in underserved areas of Arkansas may improve their chances of admission.

Admissions Requirements (Required)

MCAT Scores, Essays, Science GPA, Extracurricular activities, Non-Science GPA, Exposure to medical profession, Recommendation, Interview

Admissions Requirements (Optional)

State Residency

COSTS AND AID

Tuition & Fees

Annual tuition (in-state out-of-state)	$14,792/$29,584
Cost of books	$1,650
Fees	$773

Financial Aid

Average grant	$3,000
Average loan	$28,000
Average debt	$112,000

University of British Columbia

Faculty of Medicine

317-2194 Health Sciences Mall, British Columbia, BC V6T 1Z3 • Admission: 604-822-2421
Fax: 604-822-60617 • E-mail: ADMISSIONS.MD@UBC.CA • Website: WWW.MED.UBC.CA

Academics

The four-year leading to the M.D. degree is integrated and comprehensive, designed to take advantage of the vast resources of the Faculty of Medicine. A new case-based curriculum that emphasizes problem solving and lifelong learning was introduced during the Fall of 1998. In addition to the M.D. program, graduate programs leading to Masters, Doctorate, and combined degrees are available.

BASIC SCIENCES: Basic sciences are taught along with introductory clinical concepts during the first two years. First-year courses include Introductory Clinical Skills and Systems 1; Doctor/Dentist; Patient & Society; Family Practice Continuum; Principles of Human Biology; Host Defenses and Infection; Cardiovascular Systems; Pulmonary; and Fluids, Electrolytes & Renal. Second-year courses include Clinical Skills and Systems II; Doctor/Dentist, Patient & Society; Family Practice Continuum; Blood and Lymphatic; Musculoskeletal and Locomotor; GI/Nutrition; Metabolism and Endocrine; Integument; Brain and Behavior and Reproduction; and Growth and Development. Basic sciences are taught primarily through small group forums, through lectures, computer-based instruction and labs also utilized.

CLINICAL TRAINING

The third academic period begins with courses in Health Care Epidemiology, Radiology, and Therapeutics. Following these three courses, students enter a sequence of required clerkships. These are: Orientation (4 weeks), Anesthesia (2 weeks), Deratology (1 week), Emergency Medicine (4 weeks), Medicine (10 weeks), Ob/Gyn (8 weeks), Ophthalmology (1 week), Orthopedics (2 weeks), Pediatrics (8 weeks), Psychiatry (8 weeks), and Surgery (8 weeks). Six weeks are left open for electives during the third academic period. Sixteen weeks are left open for elecives during the fourth academic period. A portion of electives may be completed at sites outside of the network of affiliated institutions including the University Hospital, St. Paul's Hospital, British Columbia Children's Hospital, Vancouver General Hospital, British Columbia Women's Hospital and Health Center, British Columbia Cancer Center Agency, G.F.Strong Rehabilitation Center, and the Canadian Arthiritus and Rheumatism Society Center.

Students

Each entering class has about 120 students. Approximately 50 percent of students are women. Typically, all but a handful of students in each class are from British Columbia.

STUDENT LIFE

Beyond a rich academic life, medical students enjoy the resources, facilities, and surroundings of the Health Science Center, the University of British Columbia, and the city of Vancouver. The Faculty of Medicine ad greater University offer a wide range of support services including counseling, special interest clubs and organizations, resources for minorities and international students, and day-care. There are ample opportunities for athletic, social, and recreational activities on campus. Students also enjoy the cultural and recreational aspects of Vancouver.

GRADUATES

A significant number of graduates ener residency programs at hospitals affiliated with the University of British Columbia. Though most graduates enter clinical medicine, others successfully pursue research and academic medicine.

Admissions

REQUIREMENTS

Applicants should have successfully completed a minimum of 90 credits or the equivalent of three years of full-time course work in any degree program at an accredited university. A minimum of 70 percent academic average is required and all undergraduate courses are included in this average. Prerequisites are one year each of university-level Biology, Biochemistry, Chemistry, Organic Chemistry, and English Literature and Composition. The MCAT is required. The exam should be taken no later than August of the year of application.

SUGGESTIONS

There is no prefered program of study for preperation for medical school. Often, due to the large number of applicants, the competitive average for successful applicants is much higher than 70 percent. MCAT scores of a recently admitted class averaged about 10. in addition to excellent academic qualifications, admission decisions are based on spplicants' personal characteristics such as motivation and integrity. Last year, 695 applications were recieved for 120 positions.

COSTS AND AID	
Tuition & Fees	
Annual tuition	$4,000
Cost of books	$1,200
Fees	$256

University of Calgary

Faculty of Medicine

3330 Hospital Drive NW, Alberta, ON T2N 4N1 • Admission: 403-220-4262

STUDENT BODY

Type	Public
Enrollment of medical school	234
% male/female	48/52
Average age of entering class	25

ADMISSIONS

# applied	1,314

Average GPA and MCAT Scores

Overall GPA	3.5
MCAT Bio	10.7
MCAT Phys	10.5
MCAT Verbal	9.8
MCAT Essay	Q

Application Information

Regular application	11/15
Regular notification	5/14
Are transfers accepted?	Yes
Admissions may be deferred?	Yes
Admissions need-blind?	No
Application fee	$65

Academics

Medical students follow an intensive, eleven-month curriculum for a period of three years. Learning is based in part on clinical case presentations. In addition to the standard M.D. course of study, programs are offered in conjunction with the Faculty of Graduate Studies in Biomedical and Health Sciences with the objective of training clinician-scientists for academic medical research and those who will design, manage, and implement health care delivery programs. M.D./Ph.D. and M.D./M.Sc. programs are available in Biochemistry and Molecular Biology, Cardiovascular/Respiratory Sciences, Community Health Sciences, Gastrointestinal Sciences, Medical Science, Microbiology and Infectious Diseases, and Neuroscience.

BASIC SCIENCES: First year courses are based on organ systems and are taught primarily through lectures and small group discussions. Subjects are: Principles of Medicine, Blood, Muscoskeletal and Skin, Cardiovascular, Respiratory, Renal-Electrolyte, Endocrine Metabolic, Medical Skills Program, and Intergrative. The second academic period begins in July. Subjects are: Neuroscience, The Mind, Gastrointestinal, Reproduction, Human Development, and Medical Skills Program. Throughout the first and second years, students also take part in independant research projects. Courses are taught in the Calgary Health Sciences Center, about 1.5 km from the main campus of the University of Calgary. The medical library is fully computerized, receives more than 1,000 serials, and houses approximately 130,000 books. It serves medical and nursing students as well as the greater university and the medical community. Other important facilities include the Medical Learning Resource Center that houses instructional tools geared towards learning anatomical systems, and the Medical Skills Center for improving clinical skills and techniques.

CLINICAL TRAINING

Required clerkships are Anesthesia (2 weeks), Family Medicine (4 weeks), Internal Medicine (12 weeks), Ob/Gyn (6 weeks), Pediatrics (6 weeks), Psychiatry (6 weeks), and Surgery (8 weeks). Ten weeks are available for clinical electives. Training takes place primarily at the facilities of the Foothills Hospital, the Peter Lougheed Center, the Alberta Children's Hospital, and the Rockyview Hospital. In addition, the University of Calgary Medical Clinic allows medical students to learn about outpatient service delivery, preventative programs, and travel medicine.

Students

While medical students are primarily Canadian, the student body at the University of Calgary includes several hundred international students. Within the Faculty of Medicine, women compromise about 50 percent of students. The majority of medical students are from within the province of Alberta.

STUDENT LIFE

Student life is enhanced by campus activities, the resources of the community and city of Calgary, and the wide range of outdoor activities available. Nearby national parks, such as Banff and Jasper, offer skiing and hiking. The region also has vibrant wildlife and areas for fishing, swimming, and canoeing. In addition to its academic facilities, the Health Sciences Center includes a medical bookstore, exercise room, student lounge, cafeteria, and mall area. Medical students also have access to the resources of the greater university, including complete athletic and recreational facilities, intramural sports programs, outdoor programs, arts, and theatre. The University Student Union organizes events and activities and operates a bookstore, cafe, and bar, along with other services. On-campus housing is available for single and married students. An off-campus registry is managed by the student union.

GRADUATES

Though most graduates enter post graduate training that leads to careers in clinical medicine, some go on to pursue research and academic medicine. Increasingly, graduates are entering primary care fields.

Admissions

REQUIREMENTS

Students must have completed at least two full years of university education before being considered for admission. The minimum grade requirement for a Canadian citizen or landed immigrant resident of Alberta is an average of 3.0/4.0, which translates to a grade of B or at least 78 percent of each year of study. The minimum grade point average required of Canadians from other provinces is 3.5/4.0. The MCAT is required, and applicants should have at least an average score of 8. In addition to transcripts and completed application form, three letters of reference are required.

SUGGESTIONS

Although the faculty has no prescribed prerequisites, the one year of each of the following courses is strongly recommended: English, Biology, General Chemistry, Organic Chemistry, Biochemistry, Physics, Physiology, Calculus, and Pyschology/Sociology. Presently, spaces for international students are limited to those students who come from institutions and/or countries with which the Faculty of Medicine at the University of Calgary has a formal, contractional agreement. All international students must sign an acknowledgment that the M.D. program would not lead to an opportunity for post graduate training through the Canadian Resident Matching Service.

PROCESS

The application is available at www.med.ucalgary.ca/admissions. It requires information about all university courses taken, MCAT test dates/results, employment history, extracurricular activities, and an essay. The completed application is due November 15. The deadline for receipt of the three letters of reference, all official transcripts, and official MCAT scores is January 4. Applicants will be notified by March 15 whether or not they will be invited for an interview. In a recent year, there were 1,300 applicants for 100 positions.

Admissions Requirements (Required)

Interview

COSTS AND AID

Tuition & Fees

Annual tuition (in-state out-of-state)	$6,519/$30,000
Cost of books	$1,200
Fees	$333

UNIVERSITY OF CALIFORNIA—DAVIS
SCHOOL OF MEDICINE

4610 X STREET, SUITE 1202, SACRAMENTO, CA 95817 • ADMISSION: 916-734-4800 • FAX: 916-734-40507
E-MAIL: MEDADMSINFO@UCDAVIS.EDU • WEBSITE: WWW.UCDMC.UCDAVIS.EDU / MEDSCHOOL

STUDENT BODY

Type	Public
Enrollment of parent institution	33,300
Enrollment of medical school	415
% male/female	47/53
% out-of-state	1
% international	66
Average age of entering class	26

FACULTY

Total faculty	864
% female faculty	36
Student-faculty ratio	2.0:1

ADMISSIONS

# applied	5,863
% accepted	4
% enrolled	46

Average GPA and MCAT Scores

Overall GPA	3.6
MCAT Bio	10.7
MCAT Phys	10.2
MCAT Verbal	9.5

Application Information

Regular application	10/1
Regular notification	10/15
Are transfers accepted?	No
Admissions may be deferred?	Yes
Admissions need-blind?	No
Application fee	$80

Academics

The School of Medicine is well-integrated into the UC Davis Campus and benefits from the academic programs of the University. Our students have opportunity for joint-degree programs including MD/Ph.D, MD/MBA, MD/MPH, and MD/MS. Those interested in careers as physician-scientists may apply for programs leading to doctorates in the following fields: Biochemistry, Biomedical Engineering, Cell Biology, Genetics, Immunology, Molecular Biology, Neuroscience, Pathology, Pharmacology, Physiology and in the humanities or social sciences.

BASIC SCIENCES: The third year curriculum has six required clerkship rotations in Surgery, Internal Medicine, Obstetrics/Gynecology, Pediatrics, Psychiatry, and Primary Care provide comprehensive training in the major clinical disciplines. The clerkships consist of a mixture of in-patient and ambulatory rotations on various services that provide in-depth, supervised patient care experiences. Each clerkship includes required didactic sessions and case interactives. The longitudinal Doctoring curriculum runs concurrently with the clerkships. The course consists of bimonthly longitudinal small groups led by faculty members who remain with their group throughout the year as the students rotate through their clerkships. Doctoring 3 themes include advanced interviewing techniques, clinical reasoning, clinical epidemiology, evidence-based medicine, and ethics/jurisprudence. The fourth year curriculum features built-in flexibility to allow students to individualize their medical careers. The early start to the fourth year in May allows students to pursue electives for early exposure to clinical specialties or to complete clerkships which may have been deferred. All students are required to select 32 weeks of learning activities in addition to a single 4 week special study module or scholarly project. Two, 4-week acting internships and a 4-week selective covering "care of the undifferentiated patient" are strongly recommended. Students must take a comprehensive clinical skills examination at the beginning of the fourth year which features self-assessment and faculty feedback. Individual student programs are designed under the guidance of college directors, mentors and faculty advisors, with the support of the Career Advising Office. Each student's fourth year program must be approved by the Fourth Year Oversight Committee to ensure appropriate breadth, depth, and vigor. There are strict guidelines for the choices and time allowed away from the home institution. Fourth year students are required to select a single 4-week Special Study Module from a range of offerings, or they may opt to complete a Scholarly Project. The Special Study modules are designed to integrate basic sciences with clinical sciences, provide opportunities for students to practice and refine fundamental skills in critical appraisal and analysis of emerging scientific developments, and to allow students to focus in-depth on a multidisciplinary topic of special interest to the student. The Scholarly Project requires independent inquiry with faculty mentorship and leads to a publishable manuscript and student presentation of the project at a research forum held in the spring. The fourth year curriculum also provides 18 weeks of unscheduled time for electives, research, residency interviews, national board study, or vacation.

CLINICAL TRAINING

The pre-clerkship curriculum is organized around five sequentially-taught blocks to promote integration of basic sciences and clinical medicine. Five blocks of basic science and pathophysiology courses are grouped by complementary objectives, disciplines, and themes. The longitudinal Doctoring curriculum focusing on clinical skills, clinical reasoning, epidemiology, social-behavioral medicine, and biomedical ethics is woven throughout the five blocks and integrated with concurrent courses. Longitudinal courses in pathology, pharmacology, and oncology are similarly integrated with concurrent courses, beginning with the second block. Block 1: The basic science portion of Block 1 includes courses in Molecular Biology, Microscopic Anatomy, Genetics, Gross Anatomy/Embryology/Radiology, and Human Physiology. The major organizing theme is structure-function along the continuum of hierarchical biologic structure from molecule to cell, tissue and major organ systems. The three year Doctoring curriculum begins with Doctoring 1, which is presented concurrently with the other courses. The focus of Doctoring 1 in the first block is interviewing and physical examination training using standardized patients and models, correlated with concurrent gross anatomy and physiology by organ system. Cases are used in the problem-based learning approach to correlate basic science courses with concepts in clinical medicine. The course provides an introduction to epidemiology and biostatistics through didactic and small group sessions. Behavioral medicine, cross-cultural medicine, and ethics are woven into cases, workshops, and didactic presentations. Students are required to attend preceptorships in the community and participate in home visits. Block 2: The second block includes two major threads, each of which is composed of several integrated courses. The Immunology / Microbiology / Pharmacology / Pathology thread presents an introduction to host defense, infection, basic pharmacologic principles, and general pathologic processes. The Metabolism/Endocrinology/Nutrition/Reproduction (MERN) thread covers essential concepts in metabolism, basic and clinical nutrition, reproductive medicine, and clinical endocrinology. The general pathology course also includes male-female GU and endocrine pathology, and the pharmacology course covers antibiotics and endocrine pharmacology, with the goal of integration with concurrent courses. The Doctoring 1 course continues its emphasis on basic clinical skills training with a focus on interviewing skills. The course provides an introduction to behavioral medicine and human development. The problem-based learning approach is used to emphasize basic-science-clinical correlation. Preceptorships and home visits continue. Block 3 consists of an integrated neurosciences curriculum covering neuroanatomy, clinical neurology, and psychopathology. Block 4 is an integrated organ system block covering the hematopoietic-lymphoreticar, cardiovascular, respiratory, and renal-genitourinary systems. Block 5 covers gastrointestinal, musculoskeletal, and integumentary systems. Longitudinal Doctoring 2 Curriculum (Blocks 3-5): The Doctoring 2 curriculum runs throughout three blocks and focuses on advanced clinical skills, epidemiology, ethics, and problem-based assessment. History taking and physical diagnosis skills are correlated with the ongoing pathophysiology courses. Students are assigned to preceptorships where they learn how to perform and document comprehensive patient assessments. Longitudinal Pathology, Pharmacology, and Oncology Curricula: Systemic pathology and pharmacology build upon foundations presented in Block 2 during the three blocks of the second year. Oncology is presented in Blocks 4 and 5. All of these courses are designed to integrate with concurrent organ systems pathology courses, with frequent combined sessions and cases to illustrate fundamental basic science principles and their clinical applications.

Students

Located in Sacramento, the campus is part of a vibrant, metropolitan area within driving distance from tourists attractions such as San Francisco, Lake Tahoe, Reno, and Yosemite National Park to name few.

STUDENT LIFE

The UC Davis School of Medicine provides exceptional student support services including but not limited to academic services, career advising, student-interest group, student-run clinics, wellness support, and recreational opportunities. Locally, the students access to active night life and activities such as Sacramento and American River Bike Trail, professional sport events, and Second Art Saturday to name a few.

GRADUATES

Close to 45 percent of graduates enter primary care fields. The UC Davis Health System has at least 20 residency programs. Davis graduates are successful at obtaining residency position in prestigious programs all over the country.

UNIVERSITY OF CALIFORNIA—IRVINE

SCHOOL OF MEDICINE

OFFICE OF ADMISSIONS & OUTREACH, 836 HEALTH SCIENCES ROAD IRVINE, CA 92697-4089
ADMISSION: 949-824-5388 • FAX: 949-824-24857 • E-MAIL: MEDADMIT@UCI.EDU
WEBSITE: WWW.UCIHS.UCI.EDU/ADMISSIONS

STUDENT BODY

Type	Public
Enrollment of parent institution	27,792
Enrollment of medical school	430
% male/female	51/49
Average age of entering class	24

FACULTY

Total faculty	625
% female faculty	33
% part-time faculty	33
Student-faculty ratio	2.0:1

ADMISSIONS

# applied	5,380
% accepted	5
% enrolled	40

Average GPA and MCAT Scores

Overall GPA	3.7
MCAT Bio	11.3
MCAT Phys	11.1
MCAT Verbal	9.8
MCAT Essay	Q

Application Information

Regular application	11/1
Are transfers accepted?	No
Admissions may be deferred?	Yes
Admissions need-blind?	No
Application fee	$80

Academics

The UCI medical curriculum is designed to meet the changing needs of medical education within all four years of instruction. Medical students are encouraged to become participants in their education process, to be active rather than passive learners, to become lifelong learners, and to use cooperative and team-learning principles. To satisfy the requirement for the MD degree, each medical student must successfully complete the full curriculum. Students must also pass both Step 1 and Step 2 of the United States Medical Licensing Examination (USMLE) and successfully pass a Clinical Practice Examination (CPX) prior to graduation. Most students follow a four-year curriculum, throughout which the Clinical Foundations course series integrates clinical, social, and basic science concepts. Each year six students are accepted into the Medical Scientist Training Program (MSTP), leading to a combined MD/PhD degree. The PhD can be earned in a number of fields, including all of the biological sciences, engineering sciences, information and computer sciences, and physical sciences. For those who meet requirements, a joint MD/MBA program can be pursued in conjunction with UCI's Paul Merage School of Business. PRIME-LC is a dual degree program (MD/masters) and a national model for meeting the health care needs of the growing Latino population.

BASIC SCIENCES: The School has achieved vertical integration of the curriculum with the development of the Clinical Foundations course series. These courses are longitudinal multidisciplinary experiences broadly designed to prepare students for their future careers in medicine through the application of experiential and self-directed learning principles. Clinical Foundations courses utilize small group learning sessions to reinforce core concepts of patient-physician interactions and introductory clinical reasoning skill development. In addition to Clinical Foundations I, the first year curriculum includes courses in Anatomy and Embryology, Histology, Immunology, Medical Genetics, Neuroscience, Medical Biochemistry and Molecular Biology, and Medical Physiology. Second year curriculum includes Clinical Pathology, General and Systematic Pathology, Medical Microbiology, Medical Pharmacology courses. Tutorial programs, academic monitoring, and study-skills workshops promote student success in the basic sciences. The Grunigen Medical Library is located at the UCI Medical Center and meets the research, education, and patient care needs of Medical Center staff and the UCI School of Medicine. The School of Medicine is fully computerized with an internal electronic information network.

CLINICAL TRAINING

Patient contact begins during the first year with the Clinical Foundations I course and continues during the second year with Clinical Foundations II. Standardized and surrogate patients are employed throughout the four years to enhance interactive experience. During the third and fourth years Clinical Foundations III and IV explore many issues first presented during the introductory courses with greater emphasis placed on advanced skill acquisition and professional role development. Required clerkships begin in year three and include Inpatient and Ambulatory Medicine, Obstetrics and Gynecology, Surgery, Psychiatry, Family Medicine, and Pediatrics. Year four rotations include Intensive Care Unit, Neuroscience, Emergency Medicine, Radiology, a musculoskeletal elective, and Substance Abuse. The primary training sites are UCI Medical Center in the City of Orange, which includes specialized clinical and research centers; Veterans Affairs Long Beach Healthcare System; Long Beach Memorial Medical Center;

Miller Children's Hospital; Children's Hospital of Orange County; and affiliated hospitals and clinics. Affiliates are located in Orange and Los Angeles counties, serving both rural and urban communities. During the clinical years, narrative evaluations supplement the honors/pass/fail grading system.

Students

On and off campus, medical students can find a wide variety of recreational and extracurricular activities to help keep overall balance in their lives and discover new outlets for fitness and fun.

STUDENT LIFE

UCI has many student-interest groups, including those that provide support to minority students and to students with children. Other groups are geared toward volunteer and community activities. Medical students have access to a wide variety of resources at UCI, including cultural events, intramural athletics, and all facilities. On-campus, graduate-student housing is affordable, comfortable, and allows medical students to interact with students from other departments. Apartments, residence halls, and residential communities, that feature living spaces of all sizes, are available. The city of Irvine and surrounding communities, such as Newport Beach, provide recreational opportunities and attractive housing options.

GRADUATES

A large proportion of graduates enter post-graduate programs at UCI, which has one of the nation's largest residency programs in primary care disciplines and internal medicine. Most graduates enter programs in California, but seniors have been successful in obtaining residencies all over the country.

Admissions

REQUIREMENTS

The following must be completed prior to matriculation: 2 years of Chemistry (1 year of Labs, courses must include Inorganic, Organic, and Biochemistry); 1 year of Physics; 1.5 years of Biology (1 year of Labs Courses, must include 1 upper-division Biology course); 1 year of Math (courses must included Calculus and Statistics); and .5 year of English Writing/Composition. The Medical College Admission Test (MCAT) is required. An officially certified test score must be received by the Admissions and Outreach Office before a candidate's application can be considered. The MCAT must be taken within three years of application and no later than September of the year prior to matriculation.

SUGGESTIONS

Applicants are strongly encouraged to have completed their basic science requirements by the time they submit their application. No specific major is required, however, demonstrated ability in the sciences is of great importance. In addition, applicants are advised to take advantage of the intellectual maturation afforded by a well-rounded liberal arts education. English, the humanities, the social and behavioral sciences are considered particularly important. The following courses are also recommended but not required: cell biology, genetics, physical chemistry, vertebrate embryology, developmental and abnormal psychology, and Spanish.

PROCESS

The UCI Schoolof Medicine seeks to admit students who are highly qualified to be trained in the practice of medicine and whose backgrounds, talents, and experiences contribute to a diverse student body. The Admissions Committee carefully reviews all applicants whose undergraduate record and scores on the MCAT indicate that they will be able to handle the rigorous curriculum of medical school. Careful consideration is given to applicants from disadvantaged backgrounds (i.e., disadvantaged through social, cultural, and/or economic conditions).

Admissions Requirements (Required)

MCAT Scores, Essays, Science GPA, Non-Science GPA, Recommendation, Interview

Admissions Requirements (Optional)

Extracurricular activities, Exposure to medical profession, State Residency

COSTS AND AID

Tuition & Fees

Annual tuition (in-state out-of-state)	$31,134/$43,379
Room & board (on-campus off-campus)	$21,045/$15,245
Cost of books	$1,967
Fees	$4,201

Financial Aid

% students receiving any aid	88
% students receiving grants	67
% students receiving loans	68
% aid that is merit-based	0
Average grant	$11,270
Average loan	$44,000
Average total aid package	$60,163
Average debt	$150,694

UNIVERSITY OF CALIFORNIA—LOS ANGELES

DAVID GEFFEN SCHOOL OF MEDICINE AT UCLA

CENTER FOR HEALTH SCIENCES, LOS ANGELES, CA 90095-1720 • ADMISSION: 310-825-6081 • FAX: 310-825-60817
E-MAIL: SOMADMISS@MEDNET.UCLA.EDU • WEBSITE: WWW.MEDSTUDENT.UCLA.EDU

STUDENT BODY

Type	Public
Enrollment of medical school	674
% male/female	58/42
% international	30

ADMISSIONS

# applied	5,244

Application Information

Regular application	11/1
Regular notification	1/15
Early application	6/1
Are transfers accepted?	Yes
Admissions need-blind?	Yes
Application fee	$40

Academics

Each year, 10 students are admitted to an Extended Curriculum Program, which spreads the first two years of the standard curriculum over three years, creating opportunities for special projects or supplemental instruction. In each class, as many as 24 students who are interested in practicing in underserved communities spend their first two years at UCLA School of Medicine, and then complete clinical requirements at Drew University facilities. Drew University is a predominantly African American medical institution. Several joint-degree programs are offered to medical students, including an M.D./M.P.H. with the School of Public Health, an M.D./M.B.A. with the School of Management, and an M.S.T.P.-sponsored M.D./Ph.D. All entering students are required to purchase a computer because both the basic science and clinical curriculum emphasize its applications.

BASIC SCIENCES: During the first two years, students are in scheduled sessions for about 26 hours per week. In addition to required courses, Selectives give students an opportunity to explore topics of interest such as health care reform, addiction, and AIDS. Year-one courses are the following: Micro-Anatomy and Cell Biology; Topics in Physiology; Biological Chemistry; Anatomy; Organ System Physiology; Basic Neurology; Biomathematics; Doctoring I; and Clinical Applications of Basic Sciences (CAB.S.). Doctoring I is the beginning of the Doctoring Curriculum, which uses a case-based approach and addresses the interdisciplinary issues that pertain to practicing medicine. In this course, the cultural, ethical, legal, economic, and social perspectives on medicine are considered. In CAB.S., students participate in community-based, health education, or health care projects and learn to apply basic science concepts to real-life clinical problems. Year-two courses are the following: Microbiology; Pathology; Pharmacology; Pathophysiology; Psychopathology; Doctoring II; Genetics; and Clinical Fundamentals, which covers physical diagnosis and takes place largely at clinical sites. Both University-sponsored and student-initiated study and tutorial groups are available. Most classes are taught in the Health Sciences Building, a large structure on the UCLA campus in Westwood. The Biomedical Library is nearby and serves faculty, students, and the community with a collection of 500,000 volumes and 6,000 current journals. Grading is Pass/Fail, with written citations for outstanding achievement. Promotion to year three requires a passing score on the USMLE Step 1.

CLINICAL TRAINING

Outside of traditional clerkships, students gain experience with patients in Doctoring and through the extensive volunteer opportunities. Some students identify volunteer opportunities with the assistance of the Community Service Compendium, a list of community outreach sites. Formal clinical training takes place during the third and fourth years, which are treated as a continuum. Fifty-seven weeks of the third and fourth years are reserved for the following required rotations: Medicine (12 weeks); Surgery (12 weeks); Pediatrics (6 weeks); Ob/Gyn (6 weeks); Psychiatry (6 weeks); Family Medicine (6 weeks); Radiology (4 weeks); Neurology (2 weeks); and Ophthalmology (2 weeks). Clerkships take place primarily at the University Hospital (517 beds). Other affiliated sites are Harbor General (800 beds); Cedars-Sinai; Kaiser Sunset; Kaiser West LA; Kern Medical Center (Bakersfield); King/Drew Medical Center; Olive View-UCLA Medical Center (Sylmar); Sepulveda Veterans Affairs; St. Mary Medical Center (Long Beach); and West LA Veterans Affairs Medical Center. Doctoring III is taken throughout the years, occupying students for one full day every other week. This segment of the course takes students to community-based medical sites and uses a small-group format to discuss various patient problems. Twenty-seven weeks remain for electives. Some of the elective requirement may be fulfilled around the country or overseas. Grading is Pass/Fail supplemented with written evaluations. The USMLE Step 2 is required for graduation.

Students

The students reflect the multicultural population of Los Angeles, with underrepresented minorities accounting for one-third of the student body. In entering classes, the average age is 22, and there are usually no more than a few students over 28 years old. Eighty-five percent of the students are California residents. Class size is 145.

STUDENT LIFE

In addition to the beaches and beautiful weather of Southern California and Los Angeles, the UCLA campus itself offers excellent athletic facilities and plenty of entertainment. Student-led groups and activities within the medical school are numerous, ranging from the Iranian/American Medical Organization, to the Salvation Army Outreach Clinic. The medical school also sponsors activities that encourage cohesion between faculty and students. Although residence halls and married-student housing are available, most medical students opt to live off campus.

GRADUATES

Graduates are well-prepared for careers in primary care, more specialized clinical fields, and research. About half of the graduates enter primary care fields, which is roughly the current national average. Many enter residencies at UCLA or affiliated hospitals.

Admissions

REQUIREMENTS

Admissions requirements are: English (one year); college Math (one year, to include calculus and statistics); Physics (one year); Chemistry (two years, including inorganic and organic); and Biology (one year). Science courses must have associated labs, and AP credits are not counted. The MCAT is required, and scores must be no more than three years old. Generally, if a student has retaken the exam, the best set of scores is used.

SUGGESTIONS

Courses in Humanities and Social Sciences, as well as Spanish and Computer Skills are highly recommended. Undergraduate courses that overlap with those in the medical school curriculum, such as Anatomy, are not recommended. For applicants who graduated college several years ago, recent course work is expected. The April, rather than August, MCAT is advised. Extracurricular activities that are medically related, or that involve research or patient contact, are useful. UCLA is unusual among state-affiliated medical schools in California in that it welcomes applications from well-qualified, out-of-state residents.

PROCESS

Typically, 55 percent of AMCAS applicants are asked to submit supplementary information. Of those returning secondaries, about 20 percent are invited for interviews. Interviews take place from November through May and consist of one or two sessions with faculty members and/or medical students. Notification begins in January and continues until enough offers have been made to fill the class. About 25 percent of interviewees are accepted, and another group is wait-listed. Wait-listed candidates may send additional information about academic or extracurricular achievements. The UCLA/ UC Riverside Biomedical Sciences Program allows 24 admitted students to obtain both the B.S. and M.D. degrees in 7 years. In this program, students enter UCLA School of Medicine after completing 3 years of undergraduate preparation at UC Riverside.

Admissions Requirements (Required)

MCAT Scores, Science GPA, Extracurricular activities, Non-Science GPA, Exposure to medical profession, Recommendation, Interview, State Residency

Admissions Requirements (Optional)

Essays

COSTS AND AID

Tuition & Fees

Annual tuition	$12,245
Room & board (on-campus off-campus)	$4,620/$14,000
Cost of books	$4,360
Fees	$22,024

UNIVERSITY OF CALIFORNIA—SAN DIEGO

UCSD SCHOOL OF MEDICINE

9500 GILMAN DRIVE, MC 0621 LA JOLLA, CA 92093-0621 • ADMISSION: 858-534-3880 • FAX: 858-534-52827
E-MAIL: SOMADMISSIONS@UCSD.EDU • WEBSITE: MEDED.UCSD.EDU / ADMISSIONS

STUDENT BODY

Type	Public
Enrollment of parent institution	25,964
Enrollment of medical school	503
% male/female	51/49
% out-of-state	3
% international	18
Average age of entering class	23

ADMISSIONS

# applied	5,238
% accepted	6
% enrolled	42

Average GPA and MCAT Scores

Overall GPA	3.7
MCAT Bio	11.5
MCAT Phys	11.7
MCAT Verbal	10.5
MCAT Essay	Q

Application Information

Regular application	11/1
Regular notification	10/15
Are transfers accepted?	No
Admissions may be deferred?	Yes
Admissions need-blind?	No
Application fee	$60

Academics

In addition to fulfilling course requirements, students must complete an Independent Study Project to graduate. These projects allow students to explore and define their own interests, and to collaborate with faculty members who share these interests. The medical school benefits from the resources of other parts of UCSD. Joint M.D./Ph.D. programs are possible with UCSD Graduate Departments in Biochemistry, Biomedical Engineering; Biophysics, Cell Biology, Genetics, Immunology, Microbiology, Molecular Biology, Neuroscience, Pathology, Pharmacology, and Physiology. Normally, these degrees are M.S.T.P. sponsored. Students can earn an M.P.H. in conjunction with nearby San Diego State University Graduate School of Public Health.

BASIC SCIENCES: The first two years are organized into quarters. Electives are an important supplement to basic science requirements and account for about 20 percent of scheduled course time. During the fall quarter of year one, Cell Biology and Biochemistry is the principal endeavor. This lecture course is referred to as a "block," which means that the material is covered intensely during one or two quarters. Students also begin a sequence in Social and Behavioral Sciences, taught mostly through small-group sessions. Winter-quarter courses are Physiology, Pharmacology, and Introduction to Clinical Medicine, which continues throughout the basic science curriculum and prepares students for third-year rotations. The spring-quarter courses are Neurology, Pharmacology, Reproductive Biology, Metabolism, and Endocrinology, all of which are taught primarily through lectures. Year two begins with Anatomy, Histology, Biostatistics, and a Social/Behavioral Science course on Health Care Systems. Winter quarter consists of Human Disease, Psychopathology, and Hematology. The second-year, spring-quarter curriculum is Human Disease, Neurology, and Lab Medicine. During the basic science years there are, on average, 34 scheduled hours per week. Instruction takes place in the modern Basic Science Building, which is adjacent to the Biomedical Library (100,000 volumes). Computers with access to online informational services and curricular programs are available for student use in the library and in the School's Learning Resource Center. Grading uses an Honors/Pass/Fail system. The USMLE Step 1 is required for promotion to year three.

CLINICAL TRAINING

Supervised patient contact begins in January of year one, in Introduction to Clinical Medicine. The physical examination is taught in conjunction with the study of individual organ systems in the first year, and together with the history, refined in the second basic science year. In addition, a simulated-patient program provides students the opportunity to improve their history-taking and physical-examination skills, as well as to obtain feedback from faculty mentors and view videotapes of their patient interaction. Required third-year rotations are Medicine (12 weeks); Neurology (4 weeks); Ob/Gyn (6 weeks); Pediatrics (8 weeks); Psychiatry (6 weeks); Surgery (12 weeks); and Primary Care (one afternoon per week, all year). Students design their fourth-year curricula by selecting courses from within broad subject areas. Twelve weeks are selected from Direct Patient Care Clerkships, 4 weeks must be a Primary Care experience, 4 weeks Inpatient Training, and 4 weeks Outpatient Training. An additional 12 weeks of pure elective, clinical clerkships are also required. Clinical training takes place at large hospitals and small clinics including: UCSD Medical Centers (577 beds total); VA Hospital (606 beds); Navy Hospital (750 beds); Children's Hospital (154 beds); Kaiser Foundation Hospital

(1,285 beds); Sharp Memorial Community Hospital (1,415 beds); Clinica De Salubridad de Campesinos; and the U.S. Public Health Service Outpatient Clinic. Electives may be taken from the various departments of UCSD, or may be carried out in conjunction with community organizations. Most students take advantage of additional clinical training opportunities through volunteer work, some of which takes them across the border in Mexico. The USMLE Step 2 is required for graduation. UCSD students do exceptionally well on both parts of the USMLE.

Students

Students are predominantly Californians. There is a wide age range among students, and it is very common for them to have taken a year or two off after college for research or other activities. About 60 percent of incoming students in a recent class were science majors. Class size is 122.

STUDENT LIFE

On-campus housing is convenient, attractive, and popular with students. Modern apartments of all sizes are available for single and married students and for those who have children or pets. Some students rely on bicycles or shuttle buses, while others own cars. UCSD's location affords many recreational possibilities. Year-round outdoor activities include swimming, surfing, biking, sailing, rollerblading, running, and walking. Other activities are the San Diego Symphony, the zoo, and the Padres professional baseball team. Medical student organizations and events also contribute to students' extracurricular lives.

GRADUATES

Of the graduating class of 2006, the most popular fields for post-graduate training were Internal Medicine (38 graduates); Pediatrics (15); Emergency Medicine (9); Anesthesiology (8); Psychiatry (8); Ob/Gyn (8); Radiology (7); Family Medicine (6); Ophthalmology (6); General Surgery (4); Pathology (4); Orthopaedic Surgery (4); and Dermatology (3). Students also "matched" into Neurology, Urology, Otolaryngology, and Plastic Surgery. Many entered programs in San Diego, Oakland, San Jose, Los Angeles, and other California locations.

Admissions

REQUIREMENTS

One year of Chemistry, Organic Chemistry, Biology, Physics, and Math are all required. Strong written and spoken English is a requirement, and the ability to communicate in a second language is preferred. The rigor of an applicant's undergraduate institution is considered in assessing GPA. The MCAT is required, and the spring exam is advised.

SUGGESTIONS

Breadth of academic experience is important. Extracurricular activities are also important, particularly those that involve some sort of medical exposure, community involvement, or leadership.

PROCESS

About 40 percent of applicants receive a secondary application. Of those returning secondaries, between 550–600 are interviewed. Interviews take place from October through early April and consist of two one-hour sessions with faculty members. Following interviews, candidates are accepted, rejected, or put on hold for later notification. About half of those interviewed are eventually accepted. An extensive wait-list is established.

Admissions Requirements (Required)

MCAT Scores, Essays, Science GPA, Non-Science GPA, Recommendation, Interview

Admissions Requirements (Optional)

Extracurricular activities, Exposure to medical profession, State Residency

COSTS AND AID

Tuition & Fees

Annual tuition (in-state out-of-state)	$0/$12,245
Room & board (on-campus off-campus)	$11,412/$7,776
Cost of books	$2,055
Fees	$22,415

Financial Aid

% students receiving any aid	93
% students receiving grants	70
% students receiving loans	88
% aid that is merit-based	2
Average grant	$16,275
Average loan	$21,634
Average total aid package	$36,453
Average debt	$79,562

UNIVERSITY OF CALIFORNIA—SAN FRANCISCO
SCHOOL OF MEDICINE

SCHOOL OF MEDICINE ADMISSIONS, C-200, BOX 0408 SAN FRANCISCO, CA 94143-0408 • **ADMISSION:** 415-476-4044
FAX: 415-476-54907 • **E-MAIL:** ADMISSIONS@MEDSCH.UCSF.EDU • **WEBSITE:** MEDED.UCSF.EDU/ADMISSIONS

STUDENT BODY

Type	Public
Enrollment of medical school	648
% male/female	44/56
% out-of-state	5
% international	27
Average age of entering class	24

FACULTY

Total faculty	1,989
% female faculty	35
% minority faculty	19
% part-time faculty	5
Student-faculty ratio	2.0:1

ADMISSIONS

# applied	6,926
% accepted	4
% enrolled	55

Average GPA and MCAT Scores

Overall GPA	3.8
MCAT Bio	12.0
MCAT Phys	11.8
MCAT Verbal	10.6
MCAT Essay	P

Application Information

Regular application	10/15
Early application	6/1
Are transfers accepted?	No
Admissions may be deferred?	Yes
Admissions need-blind?	No
Application fee	$80

Academics

The standard curriculum for the Doctor of Medicine (M.D.) degree may be completed in four years. However, approximately 40% of UCSF students remain in school for additional time to pursue advanced studies in research or a scholarly project, international health, or additional clinical rotations. Students may spend one year in the Certificate in Biomedical Research program giving them time to complete a substantial research project and to earn the M.D. with Thesis degree. UCSF has a joint M.D.-MPH degree program with UC-Berkeley that allows up to 10 students per year to spend two semesters in Berkeley earning a masters degree from the School of Public Health. In addition, each year twelve students are admitted to the UCSF/UC-Berkeley Joint Medical Program where they complete the pre-clinical, problem-based curriculum and fulfill requirements for a masters of science degree in either public health or health & medical sciences. Upon completion, they transfer to UCSF to complete the third and fourth years. Up to 12 students enter the Medical Science Training Program (M.S.T.P.) joint Ph.D. /M.D. program yearly. Participants may earn a Ph.D. from the following UCSF programs: Biochemistry, Biophysics, Cell Biology, Developmental Biology, Endocrinology, Genetics, Immunology, Neuroscience, Cancer Biology, Stem Cell Biology, Chemistry, Vascular and Cardiac Biology, Virology and Medical Anthropology.

BASIC SCIENCES: The first two years form the "Essential Core," and they are organized into eight block courses, each about eight weeks long. These courses deal with major themes and draw together a range of interdisciplinary topics. The first year courses are Prologue; Major Organ Systems; Cancer; and Brain, Mind, and Behavior. In the second year, students take Infection, Inflammation, and Immunity; Metabolism; Life Cycle; and consolidation Cases. Essential Core lectures, labs, and small group sessions account for about 20 hours a week, and they integrate subjects from the basic, social, and clinical sciences. All courses include supplementary resources on a Web-based system that forms the e-Curriculum. The Essential Core comprises a course called Foundations of Patient Care, which offers students exposure to the clinical setting. This course also allows students to explore issues of professional development, ethics, and doctor-patient interaction.

CLINICAL TRAINING
Patient contact begins during year one in Foundations of Patient Care and in the week-long immersion in the hospital wards called the Clinical Interlude. Clinical elements are wholly integrated into the basic science curriculum, allowing for a smooth transition into the third year. Likewise, the clinical years include segments of classroom instruction that focus on basic and social science concepts. For example, the third year includes three "Intersessions," which occur between clerkship rotations, and offer lectures and small group discussions of basic science connections to the clinical experiences, ethics, evidence-based medicine, and health policy. Required third-year core clerkships are: Anesthesia (2 weeks); Family and Community Medicine (6 weeks); Medicine (8 weeks); Neurology and Psychiatry (8 weeks); Ob/Gyn (6 weeks); Pediatrics (6 weeks); Surgery (8 weeks); and Surgical Subspecialties (2 weeks). Teaching sites are primarily in San Francisco, Oakland, and Fresno and include California Pacific Medical Center; Children's Hospital; Kaiser Foundation Hospitals; UCSF Medical Center including Mount Zion Hospital; San Francisco City Clinics; San Francisco General Hospital; Veterans Affairs Medical Centers in San Francisco and Fresno; University Medical

Center-Fresno; and Langley Porter Neuropsychiatric Institute. Year four is primarily elective study, which may entail international work or research in addition to traditional advanced clinical rotations. Evaluation of students during years three and four includes an Honors/Pass/Fail system enhanced with narrative comments. Outside of clerkships, students gain clinical experience through volunteer work and community service at any number of UCSF-affiliated projects.

Students

Twenty percent of the students are out-of-state residents. Approximately 27 percent of the Fall 2012 entering class are from groups underrepresented in medicine. Virtually all undergraduate majors are represented in the student body. Class size is 141.

STUDENT LIFE

University-owned housing appropriate for both married and single students is available. Many students take part in community programs, which provide not only an opportunity to contribute, but also a chance for student-student and student-faculty interaction in an extracurricular setting. Students have access to school athletic facilities and to many local, outdoor activities including running in Golden Gate Park, surfing at Ocean Beach, mountain biking in Marin County, and skiing around Lake Tahoe, three hours away by car.

GRADUATES

Of the graduating class of 2005, the following specialties were selected by the indicated number of students: Family Practice (8); Internal Medicine (23); Internal Medicine/Primary Care (10); Pediatrics (19); Emergency Medicine (20); Psychiatry (10); Ob/Gyn (8); Surgery (7); Orthopedic Surgery (3); Neurology (3); Ophthalmology (5); Dermatology (2); Anesthesiology (12); Neurosurgery (1); Otolaryngology (3); Radiology (3); Oral Surgery (-); Pathology (4); Physical Medicine (1); Plastic Surgery (-); Radiation Oncology (4); Urology (2); and other (2). In total, 41 percent entered residencies in fields classified as Primary Care. See http://medschool.ucsf.edu/medstudents/resources/match/summary_table.html for details.

Admissions

REQUIREMENTS

To be considered for admission, applicants must complete by June of the year they expect to matriculate: General Chemistry with lab (three quarters, equal to one year); Organic Chemistry (two quarters); Physics and Biology equal to one year. Applications are welcome from candidates who have taken time off between college and applying to medical school. The MCAT is required, and the spring MCAT is strongly advised. For those who retake the test, the most recent scores are considered. MCAT scores must be no more than three years old. California residents are given preference.

SUGGESTIONS

Beyond requirements, applicants should have taken college-level Math, Humanities, and English courses. Upper-division Biology is also recommended. All extracurricular activities that reveal an applicant's interests and demonstrate his or her commitment strengthen the application. Some exposure to medical issues or to patient care is also valuable.

PROCESS

GPA, MCATs, residency, and the AMCAS application are used to screen for secondary applications. The secondary application is straightforward and does not require additional essays for the MD program. Applicants have 3 weeks from the date of receipt of the secondary application to return the secondary and have their letters of recommendation sent via the AMCAS Letter Service. Interviews take place between September and March, and consist of two one-hour blind sessions each with a faculty member or one faculty member and one student. After offers have been made to fill the class, some remaining candidates are placed on a ranked wait-list and may be offered a spot as late as August, depending on accepted students' matriculation rate.

Admissions Requirements (Required)

MCAT Scores, Essays, Science GPA, Recommendation, Interview

Admissions Requirements (Optional)

Extracurricular activities, Non-Science GPA, Exposure to medical profession, State Residency

COSTS AND AID

Tuition & Fees

Annual tuition (in-state out-of-state)	$31,134/$43,379
Room & board	$20,280
Cost of books	$1,890
Fees	$4,000

Financial Aid

% students receiving any aid	86
% students receiving grants	82
% students receiving loans	86
% aid that is merit-based	9
Average grant	$8,358
Average loan	$18,592
Average total aid package	$27,019

THE UNIVERSITY OF CHICAGO
THE UNIVERSITY OF CHICAGO PRITZKER SCHOOL OF MEDICINE

OFFICE OF MEDICAL EDUCATION BSLC 104W, 924 E. 57TH STREET CHICAGO, IL 60637-5416
ADMISSION: 773-702-1937 • FAX: 773-834-54127 • E-MAIL: PRITZKERADMISSIONS@BSD.UCHICAGO.EDU
WEBSITE: PRITZKER.BSD.UCHICAGO.EDU

STUDENT BODY

Type	Private
Enrollment of parent institution	14,721
Enrollment of medical school	451
% male/female	52/48
% underrepresented minorities	4
% out-of-state	72
% international	16
# countries represented	5
Average age of entering class	24

FACULTY

Total faculty	870
% female faculty	32
% minority faculty	24
% part-time faculty	6
Student-faculty ratio	2.0:1

ADMISSIONS

# applied	7,374
% accepted	4
% enrolled	36

Average GPA and MCAT Scores

Overall GPA	3.8
MCAT Bio	12.3
MCAT Phys	12.3
MCAT Verbal	11.1
MCAT Essay	Q

Application Information

Regular application	10/15
Are transfers accepted?	Yes
Admissions may be deferred?	Yes
Admissions need-blind?	No
Application fee	$75

Academics

Pritzker offers a curriculum best characterized as "modified traditional." Pre-clinical topics are presented in lecture, case-based methods, small group discussions and clinical exposure. For example, as students study particular parts in Anatomy, they view afflictions of that body part in a clinical setting. About 24 percent of the students in each class earn a graduate degree in addition to the M.D. degree. Some of these students are M.S.T.P. participants; others are privately funded M.D./Ph.D. students, and still others earn a J.D. or an M.B.A. along with the M.D. Pritzker students are well prepared by the curriculum as evidenced by their strong board exam performances.

BASIC SCIENCES: Chicago follows a quarter system. First-year students will begin their curriculum in August, studying Human Morphology I and II and participating in the Health Care Disparities series. First-year medical students then begin a systems-based study of basic sciences, studying Cells, Molecules and Genes and Clinical Skills 1A, which introduces students to the patient interview. During the winter, first-year students study Cell and Organ Physiology and Clinical Skills 1B, which covers social issues related to medicine (social context, medical ethics). Spring curriculum includes Response to Injury and an opportunity for elective study. Second-year, fall-quarter curriculum includes: Neuroscience, Neuroanatomy, Pharmacology and Human Behavior in Health and Illness. Winter quarter includes: Clinical Pathophysiology and Therapeutics and Clinical Skills 2A, called Physical Diagnosis. The final quarter of pre-clinical studies includes Clinical Pathophysiology and Therapeutics, more clinical skills, Review of Basic Sciences and Electives. Most students use a student-run note-taking co-op in which each participating student is responsible for providing notes on a lecture assigned to him or her. All lectures are also audio-recorded and available for download. First- and second-year students spend their time in the Biological Sciences Learning Center, which is both a center for instruction and research. Classrooms are equipped with audio/video technology, and excellent computer-based learning tools are available. The Knapp Center is a medical research facility with modern laboratory space. The Crerar Library has one of the largest science collections in the country and houses almost one million volumes. Grading is Pass/Fail although students receive graded feedback on exams. Tutoring is available for students who are in danger of failure. Passage of the USMLE is not required for promotion graduation although most students choose to take Step 1 after year two.

CLINICAL TRAINING

Students are introduced to clinical techniques and experiences during their first Autumn quarter at Pritzker, with Clinical Skills 1A. Year three is composed of a series of clerkships with short breaks between rotations. Clerkships take place at the University of Chicago Medical Center, the Comer Children's Hospital, the NorthShore University Health System and Mercy Hospital. These hospitals serve a broad community, and students learn to treat a diverse patient population. Students rotate through the following departments: Internal Medicine (3 months); Ob/Gyn (1.5 months); Psychiatry (1.5 month); Surgery (3 months); Pediatrics (2 months); and Family Medicine (1 month). During the fourth year, students choose "selectives" from the following categories: Inpatient/Subinternship, Scientific Basis of Medical Practice, Neurology, and Anesthesia. The fourth year is also an opportunity for students to pursue individual research projects or to study overseas. The University of Chicago Medical Center has expanded significantly during the past decade, suggesting a strong patient base and economic situation. Evaluation of clinical performance uses marks of Honors, High Pass, Pass, Low Pass, and Fail. Though the USMLE II is not required for graduation, it may be substituted for a comprehensive exam, which is otherwise required.

Students

Pritzker attracts a student body that is very diverse, in every sense of the word. Underrepresented minorities have accounted for 15–20 percent of the student body, and women about 50 percent. Class size is 88. The unique feature of the Pritzker School of Medicine is its integration into the rest of the University of Chicago. It is geographically, administratively and programmatically integrated. As a consequence it attracts students and faculty who have broader scholarly interests and who see the entire University as a resource for their academic goals. Over 24 percent of Pritzker's graduates leave with two degrees and Pritzker is among the top schools in training faculty for academic medicine. Pritzker students obtain additional degrees in business, law, biological sciences, physical sciences, social sciences, humanities and public health.

STUDENT LIFE

The University of Chicago is located in Chicago's Hyde Park neighborhood, a diverse and interesting community. Students are active in curriculum development and have representatives on important administrative councils. Student volunteer organizations are involved in projects such as organizing and implementing health education into public schools. Medical students take part in university-wide activities such as intramural sports. Many students also take national leadership in organizations such as SNMA and AMSA.

GRADUATES

During the past five years, the residency programs that attracted the most Pritzker graduates were: University of Chicago Hospitals; UCSF; University of Michigan; Mass General; University of Washington; University of Penn; Brigham and Women's Boston; McGaw Medical Center; Beth Israel, Boston; Barnes Hospital, Washington University and UCLA. The following specialties were the most popular within the 2006 graduating class: Internal Medicine (24); General Surgery (13); Pediatrics (13); Emergency Medicine (5); Orthopedic Surgery (4); Internal Medicine/Pediatrics (4); Psychiatry (4); Anesthesia (3); Family Practice (3); OB/Gyn (3). About 20 percent of Pritzker graduates ultimately serve as faculty members at universities.

Admissions

REQUIREMENTS

One year of lecture plus lab is required in: Biology, General Chemistry, Organic Chemistry, and Physics. Biochemistry with lab may be substituted for one semester or quarter of organic chemistry. For applicants who graduated from college more than three years prior, recent science course work is important. The MCAT is required and should be no more than three years old.

SUGGESTIONS

Biochemistry is strongly recommended, as is significant course work in social sciences and humanities. The Admissions Committee is interested in what factors motivated applicants to pursue medicine and is also concerned with demonstrated problem-solving skills, leadership, experience with persons different from themselves, and experience in research.

PROCESS

Secondary applications are available to all AMCAS applicants and should be completed as soon as possible, no later than December 1. About 15 percent of applicants returning secondaries are interviewed, with interviews held between September and February. Interviewees participate in three one-on-one sessions with faculty members, admissions staff, and medical students. Of those interviewed, about two fifths are accepted on a rolling basis. Other interviewees will be "Continued" in the process and will be re-evaluated each time the committee meets. Continued candidates are encouraged to submit information that will strengthen their application and will indicate their interest in the school. A wait-list will be created in early May.

Admissions Requirements (Required)

MCAT Scores, Essays, Science GPA, Extracurricular activities, Non-Science GPA, Exposure to medical profession, Recommendation, Interview

Admissions Requirements (Optional)

State Residency

COSTS AND AID

Tuition & Fees

Annual tuition	$37,970
Room & board	$19,868
Cost of books	$1,419
Fees	$3,379

Financial Aid

% students receiving any aid	95
% students receiving grants	80
% students receiving loans	83
% aid that is merit-based	20

University of Cincinnati
College of Medicine

Office of Admissions, P.O. Box 670552, Cincinnati, OH 45267-0552 • Admission: 513-558-7314
Fax: 513-558-11007 • E-mail: comadmis@ucmail.uc.edu • Website: www.MedOneStop.uc.edu

STUDENT BODY

Type	Public
Enrollment of parent institution	41,970
Enrollment of medical school	663
% male/female	52/48
% out-of-state	8
% international	9
Average age of entering class	22

FACULTY

Total faculty	1,837
% female faculty	37
% minority faculty	22
% part-time faculty	11

ADMISSIONS

# applied	4,439
% accepted	9
% enrolled	43

Average GPA and MCAT Scores

Overall GPA	3.7
MCAT Bio	11.2
MCAT Phys	10.9
MCAT Verbal	10.1

Application Information

Regular application	11/15
Early application	8/1
Early notification	10/1
Are transfers accepted?	Yes
Admissions may be deferred?	Yes
Admissions need-blind?	No
Application fee	$25

Academics

Students follow a four-year curriculum leading to the MD degree. There is also a combined MD/MBA program with a five-year curriculum and one year master degrees in Epidemiology, Clinical Research and Public Health. Up to seven positions a year are available in the Medical Scientist Training Program (MSTP), which is an NIH-funded, combined MD/PhD program with a seven- to eight-year curriculum. The Cincinnati MSTP is unique in that it is jointly run by the University of Cincinnati College of Medicine and Cincinnati Children's Hospital, a top-three pediatric research institution. This collaboration provides a wide range of opportunities for basic, clinical, and translational research. The PhD degree may be earned in one of the following disciplines: Cell and Cancer Biology; Environmental Health Sciences (includes clinical/genetic epidemiology); Immunobiology; Molecular, Cellular, and Biochemical Pharmacology; Molecular and Developmental Biology; Molecular Genetics, Biochemistry, and Microbiology; Neuroscience; Pathobiology and Molecular Medicine; Systems Biology and Physiology; and Biomedical Engineering. Medical students interested in shorter-term research projects may pursue them during the summer or as electives. Course grades are Honors/High Pass/Pass/Fail. Passing the USMLE Step 1 is a requirement for advancing to year three and taking and passing Step 1 and Step 2 Clinical Knowledge and Clinical Skills Exams of USMLE is a requirement for graduation.

BASIC SCIENCES: The medical school curriculum is designed to promote active learning and discovery, with an emphasis on small group activities, learning communities, and case based discussions. During the first and second years, the basic science curriculum is delivered via integrated organ system content blocks. Through an ongoing curriculum revision process, the basic sciences are being systematically woven throughout the third and fourth years. Physician & Society, which spans across all four years of the curriculum, provides in-depth learning experiences in the humanities, population health and service learning, professionalism, culture and diversity, patient safety and quality improvement, communication and teamwork, evidence based medicine, physician identity, and the business and law of medicine. Examinations during the first two years are integrated and are completed electronically. The Office of Student Affairs Academic Support Programs provide individual and group tutoring services, academic counseling and support, study skills seminars and a Student-Led Board Review Course for USMLE Step 1. Pre-clinical instruction takes place in the Medical Sciences Building, which is central to the Medical Center. The Donald C. Harrison Health Sciences Library (HSL) has a wealth of health sciences information resources. To supplement a long history of providing broad and deep collections of books and journals, collaborations with the other libraries at the University of Cincinnati (UC) and UC's participation in OhioLINK, a consortium of Ohio's college and university libraries and the State Library of Ohio, have accelerated access to electronic resources far beyond what a single library could provide. The UC libraries have a history of jointly purchasing electronic resources that benefit the entire UC community. HSL customers have access to more than 50 million library volumes, 700 research databases, 16,000 full-text electronic journals, and 68,000 electronic books.

CLINICAL TRAINING

Students complete a First Responder and BLS course in the first two weeks of medical school. After an intense history, physical exam and clinical skills course, students begin a primary care longitudinal clerkship. Medical students are paired with a community physician mentor from January of the first year through the completion of the second year. Students also participate in a year-long interprofessional clinical experience track during their first and second years. Third-year required clerkships are Internal Medicine (8 weeks); Surgery (8 weeks); Pediatrics (8 weeks); Obstetrics/Gynecology (8 weeks); Psychiatry (6 weeks); Family Medicine (4 weeks); and two Specialty electives (2 weeks each). During the fourth year, students complete an eight-week Internal Medicine acting internship, a four-week Neuroscience selective, and 24 weeks of electives, some of which must be in outpatient care. Most clinical training occurs at University Hospital, Veterans Administration Medical Center, Children's Hospital Medical Center, the Christ Hospital, the Good Samaritan Hospital, and the Jewish Hospital. Half of the elective credits may be earned at other institutions in the area, around the country, or abroad. One organized overseas program is the International Health Elective, which involves hands-on clinical experience in a UC clinic in Honduras or other international clinics.

Students

Among students in the 2012 entering class, 71 percent were Ohio residents, 10 percent were minorities, and 11 percent were 26 years of age or older at the time of application. Seventy four percent of students were science and math majors. The 2012 entering class size was 171.

GRADUATES

Of those who graduated in 2012, 27 percent entered residency programs in Cincinnati, 14 percent entered programs elsewhere in Ohio, and the remaining graduates were successful in securing positions nationwide. The most prevalent fields for post-graduate study were Emergency Medicine (14.3%), Internal Medicine (all types, 14.3%), Anesthesia (10.2%), Pediatrics and Radiology (8.2%), Surgery (7.5%), Family Medicine (5.4%), and Orthopaedic Surgery (4.8%).

Admissions

REQUIREMENTS

Candidates must submit MCAT scores that are no more than two years old at the time of application. (For example, if you are applying for the 2013 entering class, you must submit scores from the 2012, 2011, or 2010 administration). Ohio residents are given preference. Although no courses are specified, applicants are expected to have the knowledge usually gained in a one year lecture and laboratory course in Biology, General Chemistry, Organic Chemistry, Physics, and Math. Applicants are expected to have an undergraduate preparation that provides insight into behavioral, social, and cultural issues. Academically, applicants are evaluated based on the following: Overall GPA; Science GPA; MCAT scores; and undergrad, graduate, and postbacc achievement. Personal qualities are strongly considered and applicants should demonstrate motivation, maturity, coping skills, leadership abilities, interpersonal skills, compassion, sensitivity and tolerance, and good communication skills.

PROCESS

Applicants must submit an AMCAS application and complete the UC On-line Secondary Application to be considered for Admissions. Approximately 650 applicants are interviewed. Interviewees attend an informational program, eat lunch, and tour the College with current students. An interview and acceptance are given using a holistic evaluation of academic, extra-curricular activities, leadership and other personal qualities and preference is given to in state students. Notification of the Committee's decision occurs on a rolling basis, beginning on October 15th until mid March.

Admissions Requirements (Required)

MCAT Scores, Essays, Science GPA, Non-Science GPA, Recommendation, Interview

Admissions Requirements (Optional)

Extracurricular activities, Exposure to medical profession, State Residency

COSTS AND AID

Tuition & Fees

Annual tuition (in-state out-of-state)	$28,820/$46,550
Room & board	$19,015
Cost of books	$1,665
Fees	$1,804

Financial Aid

% students receiving any aid	87
% students receiving grants	30
% students receiving loans	86
% aid that is merit-based	5
Average debt	$164,625

UNIVERSITY OF COLORADO
UNIVERSITY OF COLORADO SCHOOL OF MEDICINE

MEDICAL SCHOOL ADMISSIONS, MAIL STOP C-297, PO BOX 5508 AURORA, CO 80045 • ADMISSION: 303-724-8025
FAX: 303-724-80287 • E-MAIL: SOMADMIN@UCHSC.EDU • WEBSITE: WWW.UCHSC.EDU/SOM/ADMISSIONS

STUDENT BODY

Type	Public
Enrollment of medical school	588
% male/female	50/50
% out-of-state	21
% international	11
Average age of entering class	25

FACULTY

Total faculty	1,900
% part-time faculty	0

ADMISSIONS

# applied	2,984
% accepted	9
% enrolled	56

Average GPA and MCAT Scores

Overall GPA	3.7
MCAT Bio	11.0
MCAT Phys	11.0
MCAT Verbal	10.8
MCAT Essay	Q

Application Information

Regular application	11/1
Are transfers accepted?	Yes
Admissions may be deferred?	Yes
Admissions need-blind?	No
Application fee	$100

Academics

The School of Medicine is part of the University of Colorado Health Sciences Center, which includes schools of Dentistry, Nursing, Pharmacy, and Graduate Studies. A combined M.D./Ph.D. degree through the M.S.T.P. is possible in the following fields: Biochemistry, Biophysics, Cell Biology, Immunology, Molecular Biology, Microbiology, Pharmacology, and Physiology.

BASIC SCIENCES: The first two years are organized into quarters. Throughout year one, Microanatomy, Physiology, and Foundations of Doctoring are studied. Foundations of Doctoring, which establishes one-on-one mentoring relationships between students and local practicing physicians, is the first of three segments that together constitute the curricular element of the Generalist Initiative. In addition, during the fall, students take Biochemistry and Human Anatomy. Year one, winter-quarter courses are Genetics and Neurobiology. Spring courses are Biochemistry and Nutrition, Embryology, and Ethics. Year-long courses during year two are the following: Pathology, Pharmacology, Human Behavior, and Foundations of Doctoring. Immunology and Microbiology are also taken in the fall, and Neuroscience, Pathophysiology, and Epidemiology are taken in the winter. Students spend about 28 hours per week in a structured-learning environment. About 40 percent of this time is devoted to lecture, and another 40 percent to lab. Small-group sessions are also employed as an instructional technique. Academic tutoring and counseling are available to students through a student advocacy program. Grading is Honors/Pass/Fail. Students must pass the USMLE Step 1 to begin the clinical years.

CLINICAL TRAINING
Patient contact begins in year one, when students work closely with practicing physicians and gradually gain independent responsibility. Third-year, required clerkships consist of Medicine (12 weeks); Surgery (6 weeks); Family Medicine (6 weeks); Ob/Gyn (6 weeks); Neurology (4 weeks); Pediatrics (6 weeks); and Psychiatry (6 weeks). One afternoon each week is dedicated to the continuing primary care experience as the third segment of the Foundations of Doctoring sequence. During year four, students select from Surgical Specialties (6 weeks, including one week each of Anesthesiology, Ophthalmology, Orthopedics, Otolaryngology, and Urology) and from a wide range of general electives. Most clerkships take place at University Hospital; VA Medical Center; Denver Health Medical Center; Children's Hospital; and the National Jewish Center for Immunology and Respiratory Medicine. Electives and some required clerkships may be fulfilled at community hospitals and clinics around the state, or under the supervision of affiliated private physicians in the area. Denver is a rapidly growing city with a population of over 2 million. It is an international tourist destination, making the patient population more diverse than that associated with medical schools in other predominantly rural states. Evaluation during the clinical years uses an Honors/Pass/Fail system enhanced with narratives from professors. There are opportunities for clinical experiences outside of traditional rotations, generally through outreach activities and volunteer work. Students may volunteer at clinics that provide care to Denver's homeless population or may spend time working with low-income children in need of care. The Medical Student International Program is popular, granting students credit for up to 4 months of overseas study or work. Passing the USMLE Step 2 is required for graduation.

Students

At least 85 percent of students are Colorado residents. Science and nonscience majors are equally represented. With a mean age of 26 for entering students, there is clearly a wide age range within the student body. Class size is 132.

STUDENT LIFE

Denver is a comfortable, affordable, and student-friendly place to live. It is less than an hour from perhaps the best skiing in the country. During the summer, the hiking, swimming, climbing, and mountain biking are all outstanding. Single students live off campus in apartments and shared houses. Married students can find affordable family housing in various Denver neighborhoods. On-campus activities include student-run organizations and events having either a professional or social focus. The Office of Diversity provides support for minority students.

GRADUATES

The most popular residency programs of a recent graduating class were Internal Medicine (29 students); Family Medicine (21); Surgery (9); Pediatrics (13); Emergency Medicine (4); Anesthesiology (15); Ob/Gyn (4); and Orthopedics (6). More than half of the graduates entered primary care fields. Graduates often stay in Denver for training. Other states popular for post-graduate training are Texas, Minnesota, and California.

Admissions

REQUIREMENTS

Required courses are College Mathematics (6 hours); Biology with lab (8 semester hours); Chemistry with lab (8 hours); Organic Chemistry with lab (8 hours); Physics with lab (8 hours); English Literature and English Composition or Creative Writing (9 hours). Applicants must demonstrate mathematics competency at least through college level trigonometry, either with college courses or placement test results. The MCAT is required and, if retaken, the best scores are used.

SUGGESTIONS

In addition to required courses, a course in Biochemistry is recommended. For applicants who have been out of school for a significant period of time, recent course work is suggested. Personal qualities are valued a great deal, as are extracurricular activities that involve medical research or health-related experience. As part of the Generalist Initiative, applicants from rural backgrounds are encouraged to apply.

PROCESS

All AMCAS applicants receive secondary applications. Of Colorado residents completing secondaries, 75 percent are interviewed. Less than 20 percent of out-of-state applicants are interviewed. Interviews take place on campus from September through April and consist of two sessions, each with a member of the Admissions Committee. The Admissions Committee is made up of students, faculty, and community physicians. Notification occurs on a rolling basis. About one-quarter of Colorado residents who interview are accepted, and about one-tenth of out of state interviewees are accepted. A wait list is established, from which 20–40 students are usually taken. Wait-listed candidates are not encouraged to send supplementary material.

Admissions Requirements (Required)

MCAT Scores, Essays, Science GPA, Extracurricular activities, Non-Science GPA, Exposure to medical profession, Recommendation, Interview, State Residency

COSTS AND AID

Tuition & Fees

Annual tuition (in-state out-of-state)	$23,641/$47,014
Room & board	$18,000
Cost of books	$2,230
Fees	$1,300

Financial Aid

% students receiving any aid	94
% students receiving grants	16
% students receiving loans	5
% aid that is merit-based	0
Average grant	$5,000
Average loan	$28,000
Average debt	$92,000

UNIVERSITY OF CONNECTICUT

UNIVERSITY OF CONNECTICUT SCHOOL OF MEDICINE

MEDICAL STUDENT AFFAIRS, 263 FARMINGTON AVENUE, ROOM AG-062, FARMINGTON, CT 06030-1905
ADMISSION: 860-679-3874 • FAX: 860-679-12827 • E-MAIL: SANFORD@NSO1.UCHC.EDU • WEBSITE: WWW.UCHC.EDU

STUDENT BODY

Type	Public
Enrollment of parent institution	29,383
Enrollment of medical school	331
% male/female	42/58
% underrepresented minorities	1
% out-of-state	9
% international	27
# countries represented	106
Average age of entering class	24

FACULTY

Total faculty	1,018
% part-time faculty	11

ADMISSIONS

# applied	2,919
% accepted	6
% enrolled	48

Average GPA and MCAT Scores

Overall GPA	3.7
MCAT Bio	10.9
MCAT Phys	10.4
MCAT Verbal	10.0
MCAT Essay	Q

Application Information

Regular application	12/15
Regular notification	10/15
Early application	8/1
Early notification	10/1
Are transfers accepted?	Yes
Admissions may be deferred?	Yes
Admissions need-blind?	No
Application fee	$85

Academics

In addition to the required courses, about 75 percent of students take part in a research project while in school. Grading is strictly Pass/Fail, based on the notion that, "each student is at the top of the class with regard to some important feature of skill or ability." A combined-degree program leading to both an M.D. and a Ph.D. is pursued by about five students each year in conjunction with the following Graduate Programs: Cell Biology, Genetics and Developmental Biology, Immunology, Molecular Biology and Biochemistry, Neuroscience, Skeletal, Craniofacial and Oral Biolodgy,and Cellular and Molecular Pharmacology. It is also possible for medical students to earn a Master's in Public Health or a Masters in Business Administration from the University of Connecticut's Graduate Program.

BASIC SCIENCES: The first two years cover the basic sciences, introduce clinical studies, and integrate behavioral and social aspects of medicine and health care. Instruction uses lectures, labs, case conferences, and problem-based learning. First-year courses are Human Systems, which is composed of: Human Biology; Organ Systems I (Neuroscience, Anatomy of the head and neck); Organ Systems II (Cardiovascular, Respiratory and Renal Systems, Anatomy of the thorax and abdomen); and Organ System III (Gastrointestinal, Endocrine and Reproductive, Genetics and Anatomy of the pelvis); Electives; Correlated Medical Problem Solving; and Principles of Clinical Medicine, which teaches history-taking, the physical examination, and general concepts related to clinical care. Second-year courses are Human Development and Health, which encompasses ethical, social, and legal issues; Mechanisms of Disease, which includes concepts related to Pathology; Pharmacology; Infectious Disease; Homeostasis; Oncology; Metabolism; Nervous System; Reproductive System; and Skin, Connective Tissue, and Joints; Correlated Medical Problem Solving; and Clinical Medicine. Facilities include modern lecture halls, classrooms for small-group discussions, the Lyman Maynard Stowe Library, and computer resources. Passing the USMLE Step 1 is a requirement for promotion to year three.

CLINICAL TRAINING

The third year is organized into two segments, one that involves clinical training in ambulatory settings, and the other that takes place in hospitals. The ambulatory experience is composed of the following clerkships: General Internal Medicine (7 weeks); Pediatrics (5 weeks); Psychiatry (2 weeks); Family Medicine (7 weeks); Ob/Gyn (4 weeks); and Subspecialties (3 weeks). The Hospital, or Inpatient, segment includes rotations in Medicine (4 weeks); Surgery (4 weeks); Pediatrics (2 weeks); Psychiatry (2 weeks); Obstetrics (2 weeks); and Beginning to End (2 weeks), in which students follow patients from their admittance to each diagnosis/service area that they visit in the hospital. The fourth year includes 20 weeks of electives, which may be taken at local or distant sites. Other fourth-year requirements are Advanced Inpatient Experience (4 weeks); Critical Care Experience (4 weeks); Emergency/Urgent Experience (4 weeks); and Selectives, in which students choose from rotations in research, community health, or education-related fields. Each student is paired with a faculty member of his or her choice to assist in scheduling electives and in selecting post-graduate training programs. Clinical training takes place at the University Hospital (232 beds) and at about 10 affiliated hospitals in the area. Some students gain clinical experience overseas, by participating in projects in Latin America, Asia, or Africa. Passing the USMLE Step 2 is a requirement for graduation.

Students

Underrepresented minorities, mostly African American, comprise about 15 percent of the student body. The average age of incoming students is typically about 24, with ages ranging from 21 to late 30s. About 80 percent of the students are Connecticut residents, and about 10 percent graduated from the University of Connecticut undergraduate college. Approximately 80 percent of students majored in a scientific discipline in college. Class size is about 80. Dental students participate in the basic sciences classes.

STUDENT LIFE

Life outside the classroom includes theater, concerts, and restaurants in Hartford; organized team sports on campus; and numerous clubs and groups related to professional or extracurricular interests. The Department of Health Career Opportunities provides support services throughout the academic year to minority medical students. Community-service activities, such as volunteering at homeless shelters, bring students together around important projects. Facilities such as golf courses, ski slopes, and public parks are accessible to the campus. On-campus housing is not available. Students live off campus in communities surrounding the university.

GRADUATES

Of the class that graduated in 2008, the breakdown of the most prevalent specialty choices was Internal Medicine (14%), Pediatrics (12%), OB/Gyn (12%), Surgery (9%). Approximately 30–35 percent of graduates enter residency programs in Connecticut.

Admissions

REQUIREMENTS

Requirements are one year of Chemistry, Organic Chemistry, Physics, and Biology. The MCAT is required and should be no more than three years old.

SUGGESTIONS

A broad and in-depth liberal arts education that includes English, Math, Foreign Language, Literature, History, Art, and Political Science is advised. The Admissions Committee looks very seriously at the nonacademic traits of applicants, such as their character and motivation.

PROCESS

All AMCAS applicants are sent secondary applications. About 60 percent of Connecticut applicants, and about 9 percent of out-of-state applicants are interviewed. Interviews are held from August through April and consist of two one-hour sessions with faculty, administrators, or students. Lunch and a campus tour with medical students are provided. Some candidates are accepted shortly after their interview, while others are notified later in the year. A wait-list is established in the spring. Wait-listed candidates may send supplementary information, such as transcripts.

Admissions Requirements (Required)
MCAT Scores, Essays, Science GPA, Extracurricular activities, Non-Science GPA, Exposure to medical profession, Recommendation, Interview

Admissions Requirements (Optional)
State Residency

COSTS AND AID

Tuition & Fees

Annual tuition (in-state out-of-state)	$19,833/$42,480
Room & board	$20,600
Cost of books	$3,650
Fees	$8,335

Financial Aid

% students receiving any aid	83
% students receiving grants	60
% students receiving loans	82
Average debt	$117,410

UNIVERSITY OF FLORIDA
COLLEGE OF MEDICINE

MEDICAL SELECTION COMMITTEE, BOX 100216, J. HILLIS MILLER HE, 1600 SW ARCHER ROAD, ROOM M-108
GAINESVILLE, FL 32610-0216 • **ADMISSION:** 352-273-7990 • **FAX:** 352-392-13077
E-MAIL: ADMISSIONS@UFL.EDU • **WEBSITE:** WWW.MED.UFL.EDU

STUDENT BODY

Type	Public
Enrollment of parent institution	48,000
Enrollment of medical school	458
% male/female	49/51
% out-of-state	29
% international	16
Average age of entering class	22

FACULTY

Total faculty	1,020
% part-time faculty	2

ADMISSIONS

# applied	20,079
% accepted	1
% enrolled	61

Average GPA and MCAT Scores

Overall GPA	3.7
MCAT Bio	10.8
MCAT Phys	10.6
MCAT Verbal	9.9
MCAT Essay	p

Application Information

Regular application	12/1
Are transfers accepted?	Yes
Admissions may be deferred?	Yes
Admissions need-blind?	No
Application fee	$30

Academics

Students may pursue their own interests with specialized institutes and centers, such as the Health Policy Institute, the Center for Mammalian Genetics, and the Brain and Cancer Institutes. Students with an interest in public health are encouraged to pursue the M.P.H. degree in conjunction with other academic institutions. Grading uses an A–F scale, and a ranking system. Both steps of the USMLE are required for graduation.

BASIC SCIENCES: Instructional methods include lectures, labs, and small-group sessions that together occupy 25 hours per week or less. First-year basic science courses are Biochemistry; Anatomy; Radiology; Genetics; Cell and Tissue Biology; Physiology; and Neuroscience. Integrated into basic sciences are behavioral sciences, ethical issues, and clinical training. Examples of first-year courses in these areas are Essentials of Patient Care, Keeping Families Healthy, Human Behavior, and the Preceptor Program. Second-year courses are Pathology; Oncology; Physical Diagnosis; Clinical Diagnosis; Pharmacology; Clinical Radiology; Social and Ethical Issues in Medical Practice; Public Health; and Microbiology. Classrooms, labs, and the library are in one complex. A satellite library also operates in Jacksonville.

CLINICAL TRAINING
Required third-year rotations are Medicine (8 weeks); Neurology (2 weeks); Psychiatry (6 weeks); Surgery (8 weeks); Ob/Gyn (6 weeks); Pediatrics (8 weeks); and Interdisciplinary Generalist Clerkships (10 weeks). Fourth-year clerkships are Advanced Surgery (4 weeks); Advanced Medicine, Pediatrics, or Family Medicine (4 weeks); Clinical Pharmacology (4 weeks); and Electives (28 weeks). The primary teaching hospitals are Shands Hospital (576 beds), the Gainesville Veterans Affairs Medical Center (403 beds), and the University Medical Center (528 beds). Training also takes place at outpatient clinics in nearby communities, and at clinical research facilities. Educational affiliations have been established in Tallahassee, Pensacola, Jacksonville, Leesburg, Broward County, and Orlando. With approval, up to three months of elective credits may be earned at other institutions around the country and overseas. Outside of formal rotations, students gain clinical experience through outreach projects such as Camps for Sick Kids and Care for the Homeless.

Students

About 99 percent of the students are Florida residents. Underrepresented minorities account for 11 percent of the student body, and students who have taken time off after college make up at least one-quarter of each entering class. Class size is 120.

STUDENT LIFE
Popular extracurricular activities include viewing intercollegiate sports, taking part in outdoor activities made possible by the year-round temperate climate, and occasionally going out at night to restaurants, clubs, and theaters. The University has an active student union with a theater, pool tables, a bowling alley, and a cafeteria. Athletic facilities, including a student gym, are expansive and are well-used by medical students. Outside of the classroom, students get to know each other through involvement with organizations and projects. A few examples of the numerous medical student organizations are Physicians for Social Responsibility, the Christian Medical and Dental Group, and the

Family Practice Student Organization. Service projects, such as the School of Medicine Outreach to Rural Students (S.M.O.R.S) and the EqualAccess Clinic improve students' interactive skills, and give them the opportunity to contribute to their community. There are numerous groups that devote time each year on medical missions to underserved countries.

GRADUATES

There are about 6,500 graduates of the College of Medicine, a number of whom are renowned for important contributions made in their respective fields. At University of Florida-affiliated hospitals there are 56 post-graduate programs. Many of the positions in these programs are filled by graduates of the College of Medicine.

Admissions

REQUIREMENTS

Requirements are Chemistry (8 hours); Organic Chemistry (4 hours); Biochemistry (4 hours); Biology (8 hours); and Physics (8 hours). The MCAT is required and scores must be no more than three years old from the date of expected matriculation. Generally, the best set of scores is looked at most closely.

SUGGESTIONS

Early submission, preferably by June, of the AMCAS application is advised. No undergraduate major is preferred and, science and nonscience majors are considered equally. Course work in Statistics, Biochemistry, Genetics, and Microbiology is useful. Though there is no math requirement; there is an assumption that math up through Calculus was taken as an undergraduate prerequisite for Chemistry. Extracurricular activities, non-medically related community service, health care experience and research, are import

PROCESS

Typically, the college receives 2,000 AMCAS applications for 120 available spaces. About 1,000 of the AMCAS applicants receive secondary applications, and about three hundred of those returning secondaries are invited to interview. Interviews are held on Fridays, from September through March, and consist of two sessions with faculty members. On interview day, candidates also receive lunch and tours. Interview notification occurs on a rolling basis. After their interview applicants are either accepted, rejected, or put on hold for a later decision. In April, an alternate list is established. Additional material, and updates, may be submitted by wait-listed candidates. There are two routes of admission to the College of Medicine: Junior Honors (12 places); and regular admissions (120 places). To apply for the Junior Honors program, students apply directly to the College of Medicine during their sophomore year of college. If accepted to the program, they complete a special series of seminars at the University of Florida during their junior year and begin medical school after the completion of their junior year. For Junior Honors, call 352-392-4569.

Admissions Requirements (Required)

MCAT Scores, Essays, Science GPA, Extracurricular activities, Non-Science GPA, Exposure to medical profession, Recommendation, Interview, State Residency

COSTS AND AID

Tuition & Fees

Annual tuition (in-state out-of-state)	$18,917/$46,765
Room & board (on-campus off-campus)	$9,250/$8,630
Cost of books	$2,665
Fees (in-state out-of-state)	$2,200/$3,592

Financial Aid

% students receiving any aid	89
% students receiving grants	74
% students receiving loans	82
% aid that is merit-based	1
Average grant	$1,425
Average loan	$23,352
Average total aid package	$33,359
Average debt	$96,000

UNIVERSITY OF HAWAI'I
JOHN A. BURNS SCHOOL OF MEDICINE

OFFICE OF ADMISSIONS, JOHN A. BURNS SCHOOL OF MEDICINE, 1960, 651 ILALO ST., MEB HONOLULU, HI 96813
ADMISSION: 808-692-1000 • FAX: 808-956-12517
E-MAIL: MEDADMIN@HAWAII.EDU • WEBSITE: JABSOM.HAWAII.EDU

STUDENT BODY

Type	Public
Enrollment of medical school	258
% male/female	48/52
% underrepresented minorities	3
% out-of-state	14
% international	73
# countries represented	4
Average age of entering class	24

FACULTY

Total faculty	383
% female faculty	41
% minority faculty	60
% part-time faculty	54
Student-faculty ratio	0.7:1

ADMISSIONS

# applied	1,618
% accepted	6
% enrolled	65

Average GPA and MCAT Scores

Overall GPA	3.6
MCAT Bio	11.0
MCAT Phys	10.0
MCAT Verbal	9.0
MCAT Essay	P

Application Information

Regular application	11/1
Regular notification	10/15
Early application	8/1
Early notification	10/15
Are transfers accepted?	Yes
Admissions may be deferred?	Yes
Admissions need-blind?	No
Application fee	$150

Academics

The MD curriculum is designed to provide outstanding education in the clinical and basic sciences. There is a heavy emphasis on small-group problem-based learning (PBL) in the preclinical years. Early clinical experiences and community service are also emphasized. Clinical training opportunities are available on several islands. Electives and research opportunities are offered throughout the four-year program.

BASIC SCIENCES: Instruction is through small-group problem-based learning (PBL), lectures and laboratory experiences. Opportunities for basic science research are also available.

CLINICAL TRAINING

Clinical training begins in the first year of the curriculum. Clerkships are held at various community hospitals and clinics, with opportunities on several islands. Opportunities for clinical electives are available locally, nationally and internationally.

Students

Hawaii's multi-ethnic population is reflected in the student body and faculty of the medical school. Class size is 66.

STUDENT LIFE

Although the School of Medicine is relatively small and intimate, the University of Hawaii at Manoa enrolls approximately 17,000 students. Medical students take part in campus activities but are integrated into the greater community of the city of Honolulu and the island of Oahu. Honolulu is a city with a population of about 1 million. It is a major tourist center, offering beautiful beaches in addition to many cultural, recreational, and outdoor activities.

GRADUATES

Graduates of the medical school go on to complete their residency training in some of the best programs in the country. Hawaii offers a number of excellent residency training programs and clinical fellowships.

Admissions
REQUIREMENTS

The initial screening of applicants selects those who have close ties to Hawaii and who are most likely to practice in Hawaii and in the U.S.-affiliated Pacific Islands. Applicants from Wyoming and Montana, states without medical schools who are certified by the Western Interstate Commission on Higher Education (WICHE) Program are given consideration in the screening cut-off. Requirements for application to JABSOM are: Completion of 90 semester credit hours which must include: 8 semester credit hours of Biology with Lab, 8 semester credit hours of General Physics with Lab, 8 semester credit hours of General Chemistry with Lab, 3 semester credit hours of Biochemistry (no lab required), and 3 semester credit hours of Cell and Molecular Biology (no lab required). The Medical College Admissions Test (MCAT) msut be taken within three yers of the anticipated date of matriculation to medical school. The latest MCAT scores screened/rescreened in the application process are September of the year of application (May for Early Decision).

SUGGESTIONS

Additional courses in Biological and Social Science are advised, such as Immunology, Genetics, Microbiology, Anatomy, Physiology, Embryology, Psychology, and Sociology. Experiences in health, clinical, research, human/community services are recommended for applicants to expose themselves to the health careers and to help them determine if medicine is for them. Important are personal qualities that suggest an applicant will become a humanistic physician who can relate to his/her patients.

PROCESS

Annually, about 15 to 20 percent of applicants are interviewed. Interviews are conducted from September through February and consist of two interviews with faculty members, practicing physicians, alumni, members of the health community, or fourth-year medical students. Of those interviewed, about 20 percent of in-state applicants and 5 percent of out-of-state residents are accepted. Historically, approximately 10 percent of each incoming class are non-residents. Most applicants are notified of the committee's decision in late March, though a few highly qualified applicants may hear earlier. A wait-list is established at this time. Waitlisted applicants are offered an acceptance when an accepted applicant declines or withdraws his/her application to JABSOM.

Admissions Requirements (Required)

MCAT Scores, Essays, Science GPA, Non-Science GPA, Recommendation, Interview

Admissions Requirements (Optional)

Extracurricular activities, Exposure to medical profession, State Residency

COSTS AND AID

Tuition & Fees

Annual tuition (in-state out-of-state)	$30,072/$63,312
Room & board (on-campus off-campus)	$15,682/$12,257
Cost of books	$11,617
Fees	$670

Financial Aid

% students receiving any aid	84
% students receiving grants	61
% students receiving loans	74
% aid that is merit-based	55
Average grant	$5,886
Average loan	$34,668
Average total aid package	$37,239
Average debt	$104,586

University of Illinois at Chicago
University of Illinois College of Medicine

808 S. Wood Street, Room 165 CME, M/C 783, Chicago, IL 60612 • Admission: 312-996-5635
Fax: 312-996-66937 • E-mail: MEDADMIT@UIC.EDU • Website: WWW.MEDICINE.UIC.EDU

STUDENT BODY

Type	Public
Enrollment of medical school	1,400
% male/female	52/48
% out-of-state	26
% international	28
Average age of entering class	24

FACULTY

Total faculty	1,231
% female faculty	36
% minority faculty	9
% part-time faculty	27

ADMISSIONS

# applied	4,921
% accepted	13
% enrolled	48

Average GPA and MCAT Scores

Overall GPA	3.6
MCAT Bio	10.0
MCAT Phys	10.0
MCAT Verbal	10.0
MCAT Essay	Q

Application Information

Regular application	11/1
Regular notification	6/1
Early application	8/1
Early notification	10/1
Are transfers accepted?	Yes
Admissions may be deferred?	Yes
Admissions need-blind?	No
Application fee	$70

Academics

Students participate in one of two educational tracks: 175 students complete all four years in Chicago, while 125 spend their first year in Urbana-Champaign. After the first year in Urbana-Champaign, 50 students each complete years two, three, and four in Peoria or Rockford. The remaining 25 students in Urbana-Champaign participate in the Medical Scholars Program.

BASIC SCIENCES: The first and second years include the Principles of Anatomy, Behavioral Science, Biochemistry, Genetics, Histology, Immunology, Microbiology, Neuroscience, Pathology, Pathophysiology, Pharmacology, and Physiology. All students participate in a clinical medicine course. Lectures and labs are the predominant instructional modality.

CLINICAL TRAINING
Patient contact begins in the first year when students are assigned individual physician preceptors. Students sharpen their skills in diagnosis and treatment through problem solving sessions. In the third and fourth years, students focus on patient care with a series of clerkships supplemented by conferences and lectures. The 25 affiliated facilities range from rural ambulatory healthcare centers to major metropolitan hospitals. The diverse clinical experiences prepare UIC graduates to succeed within the nation's ever-changing health care system. Required clerkships include: Family Medicine, Internal Medicine, Obstetrics/Gynecology, Pediatrics, Psychiatry, and Surgery. The elective phase provides students with the opportunity to identify special interest areas and to select educational experiences most relevant to their goals. The objective of the M.D./Ph.D. Program is to train students for careers in academic medicine and research. The Medical Scholars Program (M.S.P.), located on the Urbana-Champaign campus, permits students to integrate medicine with graduate studies in both science and non-science fields. The Independent Study Program (ISP) allows students to design their own academic programs with advice from faculty. ISP students complete an in-depth study, usually involving the basic sciences orclinical medicine. The ISP program is offered on the Chicago, Peoria, and Rockford campuses. The Rural Medical Education Program (RMED) and Rural Illinois Medical Student Assistance Program (RIMSAP) recruit students who commit to practice in medically underserved areas of Illinois.

Students

UIC is one of the most ethnically diverse medical schools in the country. Students are assigned to a faculty member who serves as an advisor. The advisor's major role is to be available to the student throughout his or her medical education for academic and personal counseling. Research interests are widely diversified and range from basic molecular biology to patient-related clinical research.

STUDENT LIFE
Students in Chicago enjoy living in one of the country's most exciting cities. In Urbana-Champaign, students benefit from a large and exciting university community. Rockford and Peoria are mid-size cities offering all students basic urban amenities. Campus housing in Chicago includes three residence halls near the college. In Urbana-Champaign, university-certified housing includes campus and private residence halls, and university apartments for family housing. In Peoria and Rockford housing is easily accessible and reasonable.

GRADUATES

UIC students undertake career specialization and training in all disciplines. Most graduates who participate in the National Residency Matching Program receive one of their top three residency choices.

Admissions

REQUIREMENTS

Only those applicants who indicate plans to obtain a baccalaureate degree prior to enrollment will be considered for admission. Major fields may be in humanities, behavioral, biological, or physical sciences. All applicants must complete: Two semesters of Introductory Biology or the equivalent with laboratory. Two semesters of General Inorganic Chemistry or the equivalent with laboratory. Two semesters of Organic Chemistry with laboratory. (Introductory Biochemistry may substitute for one semester of Organic Chemistry.) Two semesters of General Physics or the equivalent. All applicants are expected to complete three semesters of Social Science courses with an emphasis in the behavioral sciences. In addition, candidates are expected to take at least one of the following courses: Advanced-level Biology, Biochemistry, Physiology, Mammalian Histology, Comparative Vertebrate Anatomy, or Molecular Genetics. All applicants must take the MCAT no later than the fall of the year prior to enrollment and no more than three years prior to application. All applicants must complete an application to the AMCAS no later than December 31 of the year prior to enrollment. All applicants must be U.S. citizens or possess a permanent resident immigrant visa at the time of application through AMCAS. On receipt of the AMCAS application, eligible applicants will be sent a UIC Supplemental Application. Materials must be postmarked by February 15 of the year prior to enrollment. A minimum of three academic letters of recommendation or one composite recommendation from a pre-professional committee must be postmarked by February 15 of the year prior to enrollment. If you are currently enrolled in a graduate or professional school, one of your three letters of recommendation must be from a faculty member at your graduate or professional school. It is advisable that letters of recommendation be sent from the institution at which the applicant had been most recently enrolled and must be completed on official university or business letterhead. Personal letters of recommendation are not acceptable.

SUGGESTIONS

At least 90 percent of UIC students are Illinois residents. Although Illinois residents are given preference, positions are open to highly qualified nonresidents. In addition to academic strength, experience and background are considered important factors in admissions decisions.

PROCESS

About one-third of AMCAS applicants are sent a UIC Supplementary Application. Of those returning supplementals, the most highly qualified are invited to interview between September and April. The interview is a requirement and will be arranged by the Office of Medical College Admissions. Interviews are granted by invitation only. Interviews are held on all four campuses, and the interview location does not determine the campus where matriculants may attend. The interview consists of one panel interview session. Candidates have the opportunity to meet faculty members and students, receive financial aid information, tour the campus, and learn more about the College of Medicine. Interviewed candidates are accepted on a batch system. Students not immediately accepted may be put on an alternate list.

Admissions Requirements (Required)

MCAT Scores, Essays, Science GPA, Non-Science GPA, Recommendation, Interview

Admissions Requirements (Optional)

Extracurricular activities, Exposure to medical profession, State Residency

COSTS AND AID

Tuition & Fees

Annual tuition (in-state out-of-state)	$25,208/$53,262
Cost of books	$1,280
Fees	$1,574

UNIVERSITY OF IOWA
ROY J. AND LUCILLE A. CARVER COLLEGE OF MEDICINE

1213 MEDICAL EDUCATION RESEARCH FACILITY, IOWA CITY, IA 52242 • ADMISSION: 319-335-8052
FAX: 319-335-80497 • E-MAIL: MEDICAL-ADMISSION@UIOWA.EDU
WEBSITE: WWW.MEDICINE.UIOWA.EDU / MD / ADMISSIONS

STUDENT BODY

Type	Public
Enrollment of medical school	583
% male/female	52/48
% out-of-state	30
% international	22
Average age of entering class	24

FACULTY

Total faculty	837
% female faculty	27
% minority faculty	14
Student-faculty ratio	0.7:1

ADMISSIONS

# applied	3,489
% accepted	8
% enrolled	53

Average GPA and MCAT Scores

Overall GPA	3.7
MCAT Bio	11.2
MCAT Phys	10.9
MCAT Verbal	10.3
MCAT Essay	Q

Application Information

Regular application	11/1
Are transfers accepted?	No
Admissions may be deferred?	Yes
Admissions need-blind?	No
Application fee	$60

Academics

Most students at Iowa follow a four-year course of study, leading to the M.D. About 5 percent of students are M.S.T.P. participants, earning a Ph.D. concurrently with the M.D. The doctorate degree may be earned in Anatomy, Biochemistry, Microbiology, Pharmacology, and Physiology and Biophysics, among other fields. Other joint-degree programs, such as those leading to a master's degree along with the M.D., are also possible. Medical students are evaluated with near Honors/Pass/Fail for all courses except electives, which are Pass/Fail. Although the first two years are primarily devoted to basic sciences, introductory clinical training is also an important part of the curriculum. The second two years are devoted to clinical rotations.

BASIC SCIENCES: First-year courses are the following: Biochemistry; Cell Biology; Medical Genetics; Gross Anatomy; Structure and Functions of Human Organ Systems; Neuroscience; Immunology; and Foundations of Clinical Practice, which continues through the second year. This course covers topics ranging from biomedical ethics and problem-based learning to behavioral medicine, human sexuality, continuity of care, and important clinical techniques such as history-taking, the physical examination, and the doctor-patient relationship. The course Structure and Functions of Human Organ Systems covers principles of Histology and Physiology and is organized around body / organ systems. After completing their first year, many students spend the summer working and learning in an Iowa community hospital or conducting medical research projects. Second-year courses are: Principles of Infectious Diseases; Foundations of Clinical Practice; Pharmacology; Pathology. Throughout the first two years, students are in lectures, discussions, labs, or tutorials for about 23 hours per week. Basic sciences are taught in the Medical Education and Research Facility and the Bowen Science Building. The Hardin Library holds over 200,000 volumes and nearly 3,000 periodicals and is used by students, faculty, and the medical community for research and studying. It also has a .multimedia computer classroom and computer-based informational resources.

CLINICAL TRAINING

Third- and fourth-year required core clerkships are the following: Community-Based Primary Care (4 weeks); Family Medicine (4 weeks); Internal Medicine (Inpatient - 6 weeks); Internal Medicine (Ambulatory - 4 weeks); Ob/Gyn (6 weeks); Pediatrics (6 weeks); and Surgery (6 weeks). Subspecialty clerkships are Neurology (4 weeks); Psychiatry (4 weeks); two weeks of each of the following: Orthopedics and Otolaryngology; eight out of twelve weeks of the following: Dermatology (2 weeks); Ophthalmology (4 weeks); Radiology (2 weeks); Urology (2 weeks); Electrocardiography and Laboratory Medicine (2 weeks). A sub-internship, Emergency Medicine or Critical Care rotation, and at least 16 weeks of electives are also required. Clinical training takes place at the University Hospital (680 beds), the Veterans Affairs Hospital (93 beds), and various sites within the state.

Students

Each entering class has 152 students. About 70 percent of students are Iowa residents. Generally, about 30 undergraduate majors are represented in a class. Approximately 16 percent of students are underrepresented minorities. The majority of students entered medical school one year after college graduation. The Medical Education and Research facility opened for classes in the Fall of 2001. It also houses four learning communities to which each student is assigned.

STUDENT LIFE

Medical students are active in student organizations ranging from groups that support minorities to professional interest groups to a medical school singing group. The Learning Communities also sponsor activities that encourage peer-to-peer support and mentoring. Each community is staffed by a faculty director, professional and support staff with leadership provided by the elected student representatives. As part of the greater University of Iowa, medical students enjoy its facilities, resources, and sponsored events, such as Big Ten athletics. The UI campus is central to Iowa City and is convenient to restaurants, clubs, theaters, shopping areas, and parks. Though the city has a population of 60,000 people, it is relatively safe and has the feeling of a friendly small town. Just outside of the city are lakes, hiking areas, and other outdoor attractions. Urban centers such as Chicago, St. Louis, Minneapolis, Omaha, and Kansas City are within a five-hour drive. On campus housing options include coed medical fraternities with both single and double rooms, and university-owned family housing. Off-campus, reasonably priced apartments are available.

GRADUATES

Graduates are successful in entering residency programs of their choice. Iowa itself offers post-graduate training programs in about 15 fields.

Admissions

REQUIREMENTS

Prerequisites are one year each of Physics, Chemistry, Organic Chemistry, General Biology, one semester of Advanced Biology, and college-level Math or Statistics. All science courses should include laboratory instruction. The MCAT is required. All sets of scores are evaluated.

SUGGESTIONS

Though preference is given to Iowa residents, well-qualified nonresidents are also considered. Nonscience majors might benefit from additional science courses beyond requirements; specifically, biochemistry, genetics, and an anatomy course. Computer literacy, the ability to write well, strong verbal skills, and general decision-making capabilities are some of the skills sought in applicants. Also important are an applicant's personal characteristics, which are evaluated with the help of letters of reference and interviews. Some medically related experience is important.

PROCESS

Iowa participates in the AMCAS process. Most who apply through AMCAS are sent secondary applications. About one-third of Iowa residents who apply are accepted. Of the nonresident applicant pool, about 6 percent are accepted. Applicants are notified on a rolling basis and are either accepted, rejected, or wait-listed. Wait-listed candidates are not encouraged to send additional information.

Admissions Requirements (Required)

MCAT Scores, Essays, Science GPA, Extracurricular activities, Non-Science GPA, Exposure to medical profession, Recommendation, Interview

Admissions Requirements (Optional)

State Residency

COSTS AND AID

Tuition & Fees

Annual tuition (in-state out-of-state)	$26,113/$41,927
Room & board	$9,630
Cost of books	$3,414

Financial Aid

% students receiving any aid	97
% students receiving grants	62
% students receiving loans	87
% aid that is merit-based	15
Average grant	$15,766
Average loan	$34,197
Average total aid package	$43,047
Average debt	$124,440

UNIVERSITY OF KANSAS
UNIVERSITY OF KANSAS SCHOOL OF MEDICINE

3901 RAINBOW BOULEVARD, 3040 MURPHY BLDG., MAIL STOP 1049 KANSAS CITY, KS 66160
ADMISSION: 913-588-5245 • FAX: 913-588-52597
E-MAIL: PREMEDINFO@KUMC.EDU • WEBSITE: WWW.KUMC.EDU/SOM/SOM.HTML

STUDENT BODY

Type	Public
Enrollment of parent institution	29,000
Enrollment of medical school	700
% male/female	55/45
% out-of-state	13
% international	14
Average age of entering class	24

FACULTY

Total faculty	658
% female faculty	46
% minority faculty	29
% part-time faculty	18
Student-faculty ratio	1.0:1

ADMISSIONS

# applied	1,585
% accepted	14
% enrolled	76

Average GPA and MCAT Scores

Overall GPA	3.7
MCAT Bio	9.8
MCAT Phys	9.2
MCAT Verbal	9.6
MCAT Essay	Q

Application Information

Regular application	10/15
Regular notification	3/31
Are transfers accepted?	Yes
Admissions may be deferred?	Yes
Admissions need-blind?	No
Application fee	$0

Academics

In comparison to many medical schools, clinical training at the University of Kansas emphasizes rural and primary health care. Joint M.D./Ph.D. degrees are offered in the following fields: Anatomy and Cell Biology; Biochemistry and Molecular Biology; Microbiology, Molecular Genetics and Toxicology; Pathology and Oncology; Pharmacology; and Physiology. A joint M.D./M.P.H. is also offered.

BASIC SCIENCES: Basic sciences are taught in Kansas City. The facilities are modern and fully equipped with learning tools such as computers and visual-aid equipment. The School of Medicine has recently implemented a systemic methodology for teaching basic sciences. Students take part in individual and small-group projects that require initiative and problem-solving skills. First-year students take Cell and Tissue Biology; Physiology; Biochemistry; Gross Anatomy; Neuroscience; and Introduction to Clinical Medicine. Second-year students take Microbiology; Pathology; Pharmacology; and Introduction to Clinical Medicine. Tutoring is available through the Learning Resources Counseling service. A student-operated note service, in which students share note-taking, covers regularly scheduled lectures. Students are evaluated using the following descriptions: Superior, High Satisfactory, Satisfactory, Low Satisfactory, and Unsatisfactory. These marks are translated into numeric scores to determine class rank. The USMLE is required upon completion of year two. The Dykes Library of the Health Sciences supports the educational and research demands of medical students, faculty, and the public. It contains 150,000 books and offers online informational services. In addition, the Clendening History of Medicine Library has one of the top five collections of rare medical books in the country.

CLINICAL TRAINING

Patient contact begins in year one, when students take part in bi-weekly sessions with practicing physicians. Required clinical clerkships are Ambulatory Medicine/Geriatrics (6 weeks); Family Medicine (6 weeks); Ob/Gyn (6 weeks); Medicine (8 weeks); Pediatrics (6 weeks); Neuropsychiatry (8 weeks); and General Surgery (8 weeks). Year four is filled primarily with electives, from which there are many to choose including Preventive Medicine and the History of Medicine. Clinical training takes place both at the University of Kansas Hospital (464 beds), which houses nearly all the diagnostic and treatment facilities of the Medical Center, and at hospitals in Wichita. Included at the Medical Center in Kansas City are the Kansas Cancer Institute, the Burnett Burn Center, the Smith Mental Retardation Center, the Center on Aging, and the Center on Environmental and Occupational Health. Patients are drawn from Kansas, Missouri, Oklahoma, Arkansas, and Nebraska. The grading scale is the same for performance in clinical rotations as it for basic science courses. In addition to formal rotations, students gain clinical experience through volunteer activities, like the Mobile Medical Unit, which brings basic prevention and care to communities in need. Many students devote free summers to volunteer in medically related activities.

Students

About 90 percent of a typical class are Kansas residents, and most students have liberal arts backgrounds. In recent years, about 13 percent of the student body have been underrepresented minorities, mostly African and Hispanic Americans. Usually, almost a quarter of matriculants in a given year are older than 25 years of age. Class size is 175.

STUDENT LIFE

Medical students from all four classes are organized into academic societies which bring students together around academic and extracurricular activities. The Kirmayer Fitness Center is a modern facility open to all medical students. Numerous organized activities enrich the lives of medical students. Activities such as Rural Health Weekend provide opportunities for interaction with practicing physicians throughout the state. Organizations such as the Community Outreach Project provide opportunities for community service. All students live off campus.

GRADUATES

About 50 percent of graduates enter primary care fields. Graduates are successful in obtaining residency positions throughout the country. The medical school sponsors events and scholarships that encourage students and residents to consider practicing in Kansas.

Admissions

REQUIREMENTS

Required college courses are one year of Biology with lab; Chemistry with lab; Organic Chemistry with lab; Physics with lab, one year of English, and one semester of college level mathematics. A bachelors degree is required. Evaluation of GPA is irrespective of where course work was completed. The MCAT is required, with the two most recent sets of scores considered. The August MCAT is acceptable.

SUGGESTIONS

Experience in a health care setting is valued, and the breadth of an applicant's undergraduate course work is important. Demonstrated interests in rural and primary care medicine are pluses. Out-of-state residents should have particularly strong qualifications. A few students each year are accepted from the University of Kansas Postbaccalaureate Program and through the Scholars in Primary Care Program.

PROCESS

All Kansas residents are sent secondary applicants, while only about 10 percent of out-of-state applicants receive them. About 75 percent of Kansas residents and about 5 percent of out-of-state applicants are interviewed. Interviews are conducted in Kansas City, from October through March, and consist of one or two sessions each with one or two members of the interview panel. Approximately one-half of those interviewed are offered positions in the class and are notified on a rolling basis after the interview. The wait list is short, and wait-listed candidates are not encouraged to send supplementary material.

Admissions Requirements (Required)

MCAT Scores, Essays, Science GPA, Extracurricular activities, Non-Science GPA, Exposure to medical profession, Recommendation, Interview

Admissions Requirements (Optional)

State Residency

COSTS AND AID

Tuition & Fees

Annual tuition (in-state out-of-state)	$22,486/$39,878
Room & board	$9,018
Cost of books	$3,120
Fees	$2,990

Financial Aid

% students receiving any aid	85
% students receiving grants	65
% students receiving loans	80
Average grant	$2,500
Average loan	$27,500
Average total aid package	$30,000
Average debt	$90,600

UNIVERSITY OF KENTUCKY
COLLEGE OF MEDICINE

138 LEADER AVE, LEXINGTON, KY 40506-9983 • **ADMISSION:** 859-323-6161 • **FAX:** 859-323-20767
E-MAIL: KYMEDAP@UKY.EDU • **WEBSITE:** HTTP://WWW.MC.UKY.EDU/MEDICINE

STUDENT BODY

Type	Public
Enrollment of parent institution	27,000
Enrollment of medical school	479
% male/female	59/41
% underrepresented minorities	5
% out-of-state	22
% international	7
Average age of entering class	23

ADMISSIONS

# applied	2,296

Average GPA and MCAT Scores

Overall GPA	3.7
MCAT Bio	11.0
MCAT Phys	11.0
MCAT Verbal	10.0
MCAT Essay	P

Application Information

Regular application	11/1
Early application	8/1
Early notification	10/1
Are transfers accepted?	Yes
Admissions may be deferred?	Yes
Admissions need-blind?	No
Application fee	$50

Academics

The curriculum includes early patient contact and teaches lifelong learning skills, ethics, and computer-assisted learning along with traditional basic science and clinical techniques. The goal of the medical education program is to focus on principles and the organization of factual bodies of knowledge rather than on unconnected detail. Although most students complete a four-year curriculum, a few students each year enter a combined M.D./Ph.D. program. The doctorate may be earned in Anatomy, Biochemistry, Biophysics, Cell Biology, Genetics, Immunology, Microbiology, Molecular Biology, Neuroscience, Pharmacology, or Physiology. Combined M.D./M.P.H and M.D./M.B.A. programs are also available. Medical students are evaluated with letter grades and, in some cases, with Pass/Fail. Passing Step 1 of the USMLE is a requirement for promotion to year three, and passing Step 2 is a graduation requirement.

BASIC SCIENCES: During the first and second years, students are in class or other scheduled sessions for about 24 hours per week. Lectures and tutorials are the primary instructional methods. Laboratories, hands-on clinical work, and conferences are also important parts of the curriculum. The first year is devoted to basic sciences and interdisciplinary perspectives. The year is organized into blocks, each of which contains one or two courses. First-year courses are Patients, Physicians, and Society; Introduction to the Medical Profession; Human Structure/Gross Anatomy; Human Structure/Histology; Healthy Human; Cellular Structure and Function/Biochemistry; Cellular Structure and Function/Genetics; Neuroscience; and Human Function. The second year is focused on the disease process and is also broken into blocks. These are Patients, Physicians, and Society II; Introduction to the Medical Profession II; Immunity, Infection, and Disease; and Mechanisms of Disease and Treatment, which covers Pathology and Pharmacology. Students spend most of their first two years in the Medical Science Building, which houses classrooms and laboratories. Computers are important educational tools, and all incoming students are required to have their own computers. The College of Medicine has a nationally recognized program of academic computing in medical education, which provides a wide variety of services to enhance student learning. These educational support services are offered in facilities located in the College of Medicine, the Chandler Medical Center, and in the Area Health Education Centers. The library, which contains more than 150,000 volumes, is also an important resource.

CLINICAL TRAINING

Third-year required clerkships are: Women's Maternal and Child Health (12 weeks); Clinical Neuroscience (8 weeks); Principles Of Primary Care (12 weeks); and Medical and Surgical Care (16 weeks). The fourth year is comprised of a one-month acting internship selected from medical specialties (family practice, internal medicine, pediatric, neurology, psychiatry, rehabilitation medicine), a one-month acting internship selected from surgical specialties (general, subspecialty, ob/gyn), a one-month emergency medicine clerkship, one month of a clinical pharmacology and anesthesiology clerkship, and one month of a primary care or rural medicine selective. In addition, 8 weeks of electives are required. Training takes place primarily at the University of Kentucky Hospital (473 beds), although a number of affiliated hospitals and clinics are also used.

Students

Approximately 80 percent of students are Kentucky residents. About 7 percent of students are underrepresented minorities, most of whom are African American. Generally, about 25 percent of students in each class are nontraditional, having pursued other careers or interests in between college and medical school.

STUDENT LIFE

Medical students enjoy extracurricular activities associated with the main university such as attending UK basketball games. Student groups provide additional extracurricular activities, including opportunities for involvement in community service projects. They also serve as a means of interacting outside of class. Women in Science and Medicine is a group, comprised primarily of faculty and administrators, focused on improving all aspects of life for women in medicine. Lexington is an attractive and safe city with affordable housing.

GRADUATES

Graduates enter residency programs all over the United States in both primary care and specialty fields. The University of Kentucky has post-graduate training programs in more than 20 fields.

Admissions

REQUIREMENTS

One year each of Biology, General Chemistry, Organic Chemistry, Physics, and English are required. All science courses should include associated labs. The MCAT is required, and scores should be from within the past two years. For applicants who have taken the exam more than once, the most recent set of scores is weighed most heavily. Courses in Biochemistry, Cell Biology, Genetics, Statistics, Psychology, and Sociology are strongly recommended.

SUGGESTIONS

In addition to academic qualifications, UK seeks students who have the character, personality, values, and motivation for human service. Individual initiative and good judgment are important traits. Some medically related experience is important.

PROCESS

All AMCAS applicants who are Kentucky residents are sent secondary applications. Highly qualified nonresidents are also sent secondaries. Selected applicants who return secondary applications are invited to interview between September and March. On interview day, candidates also tour the campus, attend group informational sessions, and have the opportunity to meet informally with current students. Admission offers are made on a rolling basis. Others are rejected or wait-listed. Wait-listed candidates may send additional information to update their files. The class is typically full by January so early completion of both the primary and the secondary application is strongly recommended.

Admissions Requirements (Required)

MCAT Scores, Essays, Science GPA, Extracurricular activities, Non-Science GPA, Exposure to medical profession, Recommendation, Interview

Admissions Requirements (Optional)

State Residency

COSTS AND AID

Tuition & Fees

Annual tuition (in-state out-of-state)	$32,889/$60,334
Room & board	$23,161
Cost of books	$3,071

UNIVERSITY OF LOUISVILLE
SCHOOL OF MEDICINE

ABELL ADMINISTRATION CTR., RM. 413, 323 E. CHESTNUT ST. LOUISVILLE, KY 40202 • **ADMISSION:** 502-852-5193
FAX: 502-852-03027 • **E-MAIL:** MEDADM@LOUISVILLE.EDU • **WEBSITE:** LOUISVILLE.EDU

STUDENT BODY

Type	Public
Enrollment of parent institution	22,529
Enrollment of medical school	640
% male/female	56/44
% out-of-state	15
% international	28
# countries represented	95
Average age of entering class	23

FACULTY

Total faculty	887
% female faculty	37
% part-time faculty	7

ADMISSIONS

# applied	3,279
% accepted	9
% enrolled	56

Average GPA and MCAT Scores

Overall GPA	3.6
MCAT Bio	10.1
MCAT Phys	9.4
MCAT Verbal	9.7

Application Information

Regular application	10/15
Are transfers accepted?	Yes
Admissions may be deferred?	Yes
Admissions need-blind?	No
Application fee	$75

Academics

Although most students complete a four-year program leading to the M.D., a few earn a combined MD/PhD, which typically demands about seven years. Summer research scholarships allow first- and second-year students to participate in research projects alongside faculty mentors. Throughout all four years, students work closely with faculty advisers who assist with decisions related to academic and professional goals. Medical students are evaluated as Pass/Fail/Honors in both preclinical science and clinical courses. Passing Step 1 of the USMLE is a requirement for promotion to year three, and passing Step 2 Clinical Knowledge and Clinical Skills are requirements for graduation.

BASIC SCIENCES: The Core Curriculum extends over the four-year course of study and provides each student with the general education and training considered essential to all physicians. It stresses understanding concepts and general principles and provides opportunities for correlations among the sciences so that information learned in one subject reinforces ideas and builds upon concepts developed in another subject. For academic year 2014–2015, the preclinical years will consist of an integrated curriculum organized around organ systems to deliver a clinically relevant educational experience, Year One presents functional principles and anatomy of the normal human body, Year two teaches diseases and treatment. The two-year Introduction to Clinical Medicine course runs concurrently with the preclinical integrated curriculum and includes small group activities to prepare for clinical training, including the londitudinal standardized patient and preceptorship programs. The Preclinical Elective Program allows each student to customize his or her education in terms of learning experiences. Students are able to design a medical education program that best meets their needs, abilities, and goals. Studenrs are also permitted to take courses as electives in divisions of the University of Louisville other than the School of Medicine, class schedule permitting. In addition to the courses listed, students with a research interest are permitted to participate in an approved research activity for credit. Elective courses constitute an integral part of the student's total program in medical school. Second-year students take two credit hours of elective courses.

CLINICAL TRAINING
Third-year required clerkships are Internal Medicine (8 weeks); Family Medicine (6 weeks); Psychiatry (6 weeks); Basic Surgery (8 weeks); Pediatrics (6 weeks); OB/GYN (6 weeks) and Neurology (4 weeks). Fourth-year requirements are Ambulatory rotation or Longitudinal Ambouatory rotation (4 weeks); Acting Internship in Internal Medicine, Family Medicine, Pediatrics or Honors Surgery (4 weeks); Intensive Care Rotation in Internal Medicine, Pediatrics or Surgery (2 weeks); Palliative Medicine rotation (1 week); Topics in Clinical Medicine course (2 days); Clinical Electives (22 weeks with 10-12 weeks selected from the Residency Preparation Core Clinical Tracks); and Advanced Cardiac Life Support (ACLS) (1 week).

Students

In the entering class of 2013, 120 of 155 students were Kentucky residents. African Americans represented 7 percent of the class, and students older than 27 years old represented 10 percent of the class.

STUDENT LIFE

Students profit from the school's location in the center of Louisville. Louisville is the largest city in Kentucky, offering cultural and recreational activities such as orchestra, theater, ballet, opera, numerous restaurants and bars, and shopping areas. Louisville is the home of the Kentucky Derby. There is a university-owned Medical Dental Dormitory and Apartment Building, which is 2 blocks from both the School of Medicine and the university hospital. In this residential complex, there are apartments of all sizes as well as dorm rooms. Also available are varieties of housing options within 10 miles of the Health Science Campus ranging from apartments, lofts, condominiums to historic houses in Old Louisville.

GRADUATES

A large proportion of practicing physicians in Kentucky are Louisville School of Medicine graduates. At Louisville itself, at least 17 post-graduate training programs are offered.

Admissions

REQUIREMENTS

Requirements are two semesters each of Biology, Chemistry, Organic Chemistry, Physics, and 1 semester of Calculus or 2 semesters of other college-level Math. All science courses must include lab work. Two semesters of English is also required. The MCAT is required, and scores should be no more than two years old. For applicants who have retaken the exam, the most recent set of scores is considered. Thus, there is no advantage in withholding scores.

SUGGESTIONS

Approximately 75 percent of positions in each class are reserved for Kentucky residents, making out-of-state admission very competitive. Pre-medical students should develop a strong background in the Humanities, Philosophy, and the Arts. Communication and reading abilities are also important. The Committee values volunteer work, medically related experience, and evidence of strong interpersonal skills.

PROCESS

All qualified Kentucky residents and highly qualified nonresidents who submit AMCAS applications are sent secondaries. Of those returning secondary applications, about one-half of Kentucky applicants are invited to interview between August and March. Ten percent of nonresidents are invited to interview. On interview day, candidates receive two 30-minute interview sessions each with a faculty member, administrator, or medical student. In addition, interviewees have a guided campus tour, lunch, and the opportunity to meet informally with current students. About 40 percent of interviewed candidates are accepted on a rolling basis.

Admissions Requirements (Required)

MCAT Scores, Essays, Science GPA, Extracurricular activities, Non-Science GPA, Exposure to medical profession, Recommendation, Interview, State Residency

COSTS AND AID

Tuition & Fees

Annual tuition (in-state out-of-state) $33,718/$51,250

UNIVERSITY OF MANITOBA

UNIVERSITY OF MANITOBA

260-727 McDermot Avenue, Winnipeg, MB R3E 3P5 • **Admission:** 204-789-3499 • **Fax:** 204-789-39297
E-mail: ADMISSIONS@MED.UMANITOBA.CA • **Website:** WWW.UMANITOBA.CA/MEDICINE

STUDENT BODY

Type	Public
Enrollment of parent institution	28,402
Enrollment of medical school	440
% male/female	51/49
% out-of-state	10
% international	4
# countries represented	1
Average age of entering class	24

ADMISSIONS

# applied	948
% accepted	14
% enrolled	81

Average GPA and MCAT Scores

Overall GPA	4.0
MCAT Bio	10.4
MCAT Phys	10.0
MCAT Verbal	10.0
MCAT Essay	Q

Application Information

Are transfers accepted?	Yes
Admissions may be deferred?	Yes
Admissions need-blind?	No
Application fee	$95

Academics

The mission of the Faculty of Medicine is to: develop, deliver and evaluate high quality educational programs for undergraduate and postgraduate students of medicine and medical rehabilitation, for graduate students and postdoctoral fellows in basic medical sciences and for physicians to practice; to conduct research and other scholarly enquiry into the basic and applied medical sciences; and to provide advice, disseminate information to health professions and plan for the development and delivery of health care services and to help improve health status and service delivery to the Province of Manitoba and the wider community.

CLINICAL TRAINING

For information regarding curriculum, scheduling, and enrichment programs, please refer to the links posted at: www.umanitoba.ca/faculties/medicine/education/undergraduate.html

Students

STUDENT LIFE

Students are active in a number of areas, including organizing a program to help inner-city youth, coordinating an annual Medical Art Show, developing Codes of Professional Integrity, and carrying out an annual food bank drive.

Admissions

REQUIREMENTS

Applicants must have or be eligible to receive their Bachelor's degree prior to admission from a university recognized by the University of Manitoba. Applicants must have completed a full course of Biochemistry equivalent to that offered at Univesity of Manitoba and received a grade of C or higher. Two full courses in Humanities/Social Sciences are also required. The MCAT is required and should be taken within the past three years but no later than August of the year of application. Students usually prepare for the MCAT by taking university courses in Physics, Organic and Physical Chemistry, and Biology.

SUGGESTIONS

Enrolment is restricted to Canadian citizens or Permanent Residents. Priority is given to residents of Manitoba. The most successful applicants have grade point averages between 3.9 and 4.5 on a 4.5 scale and at least a 7 on each scored section of the MCAT. In addition to academic and intellectual credentials, the Admissions Committee selects applicants who demonstrate social skills, maturity, and a sense of responsibility. The Admissions Committee selects 110 students for admission out of about 900 applicants. Typically, about eleven places are offered to applicants from outside Manitoba.

PROCESS

For application material, contact the Faculty at the following email: admissions@umanitoba.ca or call: 204-474-8825. Applicants who have competitive scholastic and MCAT requirements will be invited to interview. About 350 applicants are interviewed.

Admissions Requirements (Required)

MCAT Scores, Recommendation, Interview

Admissions Requirements (Optional)

Extracurricular activities, Non-Science GPA, Exposure to medical profession, State Residency

COSTS AND AID

Tuition & Fees

Annual tuition	$7,595
Room & board (on-campus off-campus)	$10,000/$6,000
Cost of books	$4,000

Financial Aid

% students receiving any aid	35
% students receiving grants	10
% students receiving loans	35
% aid that is merit-based	10
Average grant	$1,100
Average loan	$10,615
Average debt	$46,000

UNIVERSITY OF MARYLAND
SCHOOL OF MEDICINE

COMMITTEE ON ADMISSIONS, SUITE 190, 685 W. BALTIMORE STREET BALTIMORE, MD 21201-1559
ADMISSION: 410-706-7478 • FAX: 410-706-04677 • E-MAIL: MFOXWELL@SOM.UMARYLAND.EDU
WEBSITE: MEDSCHOOL.UMARYLAND.EDU

STUDENT BODY

Type	Public
Enrollment of medical school	621
% male/female	40/60
% out-of-state	16
% international	40
Average age of entering class	24

FACULTY

Total faculty	2,600
% female faculty	45
% minority faculty	8
% part-time faculty	8
Student-faculty ratio	2.0:1

ADMISSIONS

# applied	4,166
% accepted	8
% enrolled	51

Average GPA and MCAT Scores

Overall GPA	3.7
MCAT Bio	10.5
MCAT Phys	10.0
MCAT Verbal	10.1
MCAT Essay	P

Application Information

Regular application	11/7
Early application	8/7
Early notification	10/7
Are transfers accepted?	Yes
Admissions may be deferred?	Yes
Admissions need-blind?	No
Application fee	$70

Academics

Maryland's dynamic curriculum emphasizes independent and small group learning, informatics, and the integration of basic and clinical science knowledge to produce outstanding clinicians and researchers. The traditional degree program takes students four years to complete. However, in selected cases, with permission of the dean, students may be granted extra time to complete the degree requirements. For students interested in a research career, the medical school offers a combined M.D./Ph.D. program in which the doctorate degree is offered in numerous disciplines such as Biochemistry, Biomedical Engineering, Genetics, Molecular Biology, Neuroscience, and Pharmacology. Grading is A–F. Students must sit for Step 1 of the USMLE before beginning clinical training, but must pass Step 1 within three attempts.

BASIC SCIENCES: The basic science curriculum is divided into integrated blocks and uses interdisciplinary teaching with both basic and clinical science instructors. Lectures and labs are limited to four hours per day; small-group and independent study are emphasized. Course work during the first year occupies 37 weeks and is organized into the following blocks: Structure and Development; Informatics; Principles of Human Development; Cell and Molecular Biology; Neuroscience; and Functional Systems. Introduction to Clinical Medicine runs concurrently throughout the year, covering the doctor-patient relationship, medical ethics, population medicine, and problem-based learning. The second year is particularly rigorous. Students learn pathophysiology and therapeutics by organ system, and are trained in conducting a physical diagnosis in the Introduction to Clinical Medicine course. Computers, not microscopes, are the laboratory tool of choice at Maryland. The multidisciplinary laboratories have the latest in educational technology and seat clusters of 10 to 12 students for small-group and laboratory teaching. The recently renovated library is among the largest and most accessible medical libraries in the United States, with at least 240,000 volumes, and is fully connected to the information superhighway. The Office of Student Affairs closely monitors students and provides support services. In addition, a pre-matriculation summer program allows entrants to review pre-medical course work and preview first-year material.

CLINICAL TRAINING

Year three consists of seven required rotations in Family Medicine (4 weeks); Medicine (12 weeks); Surgery (12 weeks); Pediatrics (6 weeks); Psychiatry (4 weeks); Ob/Gyn (6 weeks); and Neurology (4 weeks). The senior year includes a mandatory Area Health Education Center experience (8 weeks); two Subinternships (8 weeks); and 16 weeks of elective rotations. The majority of training takes place at University Hospital, a 747-bed tertiary care center adjacent to the Medical School. Rotations are also spent at the Baltimore VA Medical Center, Mercy Hospital, and other community hospitals. In total, 1,400 patient beds are used for teaching. One of the most unique electives is a rotation through the R Adams Cowley Shock Trauma Center. Shock Trauma was the first trauma center in America and continues to be a model for the rest of the nation.

Students

The majority of students are Maryland residents, but the Medical School attracts and accepts a significant number of out-of-state applicants. In a typical class, approximately 38 of the 150 students are from out-of-state. The student body is highly diverse, with about 20 percent of students from underrepresented minority backgrounds. More than half of our students are women. Increasingly, older students are making up a higher percentage of incoming classes. At least one-third of incoming classes took time off between college and medical school.

STUDENT LIFE

An extensive orientation program allows entering students to get to know fellow classmates, upperclassmen, and faculty advisors. Almost half of the incoming class attends. Other organized events, such as pot-luck suppers, community activities, and meetings of student organizations all serve to bring students together. Baltimore is a lively city, with interesting neighborhoods and real character. The harbor, the commercial district (Fells Point), the Orioles baseball stadium, Ravens football stadium and other attractions are accessible to the campus. The University offers athletic facilities and housing in the form of dorms. Most students find affordable, private apartments off campus. While the surrounding area has undergone a renaissance in recent years, safety remains a concern, as in most large cities.

GRADUATES

Over half of each year's graduates enter one of the primary care fields. Graduates, however, are competitive candidates for the entire range of specialties.

Admissions

REQUIREMENTS

Maryland requires one year each of Biology, General Chemistry, Organic Chemistry, Physics, and English as prerequisite courses. A grade of C or better is mandatory in each course. While the MCAT is also required, there is no set formula for determining competitive scores. Students with a wide range of scores are accepted each year. In addition, Maryland considers the best scores for those applicants who retake the exam.

SUGGESTIONS

Maryland gives clinical experience with direct patient exposure considerable weight. Research experience and service activity are also highly valued. Letters of recommendation are very important in the selection process.

PROCESS

Maryland uses the AMCAS application. Secondary applications are sent to all applicants. Of those who complete the secondary, approximately 25 percent are interviewed beginning in October. The interview day consists of a faculty interview, a medical student interview, and a casual lunch with students and a tour of the campus. Interviewed applicants normally receive a decision within a month after the interview. Half of those interviewed are accepted, and the other half are either rejected or wait-listed.

Admissions Requirements (Required)

MCAT Scores, Essays, Science GPA, Extracurricular activities, Non-Science GPA, Exposure to medical profession, Recommendation, Interview

Admissions Requirements (Optional)

State Residency

COSTS AND AID

Tuition & Fees

Annual tuition (in-state out-of-state)	$20,905/$39,140
Room & board (on-campus off-campus)	$18,490/$12,925
Cost of books	$850
Fees	$1,071

Financial Aid

% students receiving any aid	90
% students receiving grants	69
% students receiving loans	86
% aid that is merit-based	19
Average grant	$6,800
Average loan	$32,605
Average total aid package	$45,000
Average debt	$112,440

University of Massachusetts

University of Massachusetts Medical School

Associate Dean for Admissions, 55 Lake Avenue North, Worcester, MA 01655 • Admission: 508-856-2323
Fax: 508-856-36297 • E-mail: Admissions@umassmed.edu • Website: www.umassmed.edu/som/admissions

STUDENT BODY	
Type	Public
Enrollment of medical school	425
% male/female	49/51
% out-of-state	0
% international	7
Average age of entering class	24

FACULTY	
Total faculty	2,488

ADMISSIONS	
# applied	802
% accepted	23
% enrolled	56

Average GPA and MCAT Scores	
Overall GPA	3.6
MCAT Phys	10.5

Application Information	
Regular application	11/1
Regular notification	10/15
Early application	8/1
Early notification	10/1
Are transfers accepted?	Yes
Admissions may be deferred?	Yes
Admissions need-blind?	Yes
Application fee	$100

Academics

The four-year program emphasizes varied educational modalities, lifelong learning, communication skills, and a generalist approach that prepares students for all medical career paths. Ethical issues are an important aspect of the education, demonstrated by the existence of an active Office of Ethics. Year-long and summer research fellowships are available, as is a joint M.D./Ph.D. program. The doctorate degree may be earned in Biomedical Sciences, Biochemistry and Molecular Biology, Cell Biology, Cellular and Molecular Physiology, Immunology and Virology, Molecular Genetics, Microbiology, Neuroscience, and Pharmacology and Molecular Toxicology. A combined M.D./M.P.H. degree program is also offered. For pre-clinical courses, grades are Honors, Near Honors, Satisfactory, Marginal, Unsatisfactory, or Incomplete, with the exception of a few courses that are taken as Credit/No Credit. During the clinical years, ratings are Outstanding, Above Expected Performance, Expected Performance, Below Expected Performance, and Failure.

BASIC SCIENCES: First-year courses are Biochemistry/Metabolism; The Gene; Human Anatomy; Cells and Tissues; Systems I; Physiology; Immunology; Mind, Brain and Behavior I; Physician, Patient and Society (PPS); and Longitudinal Preceptor Program (LPP). PPS and LPP together introduce students to medical interviewing, physician-patient relationships, physical diagnosis, medical reasoning and decision analyses, population-based medicine, ethics, epidemiology, medical informatics, and preventive medicine. Systems I covers several body/organ systems: Hematology; Cardiovascular; Respiratory; Renal and Acid/Base; Endocrine Regulation; GI/Nutrition; and Reproduction. Second-year courses focus on the biology of disease. They are General Pathology; Neoplasia; General Pharmacology; Microbiology; Mind, Brain and Behavior II; Systems II; and a continuation of PPS and LPP. In Systems II, Dermatology, Musculoskeletal/Renal, and "Pumps, Wind and Water" are among the body systems studied. Basic sciences are taught in a wing of the School's central complex. A new Learning Center houses amphitheaters, flexible classrooms, and a video conference facility. The Lamar Soutter Library holds over 239,000 volumes, subscribes to 1,500 journals, and provides access to online search and database tools. The Library Computer Area contains personal computers and workstations for computer-assisted instruction, interactive programs, and educational databases.

CLINICAL TRAINING

Third-year required rotations are Medicine (12 weeks); Surgery (12 weeks); Family and Community Medicine (6 weeks); Ob/Gyn (6 weeks); Pediatrics (6 weeks); and Psychiatry (6 weeks). Fourth-year requirements are Neurology (4 weeks), a Subinternship in Medicine (4 weeks), and 24 weeks of elective study. Clinical training takes place at the UMass hospital (388 beds), a comprehensive facility with general and specialty services. Clinical specialties include: Cancer Center; Level I Trauma Center; Kidney-Pancreas transplantation; Children's Medical Center; Center of Stone Disease; advanced laser technology; Cardiovascular Center; Breast Center; AIDS programs; burn unit; and public sector psychiatry. UMass benefits from affiliations with hospitals in and around the Worcester area: Memorial Health Care (319 beds); Saint Vincent Hospital; and Berkshire Medical Center (330 beds).

Students

All students are Massachusetts residents. The average age of incoming students is 25, and at least half of students took some time off after college. About 60 percent of students were science majors as undergraduates. Approximately 7 percent of students are underrepresented minorities. Class size is 100.

STUDENT LIFE

Recreational and athletic facilities are conveniently located in the lower level of the basic science building. Facilities include a lounge with a TV, pool and ping pong tables, study areas, and an exercise and weight room. Students are involved in organizations focused on community service, recreational interests, and professional pursuits. Worcester is a city of nearly 200,000, offering a full range of services and activities. Students live off campus, most choosing to live in the local community. Some students rely on public transportation, while others use cars.

GRADUATES

Among a recent graduating class, the most popular fields for post-graduate training were Internal Medicine (28%); Family Practice (25%); Pediatrics (15%); Emergency Medicine (7%); Ob/Gyn (4%); and Surgery (5%). A significant proportion entered residency programs in Massachusetts.

Admissions

REQUIREMENTS

Massachusetts residency is a requirement. Prerequisites are one year each of Biology, General Chemistry, Organic Chemistry, Physics, and English. All science courses should include associated labs. The MCAT is required, and scores should be from within the past two years. For applicants who have taken the exam on multiple occasions, the best scores are weighed most heavily. Thus, withholding scores is not advantageous.

SUGGESTIONS

Applications should be submitted as early as possible. In addition to requirements, course work in Computer Science; Calculus; Statistics; Sociology; and Psychology is advised. For applicants who have been out of college for a significant period of time, some recent course work is important. Medically related experiences or research may strengthen an application.

PROCESS

All in-state AMCAS applicants are sent secondary applications. Of those returning secondaries, about half are interviewed between October and March. Interviews consist of two 30-minute sessions with faculty members and/or medical students. On interview day, candidates also have a group information session and campus tour. Approximately one-third of interviewees are accepted on a rolling basis. Wait-listed candidates may send supplementary information if it serves to update their files.

Admissions Requirements (Required)

MCAT Scores, Essays, Science GPA, Extracurricular activities, Non-Science GPA, Exposure to medical profession, Recommendation, Interview

Admissions Requirements (Optional)

State Residency

COSTS AND AID

Tuition & Fees

Annual tuition	$8,352
Cost of books	$725
Fees	$5,736

Financial Aid

% students receiving any aid	75
Average debt	$70,068

UNIVERSITY OF MIAMI
UNIVERSITY OF MIAMI MILLER SCHOOL OF MEDICINE

ADMISSIONS R-159, POB 016159 MIAMI, FL 33101 • ADMISSION: 305-243-3234 • FAX: 305-243-65487
E-MAIL: MED.ADMISSIONS@MIAMI.EDU • WEBSITE: HTTP://WWW.MED.MIAMI.EDU

STUDENT BODY

Type	Private
Enrollment of parent institution	15,500
Enrollment of medical school	753
% male/female	51/49
% out-of-state	34
% international	39
# countries represented	2
Average age of entering class	24

FACULTY

Total faculty	1,202
% female faculty	12
% minority faculty	7
% part-time faculty	0
Student-faculty ratio	0.5:1

ADMISSIONS

# applied	6,074
% accepted	5
% enrolled	63

Average GPA and MCAT Scores

Overall GPA	3.7
MCAT Bio	11.0
MCAT Phys	10.9
MCAT Verbal	10.0
MCAT Essay	P

Application Information

Regular application	12/1
Regular notification	10/15
Are transfers accepted?	No
Admissions may be deferred?	Yes
Admissions need-blind?	No
Application fee	$75

Academics

Most students follow a four-year curriculum, leading to the M.D. A number of students participate in a seven-year B.S./M.D. program organized with Miami's undergraduate college. Up to seven students each year enter a combined M.D./Ph.D. program, earning the doctorate degree in Biochemistry and Molecular Biology; Molecular, Cell, and Developmental Biology; Microbiology and Immunology; Molecular and Cellular Pharmacology; Neuroscience; or Physiology and Biophysics. Annually, 48 students will be able to participate in a 4-year, combined curriculum, MD-MPH program. Opportunities for summer research are also available to medical students. Students are graded with percentile scores during the first two years and with ratings of Honors, High Pass, Pass, and Fail during the second two years. Promotion to year three requires a passing score on the USMLE Step 1. Step 2 of the USMLE must be taken in order to graduate.

BASIC SCIENCES: The first year begins with a set of core modules designed to provide medical students with a sound working knowledge of the sciences basic to medicine. There are five modules that last for about five months: Molecular Basis of Life, Cellular function and Regulation, Host Defenses and Pathogens, Human Structure and Adaptation to Disease, Introduction to Epidemiology, and Infectious Diseases. The rest of the first two years are taught in integrated organ system modules. The second year ends with several problem-based, case-based learning sessions. Throughout the first two years, students work with practicing community physicians and learn about history-taking, how to do a physical examination and clinical diagnosis. The acquisition of clinical skills during the first two years is reinforced and broadened through interaction with clinical faculty in Academic Societies. Students are in the classroom about 20 hours per week. Lectures are the primary instructional modality, but small group discussions are also used, and are becoming more important. The basic sciences are taught in the Rosenstiel Medical Sciences Building which houses newly renovated lecture halls, teaching labs and a student computer system.

CLINICAL TRAINING

Required third-year clerkships are Introduction to Medicine (1 week); Radiology (1 week); Medicine (8 weeks); Surgery (8 weeks); Primary Care (8 weeks); Ob/Gyn (6 weeks); Psychiatry (6 weeks); Pediatrics (6 weeks); and Family Medicine (4 weeks). Fourth-year requirements are Geriatrics (2 weeks) and Neurology (4 weeks). The remainder of the fourth year is devoted to selectives, which must include at least eight weeks of Direct Patient Care, and electives which may be clinical or research-based. Clinical training takes place at: Jackson Memorial Hospital (1,567 beds); Veterans Affairs Medical Center (900 beds); Bascom Palmer/Anne Bates Leach Eye Hospital; University of Miami Hospital; Sylvester Comprehensive Cancer Center; Ryder Trauma Center; Diabetes Research Institute; and The Mailman Center for Child Development. Up to three months of the fourth year may be spent in clerkships at other institutions.

Students

A recently entering class had the following profile: age range, 18–37; women, 46 percent; underrepresented minorities, 8 percent; Florida residents, 65 percent; Science majors, 65 percent. Thirty-nine colleges and universities were represented. Class size is 150 at the Main Campus (Miami) and an additional 48 students in the combined degree MD-MPH program at the Regional Campus in Miami and Palm Beach County, Florida.

STUDENT LIFE

Although the medical campus is separate from the main campus, medical students have access to extracurricular programs and events sponsored by the greater University. In addition, the medical campus has a Wellness Center and other recreational facilities of its own. Medical students are involved in student organizations and volunteer activities in areas such as HIV/AIDS prevention, general health education, and drug-abuse counseling. Students enjoy the good weather and multicultural environment of Miami. Medical students live off campus in various parts of Miami, and usually drive to school or take Metrorail.

GRADUATES

Graduates are successful in securing residency positions nationwide. A significant proportion enter programs at Jackson Memorial Hospital, which features at least 15 post-graduate training programs.

Admissions

REQUIREMENTS

Prerequisites are one year each of Biology, Chemistry, Organic Chemistry, Physics, Math, and English. Science courses should include associated labs. Biochemistry is strongly recommended. The MCAT is required and scores must be from within the past three years. For applicants who have taken the exam on multiple occasions, the best set of scores is weighed most heavily.

SUGGESTIONS

Recommended course work includes Biochemistry, Cell and Molecular Biology, Microbiology and Immunology, Genetics, Embryology, Mammalian Physiology, and Computer Science. Students should display achievement in the humanities and social sciences as well as in the natural sciences. Beyond academic credentials, the Committee on Admissions values interpersonal skills, leadership, maturity, motivation, and compassion. Meaningful patient-contact experience is essential.

PROCESS

One-hundred percent of applicants are sent secondary applications. Approximately one-half of accepted applicants will be non-Florida residents. About 450 applicants are interviewed on campus. Interviews take place on Mondays and Fridays, between August and April, and consist of one session with a faculty member. About 60 percent of interviewed candidates are accepted, with notification occurring on a rolling basis. Approximately 25 positions in each entering class are reserved for participants in the University of Miami Honors Program in Medicine, a seven-year B.S./M.D. program.

Admissions Requirements (Required)

MCAT Scores, Essays, Science GPA, Extracurricular activities, Non-Science GPA, Exposure to medical profession, Recommendation, Interview

Admissions Requirements (Optional)

State Residency

COSTS AND AID

Tuition & Fees

Annual tuition (in-state out-of-state)	$33,587/$41,168
Room & board	$16,665
Cost of books	$9,650
Fees	$1,004

Financial Aid

% students receiving any aid	84
% students receiving grants	44
% students receiving loans	76
% aid that is merit-based	62
Average grant	$11,480
Average loan	$34,583
Average total aid package	$40,855
Average debt	$172,436

University of Michigan
Medical School

Admissions Office, M4130 Medical Science I Building, Ann Arbor, MI 48109 • Admission: 313-764-6317
Fax: 313-936-35107 • E-mail: PIBS@UMICH.EDU • Website: WWW.MED.UMICH.EDU / MEDSCHOOL

STUDENT BODY

Type	Public
Enrollment of medical school	660
% male/female	51/49
% out-of-state	55
% international	15
Average age of entering class	24

ADMISSIONS

# applied	4,931

Average GPA and MCAT Scores

Overall GPA	3.7

Application Information

Regular application	11/15
Are transfers accepted?	No
Admissions may be deferred?	Yes
Admissions need-blind?	Yes
Application fee	$50

Academics

Most students follow a four-year program leading to the M.D., although a growing number opt for combined degrees. A combined M.D./Ph.D. curriculum allows students to pursue graduate studies in numerous departments, including Anatomy and Cell Biology, Biological Chemistry, Cellular and Molecular Biology, Human Genetics, Microbiology and Immunology, Neuroscience; Pharmacology, and Physiology. Some M.D./Ph.D. students are M.S.T.P. participants, while others are funded through institutional sources. For students who are interested in research, but who are not interested in earning an additional degree, summer and year-long research fellowships are available. In addition, combined programs with Public Health and Business Administration are available. Passing Step 1 of the USMLE is a requirement for promotion to year three, and passing Step 2 is a requirement for graduation.

BASIC SCIENCES: During the first year, grading is strictly Satisfactory/Fail. This promotes student cooperation and allows for variation in the level of scientific knowledge among incoming students. Throughout the first and second years, students take Introduction to the Patient, which includes interdisciplinary perspectives and the use of simulated patients, and Multidisciplinary Conferences, which provides clinical correlations for basic science concepts. Other first-year courses are Molecular and Cell Biology; GrossAnatomy; HumanGenetics; Pathology; Embryology; Histology; Host Defenses; Microbiology; Pharmacology; and Physiology. Year two is organized around organ and body systems. These are InfectiousDiseases; Hematology; Oncology; Cardiovascular; Respiratory; Renal; Dermatology; Gastrointestinal; Neuroscience; Endocrine; Reproduction; and Musculoskeletal. The Medical School's basic science instructional facilities include recently renovated lecture halls with audiovisual and computer equipment. A Learning Resource Center is open 24 hours per day and has over 50 computers for student use. The Taubman Medical Library is one of the largest in the United States in terms of the number of volumes, journals, and electronic resources that it holds. The Office of Academic Enrichment provides academic counseling and organizes study groups and tutoring services.

CLINICAL TRAINING
During the second, third, and fourth years, students are evaluated with Honors, High Pass, Pass, and Fail. Third-year required rotations are Family Practice (4 weeks); Internal Medicine (12 weeks); Neurology (4 weeks); Ob/Gyn (6 weeks); Pediatrics (6 weeks); Psychiatry (4 weeks); Surgery (12 weeks). Students attend weekly conferences and discuss a range of topics including the ethical, social, and economic issues related to practicing medicine. Fourth-year requirements are Subinternship (8 weeks); Intensive Care Unit Experience (4 weeks); Advanced Basic Science Experience (4 weeks); and Electives (12–20 weeks), which are selected from more than 300 subjects. Clinical training takes place at the University Hospital (888 beds), St. Joseph Mercy Hospital (522 beds), the Veterans Affairs Hospital (486 beds), and at other affiliated institutions. With approval, students may earn elective credits at other academic or clinical sites in the United States and overseas.

Students

About 50 percent of students are Michigan residents, with the remainder of the student body coming from all regions of the country. Typically, at least 10 percent of entering students are older, having taken some time off after college. Approximately 15 percent of students are underrepresented minorities. Class size is 170.

STUDENT LIFE

Incoming medical students benefit from the support and advice of more senior medical students through a peer-counseling program called Big Sib, Little Sib. Students interact outside of the classroom through participation in organizations that focus on issues such as community service, support for minority and gay/lesbian students, and recreational and professional pursuits. The Furstenberg Student Study Center features a Well-Being Room for information and activities related to student health, computer stations, lounges, and quiet study rooms. Expansive sports and recreation centers also enrich student life on campus. Ann Arbor is an academic and cultural center, attracting scholars from around the world. To serve the University community, the area around the campus is filled with coffee shops, bookstores, restaurants, bars, and shops. In addition to commercial districts, Ann Arbor offers parks, lakes, theaters, farmers markets, and attractive residential areas. Although some limited campus-owned housing is available to medical students, most opt to live in privately owned apartment complexes that are within walking distance of the Medical Center.

GRADUATES

Medical students consistently score above the national average on both steps of the USMLE, contributing to their success in securing top residency positions. Among 1996 graduates, popular choices for specialty areas were Internal Medicine (23%); Pediatrics (12%); Surgery (11%); Family Practice (10%); Ob/Gyn (7%); and Emergency Medicine (6%).

Admissions

REQUIREMENTS

Prerequisites are Chemistry (8 semester hours, to include both Organic and Inorganic); Biochemistry (3 semester hours); Biology (6 semester hours); Physics (6 semester hours); and English Composition and Literature (6 semester hours). In addition, at least 18 semester hours must be completed in areas other than the natural sciences or math.

SUGGESTIONS

In addition to the required science courses, Genetics and Cell Biology are considered useful preparation for medical school. Humanities and Social Sciences course work is also important.

PROCESS

All AMCAS applicants are sent supplementary applications. Of those returning secondaries, about 15 percent are interviewed between September and March. Interviews consist of two 30-minute sessions each with a faculty member or medical student. Candidates are also given a group informational presentation, a campus tour, and lunch with medical students. About one-third of interviewees are accepted and are notified between November and May. Others are rejected or put on a wait-list.

Admissions Requirements (Required)

MCAT Scores, Science GPA, Extracurricular activities, Non-Science GPA, Exposure to medical profession, Recommendation, State Residency

Admissions Requirements (Optional)

Essays, Interview

COSTS AND AID

Tuition & Fees

Annual tuition (in-state out-of-state) $22,694/$36,018
Fees $871

UNIVERSITY OF MINNESOTA DULUTH

UNIVERSITY OF MINNESOTA MEDICAL SCHOOL—DULUTH CAMPUS

180 MEDICINE, 1035 UNIVERSITY DRIVE, DULUTH, MN 55812 • **ADMISSION:** 218-726-8511 • **FAX:** 218-726-70577
E-MAIL: MEDADMIS@D.UMN.EDU • **WEBSITE:** WWW.MED.UMN.EDU/DULUTH

STUDENT BODY

Type	Public
Enrollment of parent institution	920
Enrollment of medical school	120
% male/female	57/43
% out-of-state	13
% international	9
Average age of entering class	24

FACULTY

Total faculty	48
% female faculty	31
% minority faculty	4
% part-time faculty	6
Student-faculty ratio	2.0:1

ADMISSIONS

# applied	1,487
% accepted	6
% enrolled	69

Average GPA and MCAT Scores

Overall GPA	3.7
MCAT Bio	10.3
MCAT Phys	9.2
MCAT Verbal	9.0
MCAT Essay	Q

Application Information

Regular application	11/15
Early application	8/1
Early notification	10/1
Are transfers accepted?	No
Admissions may be deferred?	Yes
Admissions need-blind?	No
Application fee	$75

Academics

The University of Minnesota Medical School Duluth is a two-year rural program of the University of Minnesota Medical School in the Twin Cities. The basic science curriculum features system-based courses with clinical correlations and applications. Additionally, early patient contact through the Preceptorship Program in Family Practice is a hallmark of the first two years. Evaluation of medical student performance uses Honors, Pass, and No Pass. Passing Step 1 of the USMLE is a requirement for promotion to the Medical School Twin Cities.

BASIC SCIENCES: The two-year curriculum is a unique blend of basic medical and behavioral sciences and clinical "hands-on" experiences. The basic sciences, presented using an organ systems approach that begins with principles of basic science, extends to various aspects of the prevention and pathophysiology of organ system disease, and concludes with discussions of several presenting clinical symptoms and multisystems diseases. The behavioral sciences portion of the curriculum emphasizes knowledge about the psycho-social aspects of health and illness that are relevant to the clinical setting and is interwoven with the organ systems component. The clinical experience is directed by community specialists and is augmented by UMD's nationally recognized Family Practice Preceptorship program.

CLINICAL TRAINING

After successfully completing the preclinical years, students transition to the Twin Cities campus for their clinical clerkship. These are Medicine (12 weeks); Ob/Gyn (6 weeks); Surgery (6 weeks); Pediatrics (6 weeks); Psychiatry (6 weeks); Neurology (4 weeks); Surgical Specialty (4 weeks); Emergency Medicine (4 weeks); and Ambulatory Care (8 weeks). The remaining time is reserved for elective study. Clinical facilities include Abbott Northwestern Hospital, Children's Health Care, Fairview-University Medical Center, Hennepin County Medical Center, Regions Hospital, St. Luke's Hospital (Duluth), St. Mary's Medical Center (Duluth), and other sites. Each year, through the Rural Physician Associate Program, up to 40 third-year medical students study primary health care in a 9-month elective in Minnesota rural communities under the supervision of local physicians. Up to twelve weeks of clinical electives may be fulfilled at nonaffiliated institutions in other parts of the country or abroad.

Students

STUDENT LIFE

Small class size, and students' shared interest in family medicine promotes a supportive and cohesive atmosphere. University recreational events, facilities, and activities are open to medical students, including the student center, the gym, intramural sports, and student organizations. Students also take advantage of the extracurricular opportunities afforded by the school's location. Activities such as cycling, running, skiing, hiking, and camping are easily accessible within or around Duluth. Duluth functions as a cultural center for Northern Minnesota, and has a symphony, a ballet, theaters, and art museums. Affordable off-campus housing options in the immediate area are available.

GRADUATES

About 90 percent of students are Minnesota residents. About 10 percent of students are under-represented in medicine, most of whom are Native American. Class size is 60. Most graduates enter primary care fields, and most go on to practice in rural areas.

Admissions

REQUIREMENTS

Priority consideration is given to Minnesota residents who wish to become family medicine physicians in a rural Minnesota setting or American Indian community. Applicants from other states who demonstrate a high potential and motivation for practicing medicine in rural Minnesota or an American Indian community will also be considered. Applicants must have completed all requirements for a baccalaureate degree by the time of possible matriculation. Prerequisites are one Biology course with a lab, one Chemistry course with a lab, four additional science courses (two of which must be upper division), and an upper division Humanities or Social Sciences course with an extensive writing component. The MCAT is required, and scores must be no more than three years old.

SUGGESTIONS

UMD looks for applicants who demonstrate interest in entering family medicine and working with underserved rural or small town communities in Minnesota or American Indian communities.

PROCESS

Secondary applications are sent to all applicants. Of those returning secondaries, about 25 percent are invited to interview between October and April. Interviews consist of two one-hour sessions, each with a member of the Admissions Committee. Notification occurs on a rolling basis, and about 30 percent of interviewees are offered a place in the class.

Admissions Requirements (Required)

MCAT Scores, Essays, Science GPA, Extracurricular activities, Non-Science GPA, Exposure to medical profession, Recommendation, Interview, State Residency

COSTS AND AID

Tuition & Fees

Annual tuition (in-state out-of-state)	$37,128/$50,778
Room & board	$11,115
Cost of books	$2,534
Fees	$1,474

Financial Aid

% students receiving any aid	99
% students receiving grants	66
% students receiving loans	98
Average grant	$2,000
Average loan	$54,392
Average total aid package	$56,392

UNIVERSITY OF MINNESOTA, TWIN CITIES

MEDICAL SCHOOL-TWIN CITIES

OFFICE OF ADMISSIONS, BOX 293, 420 DELAWARE STREET, SE, MINNEAPOLIS, MN 55455
ADMISSION: 612-625-7977 • FAX: 612-625-82287 • E-MAIL: MEDED@UMN.EDU • WEBSITE: WWW.MEDED.UMN.EDU

STUDENT BODY

Type	Public
Enrollment of medical school	910

ADMISSIONS

# applied	3,212
% accepted	9
% enrolled	60

Average GPA and MCAT Scores

Overall GPA	3.7
MCAT Bio	11.3
MCAT Phys	11.0
MCAT Verbal	10.6
MCAT Essay	P

Application Information

Regular application	11/15
Early application	8/1
Early notification	10/1
Are transfers accepted?	Yes
Admissions may be deferred?	Yes
Admissions need-blind?	No
Application fee	$75

Academics

In addition to a four-year curriculum leading to the M.D. degree, Minnesota offers a Combined Degree MSTP M.D./Ph.D. program, leading to the doctorate degree in Biochemistry, Biomedical Engineering, Biophysics, Cell Biology, Genetics, Immunology, Microbiology, Molecular Biology, Neuroscience, Pharmacology, and Physiology. Dual degree programs are also offered—MD/MPH, MD/MBA, MD/MHI, MD/MS [BME], JD/MD. Evaluation of medical student performance in Year 1 and Year 2 is Pass/Fail, Honors. Evaluation of performance in the Year 3 and Year 4 curriculum uses grades of Honors, Excellent, Satisfactory, Incomplete, Fail. Passing both steps of the USMLE is a graduation requirement. Faculty members serve as advisors to medical students.

BASIC SCIENCES: Basic sciences are taught as part of an interdisciplinary curriculum that also includes behavioral, social, and ethical aspects of medicine in addition to introductory clinical instruction. On average, students are in class or other scheduled sessions for 24 hours per week. First-year courses are Gross Anatomy; Histology; Biochemistry, Molecular and Cellular Biology; Nutrition; Human Genetics; Physiology; Neuroscience; Microbiology; Human Behavior; Human Sexuality; General Pathology; General Pharmacology; Physician & Society; and Physician & Patient, the last of which focuses on history taking and the physical examination. Second-year curriculum is systems-based. The courses are Pharmacology; Pathology- Systemic; Pathophysiology; Physician & Society; and Physician & Patient. Second-year students participate in four six-week tutorials in Internal Medicine, Family Practice, Pediatrics, and Neurology. First- and second-year instruction takes place in the Moos Health Tower and other buildings in the basic science complex. The Bio-Medical Library contains more than 428,000 volumes, 4,393 journals, 1,194 audiovisual programs, and 223 computer programs. The reference department has over 50 computers and has access to several online databases.

CLINICAL TRAINING

Students rotate through required clerkships during their third and fourth years: Medicine (12 weeks); Ob/Gyn (6 weeks); Surgery (6 weeks); Pediatrics (6 weeks); Psychiatry (6 weeks); Neurology (4 weeks); Emergency Medicine (6 weeks); Surgical Specialty (4 weeks); and Ambulatory Care (8 weeks). The remaining time is reserved for elective study. Clinical facilities include the Fairview-University Medical Center; Variety Club Heart and Research Center; Masonic Cancer Center; Veterans of Foreign Wars Cancer Research Center; Children's Rehabilitation Center; Paul F. Dwan Cardiovascular Research Center; Hennepine County Medical Center; Regions Hospital; Abbott Northwestern Hospital; Veteran's Administration Hospital; and other hospitals and ambulatory medical facilities in the Twin Cities area. Each year, through the Rural Physician Associate Program, up to 40 third-year medical students study primary health care in Minnesota communities under the supervision of local physicians. One-quarter of clinical electives may be fulfilled at non-affiliated institutions in other parts of the country or abroad.

Students

Of the 170 students in last year's entering class, 82 percent were Minnesota residents and 24 percent were multicultural. About 12 percent were from underrepresented minority groups. Typically, the average age of incoming students is 24.

STUDENT LIFE

Some students work part-time as graduate research or teaching assistants while in medical school. These positions provide academic opportunities and a source of income or tuition reduction. The Medical Student Adytum (adytum is Greek for "innermost sanctuary") is a spacious, comfortable area reserved solely for medical students and their guests. Students use the facility for studying, socializing, eating, and relaxing. Medical students also have the opportunity to interact with other Health Sciences students at an alternate student center—Center for Health Interdisciplinary Participation. Organizations bring students together around common interests, allow them to contribute to the community, and provide extra-curricular activities. Examples of student organizations are Healthy Moms, Happy babies; Phillips Neighborhood Clinic; Medical Student Computer Group; CLARION; Confidential Peer Assistance Program; SNMA; Physicians for Human Rights; Students' International Health Committee. The medical school is part of the greater University, and medical students have access to its athletic and recreational facilities. Beyond the campus, the cities of Minneapolis and St. Paul offer a wide variety of restaurants, shopping, cultural activities, and entertainment. Housing options include residence halls, medical fraternities, and privately owned apartments that are adjacent to the Medical Center.

GRADUATES

In the 2008 graduating class, the most popular fields for residencies were Internal Medicine (19%); Family Practice (15%); Emergency Medicine (7%); Surgery (7%); Pediatrics (8%); Ob/Gyn (4%); and Orthopaedic Surgery (4%). Generally, at least half of graduates enter post-graduate programs in Minnesota.

Admissions

REQUIREMENTS

Prerequisites are Biology + (1 semester/quarters); Chemistry + lab(1 semesters/quarters); Plus four other life sciences, of which two must be upper level. We also requirement one semester of quarter of an upper level Social and Behavioral Sciences or Humanities that is also writing intensive. Advanced Placement credits cannot used to satisfy of of our requirements. The MCAT scores are required, and scores must be no more than three years old.

SUGGESTIONS

Minnesota residents are given preference. As indicated by the Social Science/Humanities requirement, breadth in undergraduate preparation is important. In addition to academic strength, applicants should demonstrate volunteer/community service activity, personal integrity, high ethical standards, motivation, intellectual curiosity, enthusiasm, dedication to lifelong learning, and the ability to work well with others. Consistent with the Medical Student Education mission, the Medical School seeks to matriculate a diverse student body. Diversity benefits the education of all students and supports the Medical School's commitment to graduate physicians who will serve the health needs of a diverse society. In evaluating an applicant's potential contribution to diversity in the Medical School, disadvantaged background, race and ethnicity, evidence of outstanding leadership, creativity, unique work or service experience, community involvement, non-educational progression and demonstrated commitment to working with diverse populations are considered.

PROCESS

Qualified applicants who submit AMCAS applications are sent secondaries. Of those returning secondaries, about 80 percent of Minnesota residents, and 30 percent of out-of-state applicants, are invited to interview. Interviews take place on campus from September through March and consist of one session with a faculty member. Of interviewed candidates, about 25 percent of Minnesota residents and 15 percent of out-of-state residents are offered a place in the class. Applicants are accepted on a rolling admission basis, October through April. Additional materials from wait-listed candidates are not accepted.

Admissions Requirements (Required)

MCAT Scores, Essays, Science GPA, Extracurricular activities, Non-Science GPA, Exposure to medical profession, Recommendation, Interview

Admissions Requirements (Optional)

State Residency

COSTS AND AID

Tuition & Fees

Annual tuition (in-state out-of-state)	$29,975/$37,508
Room & board	$11,695
Cost of books	$2,100
Fees	$2,112

Financial Aid

% students receiving any aid	95
% students receiving grants	16
% students receiving loans	79
Average grant	$2,000
Average loan	$40,500
Average total aid package	$53,080
Average debt	$174,694

UNIVERSITY OF MISSISSIPPI

UNIVERSITY OF MISSISSIPPI MEDICAL CENTER

2500 NORTH STATE STREET, JACKSON, MS 39216 • ADMISSION: 601-984-5010 • FAX: 601-984-50087
E-MAIL: ADMITMD@SOM.UMSMED.EDU • WEBSITE: SOM.UMC.EDU

STUDENT BODY

Type	Public
Enrollment of medical school	407
% male/female	59/41
% out-of-state	0
% international	14
Average age of entering class	24

FACULTY

Total faculty	590
% female faculty	24
% minority faculty	14
% part-time faculty	19
Student-faculty ratio	1.0:1

ADMISSIONS

# applied	295
% accepted	53
% enrolled	71

Average GPA and MCAT Scores

Overall GPA	3.7
MCAT Bio	9.4
MCAT Phys	8.6
MCAT Verbal	9.7
MCAT Essay	0

Application Information

Regular application	10/15
Regular notification	3/15
Early application	8/1
Early notification	10/1
Are transfers accepted?	Yes
Admissions may be deferred?	Yes
Admissions need-blind?	No
Application fee	$50

Academics

While most medical students follow a four-year curriculum leading to the M.D., some take advantage of other schools within the Medical Center and pursue joint-degree programs such as the combined M.D./Ph.D. curriculum, which leads to the doctorate in Anatomy, Biochemistry, Microbiology, Neuroscience, Pathology, and Pharmacology. Medical students receive percent scores and a class rank and may be awarded honors at the time of graduation. To be eligible for promotion, a student must achieve at least a 70 in each course, have a weighted average of 75 or higher, and attend 80 percent of the lectures and classes. Passing the USMLE Step 1 is a requirement for promotion to year three, and passing Step 2 is a requirement for graduation.

BASIC SCIENCES: The basic sciences are integrated with clinical science courses and are taught through a combination of lectures, small groups, labs, and hands-on clinical experiences. Students are in class or other scheduled activity for about 22 hours per week. First-year courses are Gross Anatomy; Histology; Neurobiology; Biochemistry; Medical Physiology; Behavioral Science and Psychiatry; and Cardiopulmonary Resuscitation. Second-year courses are Medical Microbiology; General and Systemic Pathology; Pharmacology; Biostatistics; Preventive Medicine and Public Health; Medical Genetics; Clinical Psychiatry; and Introduction to Clinical Medicine (ICM). In the ICM course students learn history-taking, examination, and diagnosis skills through classroom presentations and small-group sessions. The ICM experience helps prepare students for the clinical phase of the curriculum. Basic-science instruction facilities are central to the campus and include the Holmes Learning Resources Center, which houses the Rowland Medical Library. The library is impressive, with more than 160,000 volumes and 2,500 periodicals.

CLINICAL TRAINING
Required third-year rotations are Family Medicine (6 weeks); Medicine/Neurology (12 weeks); Ob/Gyn (6 weeks); Psychiatry (6 weeks); Pediatrics (6 weeks); and Surgery (12 weeks). The fourth year is organized into 8 month-long blocks of Selectives. Students choose specialty areas from within Internal Medicine, Ob/Gyn, Pediatrics, and Surgery. In addition, 3 blocks of Selectives in an ambulatory setting and 2 blocks in inpatient settings are required. Throughout the fourth year, students participate in a Senior Seminar, which provides a forum for interdisciplinary instruction and discussion of issues relevant to modern medical practice. Clinical training takes place at the University Hospital (593 beds); Blair E. Batson Hospital for Children; the Veterans Administration Hospital; McBryde Rehabilitation Center for the Blind; and Jackson Medical Mall ambulatory clinic, and State Health Department offices.

Students

In recent years all students have been Mississippi residents. Approximately 10 percent of students are underrepresented minorities, most of whom are African Americans. The average age of incoming students is generally around 24. Class size is 100.

STUDENT LIFE

Medical students use the resources and facilities of the University in addition to those of the greater community. As the state capital of Mississippi, Jackson offers numerous cultural and recreational attractions. Beyond clinical-care provision, the Medical School contributes directly to the community through activities such as the Base-Pair Mentorship Program, which pairs Medical School researchers and high school students and encourages them to jointly pursue academic projects. On-campus housing options include a residence hall for female students and an apartment complex with one-, two-, and three-bedroom units.

GRADUATES

Graduates are successful in securing positions in a range of specialty areas. At the University Hospital in Jackson there are more then 20 residency programs into which a number of graduates enter each year.

Admissions

REQUIREMENTS

Due to high competition in the admissions process, state residency is virtually a requirement. Required science courses are 8 semester hours each of Biology, Chemistry, Organic Chemistry, and Physics, all with associated labs. Three semester hours of college-level Algebra and three of college-level Trigonometry, or 3 semester hours of Calculus, satisfies the Math requirement. Six semester hours of English is an additional prerequisite. The MCAT is required.

SUGGESTIONS

The April, rather than August, MCAT is advised. Beyond requirements, some advanced science course work in areas such as Biochemistry, Anatomy, Embryology, Genetics, Physical Chemistry, Histology, or Advanced Physics is recommended. Other suggested courses are Advanced English, Sociology, Psychology, Philosophy, History, Geography, Foreign Language, Computer Science, and Fine Arts. Math and Science courses designed for nonscience majors are not counted toward minimum requirements.

PROCESS

All Mississippi residents who submit AMCAS applications are sent secondaries. About half of those returning secondary applications are interviewed between August and January. Candidates have three interview sessions, each with a faculty member or administrator. In addition, a tour of the campus and the opportunity to have lunch with a current medical student is provided. Among interviewees, about half are accepted with notification occurring throughout the application cycle. Wait-listed candidates may send additional information to update their files.

Admissions Requirements (Required)

MCAT Scores, Essays, Science GPA, Extracurricular activities, Non-Science GPA, Exposure to medical profession, Recommendation, Interview, State Residency

COSTS AND AID

Tuition & Fees

Annual tuition (in-state out-of-state)	$8,949/$14,327
Room & board	$12,681

Financial Aid

% students receiving any aid	96
% students receiving grants	44
% students receiving loans	85
% aid that is merit-based	20
Average grant	$7,000
Average loan	$18,500
Average total aid package	$24,349
Average debt	$22,700

UNIVERSITY OF MISSOURI
SCHOOL OF MEDICINE

MA215 MEDICAL SCIENCES BUILDING, COLUMBIA, MO 65212 • **ADMISSION:** 573-882-9219 • **FAX:** 573-884-29887
E-MAIL: MIZZOUMED@MISSOURI.EDU • **WEBSITE:** HTTP://MEDICINE.MISSOURI.EDU

STUDENT BODY

Type	Public
Enrollment of parent institution	30,000
Enrollment of medical school	387
% male/female	51/49
% out-of-state	5
% international	7
Average age of entering class	24

FACULTY

Total faculty	542
% female faculty	30
% minority faculty	14
% part-time faculty	16
Student-faculty ratio	1.0:1

ADMISSIONS

# applied	1,686
% accepted	10
% enrolled	63

Average GPA and MCAT Scores

Overall GPA	3.8
MCAT Bio	10.0
MCAT Phys	10.0
MCAT Verbal	10.0
MCAT Essay	Q

Application Information

Regular application	10/15
Regular notification	3/15
Early application	8/1
Early notification	10/1
Are transfers accepted?	Yes
Admissions may be deferred?	Yes
Admissions need-blind?	No
Application fee	$75

Academics

Although most students complete the M.D. curriculum in four years, some follow an extended program, leading to the M.S. or Ph.D. along with the M.D. Doctoral programs are available in diverse areas.

BASIC SCIENCES: Missouri is one of the leaders in the movement towards problem-based learning. Students learn in small groups and, with less than 20 hours per week in scheduled sessions, have ample time for self-study or individualized projects. The first two years are organized into eight 10-week blocks, each of which consists of eight weeks of instruction followed by one week of evaluation and one week of vacation. Each block is divided into two general instructional components, Problem-Based Learning and Introduction to Patient Care. Block one is devoted to the Structure and Function of the Human Body, covering Biochemistry, Anatomy, Histology, Embryology, and Molecular Biology and Genetics. Blocks two, three, and four each focus on a set of body/organ systems,which include the following: Cardiovascular, Respiratory, Renal, Gastrointestinal,Metabolism, Endocrine, Neuroscience, Liver, Pulmonary, Hematology, Reproductive, Immune response and Pharmacokinetics. Year two is comprised of blocks 5-8, which concentrate on Pathophysiology and Clinical Management. One of the main objectives of the second year is to prepare students for clinical rotations. Grading for the first year is Satisfactory/Unsatisfactory and for the second year is Honors/Satisfactory/Unsatisfactory. The medical library and computer facilities are comprehensive and serve as educational resources for faculty, students, and the medical community.

CLINICAL TRAINING

Year three is divided into seven blocks of required clerkships, which are the following: Child Health, Family Medicine, Internal Medicine, Ob/Gyn, Psychiatry, Neurology, and Surgery. A separate rural track offers up to six months of clinical experience in a rural community during the third year in lieu of some of the required rotations. Year four consists of twelve weeks of general electives and three 4-week advanced clinical selectives— one must be in a core medical specialty, and another must be in a core surgical specialty. Finally, fourth-year students must complete 8 weeks of advanced basic science selectives. The majority of clinical training is conducted at University Hospital and Clinics, a 288-bed tertiary care facility that draws patients from throughout central Missouri. Other training sites include Children's Hospital, Ellis Fischel Cancer Center, Columbia Regional Hospital, Truman VA Hospital and the Missouri Rehabilitation Center. In total, clinical training sites encompass over 1,000 patient beds. Grading for both of the clinical years is Honors/Letters of Commendation/Satisfactory/Unsatisfactory. Students must pass Step 1 of the USMLE to be promoted to year four and Step 2 CK and Step 2 CS in order to graduate.

Students

The University of Missouri-Columbia is a state school, and the vast majority of a recent entering students are Missouri residents. A large percentage attended the various public undergraduate colleges and universities throughout the state. Among students in the 2005 entering class, 76 percent were science majors as undergraduates. Approximately 7 percent of medical students are underrepresented minorities. The average age of incoming students is usually 24.

STUDENT LIFE

The School of Medicine is located in the heart of the University of Missouri's main campus, allowing students to take advantage of its recreational, athletic, and entertainment facilities. The curriculum gives students flexibility within their schedules, allowing them to explore both their academic and non-academic interests. Student organizations are active, particularly the local chapter of the American Student Medical Association, which coordinates academic, social, and cultural events and sponsors community-service projects. Columbia is located within a few hours of both Kansas City and St. Louis. Most medical students live in privately owned apartments, generally a short distance from campus.

GRADUATES

About half of the graduates enter residencies in one of the primary care fields. A limited number of students seeking primary care careers are selected for a program that integrates the senior year of medical school with residency training in Family Medicine, Internal Medicine, Pediatrics, or Psychiatry.

Admissions

REQUIREMENTS

The School of Medicine requires 8 credit hours each of the following courses, all of which must be taken with associated labs: Biology, General Chemistry, Organic Chemistry, and General Physics. In addition to the traditional pre-medical courses, one semester of math and two semesters of English composition are also prerequisites. The MCAT is required. If a student has taken the MCAT more than once, the highest total set of MCAT scores is considered.

SUGGESTIONS

Course work in biology and chemistry beyond requirements and biochemistry is strongly recommended. In addition, applicants are encouraged to study humanities and social sciences while in college.

PROCESS

All Missouri residents (and some residents of other states) who submit an AMCAS application receive a secondary, which should be submitted as soon as possible. Almost 50 percent of the Missouri-resident applicants and at least 50 out-of-state applicants are invited to interview between October and April. Students are interviewed one-on-one by two members of the Admissions Committee. Current medical students give a short tour of the facilities and host a lunch. About a month after interviewing, applicants may be notified of the Committee's decision. Approximately 40 percent of interviewed candidates are accepted. Wait-listed candidates are not encouraged to send supplementary information.

Admissions Requirements (Required)

MCAT Scores, Essays, Science GPA, Extracurricular activities, Non-Science GPA, Exposure to medical profession, Recommendation, Interview

Admissions Requirements (Optional)

State Residency

COSTS AND AID

Tuition & Fees

Annual tuition (in-state out-of-state)	$23,724/$47,236
Room & board	$9,808
Cost of books	$2,400
Fees	$2,243

Financial Aid

% students receiving any aid	96
% students receiving grants	72
% students receiving loans	93
% aid that is merit-based	3
Average grant	$3,120
Average loan	$32,309
Average total aid package	$39,030
Average debt	$126,986

University of Missouri—Kansas City
School of Medicine

Office of Admissions, M1-103, 2411 Holmes Street Kansas City, MO 64108-2792 • Admission: 816-235-1870
Fax: 816-235-65797 • E-mail: MEDICINE@UMKC.EDU • Website: WWW.MED.UMKC.EDU

STUDENT BODY

Type	Public
Enrollment of parent institution	14,000
Enrollment of medical school	645
Average age of entering class	18

ADMISSIONS

# applied	833
% accepted	20
% enrolled	69

Application Information

Regular application	11/1
Regular notification	4/1
Are transfers accepted?	Yes
Admissions may be deferred?	No
Admissions need-blind?	No
Application fee	$35

Academics

Founded in 1971, UMKC's School of Medicine has always been ahead of the curve in training physicians. Our combined baccalaureate/medical degree program and our docent mentoring system have expertly prepared tomorrow's physicians in unique and innovative ways.

BASIC SCIENCES: Students spend time in the first two years completing the majority of coursework towards the baccalaureate degree, while also completing a small portion of the curriculum for the MD degree. In years 3–6, the ratio will shift and the majority of coursework will be completed towards the MD degree.

CLINICAL TRAINING

Students receive clinical training beginning in the third week of the program. During the first two years, students are assigned to a docent team of 10 students. This team spends approximately three hours a week in a hospital setting learning from the docent. In years 3–6, students are assigned to a new docent team of 12 students. With this team, students spend a 1/2 day a week working in an outpatient clinic and spend two months out of the year in the last three years on Docent Rotation (the internal medicine rotation). In addition, students will complete clerkships in Surgery, Family Medicine, Emergency Medicine, Psychiatry, Pediatrics and Obstetrics/Gynecology. Students will also have elective months to complete clerkships in other specialties.

Students

The School of Medicine admits students from the state of Missouri, the regional states (Kansas, Oklahoma, Nebraska, Arkansas, and Illinois) and out-of-state. About 60 percent of the class will come from the state of Missouri.

STUDENT LIFE

Students do attend courses year-round during all six years of the program. Though students are enrolled in a year-round, intensive academic program, participation in co-curricular activities is still possible. Our students participate in medically-related clubs and organizations, Greek life, campus organizations, student senate, intramurals, etc. UMKC offers more than 300 clubs and organizations, and the School of Medicine also offers opportunities to get involved through research, international opportunities and service learning.

GRADUATES

Our graduates are successful in entering residency programs in a variety of competitive fields and programs. Our graduates enter programs both in the state of Missouri and around the country.

Admissions

REQUIREMENTS

Students must be fully admissable to UMKC in order to be considered for admission to the School of Medicine. Admission to UMKC is based on a combination of test score, class rank and completion of the core requirements. Admission to the School of Medicine is based on a holistic review of all components of a complete application: high school transcript, ACT or SAT score, essay, high school activities, health experience, references and interviews. There is no minimum ACT requirement and no minimum high school GPA requirement to be considered for admission to the School of Medicine.

SUGGESTIONS

In order to be considered for admission, students should have participated in various opportunities to investigate the profession (i.e. shadowing, volunteering at a hospital or other health care facility, participating in formal medical programs, participating in research, etc.) In addition, a student should have completed the most challenging curriculum available in high school. This may include honors, AP, IB or dual-credit courses.

PROCESS

Students may apply to the combined degree B.A./M.D. program between August 1 and November 1 of the senior year of high school. A complete application will include the general application for admission to UMKC, the supplemental application to the School of Medicine, high school transcripts, ACT or SAT scores, essay, high school activities, health experiences and a minimum of three references. The School of Medicine uses a holistic review of applications, and no one component of the application will guarantee a student an offer to interview or an offer of admission. If selected for an interview, a student must interview in person at a School of Medicine interview day between late-January and early-March. All final admissions decisions are mailed April 1.

Admissions Requirements (Required)

Essays, Extracurricular activities, Exposure to medical profession, Recommendation, Interview

Admissions Requirements (Optional)

StandardizedTest, Science GPA, Non-Science GPA, State Residency

COSTS AND AID

Tuition & Fees

Annual tuition (in-state out-of-state)	$26,000/$52,000
Room & board	$13,000
Cost of books	$2,500

Financial Aid

Average grant	$0

University of Montreal

Faculte De Medecine

CP 6128, Succursale Centre-Ville Montreal, QC H3C 3J7 • **Admission:** 514-343-6265
E-mail: FACMED@MEDDIR.UMONTREAL.CA • **Website:** WWW.MED.UMONTREAL.CA

STUDENT BODY	
Type	Public

ADMISSIONS	
# applied	1,859

Application Information	
Regular application	3/1
Regular notification	3/1
Admissions may be deferred?	No
Admissions need-blind?	No
Application fee	$45

Academics

Instruction is solely in French. Some students enter a one-year Pre-Medical program that leads into the four year M.D. curriculum, while others who qualify enter the medical curriculum directly. Although clinical exposure begins during the first year of premedical or medical training, intensive clinical training begins in the third year. The Pre-Medical program is taught through lectures. On the other hand, the majority of instruction for medical students takes place in a small-group setting. In addition to the four-year M.D. curriculum, graduate degree programs are offered in all major medical science fields. Affiliated with the School of Medicine are other health science programs in areas such as Health Administration, Public Health, Social and Preventive Medicine, Nutrition, Rehabilitation, and Speech Language Therapy.

BASIC SCIENCES: Students who enter the Pre-Medical program take courses in Genetics and Embryology, Biostatistics, Cell Biology and General Histology, General Microbiology and Virology, Clinical Immersion, Introduction to Clinical Anatomy, Cell and Molecular Biology, Nutrition and Metabolism, Cell Physiology and Pharmacology, Introduction to Physiology, Psychology and Human Behavior, Introduction to Sociology, Basic Concepts in Ethics, and an elective. First-year medical school courses are Introduction to Medical Studies; Growth, Development and Aging, General Pathology and Immunology; Infectious Diseases; Hematology; Neurological Sciences; Mind; Musculoskeletal System; Introduction to Clinical Medicine; History of Medicine; Epidemiology; and an elective. Second year studies are largely organized by anatomical systems. These are Cardiovascular, Respiratory, Kidney, Digestion, Endocrinology, and Multi-system. Second year students also take an elective and continue with Introduction to Clinical Medicine.

CLINICAL TRAINING
For clinical training, students complete a series of required clerkships that provide hands-on experience in the major medical disciplines. During the third year, required clerkships are Medicine (8 weeks), Surgery (8 weeks), Pediatrics (8 weeks), Psychiatry (8 weeks), Ob/Gyn (8 weeks), and Family Medicine (4 weeks). Third-year students also have the opportunity for a four-week clinical elective. Fourth-year clerkships are Anesthesiology (2 weeks), Ophthalmology (2 weeks), Radiology (4 weeks), Geriatrics (4 weeks), Community Medicine (4 weeks), and an elective (4 weeks). Selectives are chosen from Medical or Pediatric subspecialties (8 weeks) and from Surgical subspecialties (4 weeks). Clinical training takes place at over fifteen affiliated hospitals including Hopital Maisonneuve-Rosemont, Hopital Notre-Dame, Hopital Riviere-des-Prairies, Hopital du Sacre-Coeur de Montreal, Hopital Louis-H Lafontaine, Hopital Sainte-Justine, Hopital Saint-Luc, Hotel-Dieu de Montreal, Institute de Cardiologie de Montreal, Institut de Readaptation de Montreal, Centre Hospitalier de Verdun, Cite de la Sante de Laval, Institue de Recherches Clinique de Montreal, Institut Philppe-Pinelde Montreal, and Centre Hospitalier Cote-des-Nieges.

Students

Entering class size is 143. In a recent class, all but four students were from the province of Quebec. About 60 percent of the students are women.

STUDENT LIFE

Medical students enjoy a good quality of life. The School of Medicine is committed to its students, providing academic and nonacademic support services. Outside of the classroom, medical students interact through student groups and organized social activities. The resources of the greater university, including athletic and recreational facilities, are available to medical students as well. Finally, the city of Montreal is an internationally recognized cultural center with a wealth of activities accessible to students.

GRADUATES

Graduates enter both academic and clinical medicine. At hospitals affiliated with the University of Montreal, postgraduate medical training is available in Anesthesiology, Family Medicine, Medicine, Ob/Gyn, Ophthalmology, Pediatrics, Psychiatry, Radiology, Surgery, and many other post-graduate programs.

Admissions

REQUIREMENTS

Only Canadian citizens, landed immigrants, and highly qualified French-speaking applicants from the United States are considered for admission. Fluency in French is a requirement. Two years of college is the minimum requirement for admission to the School of Medicine. Prerequisites are Philosophy, Behavioral Sciences, Social Sciences, French, English, Mathematics (through Trigonometry), Biology, Organic Chemistry, General Chemistry, and Physics.

SUGGESTIONS

Strong preference is given to applicants from the province of Quebec. Selection is based on both records of academic performance and interviews.

PROCESS

The absolute deadline for applications is March 1. About one-third of all applicants are asked to interview, with invitations based on the candidate's academic record. The strongest candidates are then selected from those interviewed. Admissions decisions are made in the Spring, with the first acceptance notices given in May. Accepted applicants have two weeks in which to confirm their place in the entering class.

UNIVERSITY OF NEBRASKA MEDICAL CENTER

UNIVERSITY OF NEBRASKA COLLEGE OF MEDICINE

985527 NEBRASKA MEDICAL CENTER, OMAHA, NE 68198-5527 • ADMISSION: 402-559-2259 • FAX: 402-559-68407
E-MAIL: COMADMISSIONS@UNMC.EDU • WEBSITE: WWW.UNMC.EDU/COM/ADMISSIONS.HTM

STUDENT BODY

Type	Public
Enrollment of parent institution	510
Enrollment of medical school	510
% male/female	60/40
% out-of-state	12
% international	12
Average age of entering class	24

FACULTY

Total faculty	760
% part-time faculty	14

ADMISSIONS

# applied	1,568
% accepted	11
% enrolled	72

Average GPA and MCAT Scores

Overall GPA	3.7
MCAT Bio	10.5
MCAT Phys	10.2
MCAT Verbal	9.9
MCAT Essay	P

Application Information

Regular application	11/1
Early application	8/1
Early notification	10/1
Are transfers accepted?	Yes
Admissions may be deferred?	No
Admissions need-blind?	No
Application fee	$70

Academics

Most medical students complete the M.D. curriculum in four years, although some may take an additional year for research projects or other activities. A combined M.D./Ph.D. program is offered to qualified students, leading to the doctorate degree in a number of fields, including Cell Biology and Anatomy, Biochemistry and Molecular Biology, Physiology and Biophysics, Pathology and Microbiology, and Pharmacology. For medical students interested in discrete research projects, summer research stipends are available on a competitive basis. Passing the USMLE Step 1 is a requirement for promotion to year three, and all students must record a score on Step 2 in order to graduate.

BASIC SCIENCES: Throughout the first two years, basic sciences are integrated with introductory clinical instruction and topics are organized into blocks, referred to as Cores. Students are in class for about 32 hours per week, most of which is spent in lectures, small groups, or labs. During the first year, these are Structure and Development of the Human Body; Cellular Processes; Neuroscience; and Function of the Human Body. Throughout the first and second years, Integrated Clinical Experience (ICE) covers the history and physical examination, interviewing skills, behavioral sciences, ethics, preventive medicine, health care policy, and health care services research. Through ICE, students have the opportunity to work alongside primary care physicians in a longitudinal clinical experience and a summer preceptorship. Also spanning both years is Problem-Based Learning, in which students work in small groups and apply basic science concepts to clinical case studies. Second year Cores are Introduction to Disease Processes; Cardiology/Pulmonary/Endocrinology/Ear, Nose, and Throat; Neurology, Ophthalmology and Psychiatry; Hematology/Oncology/Musculoskeletal; Dermatology and Infectious Disease; and Genitourinary/Gastroenterology. Instruction takes place in the Michael F. Sorrell Center for Health Science Education. The Leon S. McGoogan Library of Medicine holds over 200,000 volumes and 2,100 current journals. Multimedia materials for computer-assisted and self-instruction are available, as are online informational systems.

CLINICAL TRAINING
Required third-year clerkships are: Internal Medicine (12 weeks); Ob/Gyn (6 weeks); Pediatrics (8 weeks); Surgery (10 weeks); Psychiatry (6 weeks); Community Preceptorship (8 weeks); Basic Science Selective (4 weeks); and a mini-clerkship in an area of choice (2 weeks). During the fourth year, a basic science selective in addition to 28 weeks of electives are required. Clinical facilities at UNMC are Nebraska Health System (650 beds); University Medical Associates, which operates over 60 primary care and subspecialty clinics throughout the greater Omaha metropolitan area; Meyer Rehabilitation Institute; Omaha Veterans Affairs Medical Center; Children's Hospital; Immanuel Hospital; and Methodist Hospital.

Students

Most students in each class are Nebraska residents. Class size is approximately 130.

STUDENT LIFE

Medical students are active in student organizations ranging from the Student Alliance for Global Health, to the Family Practice Club, to a group focused on alternative medicine. The local chapter of the American Medical Student Association is particularly active, organizing volunteer projects, film series, and opportunities for enhanced clinical exposure. Omaha is a city of 900,000, offering a symphony, theaters, art museums, shopping, restaurants, and parks, among other attractions. Students live off campus in the surrounding communities, where, for an urban area, housing is relatively inexpensive.

GRADUATES

Students are successful at securing residencies in both primary care and specialty areas. A significant percentage of graduates enter post-graduate programs at UNMC, which oversees 18 residency programs. In recent years, at least 60 percent of graduates have gone on to practice in the state of Nebraska.

Admissions

REQUIREMENTS

Prerequisites are Biology (8 semester hours); General Chemistry (8 hours); Organic Chemistry (8 hours); Physics (8 hours); Humanities and/or Social Sciences (12 hours); English Composition (3 hours); Calculus or Statistics (3 credits); Biochemistry (3 hours); and Genetics (3 hours). All science courses must include associated labs. The MCAT is required, and scores must be from 20011 or later.

SUGGESTIONS

State residents are given preference, but other highly qualified candidates are considered, particularly if they have ties to Nebraska and are interested in practicing in underserved communities in the state. Beyond required courses, the following are recommended: Molecular Biology, Immunology and Microbiology, Communications, Ethics, and Personnel Management.

PROCESS

All Nebraska residents who apply through AMCAS, and a small percentage of out-of-state applicants, are asked to submit supplementary materials and are interviewed. Interviews are conducted between October and January, and consist of a 30-minute session with a faculty member. On interview day, there is also a group information session and a campus tour. Typically, about 50 percent of Nebraska residents are accepted, with notification beginning in December.

Admissions Requirements (Required)

MCAT Scores, Essays, Science GPA, Extracurricular activities, Non-Science GPA, Exposure to medical profession, Recommendation, Interview, State Residency

COSTS AND AID

Tuition & Fees

Annual tuition (in-state out-of-state)	$27,992/$67,604
Room & board	$15,300
Cost of books	$1,800
Fees	$3,050

Financial Aid

% students receiving any aid	81
% students receiving grants	45
% students receiving loans	57
Average grant	$0
Average loan	$0
Average debt	$152,094

University of Nevada, Reno
University of Nevada School of Medicine

UNSOM Office of Admissions, 1664 N. Virginia Street, MS#0357 Reno, NV 89557-0357
Admission: 775-784-6063 • Fax: 775-784-61947
E-mail: ASA@MED.UNR.EDU • Website: WWW.MEDICINE.NEVADA.EDU

STUDENT BODY

Type	Public
Enrollment of medical school	256
% male/female	56/44
Average age of entering class	24

FACULTY

Total faculty	994
% part-time faculty	80
Student-faculty ratio	1.8:1

ADMISSIONS

# applied	948
% accepted	12
% enrolled	62

Average GPA and MCAT Scores

Overall GPA	3.7
MCAT Bio	10.5
MCAT Phys	9.9
MCAT Verbal	9.6
MCAT Essay	0

Application Information

Regular application	10/15
Regular notification	1/15
Early application	6/1
Early notification	10/1
Are transfers accepted?	Yes
Admissions may be deferred?	Yes
Admissions need-blind?	Yes
Application fee	$45

Academics

The first two years of the program are concentrated in classrooms and laboratories on the Reno campus. The curriculum emphasizes the biomedical and behavioral sciences that are foundational to the practice of medicine. Basic science disciplines are integrated with each other and with clinical problems to promote the learning of problem-solving skills. The curriculum is a systems-based, block format to further integrate the basic science disciplines with clinical problems. Early clinical training is provided for students to learn patient interviewing, doctor-patient relationship skills, and the basics of physical examination and diagnosis. Throughout the first and second years, students spend time with community physicians in and clinical settings. Opportunities to participate in basic and clinical science research throughout the curriculum are available. The third and fourth years emphasize a balance of ambulatory and inpatient medical education designed to prepare students for residency training and beyond. Third and fourth year students study clinical medicine in Reno, Las Vegas, and rural Nevada.

BASIC SCIENCES: The University of Nevada School of Medicine launched a new integrated curriculum in the fall of 2012. This exciting curriculum replaced the previous discipline-based model with integrated blocks that offer a more consistent approach to teaching science concepts within a clinical context, limited lecture hours, and an emphasis on lifelong learning strategies. Each block utilizes a "case of the week" format to align course content with clearly defined objectives that map out the work necessary for successful student learning. Each block concludes with an assessment week for clinical skills testing and a comprehensive examination. The longitudinal Clinical Skills course and Preceptorships in ambulatory care with local physicians run parallel to the blocks. In addition, the USMLE Step 1 is required passage for promotion to year three.

CLINICAL TRAINING
Our current third year curriculum consists of six clerkships—Family Medicine, Internal Medicine, Obstetrics and Gynecology, Pediatric Medicine, Psychiatry, and Surgery— which can be taken in Reno and/or Las Vegas and a longitudinal Clinical Reasoning in Medicine course which runs parallel to the primary care clerkships. Students interested in a rural medicine experience can apply to complete their Internal Medicine and Pediatrics clerkships in Elko, Nevada. The fourth year includes a mandatory 4 week Advanced Clinical Rotation in Rural Health and 32 weeks of electives. Our Institutional Objectives are based on an adapted form of the ACGME competencies for residencies. Passing the USMLE Step 2 - CK and CS is required for graduation.

Students

For current campus information, please visit: http://www.medicine.nevada.edu/dept/asa/prospective_applicants/campuses_home.htm

STUDENT LIFE

Students at UNSOM have many opportunities to participate in activities outside of the classroom to enhance their medical education. Medical students are active in all parts of the school: from participating as voting members on school committees, to providing patient care to the medically-indigent, to being student leaders in clubs and organizations. For more information on student life, please visit: http://www.medicine.nevada.edu/dept/asa/students/student_life_home.htm

GRADUATES

Graduates of UNSOM match into competitive residency specialties and programs. For more information, please visit: http://www.medicine.nevada.edu/dept/asa/students/student_life_match_home.htm

Admissions

REQUIREMENTS

The Office of Admissions coordinates the processing of all applications for admissions. Please review the requirements for admission at: http://www.medicine.nevada.edu/dept/asa/prospective_applicants/adm_home.htm

SUGGESTIONS

Please review suggestions for admissions at: http://www.medicine.nevada.edu/dept/asa/prospective_applicants/adm_home.htm

PROCESS

The admission process is coordinated by the Office of Admissions and Student Affairs. The timeline for prospective applicants can be reviewed at: http://www.medicine.nevada.edu/dept/asa/prospective_applicants/timeline.htm

UNIVERSITY OF NEW MEXICO
SCHOOL OF MEDICINE

MSC 09 5085, HSLIC ROOM #125 ALBUQUERQUE, NM 87131 • **ADMISSION:** 505-272-4766 • **FAX:** 505-925-60317
E-MAIL: SOMADMISSIONS@SALUD.UNM.EDU • **WEBSITE:** SOM.UNM.EDU / ADMISSIONS

STUDENT BODY

Type	Public
Enrollment of parent institution	29,100
Enrollment of medical school	415
% male/female	45/55
% out-of-state	1
% international	44
Average age of entering class	24

FACULTY

Total faculty	1,065
Student-faculty ratio	0.4:1

ADMISSIONS

# applied	1,153
% accepted	11
% enrolled	80

Average GPA and MCAT Scores

Overall GPA	3.6
MCAT Bio	9.9
MCAT Phys	9.1
MCAT Verbal	9.0
MCAT Essay	0

Application Information

Regular application	11/1
Regular notification	3/15
Early application	8/1
Early notification	10/1
Are transfers accepted?	No
Admissions may be deferred?	Yes
Admissions need-blind?	No
Application fee	$75

Academics

The four-year curriculum is organized into three phases, all of which involve at least some basic science instruction and clinical training. In addition, all students conduct research projects under the guidance of a faculty mentor. The complete project consists of research, presentation, and a written paper. Applicants interested in pursuing a combined M.D./Ph.D. may apply to the graduate committee at the School of Medicine in addition to completing medical school admissions requirements. The USMLE Step 1 must be passed prior to Year 3, and Step 2 must be passed in order to graduate.

BASIC SCIENCES: The first year and a half (Phase I) is organized into discrete segments, most of which focus on an organ system. During the summer following year one, students take part in a 6 week Practical Immersion Experience that involves hands-on clinical work in either a rural or urban setting. A range of learning methodologies are used, including lectures, labs, discussions, tutorials, and seminars. Concurrent to basic science instruction are weekly clinical experiences in both inpatient and ambulatory settings. Here, students learn interviewing and examination techniques, and are able to improve communication and personal interaction skills. Phase I is Credit/No Credit

CLINICAL TRAINING

Clinical rotations are accompanied by ongoing small-group sessions focused on problem solving and integrating information. Students rotate through required clerkships throughout the spring and summer of the second year and the fall and winter of the third year. Requirements are Internal Medicine (8 weeks); Surgery (8 weeks); Neurology/Psychiatry (8 weeks); Family Medicine (8 weeks); Pediatrics(8 weeks); and Ob/Gyn(8 weeks). Phase III begins in the spring of year three and is comprised entirely of selectives and electives. A month-long, community-based preceptorship, in which students work alongside a primary care physician who serves as a mentor, is also required. Clinical training takes place at the University Hospital and at several affiliated sites.

Students

At least 90 percent of students are New Mexico residents, and about half of each class graduated from UNM's undergraduate college. Class size is 100.

STUDENT LIFE

The medical school is located on the North campus of UNM, allowing students access to the resources and facilities of the University. The greater Albuquerque metropolitan area is home to nearly a third of the state's population and offers numerous cultural and recreational opportunities.

GRADUATES

About 35 percent of graduates enter residencies at UNM. Many graduates enter primary care fields.

Admissions

REQUIREMENTS

All of the prerequisites must be completed with a letter grade of C or better (C- is not acceptable). Pass/Fail (CR/NC) grading is not accepted. Prerequisites are general biology (8 semester hours), general chemistry (8 semester hours), organic chemistry (8 semester hours), physics (6 semester hours) and biochemistry (3 semester hours). Applicants must have a cumulative GPA of 3.0 or greater and an MCAT score of 22 or greater.

SUGGESTIONS

Students are selected on the basis of academic achievement, motivation for the study of medicine, problem solving ability, self-appraisal, ability to relate to people, maturity, breadth of interest and achievements, professional goals, and the likelihood of serving the health care needs of the state following postgraduate training.

PROCESS

All New Mexico AMCAS applicants that fulfill minimum GPA and MCAT requirements receive secondary applications and are invited to interview. Qualified WICHE and other out-of-state applicants who apply for early decision are also sent secondary applications and invited to interview. Interviews are conducted from August through February and consist of two one-on-one sessions with members of the Admissions Committee. On interview day, lunch and a tour of the facilities are provided. UNM SOM practices rolling admissions; candidates are notified throughout the interview season of their acceptance status.

Admissions Requirements (Required)

MCAT Scores, Essays, Exposure to medical profession, Recommendation, Interview, State Residency

Admissions Requirements (Optional)

Science GPA, Extracurricular activities, Non-Science GPA,

COSTS AND AID

Tuition & Fees

Annual tuition (in-state out-of-state)	$16,169/$46,347
Room & board	$16,193
Cost of books	$4,016
Fees	$3,224

Financial Aid

% students receiving any aid	92
% students receiving grants	62
% students receiving loans	93
% aid that is merit-based	21
Average grant	$7,836
Average loan	$36,014
Average total aid package	$37,757
Average debt	$127,491

THE UNIVERSITY OF NORTH CAROLINA SCHOOL OF MEDICINE AT CHAPEL HILL

UNC SCHOOL OF MEDICINE

121 MacNider Building, CB #9500, Chapel Hill, NC 27599 • **Admission:** 919-962-8331 • **Fax:** 919-966-99307
E-mail: ADMISSIONS@MED.UNC.EDU • **Website:** WWW.MED.UNC.EDU

STUDENT BODY

Type	Public
% male/female	54/46
Average age of entering class	24

ADMISSIONS

Average GPA and MCAT Scores

Overall GPA	3.7
MCAT Bio	10.9
MCAT Phys	10.5
MCAT Verbal	10.6

Application Information

Regular application	11/15
Early application	8/1
Admissions need-blind?	No

Academics

The core curriculum gives students the required comprehensive education needed before they embark on the next stage of their careers. In addition, many students pursue focused research training in the clinic or at the bench. Research stipends are available through training grants or individual research grants. Students with a particular interest in research may apply for the MSTP-supported MD/PhD program at UNC. Other students take the opportunity to combine an advanced degree in public health, law, or business with their medical studies. Grades of honors, pass, and fail are used to evaluate medical students in the first two years. Students must pass the USMLE Step 1 examination before promotion to the third year and pass Step 2 before graduation.

BASIC SCIENCES: The first two years are devoted primarily to studying the scientific basis of clinical practice, with emphasis on demonstrating clinical implications and correlation. Clinical instruction begins early in the first year with the two-year course introduction to clinical medicine (ICM), in which students have the opportunity to develop the clinical skills (such as history-taking, physical examination) and problem-solving abilities needed for the clinical years. ICM also serves as a forum for discussion of a wide range of crosscutting topics such as substance abuse, domestic violence, and computing in medicine. Three months of both the first and second years are spent in a community working with a physician tutor. Other first-year courses are biochemistry, cell biology, gross anatomy, histology, immunology, introduction to pathology, medical embryology, medical physiology, medicine and society, microbiology, and neurobiology. Many of the courses in the second year are organized around the pathophysiology of particular organ systems such as cardiovascular, endocrine, gastrointestinal, hematology/oncology, neurology and special senses, reproductive biology, respiratory, skin, musculoskeletal, and urinary. Closely integrated with the study of particular organ systems are courses in pathology, genetics, humanities and social sciences, and psychiatry. Throughout the first and second years, students participate in small group discussions, lectures, labs, clinical practice sessions, and real clinical experiences. The needs of the curriculum are well served by continuous training in information technology coupled with the requirement that each student have a laptop computer. The Health Sciences Library serves the Schools of Dentistry, Medicine, Nursing, Pharmacy, and Public Health and the UNC Hospitals. The library has approximately 300,000 volumes, 4,000 serial titles, and 9,000 audiovisual and microcomputer software programs.

CLINICAL TRAINING

Students rotate through six major clinical disciplines during their third year. These are medicine (twelve weeks), obstetrics/gynecology (six weeks), pediatrics (eight weeks), family medicine (six weeks), psychiatry (six weeks), and surgery (eight weeks). An additional requirement is life support skills (one week). The purpose of the fourth-year program is to offer a flexible educational experience that can be tailored to the career goals and intellectual interests of each student. Requirements are an ambulatory care selective (four weeks), an acting internship (four weeks), a neuroscience selective (four weeks), and a critical care/surgery selective. A total of twenty-eight weeks of electives is required, some of which may be completed at other universities or clinical settings, either in the United States or overseas.

Students

Approximately 90 percent of students are North Carolina residents. The School of Medicine is committed to admitting students who are representative of the diversity of the population of North Carolina. About one-third of entering students have pursued other interests or careers before applying to medical school.

STUDENT LIFE

The School of Medicine is responsive to students' needs and provides a range of support services. Faculty advisors are assigned to entering students and serve as mentors and academic counselors throughout all four years. The School of Medicine has twenty-six student organizations, including the student body government, student chapters of national medical professional organizations, community service groups, and special interest groups. Students are particularly active in outreach efforts such as Habitat for Humanity, the Domestic Violence Coalition, and Physicians for Social Responsibility and manage two community clinics. During the academic year, scheduled events bring faculty, students, families, and the community together. The university offers single room accommodations for some graduate students in a building near the medical center. Other students live off campus in surrounding neighborhoods.

GRADUATES

Among 2,000 graduates, 53 percent entered primary care fields, and 30.6 percent chose post-graduate training programs within North Carolina. Eighty-four percent of the class of 2000 matched with one of their top three choices for residency training.

Admissions

REQUIREMENTS

Prerequisites are under review and may be changed. Current prerequisites are eight semester hours of biology, at least four hours of which must be accompanied by a lab. Students are strongly encouraged to have taken at least one course in molecular and cell biology. Eight semester hours of general chemistry, organic chemistry, and physics, all with lab, are also required in addition to six semester hours of English. The MCAT is required.

SUGGESTIONS

Preference is given to residents of North Carolina. Thus, successful applicants who are not residents of North Carolina typically have outstanding qualifications.

PROCESS

Approximately 50 percent of AMCAS applicants who are North Carolina residents, and fewer than 10 percent of nonresidents, are sent secondary applications and are invited to interview. Interviews take place between August and March and consist of two sessions with faculty members, one a member of the admissions committee. On interview day, candidates also have lunch with currently enrolled medical students and go on tours of the campus.

COSTS AND AID	
Tuition & Fees	
Annual tuition (in-state out-of-state)	$8,188/$33,656
Room & board	$12,128
Cost of books	$1,050

UNIVERSITY OF NORTH DAKOTA
SCHOOL OF MEDICINE AND HEALTH SCIENCES

OFFICE OF ADMISSIONS, 501 NORTH COLUMBIA ROAD, STOP 9037, STOP 9037 GRAND FORKS, ND 58202-9037
ADMISSION: 701-777-4221 • FAX: 701-777-49427
E-MAIL: JUDE.HEIT@MED.UND.EDU • WEBSITE: WWW.MED.UND.NODAK.EDU

STUDENT BODY

Type	Public
Enrollment of parent institution	13,000
Enrollment of medical school	252
% male/female	46/54
% out-of-state	16
% international	13
Average age of entering class	24

FACULTY

Total faculty	1,442
% part-time faculty	91
Student-faculty ratio	2.0:1

ADMISSIONS

# applied	294
% accepted	28
% enrolled	77

Average GPA and MCAT Scores

Overall GPA	3.7
MCAT Bio	9.9
MCAT Phys	9.2
MCAT Verbal	9.4
MCAT Essay	N

Application Information

Regular application	11/1
Regular notification	1/15
Are transfers accepted?	No
Admissions may be deferred?	Yes
Admissions need-blind?	No
Application fee	$50

Academics

Pre-clinical instruction takes place at the University of North Dakota campus in Grand Forks, and clinical training takes place throughout the state. After students have been admitted to the MD program, they may apply to pursue a joint MD/PhD program in Anatomy and Cell Biology; Biochemistry and Molecular Biology; Microbiology and Immunology; Physiology, Pharmacology, and Therapeutics. Evaluation of students is with ratings of Satisfactory or Unsatisfactory during the first year and Honors, Satisfactory, Unsatisfactory for the final three years. Step 1 and 2 of the USMLE must be passed in order to graduate.

BASIC SCIENCES: An interdisciplinary approach is utilized to teach the basic sciences. A combination of lectures, labs, and small-group sessions are used. The curriculum puts significant emphasis on active student participation and early clinical experience. Social science courses that address topics such as statistics, human behavorial patterns, and social issues that are relevant in North Dakota and other rural areas are integrated into the basic science and clinical curriculum throughout the first and second years. The first-year courses are organized into blocks, namely: Functional Biology of Cells and Tissues; Biology of Organ Systems I; Biology of Organ Systems II; and Biology of the Nervous System. These blocks are offered in the morning. The afternoons are reserved for self-study, or Introduction to Patient Care (IPC), which is the clinical component and is also organized into blocks, such as IPC Block I-Interviewing and Professionalism. The same format continues into the second year. Second-year blocks include: Introduction to Pathobiology and Pathobiology I, II, and III. The IPC component again is covered during afternoon sessions. Students also complete their first clinical rotation, Introduction to Inpatient and Ambulatory Practice of Medicine (3 weeks). Most instruction takes place in either the Medical Sciences Building which houses administrative offices, classrooms, labs and the library or the nearby Clinical Education Center. The Harley E. French Library of the Health Sciences has over 100,000 books, periodicals, and audiovisual programs. It is fully automated, and offers computers for informational and research purposes. In addition, the library has about 18,000 electronic journals.

CLINICAL TRAINING
Third-year, required clerkships are Medicine (8 weeks); Surgery (8 weeks); Pediatrics (8 weeks); OB/GYN (8 weeks); Psychiatry (8 weeks); Family Medicine (8 weeks); and Clinical Epidemiology, which is taken throughout the year. Students are assigned to the Bismarck, Fargo or Grand Forks Campuses for the third year or they may participate in the ROME (Rural Opportunities in Medical Education) Program. ROME students are assigned to a rural practice site for seven months of the third year and to their home campus for the balance of the year. During the fourth year, students train at regional sites in Bismarck, Fargo, Minot, and Grand Forks. Each campus is affiliated with from 10 to 22 hospitals and provides health care services to anywhere from nine to 18 counties. The fourth year includes acting internships and electives. Clinical students train at sites throughout the state, including community hospitals, clinics that are part of the Indian Health Service, and physicians' offices. The University of North Dakota's Center for Rural Health focuses on policy analysis and research on rural health care delivery at the state, regional, and national level.

Students

Most students are North Dakota residents, though up to 11 students in each class may be from Minnesota, Montana, and Wyoming. Up to seven students in each class (admitted as part of INMED) are Native American. In total, underrepresented minorities account for about 14 percent of the student body. About 20 to 25 percent of an entering class is composed of older students who took time off between college and medical school. Class size is 70.

STUDENT LIFE

Grand Forks is a community of 50,000 people, located in the Red River Valley on the border between North Dakota and Minnesota. The city is affordable and safe, and offers the services that students need. Students have access to the facilities of the greater University, and are encouraged to participate in student organizations, including the local chapters of national medical student organizations. On-campus housing is available, although many students opt to live off campus. Since clinical training takes place around the state, students will experience a variety of living situations throughout their four years.

GRADUATES

About one-half of the graduates enter residency programs in primary care fields, and a significant number go on to practice in North Dakota. Post-graduate training programs are offered at all the regional training sites.

Admissions

REQUIREMENTS

State residency is a requirement, with the exception of applicants certified by the Western Interstate Commission for Higher Education (WICHE) and Native Americans, applying through the INMED Program, who must be enrolled members of a federally recognized tribe. Minnesota residents also are given some consideration. Prerequisite course work is General Chemistry (8 hours); Organic/Biochemistry (8 hours); Biology (8 hours); Physics (8 hours); Psychology/Sociology (3 hours); Language Arts (6 hours) and College Algebra (3 hours). All science coursework must be completed with the appropriate laboratory sessions. A minimum GPA of 3.0 is expected. The MCAT is required (23 minimum), and scores must be no more than three years old. For applicants who have retaken the test, the most recent set of scores is considered.

SUGGESTIONS

Preference is given to students who are broadly educated in the Sciences and Humanities. For students who have been out of college for a period of time, some recent coursework is suggested. Computer literacy also is advised.

PROCESS

North Dakota will begin participation in AMCAS for the 2013 entering class. A secondary application from screened applicants will be required. About 40 percent of applicants are invited to interview in December or January. The committee consists of basic science and clinical faculty, practicing physicians, and medical students. After interviewing, candidates are notified of the committee's decision within 4–6 weeks. About 40 percent of interviewees are accepted. Wait-listed candidates are not encouraged to send supplementary information.

Admissions Requirements (Required)

MCAT Scores, Essays, Science GPA, Extracurricular activities, Non-Science GPA, Exposure to medical profession, Recommendation, Interview, State Residency

COSTS AND AID

Tuition & Fees

Annual tuition (in-state out-of-state)	$24,722/$45,760
Room & board	$9,104
Cost of books	$2,250
Fees	$1,623

Financial Aid

% students receiving any aid	97
% students receiving grants	59
% students receiving loans	88
Average grant	$2,110
Average loan	$40,000
Average total aid package	$45,500
Average debt	$157,143

University of Oklahoma
College of Medicine

P.O. Box 26901, BSEB - 123 Oklahoma City, OK 73126 • **Admission:** 405-271-2331 • **Fax:** 405-271-88107
E-mail: AdminMed@ouhsc.edu • **Website:** www.medicine.ouhsc.edu / admissions

STUDENT BODY

Type	Public
Enrollment of medical school	601
% male/female	61/39
% out-of-state	6
% international	26
Average age of entering class	23

FACULTY

Total faculty	856
% female faculty	32
% part-time faculty	20
Student-faculty ratio	1.0:1

ADMISSIONS

# applied	1,463
% accepted	15
% enrolled	76

Average GPA and MCAT Scores

Overall GPA	3.7
MCAT Bio	10.3
MCAT Phys	10.0
MCAT Verbal	9.8
MCAT Essay	0

Application Information

Regular application	10/15
Regular notification	11/15
Are transfers accepted?	Yes
Admissions may be deferred?	Yes
Admissions need-blind?	No
Application fee	$65

Academics

All students spend their first two years on the Oklahoma City campus. On completion of year two, about 25 percent of the class enter clinical rotations at sites affiliated with the University of Oklahoma's Tulsa campus, the School of Community Medicine. Tulsa is particularly well-equipped for primary care and community-based medical instruction. Qualified students may pursue the joint M.D./Ph.D. degree from any graduate department. OUHSC also offers a joint M.D./Master's in Public Health. Medical students are evaluated on an A–F scale. They must pass Step 1 of the USMLE in order to be promoted to year three, and graduates must take, but not necessarily pass, Step 2 to earn their diploma.

BASIC SCIENCES: Basic sciences are taught through lectures, labs, computer-assisted instruction, problem based learning, and small group discussions. During the first two years, students are in class or other scheduled sessions for 20–25 hours per week, allowing ample time for self-directed study. First-year courses are Gross Anatomy, Embryology, Histology, Biochemistry/Molecular Biology, Physiology, Neuroscience, Human Behavior I, Medical Statistics, and Principles of Clinical Medicine I. Second-year courses are Microbiology and Immunology, Principles of Clinical Medicine II, Human Behavior II, Pharmacology, Introduction to Human Illness, and Professional Ethics and Professionalism. Basic sciences are taught in the Basic Sciences Education Building, which, in addition to classrooms and labs, houses a study area. The Robert Bird Library contains more than 250,000 books, journals, and audiovisuals and has two special collections—the Indian Health Collection and the Rare Book Collection. Students can access a number of online catalogs and databases from the library.

CLINICAL TRAINING

Third-year rotations are Medicine (8 weeks); Surgery (8 weeks); Ob/Gyn (6 weeks); Psychiatry (6 weeks); Pediatrics (6 weeks); Family Medicine (4 weeks); Specialty Selectives (6 weeks)and Clinical Electives (28 weeks); and Neuroscience (2 weeks). Fourth-year clerkships are: Adult Ambulatory Medicine (4 weeks); a Rural Preceptorship (4 weeks); Specialty Selectives (6 weeks); and Clinical Electives (28 weeks). Clinical affiliates and training sites are OU Medical Center; Department of Veterans Affairs Medical Center; Oklahoma Medical Research Foundation; Oklahoma City Clinic; Oklahoma Allergy Clinic; Dean A. McGee Eye Institute; Oklahoma Blood Institute; State Medical Examiner's Office; Department of Mental Health; and Oklahoma State Department of Health. Students also may do training at the Baptist Medical Center, St. Anthony Hospital and Mercy Health Center in Oklahoma City. At the Tulsa campus, clinical facilities contain more than 2,000 patient beds, and additional rural training sites are currently being developed. The Oklahoma Telemedicine Network is among the largest medical communications systems in the world, successfully bringing information and expertise to rural physicians, clinics, and hospitals.

Students

At least 75 percent of students must be Oklahoma residents, but generally only 20 to 25 students are from out of state. There is a wide age range among incoming students, and students older than 35 are not unusual. About 26 percent of students are underrepresented minorities, most of whom are Native Americans. Class size is 165.

STUDENT LIFE

Students are cohesive, both inside and outside of the classroom. A student-run note service is one example of cooperation among students. The OUHSC Student Center facilitates both social and academic interaction. It features an exercise room, study areas, computers, a food service court and common rooms. For a fee, medical students also have access to the recreational center at the nearby Healthy Living Center. Medical students are active in student organizations that offer support and focus on recreational pursuits, professional goals, and community service. Medical students are also involved in co-ed intramural football, basketball and soccer. Students are eligible for intercollegiate athletic tickets and other University-wide events. Though OUHSC has no campus housing; off-campus housing is affordable and comfortable. University-owned housing for married and single students is available on the Norman campus. Downtown Oklahoma City is 1 mile from the OUHSC campus and offers a range of activities and attractions.

GRADUATES

Typically, about half of graduates enter residencies in Oklahoma. Others are successful in securing positions nationwide. There are seven OUHSC-affiliated post-graduate programs in Tulsa, and over 25 in Oklahoma City.

Admissions

REQUIREMENTS

Prerequisites are General Zoology/Biology with lab(1 semester); Genetics, Cellular Biology, or Molecular Biology (1 semester); Inorganic Chemistry (1 year); Organic Chemistry (1 year); General Physics (1 year); English (2 semesters), and three semesters of any combination of Sociology, Psychology, Humanities; or Philosophy. The MCAT is required, and scores must be within the past two years. For applicants who have retaken the exam, the most recent set of scores is considered. Basic computer skills are required.

SUGGESTIONS

Strong preference is given to Oklahoma residents, making competition intense for out-of-state residents. Applicants are encouraged to take additional courses in Social Sciences, Humanities, Fine Arts, Computer Sciences, and English. In addition to academic achievement, a candidate's personality, maturity, and character are evaluated. Admissions decisions are made with recognition of the importance of social and cultural diversity.

PROCESS

All AMCAS applicants receive secondary applications. Of those returning secondaries, about 20 percent are interviewed. Interviews are conducted between November and January, and consist of one session with a panel of three members of the Admissions Committee. On interview day, applicants tour the campus and have the opportunity to meet informally with current students. Of interviewed candidates, about 80 percent (not including wait-listed candidates) are accepted on a rolling basis. Wait-listed candidates may send updated transcripts.

Admissions Requirements (Required)

MCAT Scores, Essays, Science GPA, Extracurricular activities, Non-Science GPA, Exposure to medical profession, Recommendation, Interview

Admissions Requirements (Optional)

State Residency

COSTS AND AID

Tuition & Fees

Annual tuition (in-state out-of-state)	$19,700/$46,170
Room & board	$124,414
Cost of books	$5,580
Fees (in-state out-of-state)	$3,299/$3,299

Financial Aid

% students receiving any aid	90
% students receiving grants	36
% students receiving loans	90
Average grant	$7,145
Average loan	$33,345
Average total aid package	$40,490
Average debt	$111,205

UNIVERSITY OF PENNSYLVANIA
SCHOOL OF MEDICINE

DIRECTOR OF ADMISSIONS, EDWARD J. STEMMLER HALL, SUITE 100, PHILADELPHIA, PA 19104
ADMISSION: 215-898-8001 • FAX: 215-573-66457
E-MAIL: ADMISS@MAIL.MED.UPENN.EDU • WEBSITE: WWW.MED.UPENN.EDU

STUDENT BODY

Type	Private
Enrollment of medical school	698
% male/female	57/43
% international	16
Average age of entering class	24

ADMISSIONS

# applied	7,465

Application Information

Regular application	10/15
Regular notification	3/1
Early application	8/1
Early notification	10/1
Are transfers accepted?	Yes
Admissions may be deferred?	Yes
Admissions need-blind?	No
Application fee	$80

Academics

The four-year curriculum is organized into five modules, some of which overlap. Patient contact begins on day one, and clinical rotations begin midway through the second year. Research and scholarly projects are encouraged, and may be pursued in a wide range of areas including biomedical science, clinical medicine, behavioral science, and public-health related fields. For qualified students, combined M.D./Ph.D. and M.D./Master's degree programs are available. Among other disciplines, graduate degrees may be earned in Cell and Molecular Biology, Neuroscience, Chemical/Structural Biology and Biophysics, Immunology, Pharmacological Sciences, Psychology, Bioengineering, Epidemiology, Health Care Systems, Public Policy and Management, History and Sociology of Science, and Philosophy. Another option is a joint M.D./M.B.A. in conjunction with the Wharton School of Business. Grading is Pass/Fail during module one and Honors/High Pass/Pass/Fail during the remaining modules.

BASIC SCIENCES: Basic sciences are taught primarily through an integrated organ/disease system model, correlated with clinical examples and hands-on experiences. Module one occupies the first semester and is devoted to Core Principles. Courses are Developmental and Molecular Biology; Cellular Physiology, Metabolism, and Pharmacological Processes; Human Body Structure and Function; Host Defenses; and Pharmacological Responses. Module two spans the second semester of the first year and the first semester of the second year. It is entitled Integrative Systems and Disease, and is organized around body or organ systems. These are Cardiology/Pulmonary; Skin/Connective tissue/Musculoskeletal/Hematology/Oncology; Gastrointestinal and Nutrition; Brain and Behavior; and Endocrinology and Reproduction. Throughout the entire first year and a half, students are introduced to clinical medicine in Module Three, The Technology, Art, and Practice of Medicine. In addition to providing training in basic clinical techniques, Module Three addresses ethics, technological issues, population-based medicine, public health, and humanistic perspectives. Classroom instruction is enhanced by various academic resources, including multimedia, video, and computerized instructional programs. The Biomedical Science Library houses over 100,000 volumes and receives more than 2,000 periodicals.

CLINICAL TRAINING

Students rotate through required clerkships during Module Four, which covers the second semester of year two and the first semester of year three. These are Internal Medicine (9 weeks); Family Medicine (3 weeks); Ob/Gyn (6 weeks); Pediatrics (6 weeks); Surgery/Anesthesia (9 weeks); Emergency Medicine (3 weeks); and Psychiatry/Substance Abuse (6 weeks); Neurology (3 weeks); and Clinical Specialists (3 weeks). Module Five begins in the second semester of year three and continues until graduation at the end of year four. It includes a subinternship, advanced electives, and a required three-month scholarly or research experience. A large portion of clinical training takes place at the Hospital of the University of Pennsylvania, also the site of research institutions and labs. Other training sites are Children's Hospital of Philadelphia; Veterans Affairs of Philadelphia Hospitals; Phoenixville Hospital; Penn Medicine at Radnor; Chestnut Hill Health Care; Chester County Hospital; Friends Hospital; Holy Redeemer Health System; and the Presbyterian-University of Pennsylvania Medical Center.

Students

The student body at UPenn is nationally represented. About 16 percent of students are underrepresented minorities, and about 20 percent of students took significant time off after college. Class size is 150.

STUDENT LIFE

Pass/Fail grading in the first semester contributes to the high degree of cooperation among students. U. Penn, a comprehensive private university, offers a wide range of extracurricular activities on and around campus, and students are involved both in school and community organizations. Medical students have access to all recreational facilities, including athletic centers. Philadelphia is an important urban center, and is also the home of a very large number of universities. The student community is vast, and the city serves the student community well. Other metropolitan areas such as New York, Baltimore, and Washington, D.C., are easily accessible by train, and mountains and beaches are a short drive. The Graduate Towers and High Rise North is a University-owned graduate student apartment complex available to medical students. However, most students choose to live off campus.

GRADUATES

During a recent three-year period, the most prevalent residency programs selected were Medicine (19% of graduates); Surgical Specialties (19%); General Surgery (6%); Pediatrics (12%); Family Practice (3%); Ob/Gyn (3%); Orthopedics (5%); Radiology (6%); Emergency Medicine (7%); and Psychiatry (4%).

Admissions

REQUIREMENTS

Applicants must complete a course of study leading to a baccalaureate degree at an accredited college or university. No prerequisites are specified, although the MCAT is required, suggesting a comprehensive science preparation. Penn recommends that applicants submit MCAT scores from the spring, but no later than the summer, of the calendar year prior to entrance.

SUGGESTIONS

Recommended undergraduate preparation includes courses in Biology, Chemistry, Organic Chemistry, Physics, Math, History, Philosophy, Ethics, Anthropology, Political Science, and Economics. For applicants who have taken time off after college, some recent course work is advised. Experience in hospitals, clinics, or community service projects is important.

PROCESS

All AMCAS applicants receive secondary applications. Of those returning secondaries, about 20 percent are interviewed between October and February. Interviews consist of two sessions, one with a student and one with a faculty member. On interview day, candidates tour the campus, attend group informational sessions, and have the opportunity to meet informally with students. Of interviewed candidates, about 20 percent are accepted. Wait-listed candidates may send additional information to update their files.

Admissions Requirements (Required)

MCAT Scores, Essays, Science GPA, Extracurricular activities, Non-Science GPA, Exposure to medical profession, Recommendation, State Residency

Admissions Requirements (Optional)

Interview

COSTS AND AID

Tuition & Fees

Annual tuition	$38,308
Room & board	$12,925
Cost of books	$3,100
Fees	$2,855

Financial Aid

% students receiving any aid	80
Average debt	$80,000

UNIVERSITY OF PITTSBURGH
SCHOOL OF MEDICINE

OFFICE OF ADMISSIONS, 518 SCAIFE HALL, 3550 TERRACE STREET PITTSBURGH, PA 15261 • ADMISSION: 412-648-9891
FAX: 412-648-87687 • E-MAIL: ADMISSIONS@MEDSCHOOL.PITT.EDU • WEBSITE: WWW.MEDSCHOOL.PITT.EDU

STUDENT BODY

Type	Public
Enrollment of parent institution	35,330
Enrollment of medical school	589
% male/female	47/53
% out-of-state	76
% international	15
Average age of entering class	23

FACULTY

Total faculty	2,262
% female faculty	35
% minority faculty	4
% part-time faculty	3

ADMISSIONS

# applied	4,912
% accepted	8
% enrolled	37

Average GPA and MCAT Scores

Overall GPA	3.7
MCAT Bio	12.3
MCAT Phys	12.1
MCAT Verbal	10.7
MCAT Essay	Q

Application Information

Regular application	10/15
Regular notification	1/31
Are transfers accepted?	Yes
Admissions may be deferred?	Yes
Admissions need-blind?	No
Application fee	$85

Academics

We seek to train tomorrow's physician-scientists, academic leaders, and finest practicing physicians. To accomplish these goals, the curriculum combines a strong foundation in basic science with early introduction to patients, small-group learning, and an emphasis on critical thinking and problem solving. Each student participates in a mentored scholarly project.

BASIC SCIENCES: During the first two years, students take classes that are grouped into blocks. Year one has five blocks: Fundamentals of Basic Science, covering the essentials of the sciences underlying physiology and medicine; Patient, Physician, and Society, covering ethical, behavioral, and sociological issues related to medicine; Introduction to Patient Care, introducing Physical Diagnosis and History-Taking; Scientific Reasoning in Medicine, focusing on analysis of medical literature; and Organ Systems, covering physiology, pharmacology, pathophysiology, and introduction to medicine, with Neuroscience and Introduction to Psychiatry in the first year. The latter four blocks continue into year two: Organ Systems includes Cardiovascular, Renal, and Pulmonary Medicine; Digestion; Hematology; Endocrinology; and Reproduction/Development, and modules on Musculoskeletal Diseases and Dermatology. The final segment of year two integrates all the organ systems in a problem-based learning format and, while doing so, revisits important points of the previous two years and challenges students to diagnose and treat clinical problems. Lectures, small-group sessions, conferences, labs, and simulations are the instructional methods used during the first two years, and students are in a structured learning environment for about 28 hours per week. Problem-based learning is used throughout the curriculum. An extensive simulation program using both mannequins and trained human patient simulators is integrated throughout all four years. A number of elective, non-credit experiences are offered during the first two years, including Medical Spanish, the Natural History of Medicine, Concepts in Human Motion, and Pandemic Preparedness, among others. With the exception of clinical work, classes meet in Scaife Hall, which houses classrooms, labs, and a library, which has state-of-the-art access to extensive online medical information services. Grades during the first two years are Honors/Pass/Fail. The USMLE Steps 1, 2CS, and 2CK are required for graduation.

CLINICAL TRAINING

Patient contact begins in year one during the Physical Exam course and the Clinical Experiences course. Students interact with patients both in the hospital as well as in ambulatory settings in years one and two. Clinical clerkships begin in mid-May of second year. The eight clerkships are Medicine (8 weeks), Surgery (8 weeks), Pediatrics (4 weeks), Obstetrics and Gynecology (4 weeks), Family Medicine (4 weeks), Specialty Care—Emergency Medicine, Ophthalmology, Otolaryngology, and Pediatric Emergency Medicine (4 weeks), Combined Ambulatory Medicine and Pediatrics (8 weeks), and Clinical Neurosciences (Psychiatry and Neurology, 8 weeks). Selected electives may be taken during third year. Fourth year requirements are an acting internship (4 weeks) and an Integrated Life Science course (4 weeks). All other weeks in fourth year are elective. Clinical training takes place in the many facilities of the internationally renowned University of Pittsburgh Medical Center (UPMC), which comprises numerous major teaching hospitals and centers including a site in Palermo, Italy. The third year is punctuated by three one week Clinical Focus Courses that prepare students for the transition to clerkships, and provide in-depth exposure to topics such as Geriatrics.

Students

About 15 percent of students are underrepresented minorities, most of whom are African American. There is also a wide spectrum of ethnic and cultural diversity within the student body, as well as a large age range as many students have taken some time off before entering medical school. Class size is 148.

STUDENT LIFE

The structure of the curriculum promotes student interaction and collegiality. In addition, medical students get to know each other through involvement in numerous organizations and extracurricular activities. Some of the many student groups on campus are the American Medical Student Association (AMSA), the Student National Medical Association (SNMA), the American Medical Association (AMA), specialty interest groups in most areas of medicine, Pitt Women in Medicine, the Global Health Interest Group, and the History of Medicine Society. Medical students have access to all facilities of the University of Pittsburgh, including athletic facilities. Pittsburgh is an accessible and exciting city, and, although on-campus housing is available, most medical students choose to live off campus.

GRADUATES

Graduates are successful in gaining admittance the most prestigious residency programs in the country.

Admissions

REQUIREMENTS

Requirements are one year each of Biology, Physics, Chemistry, and Organic Chemistry (all with associated labs), and English. In assessing grades, consideration is given to the undergraduate institution attended and the course load taken. The MCAT is required and scores must be no more than three years old prior to application.

SUGGESTIONS

Competence in science and math is valued as is evidence of success in social science and humanities courses. The University of Pittsburgh School of Medicine assesses interpersonal skills and commitment to community service in applicants. For applicants who graduated college several years ago, some recent course work is advised.

PROCESS

Secondary applications are sent to all AMCAS applicants. Interviews are conducted from August through December and consist of two sessions, one with a faculty member and one with a medical student. Notification occurs on a rolling basis. Wait-listed candidates may send additional information to strengthen their applications and to indicate interest in the school.

Admissions Requirements (Required)

MCAT Scores, Essays, Science GPA, Extracurricular activities, Non-Science GPA, Exposure to medical profession, Recommendation, Interview

Admissions Requirements (Optional)

State Residency

COSTS AND AID

Tuition & Fees

Annual tuition (in-state out-of-state)	$44,726/$45,846
Room & board	$15,795
Cost of books	$6,424
Fees	$783

Financial Aid

% students receiving any aid	86
% students receiving grants	65
% students receiving loans	68
% aid that is merit-based	28
Average grant	$23,796
Average loan	$41,672
Average total aid package	$50,836
Average debt	$146,659

UNIVERSITY OF PUERTO RICO

MEDICAL SCIENCES CAMPUS

A-878 MAIN BUILDING, PO BOX 365067 SAN JUAN, PR 00936-5067 • ADMISSION: 787-758-2525 EXT. 1800
FAX: 787-756-84757 • E-MAIL: MARRIVERA@RCM.UPR.EDU • WEBSITE: RCM.UPR.EDU

STUDENT BODY	
Type	Public
Enrollment of medical school	1,716

FACULTY	
Total faculty	189

ADMISSIONS

Application Information

Regular application	12/1
Early application	6/1
Admissions need-blind?	No
Application fee	$15

Academics

Medical training is accomplished through a variety of educational experiences, both in the classroom and at multiple service settings in the public and private sectors of Puerto Rico. Medical students benefit from the resources of other health professional schools and from interaction with students at other schools. Through the Center for International Health, medical students gain exposure to the research and policy issues surrounding global health. Grading for all courses is on an A–F scale.

BASIC SCIENCES: Basic sciences are taught using a combination of lectures, small group discussions, labs, and exposure to clinical correlates. Required first year course are: Medical Gross Anatomy, Medical Histology, Medical Embryology, Medical Neuroscience, Introduction to Biochemistry, Human Physiology, Human Development I, Public Health and Preventive Medicine I, Integration Seminar I, Behavioral Sciences, and Introduction to Clinical Diagnosis. Second year courses consist of Pathobiology-Introduction to Laboratory Medicine, Infectious Diseases, Medical Pharmacology, Fundamentals of Clinical Diagnosis, Human Development II, Public Health and Preventive Medicine II, Basic Clinical Clerkship, Mechanisms of Disease, Psychopathology, and Integration Seminar II. Outside of the classroom, students learn in the Learning Resources Center, the Standardized Patient Laboratory, and the Clinical Learning Laboratory.

CLINICAL TRAINING
The third year is comprised of clinical rotations. These are: Radiology (2 weeks), Psychiatry (4 weeks), Medicine (12 weeks), Family Medicine (4 weeks), Pediatrics (10 weeks), Surgery (10 weeks), and Ob/Gyn (6 weeks). During year four, clerkships are: Dermatology (1 week); Physical Medicine and Rehabilitation (1 week); Public Health (3 weeks); Legal, Ethical, and Administrative Aspects in Medicine (1 week); and Selective Clerkships (8 weeks). In addition, 18 weeks are open for clinical and research electives. Clinical education uses a variety of settings including University Hospital, University Pediatric Hospital, San Juan City Hospital, Veterans Administration Hospital, and the Oncology Hospital. In addition, the school uses certain private hospitals, clinics, and public health facilities. Some electives may be taken at institutions other than those affiliated with the University of Puerto Rico, such as hospitals in other regions of Puerto Rico and in other countries.

Students

Each entering class has about 100 students. Students come from foreign countries and the mainland United States as well as Puerto Rico. Fifty percent of students are women.

STUDENT LIFE

Recreational facilities on campus include the Sports and Gym Center. The medical school promotes student health through its exercise/wellness program and by sponsoring a range of student activities and events. When they have free time, medical students enjoy the city of San Juan and its surroundings.

GRADUATES

The University of Puerto Rico and its affiliated hospitals offer residency programs in most major medical fields.

Admissions

REQUIREMENTS

With few exceptions, entering students must have completed their Bachelors degree. Prerequisite courses are one year each of Biology, General Chemistry, Physics, and Organic Chemistry. The MCAT is required, and August in the year prior to admission is the latest acceptable test date.

SUGGESTIONS

Both residents of Puerto Rico and nonresidents are considered for admission. Grade point average and MCAT scores are important in admissions decisions. In addition to academic credentials, the University of Puerto Rico looks for integrity and motivation in its students.

PROCESS

All applicants are encouraged to visit the campus. Candidates for the M.D. program must submit an application by December 1. Those who qualify are invited to interview after their applications are reviewed. Final decisions and notifications are made throughout the year and are completed in the spring.

COSTS AND AID

Tuition & Fees

Annual tuition (in-state out-of-state)	$6,965/$15,000
Room & board	$4,840
Cost of books	$7,893
Fees	$1,600

UNIVERSITY OF ROCHESTER
SCHOOL OF MEDICINE AND DENTISTRY

MEDICAL CENTER BOX 601A, ROCHESTER, NY 14642 • ADMISSION: 585-275-4539 • FAX: 585-756-54797
E-MAIL: MDADMISH@URMC.ROCHESTER.EDU • WEBSITE: WWW.URMC.ROCHESTER.EDU/SMD/ADMISS

Academics

Special emphasis is placed on skills acquisition and use, with a commitment to lifelong learning. Sensitivity to the world of the patient is encompassed in the biopsychosocial integration of the curriculum and the learning experience, with mechanisms in place for continuous curricular improvement through the collaboration of students and faculty. By ensuring adequate and early electivity for students to enhance their special interests, along with rigorous training and assessment of all of the competencies demanded by modern medical practice, the curriculum generates a knowledge base characterized by depth, breadth, rigor, and flexibility. Students interested in careers in medical science may participate in the fully funded Medical Scientist Training Program (M.D./Ph.D.), or joint-degree programs including the M.P.H./M.D. and M.B.A./M.D. program in Health Care Management in conjunction with the William E. Simon Graduate School of Business Administration. Vacation and full-year fellowships facilitate student research or international medicine experiences. Evaluation of student performance uses Satisfactory/Fail, except in the required clerkships, where Honors/High Pass/Pass/Fail grades are used. Passing the USMLE is not required for promotion to the third year.

BASIC SCIENCES: An introductory module at the beginning of year one prepares students in the acquisition, management, and presentation of medical information. Students learn how to meet the challenges of active and independent learning by becoming competent in data management, information technology, and critical evaluation of the medical literature. Every course is interdisciplinary; basic sciences are integrated with one another and basic and clinical sciences are woven together as the strands of the Double Helix Curriculum throughout the four years. Clinical skills training from day one leads not to shadowing or preceptor experiences in clinics, but to real clinical work as part of the health care team while still in the first year. Not just "paper cases," but students' actual clinical cases drive the learning of science through the school-wide use of multidisciplinary problem-based learning (PBL) cases. Three two-hour PBL tutorials per week and an average of no more than 10 hours of lecture per week, with adequate time for self-study, and the use of labs, conferences, seminars, and computer-assisted learning—all these things characterize the classroom setting of the curriculum. Electives are available during all four years, including electives in Medical Humanities, International Medicine, and community outreach programs. The Edward G. Miner Library holds over 225,000 volumes and a modern, computer-based learning resource center.

CLINICAL TRAINING

Beginning in year one, students complete their introduction to clinical medicine in the fall and then participate in an Ambulatory Clerkship Experience beginning in the spring. This experience, unlike any other in the country, includes all the ambulatory components of Family Medicine, Pediatrics, Internal Medicine, Women's Health, Psychiatry, and Ambulatory Surgery, and is completed by the end of the second year. Inpatient clerkships are completed by December of the fourth year and focus on acute illness experiences in adult medicine, women's and children's health, mind/brain/behavior, and urgent/emergent care. Strong Memorial Hospital (700 beds) is the principal site for clinical teaching, along with a newly completed Ambulatory Care Center and five affiliated hospitals (2,000 beds) covering acute and chronic care.

Students

Students come from all regions of the country. About 13 percent are underrepresented minorities. The average age of incoming students is 24; one-third have majored in areas outside the sciences, and 100 students are accepted each year.

STUDENT LIFE

Most medical students have active lives outside of the classroom. Many participate in community outreach programs, international medicine electives, and student organizations and events. Students have access to resources of the University campus and athletic facilities in the medical center. Located on the southern shore of Lake Ontario, in the Finger Lakes wine-producing region of upstate New York, Rochester is a progressive, metropolitan community of more than one million people. Rochester has a rich cultural life, is an affordable and friendly city, and is a haven for boaters and other outdoor enthusiasts.

GRADUATES

Among the 2001 graduates, the most popular residencies were Internal Medicine (34%), Pediatrics (18%), Surgery (4%), Emergency Medicine (4%), Ob/Gyn (4%), Family Medicine (4%), Anesthesiology (4%), Orthopaedics (4%), ENT (4%) and Ophthamaology (4%). About 15 percent stayed in the Rochester area, while an additional 27 percent remained in New York State. The remainder went to 25 other states.

Admissions

REQUIREMENTS

Prerequisite science courses are one year of Biology, Physics, General Chemistry, and Organic Chemistry, all associated with labs. One semester of Biochemistry may be substituted for one semester of Organic. One year of English or expository writing is also required. Rochester belongs to AMCAS, and the MCAT exam is required; scores should be from the past three years. The best set of scores is considered.

SUGGESTIONS

In addition to required science courses, 12–16 credit hours in the Humanities and/or Social Sciences are required. Experiences in research, clinical settings, and the community are strongly recommended. Rochester looks for evidence of leadership, excellent interpersonal skills, a love of learning, appreciation of diversity, and outstanding scholarship.

PROCESS

Rochester is an AMCAS school. About 10 percent of applicants are interviewed between September and February. Interviews consist of two sessions with faculty, and applicants have a tour, lunch with current students, and a financial aid presentation. About 35 percent of the interviewed applicants are offered acceptance, with notification beginning in November and continuing through May. About 15 positions in each class are reserved for students from several programs, such as the Rochester Early Medical Scholar program and the Bryn Mawr post-baccalaureate program.

Admissions Requirements (Required)

MCAT Scores, Essays, Science GPA, Extracurricular activities, Non-Science GPA, Exposure to medical profession, Recommendation, Interview

Admissions Requirements (Optional)

State Residency

COSTS AND AID

Tuition & Fees

Annual tuition	$35,800
Room & board	$9,000
Cost of books	$2,060
Fees	$1,911

Financial Aid

% students receiving any aid	92
% students receiving grants	49
% students receiving loans	90
% aid that is merit-based	0
Average grant	$1,206
Average loan	$28,436
Average total aid package	$36,875
Average debt	$124,816

University of Saskatchewan

College of Medicine

5B53 Health Science Building, 107 Wiggins Road, Box 17 Saskatoon, SK S7N 5E5
Admission: 306-966-4030 • **Fax:** 306-966-26017
E-mail: MED.ADMISSIONS@USASK.CA • **Website:** WWW.MEDICINE.USASK.CA / ADMISSIONS

STUDENT BODY

Type	Public
Enrollment of parent institution	20,000
Enrollment of medical school	370
Average age of entering class	23

ADMISSIONS

# applied	806
% accepted	12
% enrolled	100

Average GPA and MCAT Scores

Overall GPA	89.5
MCAT Bio	11.0
MCAT Phys	11.0
MCAT Verbal	10.0
MCAT Essay	Q

Application Information

Regular application	10/15
Regular notification	5/13
Are transfers accepted?	No
Admissions may be deferred?	Yes
Admissions need-blind?	Yes
Application fee	$125

Academics

The goal of the College of Medicine is to enable medical students to develop the knowledge, skills, values, and attitudes that will serve as a foundation for subsequent education in primary and specialty patient care and research. In its curriculum, the College promotes the integration of basic and clinical sciences. Independent learning, problem-solving, and early patient interaction are emphasized. The curriculum is divided into four phases. For the most part, basic science instruction occurs during the first three phases. However, basic science and clinical training are integrated throughout the four-year curriculum.

BASIC SCIENCES: CLINICAL TRAINING

The College of Medicine provides an integrated four year curriculum leading to the general professional education of the physician; graduates may select careers in family medicine, specialty practice, or research. Year 1 (32 weeks) provides students with the principles of biomedical sciences appropriate to the study of medicine and the first four modules within the foundations of clinical medicine as well as professional and primary clinical skills within the context of developing the patient-doctor relationship. This first year of the program cumulates in a two-week clinical experience within one of the Saskatchewan Health Districts. Year 2 (32 weeks) continues the exploration into foundations of clinical medicine while building upon the professional and clinical skills. Early patient contact and pedagogical strategies such as effective flipped classrooms and case-based learning are integrated throughout the program. Clinical reasoning skills are embedded within each course as well as being specifically developed within the clinical integration courses. Years 3 and 4 of the program focus on clinical clerkship experiences supplemented with seminar-style classes that together will provide opportunities to apply the knowledge, skills, and attitudes students have acquired towards the management of patients within the medical environment. Specific core rotations as well as electives and selectives are available. The program concludes with a capstone course focused on ensuring students are prepared for the next phase of their training.

Students

The current size of the entering classes is 100. Typically, 90% of students are from the province of Saskatchewan.

STUDENT LIFE

With a relatively small student body and a curriculum that encourages interaction, students are generally cohesive. Between the medical school and the greater University, a wide range of extra-curricular activities and events are offered. Medical students live both on and off campus.

GRADUATES

Though research is an increasingly important activity for the College of Medicine, a large number of graduates become practicing clinical physicians in the province of Saskatchewan.

Admissions

REQUIREMENTS

Please refer to the website at www.medicine.usask.ca/admissions for most up-to-date admission requirements.

SUGGESTIONS

Criteria for selection are academic performance and personal qualities. Personal qualities are assessed primarily by the Multiple Mini Interview.

PROCESS

Application forms are available online after August 1 at www.medicine.usask.ca/admissions. Applications must be submitted by the application deadline posted on our website. Personal qualities are assessed through an interview usually held in March. Reference are also considered. All candidates are notified of their acceptance mid to late May.

Admissions Requirements (Required)

MCAT Scores, Science GPA, Non-Science GPA, Recommendation, Interview, State Residency

Admissions Requirements (Optional)

Essays, Extracurricular activities, Exposure to medical profession,

COSTS AND AID

Tuition & Fees

Annual tuition	$14,930
Room & board	$10,800
Cost of books	$1,800
Fees	$770

UNIVERSITY OF SHERBROOKE

2500, BOUL. DE L'UNIVERSITÉ, SHERBROOKE, QC J1K 2R1 • ADMISSION: 819-821-7686

STUDENT BODY

Type	Public

ADMISSIONS

Application Information

Regular application	3/1
Admissions may be deferred?	No
Admissions need-blind?	No
Application fee	$30

Academics

Sherbrooke offers a four-year curriculum leading to the M.D. degree. Educational methodology is based on small group discussions, case studies, audiovisual and computer assisted learning, and hands-on clinical experiences. Combined degree programs, such as the M.D./M.Sc. program are open to highly qualified students who have an interest in research.

BASIC SCIENCES: The first academic period begins in late August and spans 39 weeks. In general, students are in class or other scheduled session for approximately 30 hours per week. Courses are: Introduction to M.D. Program, Biological Medicine I and II, Clinical Immersion, Growth Development and Aging, Nervous System, Locomoter System, Pscyhosocial Sciences, Preventive Medicine and Community Health, Integration, and Clinical Skills. The second year is organized into blocks based on anatomical/physiological systems. These are: Cardiovascular System, Respiratory System, Urinary System, Gastrointestinal System, Hemato-Immunologic System, Infectious Disease, Endocrine System, Reproductive System, and Human Sexuality. In addition, students take part in a Rotation in Community Hospitals and a course in Clinical Skills.

CLINICAL TRAINING

The third and fourth years are organized into several components. These are: Required Courses, Required Primary Clerkships, Rotations in Community, Elective Programs, Integration Period, and Final Exam. Required Courses are: Interdisciplinary Concepts, Clinical Skills, and Introduction to Clerkships. The required Primary Clerkships are: Medicine (10.5 weeks); Surgery (7 weeks); Pediatrics (7 weeks); Psychiatry (7 weeks); Ob/Gyn (7 weeks); and Multidisciplinary—Anesthesia, Ophthalmology, Dermatology, ORL—(3.5 weeks). Rotations in Community are comprised of Family Medicine and Emergency (7 weeks) and Community Health (4 weeks). The Elective Program lasts 12 weeks, followed by the Integration Period (6 weeks) and the Final Exam Period (one week). Teaching hospitals are Cuse Fleurimont, Cuse Bowen, Hopital Charles Le Moyne, and Hopital Sainte-Croix.

Students

Each entering class has approximately 105 students. About 80 percent of students are from the Province of Quebec. Women account for 60 percent of students.

STUDENT LIFE

The University of Sherbrooke is a large university with many social, recreational and other extra-curricular activities for medical students. Medical students have both on campus and off campus housing options.

GRADUATES

Many graduates enter one of the residency programs offered at hospitals affiliated with Sherbrooke.

Admissions

REQUIREMENTS

Fluency in French is required. The minimum requirement for admissions is two years of university or a B.A. degree. Prerequisites are: General Biology (one year); General Chemistry (one year); Organic Chemistry (one year); Physics (three semesters); and Mathematics through Calculus. The MCAT is not required.

SUGGESTIONS

In addition to prerequisite courses, students should complete course work in the Humanities and in the Social Sciences. Priority is given to residents of Quebec, and 86 positions in each entering class are reserved for this group of applicants. Fifteen additional places are reserved for applicants from New Brunswick, one place is reserved for an applicant from Prince Edward Island, one from Nova Scotia, and two places are available for qualified foreign applicants. Overall, about 5% of applicants are admitted each year.

PROCESS

Applications are available from the Admissions Office at the address above. Following review of applications, qualified candidates are invited to a learning skills test (THAMUS).

COSTS AND AID

Tuition & Fees

Annual tuition (in-state
out-of-state) $3,127/$15,127

UNIVERSITY OF SOUTH ALABAMA

UNIVERSITY OF SOUTH ALABAMA COLLEGE OF MEDICINE

OFFICE OF ADMISSIONS, 241 CSAB, MOBILE, AL 36688 • ADMISSION: 251-460-7176 • FAX: 251-460-62787
E-MAIL: MSCOTT@USOUTHAL.EDU • WEBSITE: WWW.USOUTHAL.EDU/USA/DEPS-GRD.HTML

STUDENT BODY

Type	Public
Enrollment of parent institution	13,500
Enrollment of medical school	280
% male/female	49/51
% out-of-state	12
% international	11
Average age of entering class	24

FACULTY

Total faculty	300
% female faculty	30
% minority faculty	10
% part-time faculty	9
Student-faculty ratio	1.0:1

ADMISSIONS

# applied	809
% accepted	14
% enrolled	60

Average GPA and MCAT Scores

Overall GPA	3.7
MCAT Bio	11.0
MCAT Phys	10.0
MCAT Verbal	10.0
MCAT Essay	0

Application Information

Regular application	11/15
Are transfers accepted?	Yes
Admissions may be deferred?	Yes
Admissions need-blind?	Yes
Application fee	$75

Academics

The curriculum is semi-traditional, and uses a lecture format for most of the pre-clinical instruction. Although some early clinical exposure is offered, during the first two years, the program focuses on ensuring a solid understanding of the basic sciences. Combining medical and doctorate studies is possible if pursuing a Ph.D. degree in a medically related discipline. About 10 percent of the class enters the School of Medicine via a combined undergraduate-medical school program that is open to both Alabama and out-of-state high school seniors.

BASIC SCIENCES: The school operates on a quarter system. During the first year, lecture courses are Gross Anatomy, Histology, Developmental Anatomy, Physiology, Neuroanatomy, and Biochemistry. Generally, students are in lecture for about 25 hours per week. The course Medical Ethics is taught by using both lecture and small-group format. Medical Practice and Society and Physical Diagnosis use lectures and a case-based approach. During the second year, traditional lecture/lab courses include Microbiology, Pharmacology, Pathology, and Genetics. Introduction to Behavioral Sciences and a course covering principles of Public Health are also part of the curriculum. In addition, students take part in weekly sessions in clinical settings, as part of an introductory course in Clinical Medicine. Basic sciences are taught in the Medical Sciences Building, which contains administrative offices, classrooms, and laboratories. The Biomedical Library houses 65,000 volumes and offers computer and online services. Grading is AÃêF for most courses, and promotions are based not only on grades but also on faculty evaluation of students' ethical and personal maturity. Medical students are involved in the Schools' administrative affairs through an elected student governing body, which also participates in issues relating to the greater University. The schedule for the first two years is relatively firm, and students are encouraged to focus on their studies, rather than pursue employment or other activities during this period. The USMLE Step 1 is required following the basic-science portion of study.

CLINICAL TRAINING
Year three is composed entirely of required clerkships: Medicine (12 weeks); Surgery (8 weeks); Ob/Gyn (6 weeks); Psychiatry/Neurology (8 weeks); Pediatrics (8 weeks); and Family Practice (6 weeks). The fourth year is also 48 weeks but is composed of elective rather than required rotations. Students must select a one-month rotation from each broad field: Neuroscience; Surgical Subspecialties; Ambulatory Care; Primary Care; and in-house elective. Students train at University-affiliated hospitals that together constitute the largest medical complex along the Gulf Coast and that contain a total of 880 beds. All levels of trauma care and surgery are available, and patients come not only from around the state but from neighboring states as well. In downtown Mobile, the Children's and Women's Hospital offers clinical rotations in pediatric services and neonatal care. The hospital system serves managed care clients, among others, ensuring a client base. Cancer Research and Treatment, Organic Transplant, Aeromedical Transport, and Preventative Care are a few of the noteworthy services available through the University network. Students receive grades of A-F for clinical performance during required rotations and Honors/Pass/Fail during elective rotations. The USMLE Step 2 is required for graduation. A large percentage of students take part in rotations at out-of-state institutions or overseas.

Students

At least 80 percent of medical students must be Alabama residents. Reflecting the state's demographics, about 9 percent are underrepresented minorities, most of whom are African American. Each year, about 15 students enter who have taken time off after college. The student body is diverse in terms of undergraduate majors, and class size is relatively small, at 74 students.

STUDENT LIFE

Students take advantage of the University campus with its recreational facilities and activities. Students also use nearby municipal recreational facilities, which include a golf course. The School of Medicine provides opportunities for students to participate in medically related projects and events, such as volunteer activities and special seminars. The majority of students live in a variety of apartment complexes that are in close proximity to the campus. Many students find buying a house a very viable option.

GRADUATES

Of the graduating class of 70, 50 percent chose primary care specialties; 20 percent went into Internal Medicine; 5 percent into Family Medicine; into Pediatrics; and 2 chose Medicine/Pediatrics. Ob/Gyn, Pathology, Radiology, and Surgery were also popular choices.

Admissions

REQUIREMENTS

Requirements are one year each of General Chemistry, Organic Chemistry, Biology, and Physics, all with associated labs; and one year each of Math, Humanities, and English. In total, 90 semester hours of undergraduate course work are required. The quality of the undergraduate institution is considered in evaluating GPA. Generally, courses taken abroad are not counted. The MCAT is required and should be no more than three years old. The most recent score is considered, and there is no preference for the April or August MCAT.

SUGGESTIONS

Preferably, the Math requirement should be fulfilled with Calculus. Nontraditional students who have taken time off after college are advised to demonstrate recent course work, particularly in the sciences. The goal of the Admissions Committee is to select candidates who have the potential to address the wide spectrum of needs faced by the medical profession, suggesting that diverse backgrounds are valued in addition to medically related experience. Because spots are few, out-of state candidates should be competitive on a national level.

PROCESS

All Alabama residents receive a secondary application, which is sent upon receipt of the AMCAS application. About one-quarter of out-of-state residents receive a secondary. The secondary application is due on November 15, but the School of Medicine advises applicants to submit it as soon as possible. Fifty percent of Alabama residents, and about 10 percent of out-of-state residents, are interviewed. Interviews are held on campus from September through March. Students receive three half-hour interviews, which may vary in format. The interview day provides applicants and faculty an opportunity to become acquainted and is considered a two-way process. Of those interviewed, about 30 percent are accepted and 20 percent are placed on a ranked wait-list. Candidates are accepted on a weekly basis, beginning in December.

Admissions Requirements (Required)

MCAT Scores, Essays, Science GPA, Extracurricular activities, Non-Science GPA, Exposure to medical profession, Recommendation, Interview

Admissions Requirements (Optional)

State Residency

COSTS AND AID

Tuition & Fees

Annual tuition (in-state out-of-state)	$12,254/$24,508
Cost of books	$2,500
Fees	$2,197

Financial Aid

% students receiving any aid	90
% students receiving grants	40
% students receiving loans	91
Average grant	$5,000
Average loan	$22,000
Average debt	$83,762

UNIVERSITY OF SOUTH CAROLINA

UNIVERSITY OF SOUTH CAROLINA SCHOOL OF MEDICINE-COLUMBIA

ADMISSIONS OFFICE, BUILDING 3 COLUMBIA, SC 29208 • **ADMISSION:** 803-216-3625 • **FAX:** 803-216-36277
E-MAIL: ADMISSIONS@USCMED.SC.EDU • **WEBSITE:** WWW.MED.SC.EDU

STUDENT BODY

Type	Public
Average age of entering class	23

FACULTY

Student-faculty ratio	1.0:1

ADMISSIONS

# applied	1,267
% accepted	16
% enrolled	48

Average GPA and MCAT Scores

Overall GPA	3.7
MCAT Bio	9.0
MCAT Phys	8.0
MCAT Verbal	9.0
MCAT Essay	0

Application Information

Regular application	12/1
Regular notification	10/15
Early application	8/1
Early notification	10/1
Are transfers accepted?	Yes
Admissions may be deferred?	Yes
Admissions need-blind?	No
Application fee	$95

Academics

In addition to the M.D., the School of Medicine offers the M.S. and Ph.D. degrees in Biomedical Science with specialization in Anatomy, Cell Biology, Experimental Pathology, Microbiology and Immunology, Pharmacology, and Physiology. For qualified students, a combined M.D./Ph.D. program is possible. A combined M.D./M.P.H. program, offered in conjunction with the School of Public Health at USC, is available. Also offered is the M.S. in Genetics Counseling, Biomedical Science with specialization in Nurse Anesthesia, and Rehabilitation Counseling. The M.D. curriculum stresses psychological and social perspectives along with biological principles. Elective opportunities are available throughout all four years to assist students in pursuing individual interests and career goals. Medical students are evaluated with an A-F scale. Passing Step 1 of the USMLE is a requirement for promotion to year three, and passing Step 2 is a graduation requirement.

BASIC SCIENCES: Throughout the first two years, clinical case studies are correlated with basic-science material. The two-year Introduction to Clinical Practice course emphasizes active, independent, and cooperative learning and uses a small-group format. Other first-year courses are Gross Anatomy, Microscopic Anatomy, Biochemistry, Neuroanatomy, and Physiology. Second-year courses are Microbiology, Pathology/Pathophysiology, and Pharmacology. An important resource is the USCSM Library, which has a collection of more than 90,0000 volumes. Medical students also use the USC Thomas Cooper Library, which has more than 2.5 million bound volumes.

CLINICAL TRAINING

Clerkship experiences in the third year include eight week rotations in Medicine, Surgery, Ob/Gyn, Psychiatry, Family Medicine, and Pediatrics. During the fourth year, required clerkships are four weeks each in Neurology and Surgery and Medicine and a four-week acting internship. A four-week, multidisciplinary rotation concludes undergraduate clinical training and prepares students for the transition to residency and clinical practice. The remainder of the year is reserved for electives and selectives, many of which may be completed at locations around the state, at other medical schools, with federal and state agencies, and through an international elective program. While the majority of students complete core clinical training at the five affiliated hospitals in Columbia, about 15 students in each class train at the Greenville Hospital System in Greenville, South Carolina. In the Columbia area, teaching hospitals include Palmetto Richland Memorial Hospital (649 beds); Dorn Veterans Hospital (447 beds); and the William S. Hall Psychiatric Institute (270 beds).

Students

Approximately 98 percent of students are South Carolina residents. About 10 percent of students are underrepresented minorities, most of whom are African American. Typically, about 20 percent of students in each entering class are nontraditional, having taken time off or pursued other careers or interests after college.

STUDENT LIFE

Because the School of Medicine is an important component of a comprehensive research university, medical students have many opportunities for interaction with students in other disciplines and can take advantage of the numerous student organizations, intramural sporting events, and social opportunities of the main University. Medical student organizations include chapters of the AMSA and the American Medical Women's Association, in addition to professionally focused groups such as the Internal Medicine, Family Practice, Emergency Medicine, and Pediatrics Clubs and the Psychiatry/Behavioral Science Society. Medical students have initiated a number of community service activities, including participation in the Columbia Free Medical Clinic, tutoring and social events at area childrens homes, and the Health Education Leadership Program for primary school students. The School of Medicine has its own fitness center, but medical students also have access to all athletic facilities of the main campus. Columbia is a city with a population of almost 500,000, providing a wide variety of recreational and cultural activities. Both the ocean and the Great Smoky Mountains are within a few hours drive. Most students live off campus in the area adjacent to the USC campus.

GRADUATES

Two-thirds of USCSM graduates go on to practice in primary care fields, making the School of Medicine a leader among U.S. medical schools in the percentage of graduates entering primary care. Although many graduates do enter primary care, USCSM grads match in all specialties all over the U.S.

Admissions

REQUIREMENTS

Prerequisites are 8 semester hours each of General Biology or Zoology, Inorganic Chemistry, Organic Chemistry, all with associated labs. In addition, 6 semester hours of college-level Math and English are required. At least one semester of Physics is recommended. The MCAT is required, and scores must be no more than five years old. For applicants who have taken the exam more than once, the most recent set of scores is weighed most heavily.

SUGGESTIONS

A maximum of 13–15 positions in each class are open to residents of states other than South Carolina. Thus, nonresident applicants should be highly qualified. USCSM looks for applicants who are interested in primary care and who are likely to serve within the state.

PROCESS

Throughout the first two years, clinical case studies are correlated with basic-science material. The two-year Introduction to Clinical Practice course emphasizes active, independent, and cooperative learning and uses a small-group format. Other first-year courses are Gross Anatomy, Microscopic Anatomy, Biochemistry, Neuroanatomy, and Physiology. Second-year courses are Microbiology, Pathology/Pathophysiology, and Pharmacology. An important resource is the USCSM Library, which has a collection of more than 90,0000 volumes. Medical students also use the USC Thomas Cooper Library, which has more than 2.5 million bound volumes.

Admissions Requirements (Required)

MCAT Scores, Essays, Science GPA, Extracurricular activities, Non-Science GPA, Exposure to medical profession, Recommendation, Interview

Admissions Requirements (Optional)

State Residency

COSTS AND AID

Tuition & Fees

Annual tuition (in-state out-of-state)	$25,576/$61,258
Room & board	$12,613
Cost of books	$402
Fees	$800

Financial Aid

% students receiving any aid	95
Average grant	$3,000
Average loan	$25,000
Average debt	$71,352

UNIVERSITY OF SOUTH DAKOTA
SANFORD SCHOOL OF MEDICINE

OFFICE OF MEDICAL STUDENT AFFAIRS, 414 EAST CLARK STREET VERMILLION, SD 57069 • ADMISSION: 605-677-6886
FAX: 605-677-51097 • E-MAIL: MD@USD.EDU • WEBSITE: WWW.USD.EDU/MED/MD

STUDENT BODY

Type	Public
Enrollment of parent institution	10,235
Enrollment of medical school	235
% male/female	57/43
% out-of-state	9
% international	9
Average age of entering class	24

FACULTY

Total faculty	1,450
% female faculty	33
% minority faculty	11
% part-time faculty	72
Student-faculty ratio	0.2:1

ADMISSIONS

# applied	508
% accepted	13
% enrolled	82

Average GPA and MCAT Scores

Overall GPA	3.7
MCAT Bio	10.0
MCAT Phys	9.5
MCAT Verbal	9.5
MCAT Essay	0

Application Information

Regular application	11/15
Are transfers accepted?	No
Admissions may be deferred?	Yes
Admissions need-blind?	Yes
Application fee	$35

Academics

Students complete 166 credits during their four-year M.D. program. They are evaluated with letter and numerical grades. Students must pass USMLE Step 1, Step 2-CK and a school administered OSCE, and must take USMLE step 2-CS to graduate. The first 3 semesters are taught in Vermillion. For the remaining 5 semesters, about 1/2 of the class will be in Sioux Falls, 1/4 in either Rapid City or Yankton. A group of six students will have the option of training in a rural site for semesters 4 and 5.

BASIC SCIENCES: The basic biomedical sciences are taught in the Lee Memorial Medical Science Building on the USD campus in Vermillion. The Lommen Health Sciences Library is also on the Vermillion campus. The basic biomedical sciences are taught during three semeseters in an organ based system using lecture, lab, and small-group discussions utilizing team-based, case-based, or problem-based formats. Students are in class or other scheduled sessions for about 30 hours per week.

CLINICAL TRAINING
During the fourth and fifth semesters, students take all clinical rotations in a blended longitudinal integrated clerkship. All students participate in a cultural diversity experience during the year. The final three semesters include required clerkships for all students: Family Medicine (4 weeks), Emergency Room (3 weeks), a Subinternship (4 weeks) and two selectives in Surgical Specialties of two weeks each (4 weeks). Additional electives are taught throughout the state or as extramural electives at other schools. As a community based medical school, Sanford School of Medicine (SSOM) neither owns nor operates the clinical facilities utilized by SSOM for teaching. Rather, the school maintains strong affiliations with a range of health care providers throughout the state, including Rapid City Regional Hospital; Sanford Health-University of South Dakota Medical Center in Sioux Falls; Avera McKennan Hospital-University Health Center in Sioux Falls; Avera Sacred Heart Hospital and the Yankton Medical Clinic in Yankton; and Veterans Affairs Hospitals in Sioux Falls, Fort Meade, and Hot Springs.

Students

All admitted students are either South Dakota residents or have significant personal ties to South Dakota. About 5 percent of students are underrepresented minorities, most of whom are Native Americans. The average age of incoming students is about 24. Class size is 56.

STUDENT LIFE
The small class size encourages collaborations and interaction among students, as well as between faculty and students. Several student organizations give the students an opportunity to become involved in a variety of service and support activities. During the first three semeseters, students have access to the recreational and athletic facilities of the University of South Dakota as well as on-campus residence halls. During their remaining semesters, students have varied options, depending on where their clinical training takes place.

GRADUATES

Graduates are successful in securing residencies nationwide and typically choose 10-14 different specialties, and enter residencies in about 25 different states. Approximately forty percent of graduates enter primary care fields.

Admissions

REQUIREMENTS

Prerequisites are one year each of Biology, Chemistry, Organic Chemistry, Physics, and college-level Math. Advanced Placement and CLEP courses may count for fulfilling prerequisite requirements if the credits are granted on the pre-medical transcript, and there is other evidence of appropriate knowledge in the subject area. The MCAT is required, and the exam must be within three years of the application deadline. For applicants who have retaken the exam, the most recent set of scores is compared to previous scores.

SUGGESTIONS

Residents of South Dakota, nonresidents with strong personal ties to the state (for example, they graduated from high school in South Dakota, or their parents live in-state) and applicants of Native American descent who can demonstrate enrollment in federally recognized tribes in South Dakota or in border states may be invited to submit a supplemental application. In each case, the applicant must demonstrate academic qualifications on their AMCAS application before being offered a supplemental application. In addition to the academic credentials, the school highly values exposure to the medical profession, volunteer activities, interest in practicing primary care medicine, and working with underserved communities.

PROCESS

The school uses the AMCAS for initial application. Academically qualified applicants who meet South Dakota state residency criteria, or academically qualified non-residents who have completed at least three years of higher education in the state may be offered a supplemenatal application. Most of these applicants are invited to interview with the admissions committee between September and January. Interviews consist of one-to-one interviews with two faculty members who serve on the admissions committee. Of interviewed candidates, about 35 percent are accepted, with notification beginning in November. Several students are placed on an alternate list and are given a rank order for admission if vacancies occur. All accepted applicants must pass background checks prior to matriculation. SSOM does not consider applications for advanced standing.

Admissions Requirements (Required)

MCAT Scores, Science GPA, Non-Science GPA, Recommendation, Interview

Admissions Requirements (Optional)

Essays, Extracurricular activities, Exposure to medical profession, State Residency

COSTS AND AID

Tuition & Fees

Annual tuition (in-state out-of-state)	$24,580/$57,527
Room & board	$16,833
Cost of books	$3,300
Fees	$5,200

Financial Aid

% students receiving any aid	100
% students receiving grants	97
% students receiving loans	82
% aid that is merit-based	60
Average grant	$9,251
Average loan	$42,838
Average total aid package	$44,072
Average debt	$142,043

UNIVERSITY OF SOUTH FLORIDA

UNIVERSITY OF SOUTH FLORIDA—COLLEGE OF MEDICINE

ADMISSIONS/MDC-3, 12901 BRUCE B DOWNS BLVD TAMPA, FL 33612 • ADMISSION: 813-974-2229
FAX: 813-974-49907 • E-MAIL: MD-ADMISSIONS@HEALTH.USF.EDU
WEBSITE: WWW.HEALTH.USF.EDU/MEDICINE/MDADMISSIONS

STUDENT BODY

Type	Public
Enrollment of medical school	482
% male/female	48/52
% out-of-state	6
% international	10
Average age of entering class	24

FACULTY

Total faculty	449
% female faculty	40
% minority faculty	26
Student-faculty ratio	1.3:1

ADMISSIONS

# applied	2,991
% accepted	4
% enrolled	100

Average GPA and MCAT Scores

Overall GPA	3.8
MCAT Bio	11.0
MCAT Phys	10.0
MCAT Verbal	10.0
MCAT Essay	P

Application Information

Regular application	11/15
Regular notification	10/15
Early application	8/1
Early notification	10/1
Are transfers accepted?	Yes
Admissions may be deferred?	Yes
Admissions need-blind?	Yes
Application fee	$30

Academics

The four-year curriculum is designed to permit the student the learn the fundamental principles of medicine, to acquire skills of critical judgment based on evidence and experience, and to develop an ability to use principles and skills wisely in solving problems of health and disease. Medical students interested in careers in research may pursue a combined MD/PhD program, earning the doctorate in a number of biomedical fields. For students interested in public and community health issues, a combined MD/MPH program is offered in conjunction with the College of Public Health. A combined MD/MBA is available to students interested in the Business of Medicine and students interested in law can pursue a combined MD/JD program. Medical students are evaluated with Honors, Pass with Commendation, Pass, and Fail. Passing Step 1 of the USMLE is a requirement for promotion to year three, and passing Step 2 Clinical Knowledge and Clinical Skills exams is a graduation requirement.

BASIC SCIENCES: First-year students focus mainly on basic sciences and are instructed in a variety of ways including lectures, labs, small-group conferences, and interdisciplinary methods. Computers are also an important educational resource. In addition to science courses, first-year students investigate ethical and behavioral aspects of medicine in the courses Behavioral Medicine and Medical Ethics. Students also begin to learn patient-interaction skills through a Physical Diagnosis course that extends into the second year. Other first-year courses are Gross Anatomy; Biochemistry; Microscopic Anatomy; Human Embryology; Molecular Biology and Human Genetics; Medical Neuroscience; and Physiology. The second year is a continuation of basic sciences with increased emphasis on clinical correlation. The remainder of Physical Diagnosis and Introduction to Clinical Medicine further develop patient examination and evaluation skills and prepare students for the clinical phase of the curriculum. Other second-year courses are Medical Microbiology and Immunology, Pathology and Laboratory Medicine, Clinical Correlation, and Pharmacology. Students are in class or other scheduled sessions for about 25 hours per week. In between the first and second year, there are opportunities for involvement in research.

CLINICAL TRAINING
Third-year required clinical rotations are arranged in five clinical areas including: Outpatient Primary Care/Special Populations (12 weeks), Surgical Care (8 weeks), Inpatient Medicine/Pediatrics (12 weeks), Neuropsychiatry (8 weeks), Emergency Medicine/Urgent Care (4 weeks) and Maternal/Newborn (4 weeks). The fourth year is divided between four required clerkship blocks (two in Critical Care, one Oncology, one Dermatology/Musculosketal) and five electives, a portion of which may be taken at other academic or clinical institutions or locations around the state, country, or overseas. Most clinical training takes place at Tampa General Hospital (1000 beds); H. Lee Moffitt Cancer Center and Research Institute (162 beds); James A. Haley Veterans Hospital (577 beds); the USF Psychiatry Center, USF Medical Clinic; All Children's Hospital (168 beds); USF Eye Institute; University Diagnostic Institute; Shriners Hospital for Crippled Children; Bayfront Medical Center (518 beds); and Bay Pines Veterans Medical Center (520 beds). A number of community-based clinics are also used as clinical training. Pre-Clinical Training First year students focus mainly on basic sciences and are instructed in a variety of ways including lectures, labs, small-group conferences, and interdisciplinary methods. Computers are an important educational resource. Students begin year one with an introduction to medicine in the Profession of Medicine course (three weeks)

before transitioning to science courses, required as first-year students investigate ethical and behavioral aspects of medicine in the courses Behavioral Medicine and Medical Ethics. They begin to learn patient-interaction skills through Physical Diagnosis and Longitudinal Clinical Experience (LCE) courses that extend into the second year. Other first-year courses are Human Anatomy; Molecular Medicine; Medical Neuroscience; "On-Doctoring" and Physiology. The second year is an integrated presentation of basic and clinical sciences with year-long courses in Principles of Microbiology, Immunology and Infectious Diseases; Pathology and Laboratory Medicine; Pharmacology; Clinical Diagnosis and Reasoning; Evidence Based Medicine; and a problem-based learning course, Clinical Problem Solving. Students are in class or other scheduled sessions for about 32 hours per week. In between the first and second year, there are opportunities for involvement in research. The preclinical curriculum provides a solid foundation for the transition to Clinical Medicine. USF College of Medicine instituted a program of scholarly concentrations, which aims to support the educational development of medical students by providing opportunities for scholarly and leadership endeavors in areas of interest. Each concentration includes elements of course work, practical application, and scholarly presentation.

Students

Most students are Florida residents. About 13 percent of students are from those ethnic groups underrepresented in medicine, representing only a portion of the diverse cultures found among students. Although most students enter shortly after college graduation, there is a wide age range in each class. Class size is 120.

STUDENT LIFE

Students are cooperative, often studying together and interacting outside of the academic setting. The Medical School sponsors student events and organizations, and has a strong emphasis on involvement in school and community activities. The Medical School is located on the main USF campus, giving students access to the amenities of a large university. Tampa has many cultural and recreational opportunities and is generally a popular city among students. Most students live off campus where housing is relatively affordable and comfortable.

GRADUATES

Graduates are successful in securing residency positions in all specialty areas. At USF, post-graduate training programs are offered in more than 10 fields.

Admissions

REQUIREMENTS

Science requirements include one year each of basic introductory courses and laboratories in Biological Science, General Chemistry, Organic Chemistry, and Physics. One year of both English and Mathematics is also required. The MCAT is required, and at least one score must be from within the past three years. For applicants who have taken the exam more than once, the best set of scores is weighed most heavily. Thus, there is no advantage in withholding scores.

SUGGESTIONS

State residency is given preference. Courses that are recommended, but not required, include Physical or Biological Chemistry, Biochemistry, Embryology, Cell Biology, Comparative Anatomy, Genetics, Statistics, Logic, and Rhetoric. Knowledge of calculus, computer science and statistics is useful. Consideration is given to a student's participation in honors courses, independent study, and scientific research. All applicants are advised to apply as early as possible because the application process is rolling. Non-cognitive experiences (shadowing, health care experience [voluntary or paid], community service, leadership roles and research) enhance an applicants' understanding of careers in medicine.

PROCESS

All AMCAS applicants who meet minimum standards are sent secondary applications. About 15 percent of those who return secondary applications are invited to interview between September and April.

Admissions Requirements (Required)

MCAT Scores, Essays, Science GPA, Extracurricular activities, Non-Science GPA, Exposure to medical profession, Recommendation, Interview

Admissions Requirements (Optional)

State Residency

COSTS AND AID

Tuition & Fees

Annual tuition (in-state out-of-state)	$23,160/$49,355
Room & board	$11,000
Cost of books	$9,468
Fees (in-state out-of-state)	$3,673/$4,689

Financial Aid

% students receiving any aid	88
% students receiving grants	40
% students receiving loans	83
% aid that is merit-based	10
Average grant	$9,000
Average loan	$41,000
Average total aid package	$50,000
Average debt	$149,000

University of Southern California

Keck School of Medicine

1975 Zonal Avenue, KAM 100-B, Los Angeles, CA 90089-9021 • Admission: 323-442-2552
Fax: 323-442-24337 • E-mail: MEDADMIT@USC.EDU • Website: KECK.USC.EDU

STUDENT BODY

Type	Private
Enrollment of parent institution	38,000
Enrollment of medical school	700
% male/female	52/48
% underrepresented minorities	1
% out-of-state	27
% international	52
# countries represented	116
Average age of entering class	24

FACULTY

Total faculty	1,324
% part-time faculty	3
Student-faculty ratio	2.0:1

ADMISSIONS

# applied	7,747

Average GPA and MCAT Scores

Overall GPA	3.6
MCAT Bio	12.0
MCAT Phys	11.0
MCAT Verbal	10.0
MCAT Essay	Q

Application Information

Regular application	11/1
Early application	8/1
Early notification	9/1
Are transfers accepted?	No
Admissions may be deferred?	Yes
Admissions need-blind?	No
Application fee	$100

Academics

While the majority of students earn their M.D. in four years, USC offers a variety of joint-degree programs. The M.D./Ph.D. program is administered by the USC Graduate School and the Keck School of Medicine of USC, allowing students to earn their doctorate in Anatomy, Biochemistry, Biomedical Engineering, Biophysics, Cell Biology, Genetics, Immunology, Microbiology, Molecular Biology, Neuroscience, Pathology, Pharmacology, and Physiology. For those interested in more discrete research projects, the Dean's Research Scholars Program allows students to spend one year involved in research at USC or another approved institution. Students also have the option of entering a combined M.D./M.P.H. program or M.D./M.B.A. program.

BASIC SCIENCES: Lectures, labs, and small-group discussions are used during the first two years. The first year begins with introductory courses entitled Foundations of Medical Sciences, which is followed by a sequence of courses based on organ systems. They are Skin, Hematology, Neurosciences, and Musculoskeletal. Students benefit from patient contact from the very beginning in Introduction to Clinical Medicine. The second year is also organized around body/organ systems and is dedicated to studying the mechanisms of disease. They are Cardiovascular, Renal, Respiratory, Endocrine, Reproduction, and Gastrointestinal-Liver. USC's library is comprehensive and has an ample supply of computers. Computers with course material, online resources, and other study aids are also available in individually assigned laboratory spaces, which serve as student study areas. Grading for the first two years is Pass/Fail. Students must take Step 1 of the USMLE in order to be promoted to Year Three.

CLINICAL TRAINING
The clinical years are the hallmark of USC's education. The majority of teaching takes place at the LAC+ USC Medical Center. It is among the major public hospitals for Los Angeles and receives patients with every imaginable illness and injury. Students have extensive patient contact. The curriculum of required courses and electives is continuous over the third and fourth years and is individually designed. Required clerkships are Internal Medicine (6 weeks), Internal Medicine Subinternship (4 weeks), Family Medicine (6 weeks), Pediatrics (6 weeks), Obstetrics/Gynecology (6 weeks), Surgery (6 weeks), Surgical Subspecialty (4 weeks), Psychiatry (6 weeks), and Neurology (4 weeks). An additional 16 weeks of selectives and 16 weeks of electives, at approved institutions throughout the nation, and 2 weeks of Intersession are required. In addition to the LAC+USC Medical Center, clinical facilities include Children's Hospital Los Angeles, Keck Hospital of USC, and USC Norris Cancer Hospital. Grading during the clinical years is Honors/High Pass/Pass/Fail. In order to graduate, students must pass USMLE Step 1 and Step 2 (both Clinical Knowledge and Clinical Skills).

Students

Of the 186 students in each class, almost 80 percent are California residents. About 16 percent of students are underrepresented minorities. The average age of incoming students is 24, with a wide age range including significant numbers of students in their thirties.

STUDENT LIFE

The majority of students live in the communities surrounding USC. The Keck School of Medicine of USC has a cohesive and cooperative student body. Students typically study in groups, and spend time together outside of school. Keck offers a wide range of extra-curricular activities, including volunteer programs, intramural sports, and student clubs and organizations. The Health Sciences Campus recently opened a fitness center with cardiovascular and strength training equipment, a basketball court, and exercises class-es. USC's University Park campus is easily accessible by car or intercampus tram, and medical students regularly use its extensive recreational facilities as well. University-sponsored activities, such as intercollegiate sporting events, cultural events and visual arts programs, are also popular with medical students. There are several student groups on campus related to specialty interest, community service, and student government.

GRADUATES

Graduates are successful in securing positions nationwide, in both specialty and primary care fields. Most enter residency programs in California.

Admissions

REQUIREMENTS

Applicants must have completed a baccalaureate degree, or its equivalent, from an accredited college or university. International applicants must hold a degree considered equivalent to a U.S. bachelor's degree as evaluated by the USC Office of Graduate and International Admissions. The MCAT is required, and scores must be from within pre-vious three years of the date of matriculation.

SUGGESTIONS

The Admissions Committee seeks candidates with prior exposure to the field of med-icine. Applicants should demonstrate maturity, self awareness, and a commitment to patient care and service.

PROCESS

All AMCAS applicants must submit a supplemental application. The Keck School of Medicine of USC receives approximately 7,000 applications per year. Approximately 700 applicants receive interview invitations, which take place on the Health Sciences Campus. The interview day consists of a tour, lunch with medical students, and two 45-minute interviews with one faculty member and one medical student. Interviews begin in mid September and end in early March. Students receive acceptance letters beginning in October. Applicants placed on the alternate list may send additional infor-mation to update their files.

Admissions Requirements (Required)

MCAT Scores, Essays, Science GPA, Extracurricular activities, Non-Science GPA, Exposure to medical profession, Recommendation, Interview

Admissions Requirements (Optional)

State Residency

COSTS AND AID

Tuition & Fees

Annual tuition	$50,246
Room & board	$17,556
Cost of books	$3,418
Fees	$1,795

Financial Aid

Average grant	$19,166
Average loan	$46,400
Average total aid package	$50,000
Average debt	$186,000

UNIVERSITY OF TENNESSEE
MEMPHIS, COLLEGE OF MEDICINE

ADMISSIONS OFFICE, 790 MADISON AVENUE, ROOM 307, MEMPHIS, TN 38163 • ADMISSION: 901-448-5559
FAX: 901-448-17407 • E-MAIL: • WEBSITE: WWW.UTMEM.EDU/MEDICINE

STUDENT BODY

Type	Public
Enrollment of medical school	686
% male/female	61/39
% out-of-state	10
% international	15
Average age of entering class	24

FACULTY

Total faculty	1,711
% female faculty	17
% minority faculty	10
% part-time faculty	3
Student-faculty ratio	2.0:1

ADMISSIONS

# applied	1,700

Application Information

Regular application	11/15
Are transfers accepted?	Yes
Admissions may be deferred?	Yes
Admissions need-blind?	No
Application fee	$50

Academics

Most students follow a four-year curriculum, leading to the M.D. The Optional Expanded Academic Program allows students to expand the first two years into three. The Clinical Scholars Program provides special educational and financial assistance to entering students interested in careers in Family Medicine, General Internal Medicine, General Pediatrics, Medicine and Pediatrics (Med-Peds), or Ob/Gyn. Students are encouraged to pursue research, either during the summer following year one or as ongoing projects. For students interested in intensive research, an M.D./Ph.D. program is available. Medical students generally receive percentage scores on exams and are evaluated with an A-F scale. Examinations in some courses are administered by computer. Passing both steps of the USMLE is a requirement for graduation.

BASIC SCIENCES: The basic sciences are taught during the first two years primarily through lectures and lab work. Students are in class or other scheduled sessions for about 23 hours per week. First-year science courses are the following: Biochemistry; Fundamentals of Cellular and Molecular Biology; Medical Genetics; Gross Anatomy; Histology; Neuroanatomy; and Physiology. Other first-year courses are Behavioral Sciences and Preventive Medicine, both of which involve small-group discussions. Throughout the first and second years, students take Introduction to Clinical Skills, which correlates basic science concepts with actual medical cases and teaches students introductory clinical techniques. Students also participate in a longitudinal, community-based clinical program. Second-year courses are Microbiology, Neuroscience, Nutrition, Pathology, Pathophysiology, and Pharmacology. Most of the first two years is spent in the Cecil C. Humphreys General Education Building that houses classrooms, labs, and a computer center. A three-year longitudinal community program will begin in 1999 and incorporate content of five current courses: Behavorial Science, Preventive Medicine, Nutrition, and ICS and Longitudinal Community-based Clinical Program. An important educational resource is the Plane Tree Center with multimedia software technologies for learning Anatomy, Embryology, Histology, EKG readings, and lung and heart sounds. Plane Tree also provides health-oriented books, audiovisuals, and Internet connections. The Health Sciences Library is used by students both for research purposes and for studying. It is fully computerized, subscribes to approximately 1,550 current periodicals, and contains a total volume count of over 170,000.

CLINICAL TRAINING

Third-year required clerkships are two months each of the following: Family Medicine, Medicine, Ob/Gyn, Pediatrics, Psychiatry, and Surgery. The fourth year is composed of five one-month clerkships and three months of electives that provide students the opportunity to select the clinical or basic science experiences to best meet their particular career goals. Electives allow for increased responsibility in patient care as well as the opportunity to pursue areas of individual interest. Fourth-year required clerkships are Ambulatory Care Medicine, Neurology, and a Senior Clerkship in Medicine and Surgical Subspecialties. As part of a Selective requirement, one month of either Family Medicine, Medicine, Pediatrics, Ob/Gyn, Psychiatry, or Surgery is also required. All students must spend a minimum of 10 months of clerkship and elective time on the Memphis campus. This requirement allows a maximum of 10 months (excluding option months) to be spent at Knoxville, Chattanooga, and/or Nashville. Two of the 10 months away from the Memphis campus may be taken at another institution, either in the United States or overseas.

Students

At least 90 percent of students are Tennessee residents. Others are usually from the eight states contiguous to Tennessee. These are Mississippi, Arkansas, Missouri, Kentucky, Virginia, North Carolina, Georgia, and Alabama. The average age of incoming students is typically about 24 with a wide age range among students. Underrepresented minorities account for about 12 percent of students. Class size is 165.

STUDENT LIFE

Medical students are cohesive and supportive of one another. As part of the Big Sib program, incoming medical students are assigned to senior students as mentors. Typically, the Big Sibs will pass along their class notes to the new students to use as a guide during basic science lectures. Medical students are part of a larger community that includes students of all professional schools and programs. The Student Alumni Center (SAC) is the focal point of campus life, providing meeting areas, a restaurant, lounges, a television room, shopping areas, and other services. More than 35 campus-wide organizations are open to medical students. Students enjoy a fitness center that houses a multipurpose gym, a swimming pool, spa, racketball courts, and a weight room. An outdoor complex has playing fields, volleyball courts, tennis courts, golf-practice facilities, and a track. Intramural sports are popular, as is the Outdoor Adventures Program, which leads canoeing, hiking, rafting, and camping trips. Memphis is a festive city, renowned for its music scene. Other attractions include riverside areas, parks, restaurants, a lively arts community, and quiet residential neighborhoods. UT Memphis offers both residence halls and apartment-style facilities for single students. The University assists married students with finding housing in the city.

GRADUATES

Among 1999 graduates, the most popular fields for residencies were the following: Internal Medicine (31%); Pediatrics (10%); Family Practice (21%); Ob/Gyn (21%); Surgery (12%); Radiology (6%); Medicine/Pediatrics (8%). A significant proportion of graduates remains in Tennessee for post-graduate training.

Admissions

REQUIREMENTS

Prerequisite course work is 8 semester hours each of: Biology, General Chemistry, Organic Chemistry, and General Physics, all taken with associated labs. In addition, six hours of English is required. The MCAT is required and scores must be no more than 5 years old. For applicants who have taken the exam more than once, all sets of scores are considered.

SUGGESTIONS

Residents of Tennessee are given preference. Children of UT alumni are also considered, regardless of their state of residence. As a state-supported institution, no more than 10 percent of students may be nonresidents. Thus, nonresident applicants should be highly qualified. Students are encouraged to take courses in the humanities, fine arts, and social sciences. Demonstration of analytic ability and independent thinking is important.

PROCESS

All AMCAS applicants who are considered competitive are sent supplemental applications. Of those returning supplementals, approximately 400 applicants are invited to interview between October and March. The interview gives insights into the applicant's character and how well he or she has formulated plans for the study of medicine. Interviews consist of two sessions, each with a faculty member or current medical student. On interview day, applicants have lunch, attend group informational sessions, sit in on classes, and tour the campus. Of interviewed candidates, about 60 percent are accepted on a rolling basis. Others are either rejected or placed on a wait-list.

Admissions Requirements (Required)

MCAT Scores, Extracurricular activities, Exposure to medical profession, State Residency

Admissions Requirements (Optional)

Essays, Science GPA, Non-Science GPA, Recommendation, Interview

COSTS AND AID

Tuition & Fees

Annual tuition (in-state out-of-state)	$18,050/$35,440
Room & board (on-campus off-campus)	$3,600/$1,400
Cost of books	$1,600
Fees	$544

Financial Aid

% students receiving any aid	80
% students receiving loans	80
% aid that is merit-based	2
Average grant	$8,695
Average loan	$15,700
Average debt	$63,000

THE UNIVERSITY OF TEXAS
MEDICAL BRANCH AT GALVESTON SCHOOL OF MEDICINE

OFFICE OF ADMISSIONS, SUITE 1.204, ASHBEL SMITH BUILDING, 301 UNIVERSITY BLVD. GALVESTON, TX 77555-1317
ADMISSION: 409-772-6958 • FAX: 409-747-29097
E-MAIL: TSILVA@UTMB.EDU • WEBSITE: WWW.UTMB.EDU

STUDENT BODY

Type	Public
Enrollment of parent institution	2,255
Enrollment of medical school	861
% male/female	50/50
% out-of-state	5
% international	25
Average age of entering class	23

FACULTY

Total faculty	849
% female faculty	32
% minority faculty	9
% part-time faculty	6
Student-faculty ratio	1.0:1

ADMISSIONS

# applied	3,442
% accepted	8
% enrolled	78

Average GPA and MCAT Scores

Overall GPA	3.8
MCAT Bio	10.0
MCAT Phys	9.4
MCAT Verbal	9.4

Application Information

Regular application	10/1
Regular notification	11/15
Are transfers accepted?	Yes
Admissions may be deferred?	Yes
Admissions need-blind?	Yes
Application fee	$55

Academics

In addition to the standard four-year M.D. curriculum, UTMB offers a combined M.D./ Ph.D. program for students interested in training for a career in biomedical research. Generally, about five students enter this program each year and receive full funding for the duration of their studies. Summer and year-long research projects are also open to medical students. As an alternative to the primarily lecture-based basic-science curriculum, 24 incoming students each year enter an Interactive Learning Track, which relies on small-group instruction.

BASIC SCIENCES: First-year courses are the following: Gross Anatomy and Developmental Anatomy; Microanatomy; Biochemistry, Cells and Genes; Physiology and Biophysics; Neuroscience; Medical Ethics; Community Continuity Experience; and Introduction to Patient Evaluation. Second-year courses are Endocrinology; Microbiology; Pharmacology and Toxicology; Pathology; Introduction to Patient Evaluation; Immunology; Introduction to Clinical Medicine; and Community Continuity Experience. During the first and second years, students are in class or other scheduled sessions for about 30 hours per week. In addition to teaching basic-science principles, the pre-clinical curriculum involves practical problem-solving experiences and case studies that demonstrate the interrelationship between the basic and clinical sciences. The Community Continuity Experience gives first- and second-year students the opportunity to work with primary care physicians, interact with patients, and apply and expand knowledge and skills gained in the classroom. Educational support services include academic counseling, peer-tutorials, study skills workshops, and stress management workshops. An Educational Support Center provides medical students with computer-assisted educational support. For research purposes, and as a place to study, students use the Moody Medical Library, which is the oldest medical library in Texas and one of the largest medical research centers in the Southwest. Collections include nearly 250,000 volumes in addition to computerized informational services.

CLINICAL TRAINING

Third-year required clerkships are Internal Medicine (8 weeks); Surgery (8 weeks); Pediatrics (4 weeks); Ob/Gyn (6 weeks); Psychiatry (6 weeks); Family Medicine (6 weeks); and a Multidisciplinary Ambulatory Clerkship (12 weeks). Lectures in Anesthesiology, Medical Jurisprudence, Ophthalmology, and Otolaryngology are also part of the third-year curriculum. Fourth-year required clerkships are Neurology (4 weeks); Surgery (4 weeks); Emergency Medicine (4 weeks); Radiology (2 weeks); Dermatology (2 weeks); and an Acting Internship Selective (4 weeks). At least 20 weeks are reserved for elective study. Clinical training takes place primarily at UTMB hospitals and clinics. Some electives may be taken at other institutions.

Students

The University of Texas does not participate in the AMCAS system. Applications may be obtained from: The University of Texas System, Medical/Dental Application Center, Suite 6400, 702 Colorado Street, Austin, TX, 78701, Phone: 512-499-4785. Applications must be submitted between May 15 and October 15. About 1,000 applicants are invited to interview during November and December. Candidates receive two interviews, each with a faculty member. On interview day, there are also orientation sessions, a campus tour, and several opportunities to meet informally with current medical students. About

20 percent of interviewed candidates are accepted. Others are rejected or placed on a wait list and possibly accepted later in the year.

STUDENT LIFE

As a state-supported institution, UTMB gives preference to Texas residents. Applicants are encouraged to take the spring MCAT because late receipt of scores from the fall cycle may delay application processing. Medical experience, volunteer activities, and research are all helpful.

GRADUATES

A grade of at least a C must be earned in all of the prerequisite courses. These are: English (one year); Biology (two years); Math (one semester of college-level); Physics (one year); Chemistry (one year); and Organic Chemistry (one year). All science courses must include laboratory work. The MCAT is required, and scores should be from within the past year. For applicants who have taken the exam on multiple occasions, the most recent set of scores is considered.

Admissions

REQUIREMENTS

Third-year required clerkships are Internal Medicine (8 weeks); Surgery (8 weeks); Pediatrics (4 weeks); Ob/Gyn (6 weeks); Psychiatry (6 weeks); Family Medicine (6 weeks); and a Multidisciplinary Ambulatory Clerkship (12 weeks). Lectures in Anesthesiology, Medical Jurisprudence, Ophthalmology, and Otolaryngology are also part of the third-year curriculum. Fourth-year required clerkships are Neurology (4 weeks); Surgery (4 weeks); Emergency Medicine (4 weeks); Radiology (2 weeks); Dermatology (2 weeks); and an Acting Internship Selective (4 weeks). At least 20 weeks are reserved for elective study. Clinical training takes place primarily at UTMB hospitals and clinics. Some electives may be taken at other institutions. SUGGESTIONS

First-year courses are the following: Gross Anatomy and Developmental Anatomy; Microanatomy; Biochemistry, Cells and Genes; Physiology and Biophysics; Neuroscience; Medical Ethics; Community Continuity Experience; and Introduction to Patient Evaluation. Second-year courses are Endocrinology; Microbiology; Pharmacology and Toxicology; Pathology; Introduction to Patient Evaluation; Immunology; Introduction to Clinical Medicine; and Community Continuity Experience. During the first and second years, students are in class or other scheduled sessions for about 30 hours per week. In addition to teaching basic-science principles, the pre-clinical curriculum involves practical problem-solving experiences and case studies that demonstrate the interrelationship between the basic and clinical sciences. The Community Continuity Experience gives first- and second-year students the opportunity to work with primary care physicians, interact with patients, and apply and expand knowledge and skills gained in the classroom. Educational support services include academic counseling, peer-tutorials, study skills workshops, and stress management workshops. An Educational Support Center provides medical students with computer-assisted educational support. For research purposes, and as a place to study, students use the Moody Medical Library, which is the oldest medical library in Texas and one of the largest medical research centers in the Southwest. Collections include nearly 250,000 volumes in addition to computerized informational services.

PROCESS

In addition to the standard four-year M.D. curriculum, UTMB offers a combined M.D./Ph.D. program for students interested in training for a career in biomedical research. Generally, about five students enter this program each year and receive full funding for the duration of their studies. Summer and year-long research projects are also open to medical students. As an alternative to the primarily lecture-based basic-science curriculum, 24 incoming students each year enter an Interactive Learning Track, which relies on small-group instruction.

Admissions Requirements (Required)

MCAT Scores, Essays, Science GPA, Extracurricular activities, Non-Science GPA, Exposure to medical profession, Recommendation, Interview

Admissions Requirements (Optional)

State Residency

COSTS AND AID

Tuition & Fees

Annual tuition (in-state out-of-state)	$6,550/$19,650
Room & board (on-campus off-campus)	$12,240/$8,076
Cost of books	$2,720
Fees	$4,440

Financial Aid

% students receiving any aid	82
% students receiving grants	26
% students receiving loans	100
Average grant	$10
Average loan	$29,264
Average total aid package	$32,423
Average debt	$108,392

THE UNIVERSITY OF TEXAS HEALTH SCIENCE CENTER AT SAN ANTONIO
THE UNIVERSITY OF TEXAS SCHOOL OF MEDICINE AT SAN ANTONIO

7703 FLOYD CURL DRIVE, MAIL CODE 7790 SAN ANTONIO, TX 78229-3900 • ADMISSION: 210-567-6080
FAX: 210-567-69627 • E-MAIL: MEDADMISSION@UTHSCSA.EDU • WEBSITE: SOM.UTHSCSA.EDU

STUDENT BODY

Type	Public
Enrollment of medical school	900
% male/female	48/52
% out-of-state	8
% international	56
# countries represented	1
Average age of entering class	24

ADMISSIONS

# applied	3,529
% accepted	14
% enrolled	45

Average GPA and MCAT Scores

Overall GPA	3.6
MCAT Bio	10.5
MCAT Phys	9.8
MCAT Verbal	9.6
MCAT Essay	Q

Application Information

Regular application	10/15
Regular notification	11/15
Early application	5/1
Early notification	10/15
Are transfers accepted?	Yes
Admissions may be deferred?	Yes
Admissions need-blind?	Yes
Application fee	$55

Academics

Most students will follow a four-year curriculum to obtain the M.D. degree. There is a unique dual degree program, MD/MPH, where students can accomplish both degrees in four years. The MD/PhD program requires 7 years. Grading for most courses is A, B, C, F. A few courses are P/F. All students must pass Step 1 of the USMLE for promotion to the fourth year. All students must take Step 2 CK and Step 2 CS to graduate.

BASIC SCIENCES: The first and second year curriculum is organized into organ-system modules. The first year concentrates on the normal structure and function of the human body. For example, in the cardiovascular module, students will learn the anatomy, physiology, histology and relevant biochemistry of the cardiovascular system. At the same time, the On Becoming A Doctor course will teach students how to communicate with patients, appropriate questions to ask concerning the cardiovascular system and the appropriate parts of the physical exam; this is accomplished with interactions with standardized patients. The second year emphasizes the abnormal structure and function of the human body. During the cardiovascular module of second year students will learn the pathology and pathophysiology of the cardiovascular disorders, and the pharmacology of treatment. In the Advanced Clinical Evaluation Skills course students will work with actual patients to learn skills of hearing abnormal heart sounds and other physical findings in cardiovascular disorders.

CLINICAL TRAINING

Clinical training begins in the first year with the On Becoming A Doctor course. Students learn all aspects of the patient communication and physical exam with healthy standardized patients in a state-of-the-art clinical skills center. In the second year students work with real patients and discover abnormal findings in the history and physical examination. The entire third year consists of rotations in six required clerkships in the hospitals and clinics of San Antonio as well as other cities in south Texas. Students in the fourth year also spend most of the year in the clinical setting, however they can choose which specialties to work in. Many students also accomplish rotations at other institutions throughout the country and internationally as well.

Students

At least 90 percent of students are Texas residents. Underrepresented minorities account for 22 percent of the student population. Mexican-Americans are particularly well represented. The average age of incoming students is usually about 23, and about 10 percent of students in each class are in their thirties or older.

STUDENT LIFE

Medical students enjoy a collegial environment and appreciate the diversity within the student body, San Antonio, and the South Texas community. Mentoring and peer-support programs help incoming students with the transition to medical school, and the Office of Academic Enhancement assists students throughout their medical school career. Students are very active in community service, international, and research programs. A full range of student organizations, recreational sports (including a new fitness facility), and social activities is offered via the Office of Student Life. All students live off campus. San Antonio offers affordable housing accessible to the Medical Center by public transportation.

GRADUATES

More than 96% of students are successful in the initial residency Match and 100% have positions at the time of graduation. Students match into all types of specialties and 50% choose to train out of state. Many of these return to Texas.

Admissions

REQUIREMENTS

Required courses are one semester of Calculus or statistics, one year each of English and Physics, two years of Biology (three hours of which may be Biochemistry), and two years of Chemistry (which should include both Organic and Inorganic Chemistry). The MCAT is required. For applicants who have taken the exam more then once, the best set of scores is weighed most heavily. Thus, there is no advantage in withholding scores.

SUGGESTIONS

In addition to academic requirements, personal traits and an applicant's background are considered. Some type of medically related experience or voluntary service is required.

PROCESS

The University of Texas medical schools do not participate in AMCAS. Rather, applications may be obtained from: The Texas Medical and Dental Application Service, 702 Colorado, Suite 6400 Austin, Texas 78701 (https://www.utsystem.edu/tmdsas/). Applications must be completed by October 15. About one-third of applicants are interviewed between August and December. Interviews consist of two half-hour sessions with Admissions Committee members who may be faculty or senior students. Interviewers have essays only. On interview day, candidates also have lunch with students, attend group-orientation sessions, and tour the campus. The initial group of accepted candidates are notified November 15 (Texas residents). Others are notified in a match on February 1. An alternate pool of applicants is established and candidates are admitted as positions become available.

Admissions Requirements (Required)

MCAT Scores, Essays, Science GPA, Extracurricular activities, Non-Science GPA, Exposure to medical profession, Recommendation, Interview

Admissions Requirements (Optional)

State Residency

COSTS AND AID

Tuition & Fees

Annual tuition (in-state out-of-state)	$12,970/$26,070
Room & board	$16,463
Fees	$2,200

Financial Aid

% students receiving any aid	87
% students receiving grants	63
% students receiving loans	86

THE UNIVERSITY OF TEXAS HSC AT HOUSTON

THE UNIVERSITY OF TEXAS MEDICAL SCHOOL AT HOUSTON

OFFICE OF ADMISSIONS, MSB G.420, HOUSTON, TX 77030 • **ADMISSION:** 713-500-5116 • **FAX:** 713-500-06047
E-MAIL: MSADMISSIONS@UTH.TMC.EDU • **WEBSITE:** MED.UTH.TMC.EDU

STUDENT BODY

Type	Public
Enrollment of medical school	868
% male/female	54/46
% underrepresented minorities	1
% out-of-state	3
% international	27
Average age of entering class	24

FACULTY

Total faculty	870
% female faculty	37
% minority faculty	31
% part-time faculty	11
Student-faculty ratio	1.0:1

ADMISSIONS

# applied	2,922
% accepted	10
% enrolled	74

Average GPA and MCAT Scores

Overall GPA	3.7
MCAT Bio	9.7
MCAT Phys	9.2
MCAT Verbal	9.3
MCAT Essay	P

Application Information

Regular application	10/1
Regular notification	2/15
Early notification	11/15
Are transfers accepted?	No
Admissions may be deferred?	No
Admissions need-blind?	No
Application fee	$55

Academics

Although most medical students complete studies in four years, some follow an Alternate Pathway curriculum, which extends first-year courses over a two-year period and which leads to the M.D. degree in five years. Others follow a seven-year program leading to both the M.D. and the Ph.D. degrees, while others earn a Master's in Public Health along with the M.D. in five years. Summer research opportunities are available, most of which are paid. Medical students are evaluated with Honors, High Pass, Pass, Marginal Performance, and Fail. All students must take the USMLE Steps 1 and 2.

BASIC SCIENCES: First-year courses are Biochemistry, Gross Anatomy, Developmental Anatomy, Histology, Immunology, Introduction to Clinical Medicine (ICM), Microbiology, Neuroscience, and Physiology. The ICM course introduces students to interviewing, history-taking, and physical-examination skills. Instructional methods used during the first year include lectures, small-group sessions, tutorials, and labs. A problem-based learning curriculum links basic and clinical sciences and allows second-year students to begin addressing complex medical problems. Problem-based learning is an important part of the second-year curriculum, serving to integrate the various courses and provide clinical skills. Second-year courses are Behavioral Science, Genetics, Fundamentals of Clinical Medicine, Pathology, Pharmacology, Physical Diagnosis, and Reproductive Biology. During the first two years, students are in class or other scheduled sessions for about 22 hours per week. The Learning Resource Center has textbooks, audiovisuals, anatomical models, audiotapes and videotapes of lectures, computers, files of past exams, USMLE review materials, and other instructional aids. Networked computers with free access to computer-based services and instructional materials are also provided.

CLINICAL TRAINING

Third-year required rotations are Radiology (1 week); Medicine (12 weeks); Surgery (8 weeks); Ob/Gyn (6 weeks); Pediatrics (8 weeks); Psychiatry (6 weeks); Neurology (4 weeks); and Family Medicine (4 weeks). During the fourth year, required rotations are Family Practice (1 month); Medicine (1 month); and Surgery (1 month). Third and fourth-year students receive advanced technical skills training. Clinical training takes place primarily at the numerous hospitals, clinics, and care centers associated with the Texas Medical Center in Houston and in a city/county hospital in northeast Houston. There is flexibility in terms of where elective credits may be earned, and some students opt to study elsewhere in the country or at one of several international programs.

Students

At least 90 percent of students are Texas residents. Most students are recent college graduates, although there is typically a wide age range among incoming students. In terms of ethnic backgrounds, students represent the diverse population of the state.

STUDENT LIFE

There are numerous student organizations, focusing on areas such as public service projects, professional interests, religious and ethnic interests, athletics, and recreation. Houston is an exciting city for students, with a wide range of entertainment, recreational attractions, restaurants, shopping areas, and facilities for outdoor activities. The university offers apartments a short distance from school and a free shuttle runs throughout the week.

GRADUATES

Of approximately 4,200 UT Houston Medical School graduates, about 62 percent go on to practice in Texas. Among recent graduates, the most popular fields for residencies were Internal Medicine (16%); Family Practice (11%); Anesthesiology (9%); Pediatrics (9%); Surgery (8%); Emergency Medicine (6%); OB/GYN (5%); and Surgery Preliminary (4%).

Admissions

REQUIREMENTS

Prerequisites are one year of English, one semester of college-level Calculus, one year of Physics with lab, two years of Biology with lab, one year of General Chemistry with lab, and one year of Organic Chemistry with lab. The MCAT is required, and scores should be from within the past 5 years. For applicants who have retaken the exam, the last three scores will be reviewed.

SUGGESTIONS

No more than 10 percent of students may be nonresidents; thus, admission is very competitive for nonresidents. A liberal arts background is important and, as long as science requirements are fulfilled, students are encouraged to pursue a major in their area of interest while in college. Important traits include intellectual capacity, interpersonal and communication skills, breadth and depth of pre-medical educational experience, potential for service to the State of Texas, motivation, and integrity.

PROCESS

The University of Texas does not participate in the AMCAS system. Applications may only be made online at the Texas Medical and Dental Schools Application Service website: www.utsystem.edu/tmdsas Applications must be submitted between May 1 and October 15. Additional information about the admissions process may be obtained from: Texas Medical and Dental Schools Application Service, 702 Colorado Street, Suite 6400, Austin, TX 78701, Phone: 512-499-4785. About 1,200 applicants are interviewed at UT Houston between August and January. Applicants generally receive two one-on-one interviews, each with a faculty member. On interview day, candidates also have lunch with medical students and faculty, tour the campus, and attend group orientation sessions. About one-fifth of interviewees are accepted, with notification occurring via the TMDSAS website on February 1. Some wait-listed candidates are accepted later in the spring and summer.

Admissions Requirements (Required)

MCAT Scores, Essays, Science GPA, Extracurricular activities, Non-Science GPA, Exposure to medical profession, Recommendation, Interview

Admissions Requirements (Optional)

State Residency

COSTS AND AID

Tuition & Fees

Annual tuition (in-state out-of-state)	$9,775/$22,875
Room & board	$13,360
Cost of books	$2,000
Fees (in-state out-of-state)	$1,908/$1,908

Financial Aid

% students receiving any aid	99
% students receiving grants	42
% students receiving loans	99
% aid that is merit-based	0
Average grant	$2,539
Average loan	$10,012
Average total aid package	$32,271
Average debt	$98,345

THE UNIVERSITY OF TEXAS SOUTHWESTERN MEDICAL CENTER

UT SOUTHWESTERN MEDICAL CENTER AT DALLAS

5323 HARRY HINES BOULEVARD, DALLAS, TX 75390-9162 • ADMISSION: 214-648-5617 • FAX: 214-648-32897
E-MAIL: ADMISSIONS@UTSOUTHWESTERN.EDU • WEBSITE: WWW.UTSOUTHWESTERN.EDU

STUDENT BODY

Type	Public
Enrollment of medical school	940
% male/female	54/46
% underrepresented minorities	3
% out-of-state	9
% international	44
# countries represented	21
Average age of entering class	23

FACULTY

Total faculty	2,219
% female faculty	39
% minority faculty	18
% part-time faculty	23
Student-faculty ratio	1.0:1

ADMISSIONS

# applied	3,927
% accepted	11
% enrolled	55

Average GPA and MCAT Scores

Overall GPA	3.8
MCAT Bio	11.6
MCAT Phys	11.5
MCAT Verbal	10.4

Application Information

Regular application	10/1
Regular notification	11/15
Are transfers accepted?	Yes
Admissions may be deferred?	Yes
Admissions need-blind?	No
Application fee	$140

Academics

The vast majority of students follow a four-year path leading to the M.D. degree. A small number of students each year enter a joint M.D./Ph.D. program in conjunction with the Southwestern Graduate School of Biomedical Sciences. Grading is a combination of Pass/Fail and letter grades (A–F, C is minimum pass. First semester of year 1 and 4th year are Pass/Fail. No normative grading.

BASIC SCIENCES: During the first two years, a variety of teaching/learning formats are used, including lectures, small-group, problem-based learning, computerized curriculum, and standardized patient interviews. First-year courses include Anatomy; Biochemistry; Cell Biology; Embryology; Genetics; Human Behavior; Immunology; Neuroscience; and Physiology. In addition, Clinical Ethics in Medicine and Colleges expose first-year students to the ethical, behavioral, and clinical perspectives of medicine in a problem-based learning format. During the 10-week period between the first and second years, numerous clinical and research opportunities are available for students who wish to participate. Clinical exposure continues in the second year through Clinical Medicine: Principles and Practice when students learn about the physical examination and experience direct, one-on-one, patient contact. Second-year courses also include Medical Microbiology; Anatomic and Clinical Pathology; Medical Pharmacology; and Psychopathology. Colleges continues in the second year. On average, students are in scheduled sessions for 25–30 hours per week. The campus where pre-clinical instruction takes place is also part of a large medical complex that includes several hospitals, research centers, and the medical school library, which holds more than 229,000 volumes and currently subscribes to almost 2,000 journals. Passing the USMLE Step 1 is required in order to progress to the fourth year.

CLINICAL TRAINING

Clinical training begins in the first year with the Colleges, pairing faculty with small groups of students to mirror the professional clinical skills, behaviors, and attitudes of a physician through clinical skills taught at the bedside and discussions of clinical medicine, clinical reasoning, ethics, professionalism, and human behavior. Building upon the clinical experiences in the first two years, the third and fourth years offer intense clinical experiences involving medical students in direct patient care. Third-year required clinical rotations are Surgery (8 weeks); Pediatrics (8 weeks); Obstetrics and Gynecology (6 weeks); Internal Medicine (12 weeks); Psychiatry (6 weeks); and Family Practice (4 weeks). The fourth year is organized into 4-week periods filled with electives, selectives, and a few remaining required rotations. Requirements include Neurology (4 weeks);Internal Medicine (4 weeks of a subinternship and 4 weeks of ambulatory care); and Women's Health Care (4 weeks). Four 4-week periods remain, two of which are for selectives and two of which are reserved for electives. Clinical training takes place at University sites and affiliated institutions, including Parkland Memorial Hospital; the James Aston Ambulatory Care Center; Zale Lipshy University Hospital; Children's Medical Center; Dallas Veterans Affairs Medical Center; Southwestern Institute of Forensic Sciences; Baylor University Medical Center; Presbyterian Hospital of Dallas; Methodist Hospitals of Dallas; St. Paul Medical Center; Texas Scottish Rite Hospital for Children; and John Peter Smith Hospital in Fort Worth. Students may fulfill many of their senior rotations at academic or medical institutions in other parts of the state, the country, or the world.

Students

At least 90 percent of the student body are Texas residents. Underrepresented minorities account for about 10 percent of the population. The average age of incoming students is usually 23; the range of ages is typically 20 to 45. Incoming class size at UT Southwestern is 230 students.

STUDENT LIFE

The Bryan Williams, M.D. Student Center has exercise and recreational facilities and offers students a convenient place to relax and socialize. Dynamic campus activity programming includes intramural sports, special-interest organizations, recreational and cultural events, and parties. Students also join groups based on professional and academic interests or participate in community service projects. Dallas is an exciting city with a diverse population and many kinds of cultural, recreational, and entertainment activities. All students live off campus, and most students own cars.

GRADUATES

Graduates are successful in securing residencies at prestigious institutions all over the country. The majority of graduates go on to become practicing physicians, typically with a large percentage choosing primary care specialties. Some go into academic medicine or research.

Admissions

REQUIREMENTS

Prerequisite courses include one semester of Calculus or statistics, two semesters of English, two semesters of Physics (with lab), four semesters of Biology (two of which should be with lab and one of which may be Biochemistry), and four semesters of Chemistry (with lab), which should be equally divided between Organic and Inorganic Chemistry. The MCAT is required, and scores must be no more than five years old. For applicants who have retaken the exam, the best set of scores is used.

SUGGESTIONS

Admission for out-of-state applicants is highly competitive, as Texas law requires that no more than 10 percent of each class be nonresidents. In addition to academic credentials (GPA, MCAT score, relative rigor of the undergraduate curriculum, letters of recommendation), the Admissions Committee considers extracurricular activities, socioeconomic background, any time spent in outside employment, personal integrity and compassion for others, the ability to communicate in English, motivation for a career in medicine, and other personal qualities and individual factors such as leadership, insightful self-appraisal, determination, social/family support, and maturity/coping capabilities. Applicants are also evaluated for the demonstration of significant interest and experiences that parallel the mission of UT Southwestern.

PROCESS

UT Southwestern does not participate in the AMCAS system. A common application is available for the University of Texas System medical schools (Southwestern at Dallas, Galveston, Houston, and San Antonio), Texas A&M University College of Medicine, and Texas Tech University School of Medicine, and the Paul Foster School of Medicine. An online application is available at http://www.utsystem.edu/tmdsas/. Applications must be submitted between May 1 and October 1. About one-quarter of the applicants are invited to interview, with interviews taking place between September and December. Interviews consist of two sessions with individual faculty members. About 40 percent of interviewed candidates are accepted, with notification beginning on in mid-November.

Admissions Requirements (Required)

MCAT Scores, Essays, Science GPA, Extracurricular activities, Non-Science GPA, Exposure to medical profession, Recommendation, Interview

Admissions Requirements (Optional)

State Residency

COSTS AND AID

Tuition & Fees

Annual tuition (in-state out-of-state)	$16,413/$29,513
Cost of books	$2,040
Fees	$1,430

Financial Aid

% students receiving any aid	88
% students receiving grants	63
% students receiving loans	79
% aid that is merit-based	5
Average grant	$4,500
Average loan	$18,700
Average total aid package	$24,500
Average debt	$90,000

THE UNIVERSITY OF TOLEDO

UNIVERSITY OF TOLEDO COLLEGE OF MEDICINE AND LIFE SCIENCES MEDICAL SCHOOL

3000 ARLINGTON AVE. MS#1043, MULFORD LIBRARY, OFFICE 136 TOLEDO, OH 43614 • **ADMISSION:** 419-381-4229
FAX: 419-381-33227 • **E-MAIL:** MEDADMISSIONS@UTNET.UTOLEDO.EDU
WEBSITE: WWW.UTOLEDO.EDU / MED / MD / INDEX.HTML

STUDENT BODY

Type	Public
Enrollment of medical school	701
% male/female	55/45
% out-of-state	30
% international	4
Average age of entering class	22

FACULTY

Total faculty	354
% female faculty	30
% minority faculty	7
% part-time faculty	12
Student-faculty ratio	2.0:1

ADMISSIONS

# applied	4,054
% accepted	4
% enrolled	100

Average GPA and MCAT Scores

Overall GPA	3.7
MCAT Bio	10.6
MCAT Phys	10.2
MCAT Verbal	9.3
MCAT Essay	Q

Application Information

Regular application	11/1
Regular notification	10/15
Are transfers accepted?	Yes
Admissions may be deferred?	Yes
Admissions need-blind?	No
Application fee	$65

Academics

The UTCOM is a four year program that consists of a two year pre-clinical educational curriculum followed by two years clinical training. Upon successful completion of the four year program, a M.D. degree is conferred.

BASIC SCIENCES: The first two years are devoted to an integrated approach to the basic sciences, behavioral sciences, primary care preceptorships, introductory clinical experiences, and problem-based learning (PBL) for all students. First-year courses are the following: Cellular and Molecular Biology; Human Structure and Development; Neuroscience and Behavioral Science; Integrated Pathophysiology I (PBL); and Physician, Patient, and Society I. During the first year, students are in class for about 30 hours per week, most of which is either lecture or lab periods. Second-year courses are Introduction to Primary Care; Immunity and Infection; Organ Systems; Integrated Pathophysiology II (PBL); and Physician, Patient, and Society II. Physician, Patient, and Society includes Introduction to Primary Care; Introduction to Clinical Medicine; and a series of courses that address topics in medical ethics, managed care, medical decision-making, nutrition, geriatrics, and substance abuse disorders. The ICM course covers practical skills such as taking patient histories and conducting physical examinations. It also serves as a forum for correlating basic science principles with clinical case studies and for discussing ethical issues related to practicing medicine. Second-year students are in class for about 20 hours per week. Basic science instruction takes place in the Health Sciences Teaching and Laboratory Building and the Health Education Building. The Mulford Library holds 125,000 volumes and 1,800 journals and, along with the Computer Learning Resource Center, provides educational and informational resources to students.

CLINICAL TRAINING

Third-year required clerkships are the following: Medicine (12 weeks); Surgery (12 weeks); Pediatrics (6 weeks); Psychiatry (6 weeks); Family Medicine (6 weeks); and Ob/ Gyn (6 weeks). During the fourth year, one Basic Science Selective (4 weeks) and one Neurology clerkship (4 weeks) are required. The remaining 28 weeks are reserved for elective study. Students also receive clinical training during their clerkships with other area hospitals that have educational agreement with UTCOM; including Promedica; Flower Hospital; and St. Vincent Mercy Hospital. Through the Area Health Education Center clerkships, UTCOM students also have the opportunity to train in rural and inner-city communities.

Students

At least 35 percent of students are Ohio residents although many attended undergraduate institutions outside of the state. Underrepresented minorities, mostly African Americans, account for approximately 10 percent of the student body. Typically, about 80 percent of medical students were science majors in college.

STUDENT LIFE

In addition to providing academic resources, the Office of Student Affairs supports students in and outside of the classroom, organizing events such as an annual orientation for incoming students. There are countless student associations, ranging from one that administers a community care clinic, to a student-to-student support group, to organizations focused on personal, recreational, religious, cultural, and professional interests. UTCOM is situated on 475 acres of land, with ponds, streams, trees, and open areas. The campus offers extensive athletic and recreational facilities. Major attractions in Toledo are easily reached on public transportation and include riverside restaurants and bars, museums, parks with golf courses and other facilities, a zoo, theaters, and shopping areas. Further attractions are found in Detroit, Cincinnati, Pittsburgh, Cleveland, and Chicago all of which are in driving distance of UTCOM. Students live off campus, usually in the surrounding residential neighborhood.

GRADUATES

Out of the UTCOM class, 57 percent of the students were accepted into Residency programs in Ohio. Total number of the students accepted in Residency Primary Care Specialities was 58 percent.

Admissions

REQUIREMENTS

Prerequisites are one year each of Biology, General Chemistry, Organic Chemistry, Physics, Math, and English. All science courses must include labs. The MCAT is required. For applicants who have retaken the exam, the best set of scores is weighted most heavily. Thus, withholding scores is not advantageous.

SUGGESTIONS

As a state-supported institution, UTCOM gives preference to Ohio residents. Additional preparation in Biology is recommended as are courses in the Humanities and Social Sciences. For students who have been out of school for a significant period of time, some recent course work is advised. Community service and medically related experience involving patient contact are both considered valuable.

PROCESS

About 80 percent of AMCAS applicants are sent secondary applications. Of those returning secondaries, about 27 percent of Ohio residents and 73 percent of nonresidents are invited to interview. Interviews take place between October and April and consist of two hour-long sessions each with a faculty member, medical student, or school administrator. Also on interview day, candidates tour the campus, hear group informational sessions, and have the opportunity to meet informally with current students. About one-third of interviewees are accepted, with notification occurring throughout the year. Wait-listed candidates may send additional information, such as transcripts and test scores, to update their files.

Admissions Requirements (Required)

MCAT Scores, Essays, Science GPA, Extracurricular activities, Non-Science GPA, Exposure to medical profession, Recommendation, Interview, State Residency

COSTS AND AID

Tuition & Fees

Annual tuition (in-state out-of-state)	$29,797/$60,001
Room & board	$12,468
Cost of books	$6,865
Fees	$1,390

Financial Aid

% students receiving any aid	84
% students receiving grants	18
% students receiving loans	82
Average grant	$7,739
Average loan	$54,061
Average total aid package	$53,945
Average debt	$177,948

University of Toronto

Faculty of Medicine

315 Bloor Street West, Toronto, ON M5S1A3 • Admission: 416-978-2190 • Fax: 416-978-70227
Website: www.utoronto.ca

STUDENT BODY	
Type	Public

ADMISSIONS	
# applied	1,731

Application Information	
Regular application	10/15
Regular notification	5/31
Are transfers accepted?	No
Admissions may be deferred?	Yes
Admissions need-blind?	No
Application fee	$75

Academics

The curriculum is based on four guidelines: Patient-Centered Learning, Integrated and Multidisciplinary Content, Student-Motivated Learning, and Structured Problem-Based Learning. In addition to the four-year program leading to an M.D., a six-year M.D./Ph.D. program is offered jointly by the Faculty of Medicine and the School of Graduate Studies.

BASIC SCIENCES: The initial phase of the undergraduate medical program spans approximately 82 weeks. The curriculum consists of the following sequential blocks or units which focus on principles of medicine: Art and Science of Clinical Medicine; Brain and Behavior; Metabolism and Nutrition; Determination of Community Health; Structure and Function; Pathobiology of Disease; and Foundations of Medical Practice. Students meet actual as well as simulated patients, and are introduced to clinical medicine by faculty members in teaching hospitals. The emphasis is on student-centered, self-directed work and small group tutorials. Students are in scheduled sessions for approximately 35 hours per week. Most learning takes place in small group settings. Independent study is also important.

CLINICAL TRAINING

The third and fourth academic periods are comprised mainly of six-week clinical clerkships. These are: Medicine, Surgery, Ob/Gyn, Pediatrics, Family and Community Medicine, Psychiatry, Specialty Medicine, Specialty Surgery, Emergency Medicine and Anesthesia, Ambulatory and Community Experience, and three electives. Training takes place at a network of teaching hospitals and community-based health agencies. Affiliated hospitals include Baycrest Centre for Geriatric Care, Centre for Addiction and Mental Health (formerly Addition Research Foundation and the Clarke Institute of Psychiatry), The Hospital for Sick Children, Mount Sinai Hospital, St. Michael's Hospital, Toronto Rehabilitation Institute (formerly Hillcrest Hospital and Queen Elizabeth Hospital), Sunnybrook and Women's College Health Science Centre, The Toronto Hospital (formerly the Toronto Hospital and the Ontario Cancer Institute/ Princess Margaret Hospital. Students are also able to learn in the community through participation in settings such as teaching health units and physicians' offices.

Students

About 15 percent of students are from outside of the province. Approximately 40 percent of students are women. Class size is 177.

STUDENT LIFE

One of the advantages of attending medical school at the University of Toronto is the City itself. The university campus is located within easy walking distance of the attractions and facilities of Toronto. Students enjoy clubs, concerts, museums, major league sporting events, and shopping. Just outside of the city, skiing and other outdoor sports are readily accessible. On-campus activities include pubs, concerts, special lectures, theaters, intramural sports, student government, special interest clubs, and the Medical Journal. Medical students benefit from the large campus of 55,000 students and its resources. Student support includes health services and a housing office that coordinates both on- and off-campus housing. Residence halls with meal plans are one of many housing options.

GRADUATES

A key aspect of the program is that it provides exposure to all medical career options. Graduates enter primary care fields, specialties, academic medicine, research, and leadership positions.

Admissions

REQUIREMENTS

Academic achievement is measured by grades and MCAT results. Prerequisite courses are at least two full course equivalents in Life Sciences and at least one full course equivalent in Humanities, Social Sciences, or Languages. These courses should provide applicants with an understanding of the basic principles and vocabulary of physics, chemistry, and biology, a working knowledge of statistics, and the ability to gather, interpret, and present information from complex texts both in writing and orally. Students must be in their third year or higher of university to be considered for admission.

SUGGESTIONS

Students from social sciences, humanities, and physical and life sciences are encouraged to apply. Demonstrated high-level proficiency in oral and written English is considered essential for success in the curriculum and in practice, and applicants are encouraged to have completed at least two full equivalents in course that require expository writing. Generally, minimum requirements are an average grade point average of 3.6/4.0 and a minimum of 8 on each section of the MCAT. Desired personal characteristics include a perceptive nature, strong commitment, high personal standards, and a history of academic and personal achievement.

PROCESS

Applications for admission to the medical school must be submitted by October 15 to: OMSAS, Ontario Universities Application Center, PO Box 1328, Guelph, Ontario N1H 7P4. The Faculty will invite selected applicants for an interview. Notices of acceptance are sent to students in the spring or summer prior to the proposed date of enrollment.

Admissions Requirements (Required)

Interview

COSTS AND AID

Tuition & Fees

Annual tuition (in-state
  out-of-state) $14,000/$23,750
Fees (in-state
  out-of-state) $919/$1,498

UNIVERSITY OF VERMONT

THE UNIVERSITY OF VERMONT COLLEGE OF MEDICINE

89 BEAUMONT AVENUE, E215 GIVEN BUILDING, BURLINGTON, VT 05405 • ADMISSION: 802-656-2154
FAX: 802-656-96637 • E-MAIL: MEDADMISSIONS@UVM.EDU • WEBSITE: WWW.MED.UVM.EDU

STUDENT BODY

Type	Public
Enrollment of parent institution	10,096
Enrollment of medical school	404
% male/female	41/59
% underrepresented minorities	6
% out-of-state	66
% international	20
# countries represented	14
Average age of entering class	24

FACULTY

Total faculty	1,806
% female faculty	30
% minority faculty	10
% part-time faculty	10

ADMISSIONS

# applied	5,770
% accepted	4
% enrolled	50

Average GPA and MCAT Scores

Overall GPA	3.6
MCAT Bio	10.0
MCAT Phys	10.0
MCAT Verbal	10.0
MCAT Essay	Q

Application Information

Regular application	11/1
Regular notification	10/15
Are transfers accepted?	Yes
Admissions may be deferred?	Yes
Admissions need-blind?	No
Application fee	$85

Academics

The Vermont Integrated Curriculum, fully launched in Fall 2003, progresses through three levels of increasing competency. Block courses in Level I/Foundations provide students with a fundamental understanding of the basic biology of health and illness within systems ranging from genes to organs to individuals to populations. A comprehensive assessment of integrated knowledge and skills takes place at the end of the first year and again at the completion of the level mid-way through the second year of school. Level II/ Clinical Clerkships focuses on the student's development of clinical skills, decision-making skills, and application of foundational sciences. It consists of seven clerkships with a longitudinal "bridge" curriculum of advanced sciences and clinical skills over a period of 13 months. Clinical training takes place primarily at adjacent teaching hospital Fletcher Allen Health Care, an integrated health care delivery system located in Burlington, which serves the State of Vermont and beyond, attracting patients from New York and around New England. Students advance to Level III/Advanced Integration after successful achievement on a clinical competency exam. During the final 15 months of Advanced Integration, the student gains an understanding of the impact of economic, social, and political systems on the health care environment. This level includes acting internships, an emergency medicine rotation, a teaching practicum and scholarly project. During this section, there is flexibility in how students may earn elective credit. Many rotate to hospitals outside of the state, some work on Indian reservations, and others head overseas. Throughout the College's curriculum, complementary curricular themes aim to teach the student to take an integrated approach to patient care and responsibility for their own professional development. Student leadership groups provide the student with an opportunity to collaborate with classmates, a faculty facilitator and various "family faculty" members from the community. These groups, which begin the first week and continue through the curriculum, support such efforts as public health research projects, individual scholarly projects and teaching requirements and statewide health education and health-delivery programs. The M.D.-Ph.D. program is designed to train future physician-scientists through a curriculum that integrates clinical care with basic research. The M.D.-PhD. Degree is awarded by the joint efforts of The College of Medicine and the Graduate College. Award of the M.D. degree requires completion of the entire medical curriculum. Award of the Ph.D. degree requires fulfillment of the requirements of any of the basic science graduate programs, which include Anatomy and Neurobiology, Biochemistry, Microbiology and Molecular Genetics, Molecular Physiology and Biophysics and Pharmacology, or those of the multi-disciplinary program in Cell and Molecular Biology. It is anticipated that a period of seven years will be necessary to complete the combined program. Four students are chosen yearly for this program. Students enrolled in the program will receive financial support that includes full graduate school tuition remission Medical students use Dana Medical Library to study in and to conduct research. Computer technology is widely used by the Medical School, and all students receive laptop computers upon matriculation. Students use COMET, a web-based UVM-designed integrated teaching and learning environment, during all phases of the curriculum. UVM is known for health information systems that it has developed, such as the Vermont Oxford Neonatal Network Database, which is in operation nationwide. The Academic Medical Center opened a new educational center in Fall 2005, housing the Dana Medical Library, 16 classrooms and a large lecture hall, all equipped with state-of-the-art technology to support interactive learning. An ambulatory center also opened adjacent to the campus in Fall 2005. A student assessment center is home to a well-established standardized patient program. The Academic Medical Center, along with the rest of the University of Vermont campus, is located in picturesque Burlington. The city is safe, affordable, and comfortable.

Students

Approximately 40% of students are residents of Vermont, 10% are from Maine, and the remainder come from out of area. In the class entering in 2008, the average age was 24. Students came from 64 different universities, 6 countries and a variety of academic backgrounds. Class size is 114.

STUDENT LIFE

Students have access to all of the University's athletic facilities. In addition, Burlington and the surrounding area offer excellent skiing, hiking and mountain biking. The campus is integrated into the city, which is safe, friendly and student-oriented. Housing options on-and off-campus are good. On-campus choices include UVM's married-student housing, about four miles from campus, and nearby apartments and residence halls. Group houses or shared apartments in walking or biking distance from school are popular off-campus choices.

GRADUATES

Graduates are successful in obtaining residencies at strong programs nationwide. In 2008, about half of the graduates entered primary care residencies. Favored specialties include: Internal Medicine (23%); Emergency Medicine (12%), Pediatrics (16%); Anesthesiology (10%).

Admissions

REQUIREMENTS

One year each of Biology, Chemistry, Organic Chemistry and Physics, all with associated labs are required. The MCAT is required, and all sets of scores are considered.

SUGGESTIONS

We recommend one course in biochemistry or molecular genetics be taken. We recommend that the MCAT be taken no later than September of the application year to facilitate timely review of the entire application file. We encourage students who have a broad and balanced educational background during their undergraduate years. In addition to prerequisite courses in the sciences, recommended areas of study include literature, mathematics, behavioral sciences, history, philosophy and the arts. College work must demonstrate intellectual drive, independent thinking, curiosity, and self-discipline. A career in medicine calls for excellent oral and written communication skills. Applicants should seek out opportunities to develop such skills during their college years. Successful applicants often have a history of service to community. We encourage students who have a broad and balanced educational background during their undergraduate years. In addition to prerequisite courses in the sciences, recommended areas of study include literature, mathematics, behavioral sciences, history, philosophy and the arts. College work must demonstrate intellectual drive, independent thinking, curiosity, and self-discipline. A career in medicine calls for excellent oral and written communication skills. Applicants should seek out opportunities to develop such skills during their college years. Successful applicants often have a history of service to community.

PROCESS

All AMCAS applicants receive a supplemental application. All well-qualified VT residents who apply are interviewed. Approximately 10 percent of out-of-state applicants are interviewed. Interviews take place from September through March, and consist of a meeting with a faculty member of the admission committee. Decisions are made on a rolling basis, and applicants are notified of their status—accept, reject, or wait list—shortly after the interview. Wait-listed candidates should indicate if UVM is their first choice.

Admissions Requirements (Required)

MCAT Scores, Essays, Science GPA, Extracurricular activities, Non-Science GPA, Exposure to medical profession, Recommendation, Interview

Admissions Requirements (Optional)

State Residency

COSTS AND AID

Tuition & Fees

Annual tuition (in-state out-of-state)	$23,080/$40,390
Room & board	$9,392
Cost of books	$8,000
Fees	$1,287

Financial Aid

% students receiving any aid	91
% students receiving grants	65
% students receiving loans	84
% aid that is merit-based	1
Average grant	$15,272
Average loan	$37,576
Average total aid package	$46,465
Average debt	$130,914

UNIVERSITY OF VIRGINIA

U. VIRGINIA SCHOOL OF MEDICINE

BOX 800725, CHARLOTTESVILLE, VA 22908 • ADMISSION: 804-924-5571 • FAX: 804-982-25867
E-MAIL: BAB7G@VIRGINIA.EDU • WEBSITE: WWW.MED.VIRGINIA.EDU/HOME.HTML

Academics

Most medical students follow a four-year, highly integrated curriculum leading to the M.D. Each year six students enter a combined M.D./Ph.D. curriculum. Training for the Ph.D. degree is usually in one of the Biomedical Science programs, which include Anatomy, Biochemistry, Microbiology, Pharmacology, Physiology, Biophysics, and Neuroscience. A Generalist Scholars Program supplements the medical education of students with special opportunities in the area of primary care. Students who participate in this program work closely with a faculty mentor and complete a thesis as part of their graduation requirements. Medical students are evaluated in a variety of ways including both Pass/Fail and letter grades.

BASIC SCIENCES: First-year courses are Biochemistry; Cell and Tissue Structure; Gross Anatomy; Physiology; Human Behavior; Neuroscience; Genetics; Physical Diagnosis; Medical Ethics; and The Practice of Medicine, in which topics such as human behavior and medical ethics are discussed. Basic clinical skills such as the patient interview are also introduced. Second-year courses are Microbiology; Pathology; Pharmacology; Psychiatric Medicine; Psychopathology; Clinical Epidemiology; Community Preceptorship; and Introduction to Clinical Medicine (ICM). Basic-science concepts are coordinated with the ICM course, which involves discussion of clinical cases in small-group tutorials. In the spring of the second year, each student completes a one-month community medicine preceptorship that provides hands-on primary care experience and serves as a transition to third-year clinical rotations. Instruction takes place at the Harvey E. Jordan Hall, a seven-story structure that houses lecture halls and laboratories. First- and second-year students also use the School of Medicine Learning Center, which contains conference rooms, tutorial rooms, and a student lounge. The Claude Moore Health Sciences Library is a modern, fully computerized facility with almost 79,000 books, 3,000 periodicals, and 4,000 audiovisual titles.

CLINICAL TRAINING
Third-year required rotations are Medicine (12 weeks); Surgery (12 weeks); Psychiatry (6 weeks); Family Medicine (4 weeks); Pediatrics (8 weeks); Neurology (4 weeks); and Obstetrics (6 weeks). Clinical training takes place primarily at the University of Virginia Medical Center University Hospital (552 beds); Kluge Children's Rehabilitation Center; and at 40 outpatient clinics associated with the Medical Center. Students also train at affiliated hospitals, which include The Community Hospital of Roanoke Valley (400 beds); Roanoke Memorial Hospital (677 beds); and the Veterans Affairs Medical Center (750 beds). Electives may be taken at other academic or clinical institutions in other parts of the country or abroad.

Students

About 90 of the 139 students in each class are Virginia residents. Underrepresented minorities account for approximately 10 percent of the student body. There is typically a wide age range among incoming students, with at least a few students in their thirties.

STUDENT LIFE

Students are highly active in on-campus activities and events. Many are involved in community activities such as Service, Humanity, Action, Responsibility, Education (SHARE), which initiates health education projects and other service-oriented activities. Support groups for minority students are available, as are clubs focused on professional interests and recreational pursuits, such as singing. UVA also has local chapters of national medical student organizations. Medical students enjoy Charlottesville, a thriving tourist and cultural center located at the foot of the Blue Ridge Mountains and close to the Shenandoah Valley. The city of Richmond, Virginia, is an hours drive, and Washington, D.C. is just two hours away.

GRADUATES

Graduates are successful in securing top residency positions in all regions of the country. A significant number stay on to do post-graduate training at UVA-affiliated hospitals.

Admissions

REQUIREMENTS

Prerequisites are one year each of Biology, General Chemistry, Organic Chemistry, and Physics, all with associated labs. The MCAT is required, and scores must be no more than three years old at the time of matriculation. For applicants who have taken the exam more than once, the best scores are considered. Thus, there is no advantage to withholding scores.

SUGGESTIONS

State residency is a factor in admissions decisions as about 65 percent of positions in a class are reserved for Virginia resident applicants. The Admissions Committee looks for students who will make significant contributions to society as members of the medical profession. Factors such as depth of motivation and commitment to medicine are evaluated. Some medically related experience that involves patient contact is considered important.

PROCESS

AMCAS applicants are sent secondary applications. About 25–30 percent of Virginia resident applicants are interviewed, while only about 10 percent of nonresidents make it to the interview stage. On interview day, applicants have two interviews, each with a member of the Admissions Committee. Candidates also attend a group orientation session and have the opportunity to tour the campus and eat lunch with current medical students. Notification begins after October 15, and continues on a rolling basis until the class is filled. Wait-listed candidates may send additional information to update their files.

Admissions Requirements (Required)

MCAT Scores, Essays, Science GPA, Extracurricular activities, Non-Science GPA, Exposure to medical profession, Recommendation, Interview

Admissions Requirements (Optional)

State Residency

COSTS AND AID

Tuition & Fees

Annual tuition (in-state out-of-state)	$30,100/$40,100
Room & board	$12,000
Cost of books	$1,000

Financial Aid

% students receiving any aid	85
% students receiving grants	85
% students receiving loans	85
% aid that is merit-based	3
Average grant	$12,000
Average loan	$18,000
Average debt	$82,000

University of Washington

University of Washington School of Medicine

Admissions Office, A-300 Health Sciences, Box 356340 Seattle, WA 98195-6340 • Admission: 206-543-7212
Fax: 206-616-33417 • E-mail: askuwsom@uw.edu • Website: www.uwmedicine.org/admissions

STUDENT BODY

Type	Public
Average age of entering class	24

ADMISSIONS

# applied	4,962
% accepted	6
% enrolled	79

Average GPA and MCAT Scores

Overall GPA	3.7
MCAT Bio	10.7
MCAT Phys	10.3
MCAT Verbal	10.0
MCAT Essay	Q

Application Information

Regular application	10/15
Regular notification	10/15
Are transfers accepted?	Yes
Admissions may be deferred?	Yes
Admissions need-blind?	No
Application fee	$35

Academics

Students who enter UW as residents of Wyoming, Alaska, Montana, and Idaho spend their first year at the University site in their home state. Twenty Washington students begin medical studies at Washington State University in Pullman and then transfer to the UW campus after completion of their first year. Other students complete a four-year program based in Seattle. From 8 to 10 students each year enter the M.S.T.P. M.D./Ph.D. program. The doctorate degree may be earned in Biochemistry, Bioengineering, Biomathematics/Biostatistics, Biological Structure, Epidemiology, Environmental Health, Genetics, Immunology, Microbiology, Molecular Biotechnology, Pathology, Pharmacology, Physiology, Biophysics, and Zoology. Medical students are evaluated with Honors, Satisfactory, and Not Satisfactory. Passing Step 1 of the USMLE is a requirement for promotion to year three and passing Step 2 is a requirement for graduation.

BASIC SCIENCES: First-year courses at the UW campus are Microscopic Anatomy; Gross Anatomy and Embryology; Mechanisms in Cell Physiology; Biochemistry; Cell and Tissue Response to Injury; Natural History of Infectious Diseases and Chemotherapy; Introduction to Immunology; Systems of Human Behavior; Epidemiology; Head, Neck, Ear, Nose and Throat; and Nervous System. Most second-year topics are organized around body/organ systems, which are Cardiovascular; Complementary Medicine; Respiratory; Pharmacology; Endocrine; Systemic Pathology; Gastrointestinal; Hematology; Musculoskeletal; Genetics; Urinary; Reproduction; Skin; and Nutrition. Other courses are Introduction to Clinical Medicine and Medicine, Health, and Society. The Rural/Underserved Opportunities Program enables first-year medical students to work with practicing physicians in small towns or inner-city neighborhoods and to learn first-hand about working with underserved communities.

CLINICAL TRAINING

The clinical curriculum covers the third and fourth years and includes clerkships in Medicine (12 weeks); Ob/Gyn (6 weeks); Pediatrics (6 weeks); Psychiatry (6 weeks); Surgery (6 weeks); Family Medicine (6 weeks); Emergency Medicine (4 weeks); and Rehabilitation (2 weeks). An additional 24 weeks of electives are required. Selected third-year students participate in an alternate, rural training program, which involves six months in a rural, primary care practice. In its teaching, patient care, and research programs, the School of Medicine is affiliated with Children's Hospital, Harborview Hospital (411 beds), UW Medical Center (450 beds), Seattle Veterans Affairs Hospital, Fred Hutchinson Cancer Research Center, Boise Veterans Affairs Hospital, Providence Hospital, Swedish Hospital, Madigan Hospital, and the Group Health Cooperative. Additional affiliations across the Pacific Northwest enable medical students to train in more than 75 communities in Washington, Alaska, Montana, and Idaho. The International Medical Education Office organizes a range of activities including exchange programs that allow UW medical students to participate in clinical electives overseas.

Students

About 93 percent of the 176 students in each class are residents of Washington, Alaska, Montana, Wyoming or Idaho. Out-of-region students, who comprise a total of about 10 percent of the student body, which includes M.D./Ph.D. students. There is a wide age range among medical students, with significant numbers of entrants in their late twenties and thirties.

STUDENT LIFE

UW offers countless extracurricular opportunities and attractions, including cultural programs, student groups, intercollegiate sporting events, and social functions. Medical students take advantage of these opportunities and the tremendous resources afforded by UW and its student community. Seattle is an ideal city for students, offering outstanding daytime and outdoor activities and an excellent nightlife. Around the city are beautiful areas suitable for hiking, camping, mountain climbing, running, biking, swimming, and skiing. Most students live off campus.

GRADUATES

Of the roughly 5,000 UW School of Medicine alumni, about 50 percent are practicing or training in fields designated as physician-shortage specialties, which include family physicians, general internists, general pediatricians, psychiatrists, general surgeons, and general practitioners.

Admissions

REQUIREMENTS

Prerequisites are Biology (8 semester hours), Chemistry (12 semester hours, which can be satisfied by any combination of Inorganic, Organic, Biochemistry, or Molecular Biology courses), and Physics (4 semester hours). In addition the understanding of basic biochemistry molecular biology concepts is required. An additional 8 semester hours of unspecified science course work is required. This requirement can be met by taking other courses in any of the above three categories. The MCAT is required, and scores must be from within three years of application.

SUGGESTIONS

Preference is given to legal residents of Washington, Wyoming, Alaska, Montana, and Idaho. Applicants from disadvantaged backgrounds or who are willing to serve the underserved are also considered. Candidates should be proficient in the use of the English language and in basic mathematics and are expected to have an understanding of personal computing and information technologies. Some Biochemistry or Molecular Biology is also recommended.

PROCESS

All Washington residents and a limited number of highly qualified, nonresidents are sent secondary applications and invited to interview. Interviews take place between October and April and consist of one session with a panel of interviewers. Also on interview day, candidates have the opportunity to meet with current students and to tour the campus. About 30 percent of interviewed candidates are accepted. Others are rejected or put in a hold category.

Admissions Requirements (Required)

MCAT Scores, Essays, Exposure to medical profession, Recommendation, Interview

Admissions Requirements (Optional)

Science GPA, Extracurricular activities, Non-Science GPA, State Residency

COSTS AND AID

Tuition & Fees

Annual tuition (in-state out-of-state)	$15,347/$37,169
Cost of books	$0
Fees	$525

Financial Aid

% students receiving any aid	83
Average grant	$0
Average loan	$0

UNIVERSITY OF WESTERN ONTARIO
ADMISSIONS & STUDENT AFFAIRS

HEALTH SCIENCES BUILDING, LONDON, ON N6A 5C1 • **ADMISSION:** 519-661-3744 • **FAX:** 519-661-37977
E-MAIL: ADMISSIONS@SCHULICH.UWO.CA • **WEBSITE:** WWW.SCHULICH.UWO.CA

STUDENT BODY

Type	Public
Enrollment of medical school	534
% male/female	55/45
% international	0
Average age of entering class	23

ADMISSIONS

# applied	1,872
% accepted	7
% enrolled	100

Average GPA and MCAT Scores

Overall GPA	3.7
MCAT Bio	10.0
MCAT Phys	9.0
MCAT Verbal	10.0
MCAT Essay	P

Application Information

Regular application	10/15
Regular notification	5/15
Early application	10/15
Early notification	5/15
Are transfers accepted?	No
Admissions may be deferred?	No
Admissions need-blind?	Yes
Application fee	$175

Academics

The Faculty of Medicine and Dentistry, along with the Faculty of Graduate Studies, has established a combined M.D.-Ph.D. program in which the research curriculum of the graduate program is integrated into the M.D. program. Applicants must be accepted to the medical school as M.D. candidates before entering the combined program.

BASIC SCIENCES: Year 3 During the third year integrated Clerkship, the student will become an active member of clinical care teams in the following medical disciplines: family medicine, medicine, obstetrics and gynaecology, pediatrics, psychiatry, and surgery. Under the supervision of faculty and more senior house staff, clerks will be given graded responsibility in the investigation, diagnosis, and management of patients in hospital and outpatient settings. The Clerkship year incorporates rural experiences throughout Southwestern Ontario. Some students will be placed outside London for the entire Clerkshiip year. Year 4 Beginning in Year 4, clinical electives will be arranged by the student in any area of medicine, at U.W.O. or other approved centres. For students wishing to arrange electives in developing countries, we have a Medical Electives Overseas Officer who advises and assists students in making their arrangements. After completion of the clinical electives, students will return to the U.W.O. in February for the Transition Period which includes: Advanced Basic Sciences (eg. Surgical Anatomy, Medical Physiology), Advanced Communication Skills, General Review, Health Care Systems, etc. This will permit students to further integrate the basic and clinical aspects of medicine in light of their clinical experience.

CLINICAL TRAINING

Years 1 and 2 The first two years of the new curriculum will provide students with a solid grounding in the basic and clinical sciences. These two years are each divided into a series of six blocks. Within each block various subject areas are presented which integrate the basic and clinical sciences. The blocks are: Introduction to Medicine; Heart & Circulation; Digestive Systems & Nutrition; Endocrine & Metabolism; Genito-urinary System; Immunology & Skin; Life Cycle; Musculoskeletal; Neurosciences; Eye & Ear; Psychiatry & Behavioural Sciences; Reproduction; Respiration & Airways. During each week or block, the case of a single patient will be discussed. A facilitator will help students determine the biological, behavourial and population issues that are pertinent to the patient, and the objectives for the week's instruction will be described. Students will then receive instruction throughout the week relevant to the patient's case using a variety of teaching methods such as lectures, small group sessions, and labs. Students will also be expected to obtain information pertinent to the case objectives. The Faculty has excellent library and resource facilities to support self study. In the middle of the week, students will meet to review the instruction to date and relate it to the patient case. At the end of the week, the students will meet in a plenary session to discuss the case of the week. A particular strength of our program will be the opportunity for early patient contact. Patient-centered care recognizes the need to see the health concerns of a patient "through the patient's eyes". The illness experience differs, markedly from the traditional teaching in medical schools where the emphasis has been on teaching about the disease only and not on the experiences of the patient with that disease. In the patient-centered approach, the emphasis is on defining the unique illness experience of the patient and his or her relation to family and community in economic, social and environmental dimensions. The first two years of the program provide a variety of opportunities for students to better understand the relationship between health care and the community.

Students

Class size is 133.

STUDENT LIFE

The University of Western Ontario offers students a rich lifestyle. School-sponsored events and countless clubs and organizations are offered on campus. London is a small city of about 300,000 with a range of cultural and recreational activities. Both on- and off-campus housing is available.

GRADUATES

The curriculum is designed to allow graduates to enter any clinical or medical research field. A significant portion of graduates enter residency programs at hospitals affiliated with the University of Western Ontario.

Admissions

REQUIREMENTS

Enrollment is limited to Canadian citizens and permanent residents of Canada. Those who are in the third year or have successfully completed three full years of study in any degree program at a recognized university are eligible to apply. A minimum of five full or equivalent courses must be included in the final undergraduate year (September to April year only). Science prerequisites are one full course in Biology, one full course in Organic Chemistry, and one additional full science course. Nonscience prerequisites are two full nonscience courses from different disciplines and one senior-level course in one of these two subjects. Interested applicants should contact the Faculty for more detailed course requirements. The MCAT is required. The latest date that applicants should take the exam is August in the year of application. Only applicants who have achieved a certain grade point average and MCAT scores will be considered for admission. Typically, the minimum GPA is 3.50 and minimum MCAT scores are a 9 on Biological Sciences, an 8 on Physical Sciences, a 9 on Verbal Reasoning, and a Q on the Writing Sample. English proficiency is a requirement.

SUGGESTIONS

Admission is competitive. Apart from science prerequisites, there is no prescribed pre-med program. Students at Western Ontario come from a variety of undergraduate programs and a wide range of disciplines. For those who have taken the MCAT more than once, only the most recent scores is used.

PROCESS

The deadline for application is October 15 for the following September. Applicants now apply on-line at: www.ouac.on.ca/omsas/. Those applicants who satisfy the course load, GPA, and MCAT requirements will generally be invited for an interview. Letters indicating admissions decisions are sent to applicants beginning in the end of May and continuing until the class is full.

Admissions Requirements (Required)

MCAT Scores, Science GPA, Non-Science GPA, Recommendation, Interview, State Residency

Admissions Requirements (Optional)

Essays, Extracurricular activities, Exposure to medical profession

COSTS AND AID

Tuition & Fees

Annual tuition	$14,566
Room & board	$13,000
Cost of books	$2,200
Fees	$863

Financial Aid

% students receiving grants	48
% aid that is merit-based	25
Average grant	$0
Average loan	$0

UNIVERSITY OF WISCONSIN

UNIVERSITY OF WISCONSIN SCHOOL OF MEDICINE AND PUBLIC HEALTH

2130 HEALTH SCIENCES LEARNING CENTER, 750 HIGHLAND AVE MADISON, WI 53705 • **ADMISSION:** 608-263-4925
FAX: 608-262-42267 • **E-MAIL:** MEDADMISSIONS@MED.WISC.EDU • **WEBSITE:** WWW.MED.WISC.EDU

STUDENT BODY

Type	Public
Enrollment of parent institution	43,275
Enrollment of medical school	676
% male/female	51/49
% out-of-state	20
% international	12
Average age of entering class	25

FACULTY

Total faculty	1,386

ADMISSIONS

# applied	3,859
% accepted	7
% enrolled	62

Average GPA and MCAT Scores

Overall GPA	3.7
MCAT Bio	10.9
MCAT Phys	10.8
MCAT Verbal	10.0
MCAT Essay	P

Application Information

Regular application	11/1
Are transfers accepted?	Yes
Admissions may be deferred?	Yes
Admissions need-blind?	No
Application fee	$56

Academics

The UW School of Medicine and Public Health offers an MD degree and a dual degree (MD/PhD) option. In addition, flexibility exists to allow for combining training for the MD degree with earning a Master's Degree in Public Health. Medical students are evaluated with pass/fail grades in year 1 followed by letter grades in the following years. Students must pass Step 1 of the USMLE for promotion to year three and Step 2 must be taken to graduate.

BASIC SCIENCES: First- and second-year courses provide an optimal balance between hands-on and didactic/independent learning, featuring a lively and varied educational experience through multiple teaching formats. These include lectures, small group discussions, labs, case-based learning, interdisciplinary approaches and adaptation of Web-based materials. An important component of the Patient, Doctor and Society course is the Generalist Partners Program (GPP) which matches first-year medical students with primary care physicians who practice in the community and who serve as teachers and mentors to students. Through GPP, students learn first-hand about generalist medicine, and enjoy early patient-care opportunities. Other first-year courses are Human Biochemistry, Cell Structure & Function, Molecular & Medical Genetics,Population Medicine and Epidemiology, Integrated Medical Anatomy, Human Physiology. The second-year Pathophysiology courses are organized around body/organ systems, including Hematology, Cardiovascular, Renal, Respiratory, Neoplastic Disease, Endocrine, Gastrointestinal, and Hepatic. Other courses are Foundations of Medicine and Patient, Doctor and Society. The Ebling Medical Library is used by students for research and for studying. It houses more than 330,000 volumes and 3,000 publications.

CLINICAL TRAINING

The third- and fourth-year clerkships expose students to a wide variety of clinical settings (outpatient, inpatient, community based, rural, and urban). Training takes place at University Hospitals in Madison as well as affiliated sites such as Milwaukee, La Crosse and Marshfield. Third-year required clerkships are Medicine (8 weeks); Primary Care (8 weeks); Surgery (8 weeks); Pediatrics (6 weeks); Ob/Gyn (6 weeks); Anesthesia (2 weeks); Neuroscience (6 weeks); Psychiatry (4 weeks); and Radiology (2 weeks). During the fourth year, students complete an Acting Internship in Medicine (4 weeks); an advanced Surgery Clerkship (4 weeks); a Preceptorship (6 weeks); and 18 weeks of electives. A portion of electives may be taken at other academic and clinical institutions, both in the United States and overseas.

Students

Each class is comprised of 150 students, plus 25-26 students in the rural medicine program. Approximately 75 percent of students are Wisconsin residents, and during the past four years, about 40 percent of students attended UW-Madison for their undergraduate education. About 9 percent of students are underrepresented minorities. About 10 or more students in each class are in their late twenties or thirties.

STUDENT LIFE

The School of Medicine and Public Health benefits from the resources of one of the nation's top public universities. Medical students have access to the facilities of the large campus and enjoy the lively environment of a popular college city. Students are active in community service projects such as volunteering at homeless shelters and clinics, and organizing AIDS or other education projects. On-campus housing, including married-student facilities, is available. However, most students prefer to live in shared apartments off campus. Madison is a medium-sized city, organized around three lakes, which provide many opportunities for outdoor recreation.

GRADUATES

Graduates are successful in securing residency positions at prestigious institutions nationwide and within Wisconsin.

Admissions

REQUIREMENTS

Minimum science requirements are General Biology with lab (1 semester); Advanced Biology (1 semester); Biochemistry (1 semester); General Chemistry with lab (1 year); Organic Chemistry (1 semester); General Physics with lab (1 year); Mathematics (1 semester); and Statistics (1 semester). The MCAT is required, and for the 2015 entering class, scores must be from 2011 or later.

SUGGESTIONS

UW gives preference to residents of Wisconsin. Each incoming class consists of about 25% nonresidents. A sound liberal arts education, including both humanities and social sciences, is considered important. While specific courses are not required, the applicant's preparation should include courses in those areas that prepare for the social, psychological, and economic aspects of medical practice. The Admissions Committee members rely heavily on the applicants' essays, letters of recommendation, and the personal interviews to assess motivation and personal character. Community service and exposure to medicine and patient care is needed.

PROCESS

Upon receipt of the AMCAS application, the UW Secondary Application, is sent to selected applicants who meet the minimal academic thresholds (GPA > 3.00, MCATS > 7,8,8). Upon further review, selected applicants are invited to interview. Interviews take place between September and March and consist of one session with a faculty member and one with a small group of medical students and applicants. Interview day activities include group informational sessions, tours, and opportunities to interact with current medical students.

Admissions Requirements (Required)

MCAT Scores, Essays, Science GPA, Extracurricular activities, Non-Science GPA, Exposure to medical profession, Recommendation, Interview

Admissions Requirements (Optional)

State Residency

COSTS AND AID

Tuition & Fees

Annual tuition (in-state out-of-state)	$23,825/$33,721
Room & board	$19,719
Cost of books	$2,090
Fees	$1,111

Financial Aid

% students receiving any aid	81
% students receiving grants	34
% students receiving loans	76
% aid that is merit-based	12
Average grant	$12,396
Average loan	$36,923
Average total aid package	$41,146
Average debt	$136,285

VANDERBILT UNIVERSITY

VANDERBILT UNIVERSITY SCHOOL OF MEDICINE

303 LIGHT HALL, VANDERBILT UNIVERSITY SCHOOL OF MEDICINE NASHVILLE, TN 37232 • ADMISSION: 615-322-2145
FAX: 615-343-23127 • E-MAIL: JENNIFER.S.KIMBLE@VANDERBILT.EDU
WEBSITE: HTTPS://MEDSCHOOL.VANDERBILT.EDU/ADMISSIONS/MD-ADMISSIONS

STUDENT BODY

Type	Private
Enrollment of parent institution	12,721
Enrollment of medical school	436
% male/female	50/50
% underrepresented minorities	8
% out-of-state	70
% international	34
# countries represented	112
Average age of entering class	23

FACULTY

Total faculty	2,398
% female faculty	40
% minority faculty	19
% part-time faculty	4
Student-faculty ratio	5.0:1

ADMISSIONS

# applied	5,397
% accepted	5
% enrolled	37

Average GPA and MCAT Scores

Overall GPA	3.8
MCAT Bio	11.9
MCAT Phys	11.5
MCAT Verbal	10.5
MCAT Essay	Q

Application Information

Regular application	11/1
Are transfers accepted?	No
Admissions may be deferred?	Yes
Admissions need-blind?	No
Application fee	$50

Academics

Unique assessment and advising systems track student progress across multiple domains of performance throughout all years of training. Meaningful feedback, coaching from mentors, Personalized Learning Plans and deliberate practice help all students continually grow. This structure is designed to foster skills in informed self-assessment and continual improvement that are essential throughout one's ensuing career.

BASIC SCIENCES: During the first phase (13 months), VUSM provides a strong foundation in the basic sciences, humanities, and behavioral and social sciences. All students participate in meaningful clinical work during this phase to initiate development as professionals, to provide clinical relevance for the foundational coursework, and to provide an early understanding of healthca.

CLINICAL TRAINING

The Vanderbilt Core Clinical Curriculum (VC3) is based upon a set of 25 common presenting complaints. The VC3 topics are introduced in the first year; core clerkships provide specific teaching activities in multiple settings. An electronic portfolio allows each student to track experience caring for patients with VC3 complaints. Centralized assessment events intermittently test student competence with VC3 problems.

Students

The 2012 entering class came from 31 states and 3 foreign countries. Fifty-three undergraduate institutions were represented. The age range was 21–30, 16 percent of students were underrepresented minorities, and 58 percent were females.

STUDENT LIFE

Vanderbilt's attractive campus provides a focal point for student life and promotes cohesiveness within the student body. Students interact in common areas, such as dining halls, cafes, study areas, and the student center. Athletic facilities include fitness centers, indoor and outdoor tracks, a tennis center, playing fields, a swimming pool, basketball, racquetball and squash courts, and a rock-climbing wall. Medical students join other graduate and professional students for intramural sports, fitness classes, and recreational clubs. In addition to being a world-renowned hub for live music, Nashville offers many attractions including a historic riverfront district, many restaurants, brew pubs, coffeehouses, nightclubs, bookstores, seasonal street fairs, farmers markets, museums, and a large performing arts center. Nashville is also an academic center and is home to more than a dozen colleges and universities. Conveniently located, University-owned apartments are available to single and partnered students and to students with larger families. In addition, off-campus housing is readily available.

GRADUATES

Students perform exceptionally well on the USMLE, contributing to their success in securing residency positions at prestigious institutions nationwide.

Admissions

REQUIREMENTS

Required coursework should be completed by the end of the fall semester (or fall because we have applicants with gap years) in the year applying. Prerequisites include eight semester hours each (with laboratories) of Biology, Chemistry, Organic Chemistry, and Physics along with six semester hours of English. No AP, PASS/FAIL, or CLEP credit is accepted for required courses although advanced classes in these specific areas may be considered as alternatives. An MCAT score from the last three years is required. For individuals who have taken the examination more than once, the highest score in each section is considered in review.

SUGGESTIONS

Students with strong records in diverse areas of scholarship are sought. Research experience in any area of interest is also viewed positively. Evidence of leadership activities has a positive impact for applicants as does involvement in extracurricular activities. Applicants are encouraged to seek out hospital and medical experiences.

PROCESS

Secondary applications will be sent only to those granted an interview. Interviews are conducted between late August and March and consist of one session with a faculty member or administrator. On interview day, applicants also take part in a group orientation session, lunch with students, and a tour of the campus. About 25 percent of interviewees are accepted with notification occurring on a rolling basis. Wait-listed candidates may send supplementary information to update their files.

Admissions Requirements (Required)

MCAT Scores, Essays, Science GPA, Non-Science GPA, Recommendation, Interview

Admissions Requirements (Optional)

Extracurricular activities, Exposure to medical profession, State Residency

COSTS AND AID

Tuition & Fees

Annual tuition	$44,030
Room & board	$18,158
Cost of books	$1,842
Fees	$3,433

Financial Aid

% students receiving any aid	94
% students receiving grants	89
% students receiving loans	64
% aid that is merit-based	38
Average grant	$23,565
Average loan	$34,515
Average total aid package	$45,757
Average debt	$124,236

VIRGINIA COMMONWEALTH UNIVERSITY
SCHOOL OF MEDICINE

Box 980565, RICHMOND, VA 23298 • **ADMISSION:** 804-828-9629 • **FAX:** 804-828-12467
E-MAIL: SOMUME@VCU.EDU • **WEBSITE:** WWW.MEDSCHOOL.VCU.EDU

STUDENT BODY

Type	Public
Enrollment of parent institution	32,000
Enrollment of medical school	791
% male/female	54/46
% out-of-state	42
% international	10
# countries represented	108
Average age of entering class	25

FACULTY

Total faculty	1,421
% female faculty	37
% minority faculty	7
% part-time faculty	8
Student-faculty ratio	1.0:1

ADMISSIONS

# applied	6,451
% accepted	6
% enrolled	48

Average GPA and MCAT Scores

Overall GPA	3.6
MCAT Bio	10.4
MCAT Phys	10.1
MCAT Verbal	9.3
MCAT Essay	Q

Application Information

Regular application	10/15
Early application	7/1
Early notification	10/1
Are transfers accepted?	Yes
Admissions may be deferred?	Yes
Admissions need-blind?	No
Application fee	$80

Academics

The M.D. Degree program is four years in length. A combined M.D./Ph.D. program is also offered and generally takes seven years to complete. Medical students can pursue an MD/MPH or MD/MHA degree. A fellowship program gives medical students the opportunity to participate in research projects, during summers, a year out or throughout the school year. Grades assigned in the M1 and M2 year will be competencies achieved and competencies not yet achieved (C/CN).

BASIC SCIENCES: Although the emphasis is on the basic sciences, behavioral science, preventive medicine, epidemiology, and public health are also taught during the first two years. Laboratory and classroom time is supplemented by a longitudinal experience designed to give students early clinical exposure. First-year courses are the following: Cell Biology; Biochemistry; Anatomical Sciences; Physiology; Behavioral Sciences; Human Genetics; Population Medicine/Biostatistics; Neuroscience; Pathogenesis; Immunology; Ethics; and Foundations of Clinical Medicine, which meets two half-days per week, uses community physicians as mentors, and teaches the basics of patient interviewing and physical diagnosis. The second-year curriculum is organized largely by body/organ systems. Courses are the following: Autonomic Pharmacology; Microbiology/Infectious Diseases; Preventive Medicine; Hematology/Oncology; Central Nervous System; Gastroenterology; Behavioral Science; Respiratory; Cardiovascular; Musculoskeletal/Dermatology; Renal; Endocrine; Reproduction; and continuation of Foundations of Clinical Medicine. Two libraries, the University Library and the Tompkins-McCaw Library, support the research needs of students and faculty. Another important educational resource is the computer-based instructional laboratory, which features computer workstations and audiovisual equipment.

CLINICAL TRAINING

Third-year required clerkships are the following: Medicine (12 weeks); Surgery (8 weeks); Psychiatry (6 weeks); Ob/Gyn (6 weeks); Pediatrics (8 weeks); Family Practice (4 weeks); and Neurology (4 weeks). An additional requirement is one week of a workshop that covers topics such as nutrition, ethics, legal medicine, health economics, and clinical pharmacology. Fourth-year requirements are an acting internship and a critical care month, and a clinical update course, and 24 weeks of electives. For training purposes, medical students have access to approximately 1,000 beds at MCV hospitals. A Level I trauma center, a transplant center, and one of the nation's most prominent head injury centers are among MCV's clinical facilities along with the new critical care tower. Students also have contact with outpatients at McGuire Veterans Administration Medical Center and 24 third year students spend their third and fourth year at Inova Fairfax Hospital in Northern Virginia.

Students

Approximately 70 percent of students are Virginia residents. The average age of incoming students is usually 24.5, and each year about 30 students in their late twenties and thirties enter VCU. Underrepresented minorities account for about 10 percent of the student body. Class size is 200.

STUDENT LIFE

VCU has at least 30 student organizations. These include groups focused on professional pursuits, community service, and religious interests. A variety of facilities, services, and programs designed to meet the leisure and health needs of students are coordinated by the recreational sports staff. The Cary Street Recreation complex and the Larrick Student Center offer fitness facilities including a pool, weight rooms, areas for fitness classes and squash, tennis, and basketball courts. Students have the opportunity to interact outside of class in the Hunton Hall student lounge and in other common areas. Richmond offers many recreational attractions such as parks, museums, historical centers, and shopping areas. While some medical students live in campus residence halls, most live in nearby restored neighborhoods or in the surrounding suburban areas.

GRADUATES

MCV students score above the national average on the USMLE, contributing to their success in obtaining post-graduate positions. About 25 percent of each graduating class enters residency programs administered by MCV Hospitals, while others are successful at securing positions in other parts of the state and country. VCU alumni sponsor a unique bed-and-breakfast program, whereby members of the alumni host medical students when they travel for residency interviews.

Admissions

REQUIREMENTS

The prerequisites for admission are eight semester hours each of Biology, Chemistry, Organic Chemistry, and Physics all with associated labs. Two semesters of English and two semesters of college-level Math are also required. The MCAT is required and must have been taken within 3 years of the year in which an applicant would matriculate. For applicants who have taken the exam more than once, the total scores of each exam are averaged.

SUGGESTIONS

Students are encouraged to pursue their own intellectual interests in college. VCU recognizes that studying medicine requires commitment, strong analytical abilities, good judgment, and sound communication skills. In addition to academic abilities, the Admissions Committee looks for important attributes of character and personality.

PROCESS

About 75 percent of AMCAS applicants who are Virginia residents are sent secondary applications, and about 35 percent of nonresidents are sent secondaries. Applicants returning secondary applications are further screened, and some are invited to interview on campus. Interviews take place between August and March, and consist of one session with a faculty member, medical student, or administrator. On interview day, students also attend group informational sessions, have lunch with current medical students, and tour the campus. Notification occurs on October 15, in mid-December, and in mid-March.

Admissions Requirements (Required)

MCAT Scores, Essays, Science GPA, Extracurricular activities, Non-Science GPA, Exposure to medical profession, Recommendation, Interview

Admissions Requirements (Optional)

State Residency

COSTS AND AID

Tuition & Fees

Annual tuition (in-state out-of-state)	$27,345/$41,273
Room & board	$14,000
Cost of books	$3,970
Fees (in-state out-of-state)	$2,429/$3,005

Financial Aid

% students receiving any aid	96
% students receiving grants	56
% students receiving loans	93
% aid that is merit-based	11
Average grant	$9,000
Average loan	$41,000
Average total aid package	$63,000
Average debt	$157,000

WAKE FOREST UNIVERSITY
WAKE FOREST SCHOOL OF MEDICINE

OFFICE OF ADMISSIONS, MEDICAL CENTER BOULEVARD, WINSTON-SALEM, NC 27157-1090 • **ADMISSION:** 336-716-4264
FAX: 910-716-95937 • **E-MAIL:** MEDADMIT@WAKEHEALTH.EDU • **WEBSITE:** WWW.WAKEHEALTH.EDU

STUDENT BODY

Type	Private
Enrollment of medical school	469
% male/female	54/46
% out-of-state	58
% international	30
Average age of entering class	24

FACULTY

Total faculty	1,168
% female faculty	32
% minority faculty	22
Student-faculty ratio	1.0:1

ADMISSIONS

# applied	7,432
% accepted	4
% enrolled	42

Average GPA and MCAT Scores

Overall GPA	3.6
MCAT Bio	10.6
MCAT Phys	10.0
MCAT Verbal	10.7
MCAT Essay	P

Application Information

Regular application	11/1
Early application	8/1
Early notification	10/1
Are transfers accepted?	No
Admissions may be deferred?	Yes
Admissions need-blind?	No
Application fee	$100

Academics

The curriculum combines features of traditional and problem-based learning methodologies. For details about the curriculum, contact the admissions office. Joint-degree programs include the M.D./M.S.; M.D./M.A. in Bioethics; and the M.D./Ph.D in conjuction with the Graduate School. The Ph.D. degree is offered in the following fields: Anatomy, Biochemistry, Genetics, Immunology, Microbiology, Molecular Biology, Neuroscience, Pathology, Pharmacology, and Physiology. Students are evaluated using a 0-4 scale, and both steps of the USMLE are required for graduation.

BASIC SCIENCES: The pre-clinical curriculum emphasizes self directed and lifelong learning skills, core biomedical science knowledge, problem solving/reasoning, interviewing and communication skills, information management, and professional attitudes and behavior. The course Foundations of Clinical Medicine is taken throughout year one and two, and provide instruction in interviewing and physical examination skills. First year courses provide a foundation in the core biomedical sciences and second-year courses are organized around body/organ systems. The course, Being a Physician, develops the concept of medical professionalism into a clearly definded and utilitarian set of guiding principles assessed through observations of personal behaviors and attitudes. Most pre-clinical instruction takes place in the Hanes Research Building.

CLINICAL TRAINING
Third-year required rotations are: Inpatient Medicine (8 weeks); Surgery (8 weeks); Ob/Gyn (6 weeks); Pediatrics (8 weeks); Neurology/Rehibilitation Medicine (4 weeks); Anesthesiology (1 week); and Radiology (1 week). Required Outpatient clerkships are: Internal Medicine (4 weeks), Ob/Gyn and Women's Health (6 weeks); Family Medicine (4 weeks). During the fourth year, students fullfill the remaining requirements, which are Emergency Medicine (4 weeks); Intensive Care (4 weeks); 8 weeks of required Advancement Patient Management Clerkships; and Electives (24 weeks). Training takes place at North Carolina Baptist Hospital (806 beds) which includes a children's Hospital and a rehibilitation unit, among other specialty facilities. Other sites used for instruction, located in both rural and urban areas include Forsyth Medical Center and the Downtown Health Plaza.

Students

Approximately 30-40 percent of each class is made up of North Carolina residents, and about 10 percent are from Wake Forest's undergraduate program. The remainder represent up to 100 different colleges. About 14 percent of students are underrepresented minorities, most of whom are African American. Class size is 120.

STUDENT LIFE

A Student Life and Fitness Center gives students the opportunity to work out, study, gather, or simply relax. The fitness center includes Nautilis equipment, free weights, showers and a steam room. Other features are a quiet, 24-hour study area, vending machines, a TV lounge, and rooms suitable for small-group discussions. The School of Medicine is located on the Bowman Gray campus, about four miles from the Reynolda campus of Wake Forest, where many academic and cultural events take place. Two state parks are within an hour's drive of Wake Forest, and the Carolina beaches are about four hours away. There is no campus housing, but apartments and rooms are readily available in the surrounding area.

GRADUATES

Wake Forest's reputation, coupled with its students above-average scores on national boards, allows graduates to enter competitive residency programs all over the country.

Admissions

REQUIREMENTS

Ninety semester hours (3 years) of undergraduate course work including eight semester hours each of Biology, Chemistry, Organic Chemistry, and Physics. The MCAT is required and scores must be no more than three years old. For applicants who have retaken the exam, the best set of scores is considered.

SUGGESTIONS

A well-rounded academic experience, including courses in the humanities, is strongly advised. For students who have taken significant time off after college, recent course work is suggested. Early, rather than the later MCAT is recommended, as it allows applicants to retake the exam if necessary in the same application year. Medically related or community-service experiences are considered valuable. Most entering students have four year degrees.

PROCESS

Approximately two thirds of AMCAS applicants are sent secondary application materials. About 10 percent of those returning secondary applications are invited to interview sometime between September and March. Interviews are one on one, and consist of three 15–20 minute sessions with faculty and/or Admissions Committee members. On interview day, candidates also receive a tour and a group orientation. Notification occurs on a rolling basis, the possible outcomes being accept, reject, or wait-list. Wait-listed candidates are generally not encouraged to submit supplementary materials. An alternate path to admissions is through an early assurance program for Wake Forest undergrads only which accepts competitive college juniors without the MCAT. If successful, these students complete their senior year knowing that they have been admitted to medical school for the year following college graduation.

Admissions Requirements (Required)

MCAT Scores, Essays, Science GPA, Extracurricular activities, Non-Science GPA, Exposure to medical profession, Recommendation, Interview

Admissions Requirements (Optional)

State Residency

COSTS AND AID

Tuition & Fees

Annual tuition	$46,484
Room & board	$21,968
Cost of books	$1,790
Fees	$1,788

Financial Aid

% students receiving any aid	88
% students receiving grants	44
% students receiving loans	73
% aid that is merit-based	34
Average grant	$21,072
Average loan	$48,894
Average total aid package	$52,580
Average debt	$150,301

WASHINGTON UNIVERSITY IN ST. LOUIS

WASHINGTON UNIVERSITY SCHOOL OF MEDICINE

OFFICE OF ADMISSIONS, CAMPUS BOX 8107, 660 SOUTH EUCLID AVEN, ST. LOUIS, MO 63110
ADMISSION: 314-362-6848 • FAX: 314-362-46587
E-MAIL: WUMSCOA@MSNOTES.WUSTL.EDU • WEBSITE: MEDSCHOOL.WUSTL.EDU/ADMISSIONS

STUDENT BODY

Type	Private
Enrollment of parent institution	12,003
Enrollment of medical school	578
% male/female	55/45
% international	40
Average age of entering class	23

FACULTY

Total faculty	2,787
% female faculty	26
% minority faculty	10
% part-time faculty	41
Student-faculty ratio	2.0:1

ADMISSIONS

# applied	3,733
% accepted	9
% enrolled	36

Average GPA and MCAT Scores

Overall GPA	3.8
MCAT Bio	12.5
MCAT Phys	12.6
MCAT Verbal	11.3
MCAT Essay	Q

Application Information

Regular application	12/1
Are transfers accepted?	Yes
Admissions may be deferred?	Yes
Admissions need-blind?	No
Application fee	$50

Academics

In addition to the four-year M.D. program, students may apply for a five-year combined M.A./M.D. program, which involves a year of funded research and the completion of a thesis. The MSTP-sponsored M.D./Ph.D. program is one of the largest in the country, with up to 23 positions available each year. During the first year, students are graded using a Pass/Fail system, but grades of Honors/High Pass/Pass/Fail are used from the second year onward.

BASIC SCIENCES: During the first two years, students are in class for about 20 hours per week. Scheduled sessions are divided among lectures, labs, and problem-based sessions conducted in small groups. Topics covered in lectures are documented by a transcript service, to which most students subscribe. Most first-year courses address normal human structure and function. They are Anatomy, the Molecular Foundations of Medicine, Cell and Organ Systems Biology, Immunology, Genetics, and Neuroscience. The course Physicians, Patients, and Society offers first-year students a multidisciplinary perspective on practicing medicine, and continues into the second year. Patient contact begins in the first year, in Introduction to Clinical Medicine. Second-year courses focus on the effects of disease and are organized into blocks, most of which are defined by body systems or physiological concepts. These are Cardiovascular; Clinical Epidemiology; Dermatology; Nervous System; ENT; Endocrinology and Metabolism; Gastrointestinal and Liver Disease/Nutrition; Hematology and Oncology; Infectious Disease; Ob/Gyn; Ophthalmology; Pathology; Pediatrics; Nervous System; Pulmonary; Renal and Genitourinary; and Rheumatology. Clinical experience is expanded and integrated into Pathology, Pathophysiology, and Pharmacology. Students have significant input in curriculum development and revision. The library is extensive, housing about 300,000 volumes and equipped with computer and Internet facilities. The gross anatomy lab is particularly renowned.

CLINICAL TRAINING

The third year is reserved for core, required clerkships, which are: Medicine (12 weeks); Surgery (12 weeks); Neurology (4 weeks); Psychiatry (4 weeks); combined Ob/Gyn and Pediatrics (12 weeks); and Ambulatory Care, which involves Emergency Medicine, Family Practice, and Psychiatric Consultation (12 weeks). The fourth year (44 weeks) is reserved entirely for electives, which may be in clinical and/or basic science departments. Students are permitted to fulfill up to 12 weeks of clinical clerkships at nonaffiliated institutions. While many other academic health care institutions are struggling, Washington University's Medical Center and their other Barnes-Jewish associated hospitals and clinics are thriving and expanding. Children's Hospital ranks as one of the premier pediatric hospitals in the country. In total, affiliated hospitals provide over 2,000 patient beds. Students are exposed to a local population in need of basic care and to patients who have come from around the world for the most advanced treatments. The School of Medicine expects students to play important roles in the provision of patient care.

Students

The current student body represents 43 states and 21 foreign countries. Although most are recent college graduates with degrees in one of the hard sciences, there is tremendous diversity in terms of age and undergraduate background. Class size is 120.

STUDENT LIFE

Since most students come from out-of-state (and country), they are eager to get to know each other and tend to form a coherent group quickly. An extensive orientation session at the beginning of the year aids in this process. Student groups are extremely active, and range from those that focus on community service projects, such as operating a free clinic on weekends, to intramural sports clubs, to Hot Docs (a musical group). Well-used, on-campus facilities include the Hilltop Campus Athletic Facility, which is a comprehensive gym and sports center. Social life often centers on the restaurants and bars of the Central West End and the tree-lined paths of Forest Park. Campus housing is available adjacent to the Medical School, but many students prefer to live in the surrounding areas, where housing is affordable and attractive.

GRADUATES

Graduates gain acceptance to the nation's most competitive residency programs. About half enter a primary care field.

Admissions

REQUIREMENTS

Washington University expects applicants to have completed one year of Biology, General Chemistry, Organic Chemistry, and Physics, in addition to Math through the Calculus level. The MCAT is required, and scores must be no more than three years old.

SUGGESTIONS

The Admissions Committee looks favorably on those who have pursued in-depth study of a particular subject, whether in the natural sciences, social sciences, or humanities. Successful applicants also demonstrate commitment and leadership through their extracurricular activities. Since the Medical School offers rolling admissions beginning October 15, applicants should make every attempt to complete materials early.

PROCESS

About 20 percent of AMCAS applicants are interviewed, with interviews taking place between September and March. Interviews consist of one session with a member of the School's Faculty or Administration. Notification occurs on a rolling basis, and about one-third of interviewees are accepted. Wait-listed candidates are not ranked and are generally not encouraged to send supplementary material.

Admissions Requirements (Required)

MCAT Scores, Essays, Science GPA, Non-Science GPA, Recommendation, Interview

Admissions Requirements (Optional)

Extracurricular activities, Exposure to medical profession, State Residency

COSTS AND AID

Tuition & Fees

Annual tuition	$41,910
Cost of books	$1,613
Fees	$0

Financial Aid

% students receiving any aid	72
% students receiving grants	72
% students receiving loans	53
% aid that is merit-based	30
Average grant	$27,192
Average loan	$25,264
Average debt	$49,905

WAYNE STATE UNIVERSITY

WAYNE STATE UNIVERSITY SCHOOL OF MEDICINE

ADMISSIONS, 540 EAST CANFIELD , STE. 1310, DETROIT, MI 48201 • ADMISSION: 313-577-1466
FAX: 313-577-94207 • E-MAIL: ADMISSIONS@MED.WAYNE.EDU • WEBSITE: WWW.MED.WAYNE.EDU / ADMISSIONS

STUDENT BODY

Type	Public
% male/female	100/0
% out-of-state	0
% international	0
Average age of entering class	24

ADMISSIONS

# applied	2,722
% accepted	19
% enrolled	51

Average GPA and MCAT Scores

Overall GPA	3.5
MCAT Bio	9.8
MCAT Phys	9.5
MCAT Verbal	8.8
MCAT Essay	0

Application Information

Regular application	12/15
Regular notification	10/15
Early application	8/1
Early notification	10/1
Are transfers accepted?	Yes
Admissions may be deferred?	Yes
Admissions need-blind?	No
Application fee	$50

Academics

The School of Medicine administers academic programs leading to the M.D., M.S., and Ph.D. Some medical students pursue a combined M.D./Ph.D., leading to the doctorate degree in Anatomy and Cell Biology, Cellular and Clinical Neurobiology, Immunology/Microbiology, Medical Physics, Molecular Biology and Genetics, Pathology, Pharmacology, and Physiology. Other students earn an M.S. in biomedical or behavioral sciences along with the M.D. The standard medical curriculum consists of two years of basic sciences, a year of clinical clerkships, and a year of clinical electives. Evaluation of medical student performance uses Honors, Pass, and Fail. Promotion to year three requires passing Step 1 of the USMLE. In order to graduate, all students must record a score on Step 2 of the USMLE.

BASIC SCIENCES: Basic-science courses are taught primarily in a lecture/lab format, with some use of small-group sessions. Students are in class for about 20 hours per week. This schedule gives students the time they need to study, pursue independent projects, and take part in community service or other extracurricular activities. During year one, students learn about the normal functions of the human body. Courses are Anatomy, Histology, Embryology, Evidence Based Medicine, Physiology, Biochemistry, Genetics, Neuroscience, Clinical Nutrition, Introduction to the Patient, Human Sexuality, and Behavioral Medicine. Second-year courses focus on the effects of disease and the principles of drug action and therapy. The Pathophysiology course is organized by body/organ systems, which are Connective Tissue, Cardiovascular, Hematology, Pulmonary, Renal, Endocrine, Gastrointestinal, and Neuroscience. Other courses are Pathology, Microbiology, Psychiatry, Pharmacology, Public Health and Preventive Medicine, Physical Diagnosis/Interviewing, Introduction to the Patient, Medical Ethics, and Human Sexuality. The majority of first- and second-year classes are conducted in Scott Hall, a modern building that houses laboratories, lecture halls, and faculty offices. The Shiffman Medical Library has more than 150,000 volumes, computer facilities, and ample space for studying. Students can view recorded lectures and take advantage of other audio-visual study aids in the Self-Instruction Center.

CLINICAL TRAINING

During the third year, students complete 8-week, required clerkships in Internal Medicine, Surgery, Pediatrics, and Ob/Gyn. There are also 4-week clerkships in Family Medicine, Neurology, and Psychiatry. During the fourth year, Selectives in Ambulatory Medicine (4 weeks) and Emergency Medicine (4 weeks), in addition to a Subinternship (4 weeks), are required. Five months of electives are also required, a significant portion of which may be taken at other institutions. Clinical training takes place at the Detroit Medical Center (DMC) which is comprised of numerous hospitals, institutes, and care centers and has, in total, over 2,400 beds. DMC includes Harper Hospital; Grace Hospital; Hutzel Hospital; Children's Hospital of Michigan; Rehabilitation Institute of Michigan; Detroit Receiving Hospital/University Health Center; Gershenson Radiation Oncology Center; Kresge Eye Institute; and Huron Valley Hospital. Medical students also rotate to affiliated hospitals in suburban areas.

Students

About 90 percent of the 256 students in each class are Michigan residents. Approximately 12 percent of students are underrepresented minorities, most of whom are African American. Although a few students are older or nontraditional, most entering students are in their early twenties.

STUDENT LIFE

Medical students are involved in chapters of national organizations such as the American Medical Student Association, professionally oriented groups such as the Family Medicine Interest Group, production of a student newspaper, and numerous community service projects. Volunteer activities involve working with the city's youth, elderly, under- and non-insured populations. Medical students also enjoy the extensive extracurricular offerings of Wayne State University, as well as the diverse culture of Detroit. Students live off campus, usually in apartments in the Detroit metropolitan area or in surrounding suburbs. Parking is available on campus, and most students own cars.

GRADUATES

About 65 percent of graduates chose residency programs in Michigan hospitals, with more than 50 percent staying in the Detroit area. In recent years, more than half of graduates entered primary care fields.

Admissions

REQUIREMENTS

One year each of Biology, Chemistry, Organic Chemistry, and Physics, all with associated labs, is required. The MCAT is required, and scores should be from the spring or fall of the year prior to entrance. For applicants who have retaken the exam, the most recent set of scores is weighed most heavily. Thus, there is no advantage in withholding scores.

SUGGESTIONS

Although most positions are reserved for Michigan residents, well-qualified, non-residents are also considered. In addition to academic credentials, the Admissions Committee is interested in extracurricular activities and work. Health-related volunteer work and research are valuable.

PROCESS

About 50 percent of AMCAS applicants are sent secondary applications. Of those returning secondaries, about 20 percent are interviewed between September and April. The interview consists of one session with a member of the Admissions Committee. Candidates also receive a tour and have the opportunity to meet with current students. About one-third of interviewed candidates are accepted and are notified shortly after the interview. Wait-listed candidates are generally not encouraged to send additional information.

Admissions Requirements (Required)

MCAT Scores, Essays, Science GPA, Extracurricular activities, Non-Science GPA, Exposure to medical profession, Recommendation, Interview

Admissions Requirements (Optional)

State Residency

COSTS AND AID

Tuition & Fees

Annual tuition (in-state out-of-state)	$22,953/$47,765
Cost of books	$1,000
Fees	$1,651

Financial Aid

% students receiving any aid	83
% students receiving grants	44
% students receiving loans	79
% aid that is merit-based	1
Average grant	$5,452
Average loan	$22,649
Average total aid package	$24,385
Average debt	$62,468

WEST VIRGINIA UNIVERSITY

WEST VIRGINIA UNIVERSITY SCHOOL OF MEDICINE

ROBERT C. BYRD HEALTH SCIENCES CENTER, P.O. BOX 9111 MORGANTOWN, WV 26506 • **ADMISSION:** 304-293-2408
FAX: 304-293-78147 • **E-MAIL:** MEDADMISSIONS@HSC.WVU.EDU • **WEBSITE:** WWW.HSC.WVU.EDU/SOM

STUDENT BODY

Type	Public
Enrollment of parent institution	32,731
Enrollment of medical school	424
% male/female	62/38
% out-of-state	38
% international	4
# countries represented	103
Average age of entering class	22

FACULTY

Total faculty	676
% female faculty	30
% part-time faculty	7
Student-faculty ratio	0.6:1

ADMISSIONS

# applied	2,531
% accepted	6
% enrolled	65

Average GPA and MCAT Scores

Overall GPA	3.8
MCAT Bio	9.8
MCAT Phys	9.5
MCAT Verbal	9.2
MCAT Essay	0

Application Information

Regular application	11/1
Early application	8/1
Early notification	10/1
Are transfers accepted?	Yes
Admissions may be deferred?	Yes
Admissions need-blind?	Yes
Application fee	$100

Academics

While most medical students follow a four-year curriculum and earn the M.D. degree, three or four medical students each year pursue joint M.D./Ph.D. degrees. This track leads to the doctorate in Anatomy, Biochemistry, Medical Technology, Microbiology, Pathology, Pharmacology and Toxicology, and Physiology. Medical students are graded with Honors, Satisfactory, or Unsatisfactory. A narrative accompanies the grades for all courses and clerkships. All students must pass Step 1 of the USMLE to be promoted to year three of the curriculum. Passing Step 2CK and CS are graduation requirements.

BASIC SCIENCES: All first-year courses are all held on the Morgantown campus. These classes include Human Function (Physiology, Biochemistry, Genetics; Human Structure (Gross Anatomy, Microanatomy, Embryology); Public Health; Neurobiology; Physical Diagnosis and Clinical Integration (PDCI); and Problem Based Learning (integrates clinical correlation to the basic sciences). The second-year courses are also on the Morgantown Campus. They are integrated Pathology, Microbiology and Immunology, Pharmacology, and Physical Diagnosis and Clinical Integration, and Behavioral Medicine and Psychiatry. All class work and testing is done on laptop computers.

CLINICAL TRAINING

Clinical training takes place on one of three campuses: Morgantown, Charleston or Eastern Division. About one-third of the third year students enter a clinical training program at University-affiliated hospitals in Charleston, WV. Approximately ten students will complete their third year curriculum at the Eastern campus. The remaining students stay on the Morgantown campus. Required third-year clerkships are eight weeks each in the following: Medicine; Surgery; Behavioral Medicine and Psychiatry; Ob/Gyn; Pediatrics; and Family Medicine. A portion of the Family Medicine rotation includes a rural rotation with an affiliated clinician. Year four requirements include one month of a sub-internship in one of the following: Internal Medicine, Pediatrics, or Family Medicine. Half month rotations in critical care and anesthesiology; and two months of a Rural Primary Care experience. Half of the fourth year is reserved for electives. The aforementioned requirements must be successfully completed at one of the three WVU sites. This leaves ample opportunity for students to rotate in other academic institutions. All students have the opportunity to rotate at any of the affiliated facilities that are part of a large network of physicians and hospitals located in rural areas of West Virginia.

Students

About 80% of our students are West Virginians, and more than one-third attended WVU for undergraduate studies. During the first and second years, all students are on the Morgantown Campus. Morgantown is a small college town that has been ranked as one of the best small towns in America. During the 3rd year, students on the Charleston Campus live in the capital of the state. The Eastern Campus is approximately 1.5 hours from Washington, DC and affords the student a lifestyle that includes the small town feel with close proximity to our Nation's capital. Regardless of campus, the student is part of the tight Mountaineer family and all that it encompasses.

STUDENT LIFE

With more than 1,900 students enrolled in programs at the Health Sciences Center, camaraderie exists among WVU students pursuing a career in the sciences. The medical school class size of 110 promotes class cohesion and cooperation amongst colleagues. Student organizations include local chapters of national medical student organizations, community service-based groups, and clubs focused on professional interests. Morgantown and the two other campuses offer a safe and culturally rich environment.

GRADUATES

About one-third of the practicing physicians in the state of West Virginia are graduates of WVU School of Medicine. At least half of our graduates enter primary care fields such as Family Medicine, Internal Medicine, Pediatrics, and Ob/Gyn. While the emphasis is on primary care, students are encouraged to pursue sub-specialties, if that is their intended medical career.

Admissions

REQUIREMENTS

Prerequisites are: one year each of English, Social Sciences, Biology, General Chemistry, Organic Chemistry, and Physics. One semester of Organic Chemistry may be substituted with Biochemistry. All science courses must include lab work. The MCAT is required and is used, along with undergraduate transcripts, to assess academic achievement. For applicants with multiple MCAT scores, all are considered but with emphasis on the most recent score.

SUGGESTIONS

State residents are given strong preference in admission. A limited number of highly qualified nonresidents may also be admitted. Beyond required coursework, HIGHLY RECOMMENDED courses are Biochemistry, Advanced Cellular and Molecular Biology and upper level Physiology coursework. The Admissions Committee expects strength in the sciences but gives no preference to any particular major. Previous medical experience and community service are HIGHLY PREFERRED as a demonstrated understanding of the medical profession is important. Previous work or research experience is a plus.

PROCESS

All qualified West Virginia resident applicants and highly qualified nonresidents are sent secondary applications after an initial screening process. Approximately one third of the non-resident applicants are offered a secondary and the vast majority of those who return the secondary will be offered an interview. Of the in-state applicant pool, approximately 75% are offered a secondary and the vast majority of those who return the secondary are offered and interview. An interview generally consists of one interviewee and two interviewers. The interviewers are medical school basic science and clinical faculty, fourth-year students, or administrators. During the day of their interview, candidates tour the campus and have lunch with current students. Approximately one-third of interviewed candidates are accepted on a rolling basis; the remaining candidates are either rejected or wait-listed. Qualified West Virginia residents on the wait list have a reasonable chance of being accepted later in the spring.

Admissions Requirements (Required)

MCAT Scores, Essays, Science GPA, Extracurricular activities, Non-Science GPA, Recommendation, Interview

Admissions Requirements (Optional)

Exposure to medical profession, State Residency

COSTS AND AID

Tuition & Fees

Annual tuition (in-state out-of-state)	$23,070/$51,010
Room & board	$10,188
Cost of books	$4,660
Fees	$1,178

Financial Aid

% students receiving any aid	86
% students receiving grants	47
% students receiving loans	75
% aid that is merit-based	47
Average grant	$11,728
Average loan	$41,440
Average total aid package	$42,322
Average debt	$156,579

WRIGHT STATE UNIVERSITY

BOONSHOFT SCHOOL OF MEDICINE

WRIGHT STATE UNIVERSITY, OFFICE OF STUDENT AFFAIRS, P.O. BOX 1751 DAYTON, OH 45401-1751
ADMISSION: 937-775-2934 • FAX: 937-775-33227
E-MAIL: SOM_SAA@WRIGHT.EDU • WEBSITE: WWW.MED.WRIGHT.EDU

STUDENT BODY

Type	Public
Enrollment of parent institution	17,595
Enrollment of medical school	423
% male/female	51/49
% out-of-state	4
% international	10
Average age of entering class	24

FACULTY

Total faculty	1,654
% part-time faculty	75
Student-faculty ratio	4.0:1

ADMISSIONS

# applied	3,552
% accepted	6
% enrolled	52

Average GPA and MCAT Scores

Overall GPA	3.6
MCAT Bio	10.0
MCAT Phys	9.6
MCAT Verbal	9.6

Application Information

Regular application	10/15
Regular notification	10/15
Early application	8/1
Early notification	10/1
Are transfers accepted?	Yes
Admissions may be deferred?	Yes
Admissions need-blind?	No
Application fee	$60

Academics

Although most students complete the MD curriculum in four years, a few enter the MD/PhD, MD/MBA, or MD/MPH program which requires additional course work. Graduate degrees are offered in most Biomedical Sciences including Anatomy, Physiology, Biochemistry, Pathology, and Pharmacology. Students are evaluated with percent scores and a Pass/Fail designation. Students take the USMLE Step 1 after completion of year-two and Step 2 after the completion of year-three. Over 60 two-week clinical enrichment electives are available in the first two years.

BASIC SCIENCES: Basic-science instruction includes use of small-groups, clinical case studies, team-based learning, and computer-aided instruction. First-year courses are Human Structure, Human Development, Introduction to Clinical Medicine, Molecular Basis of Medicine, Cell and Tissue Organ Systems, Social and Ethical Issues in Medicine, Biostatistics, and Principles of Disease. The second year is organized around organ/body systems. These are Clinical Decision Making; Pathobiology and Therapeutics, Medical Neuroscience, The Mind, Hematology, Cardiovascular, Endocrine, Gastrointestional, Musculoskeletal and Integument, Renal, Reproduction, Respiratory, and Introduction to Clinical Medicine II. The ICM course provides patient exposure from the very first week of class. In this series, students learn to take medical histories, conduct physical exams and to identify common diseases. Two two-week enrichment elective periods during the first two years give students the opportunity to immerse themselves in a specialty of medicine. Students study in White Hall and the main university's library. The Interdisciplinary Teaching Laboratory enhances learning through the use of audio-visual equipment, hard-wired labs, and medical software. Audio recordings, Power Point slides, and video from lectures are available from a pass word protected web site. All exams in the first two years are computer-based and resemble the USMLE testing format.

CLINICAL TRAINING

Third-year required rotations are: Family Medicine (6 weeks); Internal Medicine (12 weeks); Women's Health (8 weeks); Pediatrics (8 weeks); Psychiatry (6 weeks); and Surgery (8 weeks). Fourth-year requirements are Emergency Medicine (4 weeks), Neurology (4 weeks), and electives (7 months, students may choose from 150 plus). Training takes place at Children's Medical Center (155 beds); Dayton Veterans Affairs Medical Center (120 beds); Good Samaritan Hospital and Health Center (520 beds); Greene Memorial Hospital (199 beds); Kettering Medical Center (545 beds); Miami Valley Hospital (865 beds); Wright-Patterson Air Force Base Medical Center (60 beds), and Mount Carmel Hospital (Columbus, 233 beds). Some students participate in international electives as part of individually designed or faculty-led electives.

Students

About 80 percent of entering students are Ohio residents. Nonresidents, disadvantaged applicants, and nonscience majors are strongly encouraged to apply. Approximately 10% of entering students are minorities. Students are admitted without regard to race, color, religious beliefs, national origin, gender, age, ability, sexual orientation, or socio-economic status. Typically, about 10 percent of entering students took significant time off between college and medical school. The class size is 105.

STUDENT LIFE

Students have active extracurricular lives, taking advantage of the offerings of the medical school, the main University, and a variety of cultural and outdoor activities in the Dayton and greater Dayton areas. Students are involved in community service organizations and projects such as Student-to-Student and the Center for Healthy Communities, which provides health education services to the Dayton community. Other student organizations are chapters of state and national medical organizations, honor societies, support groups, and clubs focused on professional or recreational interests. Athletic facilities on campus include racquetball, squash, basketball and tennis courts, indoor and outdoor tracks, soccer, softball, football, a climbing wall, and several state-of-the-art fitness centers. The University's 200 acres of woods are used for walking, jogging and environmental study. The University main campus is located 12 miles northeast of downtown Dayton. Dayton and the greater Dayton area have a population of approximately 1 million residents. Students live in privately owned apartments, condominiums, and homes. All are generally affordable, conveniently located, and safe for students.

GRADUATES

Typically about 50 percent of graduates enter primary care residencies, including Family Medicine, Internal Medicine, Pediatrics and IM/Peds. Remaining students enter all other specialties. Our graduates pursue residency training throughout the US.

Admissions

REQUIREMENTS

Prerequisites are one year each of Biology, Chemistry, Organic Chemistry, and Physics, all with associated labs. In addition, one year each of English and Mathematics are required. The MCAT exam is required and scores should be from within the past three years. For applicants who have retaken the exam, all scores are considered.

SUGGESTIONS

Ohio residents as well as nonresidents from the entire US are strongly encouraged to apply. In addition to academic qualifications, selection is based on dedication to human concerns, communication skills, maturity, and motivation. Some hospital or other medically related experience is strongly recommended.

PROCESS

All AMCAS applicants receive secondary applications. About 17 percent of those returning secondaries are invited to interview between September and February. Interviews consist of two sessions, each with a member of the admissions committee. On the interview day, students attend group information presentations, have lunch with students, tour the campus, and receive financial aid information. About 45 percent of interviewed candidates are accepted on a rolling basis. Others are put on an alternate list or not accepted. Alternate list candidates are not encouraged to send additional information. For accepted applicants, there is no deposit to hold a place in the class.

Admissions Requirements (Required)

MCAT Scores, Essays, Science GPA, Extracurricular activities, Non-Science GPA, Exposure to medical profession, Recommendation, Interview

Admissions Requirements (Optional)

State Residency

COSTS AND AID

Tuition & Fees

Annual tuition (in-state out-of-state)	$30,842/$47,502
Room & board	$15,884
Cost of books	$1,757
Fees	$2,612

Financial Aid

% students receiving any aid	90
% students receiving grants	51
% students receiving loans	87
% aid that is merit-based	7
Average grant	$7,695
Average loan	$56,385
Average total aid package	$58,821
Average debt	$191,779

YALE UNIVERSITY
SCHOOL OF MEDICINE

OFFICE OF ADMISSIONS, 367 CEDAR STREET, NEW HAVEN, CT 06510 • **ADMISSION:** 203-785-2643 • **FAX:** 203-785-32347
E-MAIL: MEDICALSCHOOL.ADMISSIONS@QUICKMAIL.YALE.EDU
WEBSITE: INFO.MED.YALE.EDU / EDUCATION / ADMISSIONS / INDEX.HTML

STUDENT BODY

Type	Private
Enrollment of medical school	479
% male/female	51/49
% international	18
Average age of entering class	24

ADMISSIONS

# applied	3,093

Application Information

Regular application	10/15
Are transfers accepted?	Yes
Admissions may be deferred?	Yes
Admissions need-blind?	No
Application fee	$60

Academics

Although most students complete courses, clerkships, and a thesis in four years, about 30-50 percent of students extend their studies over a five-year period at no extra cost. Some students take an extra year to earn a M.P.H. along with the M.D. Other combined degree programs offered are the M.D./J.D., M.D./M.Div, and M.D./Ph.D. Entering students are assigned a clinical tutor who serves as a mentor during all four years. Also throughout all four years, students take a series of lectures, workshops, and clinical discussion under the broad topic of Medicine, Society and Public Health. Evaluation of students is strictly Pass/Fail. Passing Steps 1 and 2 of the USMLE is a graduation requirement.

BASIC SCIENCES: The first two years are spent building a foundation in the basic sciences as well as learning skills and techniques for training in clinical responsibilities. Year one is devoted to understanding normal relevant biological form and function. Year two concentrates on the study of disease. Formats include lecture, small group discussion, laboratories, demonstrations, and individual tutorials; many of these involve patients, both at the bedside and in the classroom. First year students must pass the following courses: Cellular and Physiologic Basis of Medicine (Physiology and Cell Biology), Human Genetics, Human Anatomy and Development, Molecular Foundations of Medicine (Biochemistry), Neurobiology, Psychological Basis of Medical Practice, Biological Basis of Behavior, and Aspects of Child and Adolescent Development. In addition there is an umbrella course called Medicine, Society and Public Health that includes related but distinct subcourses: Biostatistics, History of Medicine, Professional Responsibility, and Health Policy. Pre-clinical training is included in the course The Doctor/Patient Encounter. The major, second-year course is called Mechanisms of Disease and is organized into two segments. The initial offering, called Basic Principles, includes Immunobiology, Pathology, Pharmacology, Microbiology, and Basics of Diagnostic Radiology, and Laboratory Medicine. The second segment is called Mechanisms of Disease: Organs/Systems. Each integrated module, organized around body systems or organs, includes Pathology, Pharmacology, Pathophysiology, Diagnostic Radiology, Laboratory Medicine, and Prevention. The modules are Blood/Hematology; Neoplasias/Oncology; Cardiovascular System; Respiratory System; Digestive System; Musculoskeletal System; Renal, Urinary Tract and Male Reproductive System; Female Reproductive System; Endocrine Systems; Skin; Clinical Neuroscience; and Psychiatry. Medicine, Society and Public Health continues, offering Epidemiology and Public Health in the first semester, and relevant Prevention during the modules. The Doctor/Patient Encounter course also continues, building as it progresses.

CLINICAL TRAINING

There are seven required clerkships in the third year, one of which may be completed early in the fourth year. These are Internal Medicine (12 weeks); General Surgery/Surgical Subspecialties (12 weeks); Pediatrics (8 weeks); Psychiatry (6 weeks); Ob/Gyn (6 weeks); and Clinical Neuroscience (4 weeks). During the fourth year, an Integrated Clinical Medicine Clerkship (3 weeks) and a Primary Care Clerkship (4 weeks) are required. The Primary Care Clerkship takes place in a variety of community- and practice-based sites. Most clinical rotations are completed at the Yale New Haven Hospital and the West Haven Veteran's Administration Hospital. Other affiliated hospitals are Bridgeport Hospital; Danbury Hospital; Greenwich Hospital; Griffin Hospital in Derby; Hospital of Saint Raphael; Lawrence and Memorial Hospital; Norwalk Hospital; Saint Mary's Hospital in Waterbury; Saint Vincent's Medical Center in Bridgeport; and Waterbury Hospital. Several clinics and mental health centers are also used for training. Although some students begin working on their thesis early in medical school, the majority of research and writing takes from four to seven months and is completed in the fourth year. Some students publish their work, while others continue developing their research post-graduation.

Students

Yale attracts students from all regions of the country. Approximately 15-20 percent of entering students are underrepresented minorities. The age range of the student body is considerable, with an average of 24. Class size is 100.

STUDENT LIFE

The School of Medicine is a short walk from the University's main campus. This gives medical students access to athletic facilities, student meeting areas, libraries, and university-sponsored events. Medical students participate in intramural sports, competing against other graduate and professional school teams. About three-quarters of medical students are involved in community service activities such as STATS (Students Teaching AIDS to Students), the Prenatal Care Project, and ASAP (the Adolescent Substance Abuse Prevention Project). The Office for Women in Medicine is the oldest of its kind in the nation and provides support, guidance, and special programs of interest for women medical students. The Office for Multicultural Affairs recruits and supports minority students, serves as a link between the school and its surrounding community, and sponsors various cultural events and centers. The Edward S. Harkness Memorial Hall is a residence hall for medical, physician associate, nursing, public health, and other graduate students. Both dormitory-style rooms and apartments are available.

GRADUATES

Among recent graduates, the most popular areas for residency training were Internal Medicine (40%); Pediatrics (12%); Surgery (5%); Diagnostic Radiology (1%); Orthopedics (8%); Plastic Surgery (4%); Dermatology (3%); and Otolaryngology (5%).

Admissions

REQUIREMENTS

Prerequisites are one year each of General Biology or Zoology, General Chemistry, Organic Chemistry, and General Physics, all taken with associated labs. The MCAT is required, and scores should be from within the past four years. For applicants who have retaken the exam, the best set of scores is considered.

SUGGESTIONS

In addition to academic credentials, the Committee on Admissions looks for intelligent, mature, and highly motivated students who possess integrity, common sense, personal stability, dedication to service, and the ability to inspire and maintain confidence.

PROCESS

Yale does not participate in AMCAS. Applications should be requested from the address above, or downloaded from info.med.yale.edu/medadmit. About 25 percent of applicants are interviewed between October and February. Interviews consist of two sessions, each with a faculty member or medical student committee member. Candidates attend group information sessions and have the opportunity to eat lunch and tour the campus with current medical students. About 15 percent of interviewed candidates are accepted. Notification occurs in mid-March.

Admissions Requirements (Required)

MCAT Scores, Essays, Extracurricular activities, Exposure to medical profession, State Residency

Admissions Requirements (Optional)

Science GPA, Non-Science GPA, Recommendation, Interview

COSTS AND AID

Tuition & Fees

Annual tuition	$39,150
Room & board	$9,650
Cost of books	$1,700
Fees	$375

Financial Aid

% students receiving any aid	2
% students receiving grants	2
% students receiving loans	2
% aid that is merit-based	2

Yeshiva University

Albert Einstein College of Medicine

Jack and Pearl Resnick Campus, 1300 Morris Park Avenue, 1300 Morris Park Avenue Bronx, NY 10461
Admission: 718-430-2106 • Fax: 718-430-88257
E-mail: ADMISSIONS@AECOM.YU.EDU • Website: WWW.AECOM.YU.EDU

STUDENT BODY

Type	Private
Enrollment of medical school	724
% male/female	51/49
% underrepresented minorities	2
% out-of-state	51
% international	7
Average age of entering class	23

FACULTY

Total faculty	3,510
% female faculty	35
% part-time faculty	42
Student-faculty ratio	1.0:1

ADMISSIONS

# applied	5,943
% accepted	9
% enrolled	35

Average GPA and MCAT Scores

Overall GPA	3.6
MCAT Bio	10.6
MCAT Phys	10.5
MCAT Verbal	9.4
MCAT Essay	P

Application Information

Regular application	12/31
Regular notification	1/15
Early application	8/15
Are transfers accepted?	No
Admissions may be deferred?	Yes
Admissions need-blind?	No
Application fee	$90

Academics

In addition to the requirements described below, all students conduct research projects through the Independent Scholars Program. Such research often leads to publication or to distinction at the time of graduation. Projects involve a faculty mentor, and can be in traditional or nontraditional medical science fields. Students may apply for joint Ph.D./ M.D. programs at the time of initial application or while enrolled in the M.D. program. Those accepted into this program receive stipends, either through the M.S.T.P. program or from institutional sources. The Ph.D. may be earned in the following fields: Anatomy, Biochemistry, Biophysics, Cell Biology, Genetics, Immunology, Microbiology, Molecular Biology, Neuroscience, Pathology, Pharmacology, and Physiology. Evaluation of student performance uses Honors, Pass, and Fail. Passing the USMLE Steps 1 and 2 are requirements for graduation.

BASIC SCIENCES: Throughout the first and second years, Introduction to Clinical Medicine complements the basic science curriculum by addressing practical and personal issues related to the patient interview and examination. About forty entering students participate in a Generalist Mentorship program, which involves shadowing a primary care physician. First-year courses, taught primarily with lectures and labs, are: Histology, Anatomy, Cardiovascular Physiology, Principles of Pharmacology, and Disease Mechanisms. The course Molecular and Cellular Foundations of Medicine uses both lectures and small group sessions. During the second part of year one, and throughout all of year two, instruction is organ-based, is carried out in small groups, and uses a case-based approach. Courses are Renal Physiology and PathoBiology; Nervous System and Behavior; Endocrine System; Reproductive System and Human Sexuality; Cardiovascular System; Respiratory System; Gastrointestinal System and Liver; Hematology; and Rheumatologic and Orthopedic Disease. Other second-year courses are Microbiology and Infectious Disease and Parasitology. On average, students spend about twenty hours per week in class. A Cognitive Skills Program offers reviews for the USMLE and tutoring for students who will benefit from it. Basic science instruction takes place in the Arthur B. and Diane Belfer Educational Center for Sciences, which is open 24 hours a day and contains classrooms, laboratories, study areas, a student bookstore, and computer rooms. The D. Samuel Gottesman Library has 250,000 volumes, 2,400 journal subscriptions, computer databases, and other informational technology. Electronic search mechanisms allow easy access to several large collections in the New York area.

CLINICAL TRAINING
Third-year required clerkships are Medicine (11 weeks); Pediatrics (7 weeks); Psychiatry (6 weeks); Ob/Gyn (6 weeks); Surgery (8 weeks); Family Medicine (6 weeks); Geriatrics (2 weeks); and Neurology (2 weeks). During the fourth year, two months of a subinternship in either Medicine or Pediatrics is required, as are two months in an ambulatory care program. For clinical training, Einstein students have access to six prominent hospitals in New York, comprising a total of 6,988 beds. These are Jacobi Medical Center (537 beds); Montefiore Medical Center (745 beds); Long Island Jewish Medical Center (829 beds); Beth Israel Medical Center (212 beds); and the Bronx-Lebanon Medical Center (two centers, 540 beds). Training also takes place at mental health facilities and long-term care centers primarily for older populations. Several nationally recognized research

institutes are part of Einstein's resources and provide further opportunities for students. Fellowships are available for up to 20 fourth-year students, enabling them to fulfill elective requirements overseas. Numerous organized exchange programs also exist, with countries such as Germany, Sweden, Israel, France, Japan, and Cuba.

Students

Students come from around the country. Undergraduate institutions that are particularly well represented are Yeshiva, State Universities of New York, private northeastern colleges and universities, and public universities in California. In a typical entering class, about 9 percent of students are minorities, most of whom are African American. Students who have taken time off after college account for about one-third of entering classes, and those over 30 years old account for about 5–10 percent. Class size is 180.

STUDENT LIFE

Central meeting areas, such as the Lubin Student Lounge and the Max and Sadie Friedman Lounge, feature music, food, television, and an opportunity for interaction outside of the academic environment. There are full athletic facilities for student use. School-sponsored activities include class parties, clubs focused on films or the outdoors, and organizations based on cultural, religious, or ethnic affiliations. Einstein has its own symphony orchestra. The beaches of Long Island and the culture, entertainment, and excitement of Manhattan are easily accessible by car or public transportation. Most students live on campus, in the Eastchester Road or Rhinelander Residences, where studios and one- and two-bedroom apartments are available.

GRADUATES

Among recent graduates, the predominant residency choices were Internal Medicine (45%); Pediatrics (12%); Surgery or General Surgery (10%); Ob/Gyn (6%); Emergency Medicine (6%); Psychiatry (5%); Family Practice (4%); and Ophthalmology (3%). Einstein has the largest post-graduate training program in the country, and is the destination of about 40 percent of Einstein School of Medicine graduates. Programs at other New York institutions, in the Philadelphia area, and in California are also popular choices.

Admissions

REQUIREMENTS

Requirements are Biology (8 semester hours); Chemistry (8 hours); Organic Chemistry (8 hours); Physics (8 hours); College Math (6 hours); and English (8 hours). The MCAT is required and should be no more than 3 years old. For those who have retaken the MCAT, the best score is counted. Thus, there is no advantage to withholding scores.

SUGGESTIONS

College students should pursue studies in their area of interest, as no particular major is considered more appropriate than the next. Course work in the Humanities and Social Sciences is important. Statistics is useful, and computer literacy is necessary. Einstein looks closely at the personal interaction skills of its applicants and at their ability to work with people from diverse backgrounds.

PROCESS

All AMCAS applicants are sent secondary applications. Of those returning secondaries, about 20 percent are invited to interview. Interviews are with faculty members, last for about an hour, and take place between August and May. On interview day, there is a tour of the campus, and a lunch period with current Einstein students. Notification begins in January, at which point applicants are accepted, wait-listed, or rejected. Wait-listed candidates may submit additional material.

Admissions Requirements (Required)

MCAT Scores, Essays, Science GPA, Extracurricular activities, Non-Science GPA, Exposure to medical profession, Recommendation, Interview

Admissions Requirements (Optional)

State Residency

COSTS AND AID

Tuition & Fees

Annual tuition	$39,450
Room & board (on-campus off-campus)	$7,000/$4,000
Cost of books	$1,600
Fees	$2,250

Financial Aid

% students receiving any aid	75
% students receiving grants	25
% students receiving loans	80
% aid that is merit-based	5
Average grant	$8,500
Average loan	$20,000
Average total aid package	$12,000
Average debt	$65,00

8 Naturopathic Profiles

BASTYR UNIVERSITY
SCHOOL OF NATUROPATHIC MEDICINE

14500 JUANITA DR NE, KENMORE, WA 98028 • ADMISSION: 425-602-3330 • FAX: 425-602-3090
E-MAIL: ADMISSIONS@BASTYR.EDU • WEBSITE: WWW.BASTYR.EDU

STUDENT BODY

Type	Private
Enrollment of parent institution	1,123
Enrollment of medical school	591
% male/female	21/79
% underrepresented minorities	8
% out-of-state	29
% international	38
# countries represented	30
Average age of entering class	29

FACULTY

Total faculty	30
% female faculty	60
% part-time faculty	64
Student-faculty ratio	9.0:1

ADMISSIONS

# applied	370
% accepted	68
% enrolled	95

Average GPA and MCAT Scores

Overall GPA	3.3

Application Information

Regular application	2/1
Regular notification	4/15
Early application	11/1
Early notification	2/1
Are transfers accepted?	Yes
Admissions may be deferred?	Yes
Admissions need-blind?	No
Application fee	$75

Academics

Bastyr University's fully accredited naturopathic doctor (ND) program is internationally renowned for the quality of its curriculum, clinical training and research. The University's faculty use a distinct multidisciplinary, science-based teaching approach and emphasize the inter-relation of mind, body, spirit and nature. This prepares future naturopathic physicians to become leaders and successful clinicians either in private practice or in integrative health care settings. A pioneer in natural medicine since its inception, the University designs innovative models for 21st-century medicine.

BASIC SCIENCES: Students receive a thorough foundation in the basic medical sciences along with instruction in naturopathic medicine, clinical and laboratory diagnosis, nutrition, and counseling. Anatomy, physiology, and biochemistry serve as the foundation for further basic science courses and all chemical courses. Further courses include pathology, immunology, infectious diseases, embryology and research methods. Problem-solving, clinical cases and examples are an integral part of the basic science curriculum.

CLINICAL TRAINING

Clinical training at Bastyr University focuses on clinical diagnosis and therapeutics, including clinical studies in nutrition, botanical medicine, homeopathy, obstetrics, pediatrics, geriatrics and other specialty areas. Students receive their clinical education through supervised internships at the University's own teaching clinic, Bastyr Center for Natural Health, as well as at numerous off-site clinic placements. All ND students must accrue 132 hours in preceptorships. These hours are spent observing and "shadowing" health-care professionals in their practices. Bastyr ND students receive a minimum of 1,200 clinical training hours. Those hours must include a minimum of 350 direct patient contacts in order to graduate. Most of our students average 600 patient contacts by the time they earn their degree. Students in the ND/acupuncture and Oriental medicine (AOM) dual program are eligible to participate in clinical internships in China—either at Chengdu University of TCM or Shanghai University of TCM. Chengdu University has been Bastyr's sister college since 1993 and is one of the four colleges approved by the State Council in 1956.

Students

Bastyr University's campus is in Kenmore, just north of Seattle in the beautiful Pacific Northwest. The 186,000 square-foot facility rests on 51 acres of fields and woodlands on the northeast shore of Lake Washington. Built in 1959 as a Catholic seminary, the building houses the University's classrooms, laboratories and research facilities, library and reading room, bookstore, conference and seminar space, administrative offices, dining commons, chapel, and eco-friendly dorms. A variety of off-campus apartments and rental homes are available in Seattle and the Juanita, Mountlake Terrace, Bothell and Kenmore areas. Bastyr students thrive in our close-knit and nurturing community, enjoying a campus surrounded by forest—a peaceful setting for the study and celebration of nature. At Bastyr you will be part of a community that thrives on diversity and the free exchange of ideas. Bastyr also opened a campus in San Diego, California, in fall 2012. Bastyr University California offers the naturopathic medicine program with the same classroom and clinical training as the Kenmore program.

STUDENT LIFE

Bastyr students participate in a wide variety of activities on campus. Students are involved in the governance system of the University through the Student Council. Others volunteer in the medicinal and culinary herb garden and on various clubs and committees: Herbal Ways, Nutrition Advisory Committee, American Psychological Association, Aikido, African-American Support Group, Student Dietetics Association, Supper Club, Student Chapter of Physicians for Social Responsibility, various spiritual groups, and various athletic groups. Students benefit from the multidisciplinary curriculum and can take advantage of visiting speakers and weekend workshops on a wide range of natural health topics, including ayurvedic and Oriental medicine and craniosacral massage. Numerous special events throughout the year help create a sense of school identity and a feeling of community.

GRADUATES

Graduates of Bastyr's ND program are qualified primary health care practitioners who diagnose and treat disease with a focus on treating the whole person. Their scope of practice includes all aspects of family care, from pediatrics to geriatrics, and relies on a broad spectrum of modalities, including botanical medicine, nutrition, hydrotherapy, naturopathic manipulation and psychological counseling. Graduates leave Bastyr qualified to pass professional licensure exams and prepared to set up and maintain private practices or join integrative health care practices.

Admissions

REQUIREMENTS

Applicants must submit the following credentials: all official transcripts, two letters of recommendation, a completed application form and a $75 application fee. Required coursework includes a bachelor's degree, one course in college-level algebra or precalculus, four courses in chemistry (including a two-term sequence of organic with labs), three quarters or two semesters of biology with labs (must include work in cell biology and genetics), at least one course in physics (must include mechanics, optics, electricity and magnetism), and one course in psychology. Courses earning a C- or below are not accepted for prerequisite consideration. Required chemistry and biology courses not taken within seven years of matriculation into the program are subject to review by the admissions committee. Additional coursework may be required. Applicants who meet the basic admission standards may be invited to an interview.

SUGGESTIONS

For priority consideration, applications should be received by February 1 for admission the following fall. Late applications are considered on a space-available basis. When requesting an application or program information, please indicate the specific program of interest and materials of interest.

PROCESS

Admission is based on academic achievement, personal and social development, relevant experience and demonstrated humanistic qualities.

Admissions Requirements (Required)

Essays, Science GPA, Non-Science GPA, Exposure to medical profession, Recommendation, Interview

Admissions Requirements (Optional)

StandardizedTest, Extracurricular activities, State Residency

COSTS AND AID

Tuition & Fees

Annual tuition	$31,789
Room & board	$21,600
Cost of books	$3,725
Fees	$75

Financial Aid

% students receiving any aid	90
% students receiving grants	27
% students receiving loans	83
Average grant	$2,460
Average loan	$56,062
Average total aid package	$53,710
Average debt	$252,279

BOUCHER INSTITUTE OF NATUROPATHIC MEDICINE

BOUCHER INSTITUTE OF NATUROPATHIC MEDICINE

300-435 COLUMBIA STREET, NEW WESTMINSTER, BC V3L 5N8 • ADMISSION: 604-777-9981 • FAX: 604-777-9982
E-MAIL: INFO@BINM.ORG • WEBSITE: WWW.BINM.ORG

STUDENT BODY

Type	Private
Enrollment of medical school	154
% male/female	16/84
Average age of entering class	26

FACULTY

Total faculty	50
% part-time faculty	40
Student-faculty ratio	3.2:1

ADMISSIONS

# applied	107
% accepted	56
% enrolled	62

Average GPA and MCAT Scores

Overall GPA	3.4

Application Information

Regular application	3/1
Early application	11/30
Are transfers accepted?	Yes
Admissions may be deferred?	No
Admissions need-blind?	Yes
Application fee	$150

Academics

The academic philosophy as evidenced by the Institute's curriculum design strives to incorporate principles of both proven conventional academic wisdom and a mentorship program. BINM's commitment to small class size allows maximum flexibility in the incorporation of various educational methodologies including hands-on situational learning. Thirty-five hundred hours of instruction are divided among the five basic categories of courses which constitute the Naturopathic Medical Program academic curriculum: Biomedical Sciences; Professional Development; Naturopathic Therapeutic Modalities; Clinical Science; Clinical Practice and Integration.

BASIC SCIENCES: Anatomy (plus dissection lab); Biomedicine –Biochemistry; Laboratory Diagnosis; Pathology; Pharmacology; Physiology; Diagnostic Imaging; Differential Diagnosis; Microbiology; Neuroanatomy; Oncology; Physical Clinical Diagnosis

CLINICAL TRAINING

Twelve hundred hours are spent on the clinical component of the education, with an additional 300 preceptorship hours spent in the offices of practicing physicians.

Students

The Boucher Institute of Naturopathic Medicine is located in the 46,000-square-foot Boucher Centre in New Westminster, BC, Canada and houses a busy Sky Train Station, part of the region's rapid transit system, and provides a view of the mighty Fraser River. The Boucher Institute currently occupies approximately 25,000-square-foot in the building, including classrooms, administrative offices, an active teaching clinic of twelve treatment rooms and plenty of room to grow. Established in 2001, the Boucher Institute is Western Canada 's only accredited college of naturopathic medicine, offering both a four-year full-time program of study and an innovative six-year part-time program culminating in a Doctor of Naturopathic Medicine diploma.

STUDENT LIFE

Student life involves a deep connection with classmates in the small classes at BINM. The Boucher Naturopathic Students Association is an active member of campus life, ensuring a variety of social activities to balance the intense academic load. An elected representative sits as a full voting member of the Board of Governors. Students work together and help one another to achieve a high standard of learning. Collaborative projects begin in the first week of school and continue throughout. Students live anywhere in the Lower Mainland and enjoy access within minutes of the school to downtown Vancouver, the snow-capped coastal mountains, fertile farmlands, and the shoreline of the Pacific Ocean.

GRADUATES

Graduates are currently practicing in BC, Alberta, New Brunswick, Nova Scotia, Ontario, California, Hawaii, Australia and Saudi Arabia. Several alumni have return to BINM as instructors and clinic supervisors.

Admissions

REQUIREMENTS

A University bachelor's degree in any field is required from a recognized post-secondary institution or the equivalent for entry into the program. For credentials earned outside of the USA and Canada a "comprehensive evaluation" must be completed from ICES or from

WES and sent directly to the Admissions Office prior to the admissions deadline. Potential students may apply for admission in the final year of study if they will be able to provide an official transcript showing the degree conferred date no later than two weeks prior to matriculation. Credentials obtained at a foreign institution require further evaluation on a course by course basis. Prerequesites: The following specific courses are required prerequisites and must show a minimum final grade of 60% or 'C'. Prerequisite courses must be taken at a recognized post-secondary institution, either on-site or on-line. Boucher Institute does not require the separate lab courses as a prerequisite. Lab courses may not be used to fulfil the number of required prerequisite credit hours or be included in calculating prerequisite grades. Biochemistry: half-year (3 credit hours); Biology: one full-year (6 credit hours). This may be fulfilled either by one year of general biology or by one semester of cell biology plus one semester of an appropriate biology, such as botany, ecology, genetics, microbiology or zoology. Please note: anatomy and physiology courses may not satisfy the biology requirement. General Chemistry: one full-year (6 credit hours); English/Humanities: one full year (6 credit hours). This requirement may be fulfilled by courses such as: academic writing, anthropology, history, literature, philosophy, sociology, women's studies, written communication, or similar courses. Coursework must include a significant essay-writing component. Applicants may be required to write a short essay at the time of interview. Second language courses (Spanish, French etc.) and courses taught in a language other than English may not be used to satisfy this requirement. Organic Chemistry: half-year (3 credit hours); Psychology: half-year (3 credit hours). This requirement may be filled by courses such as: behavioural, cognitive, developmental, introductory and learning psychology. Please note: According to both PCTIA bylaws and BINM policy, minimum program admission requirements may not be waived. A passing mark of 60% or 'C' is the absolute minimum grade required for all prerequisites and for any additional courses (as above) to be considered. It is recommended that an overall cumulative grade-point average of 3.0 on a four-point scale (i.e. 75%) be attained for the applicant to be competitive for the limited seats available. However, students with lower cumulative GPAs may also be accepted. Credit may or may not be given for courses completed more than 10 years prior to application for admission, at the discretion of the Admissions Committee. Students should be prepared to show that they have kept themselves up-to-date in the sciences. BINM may at its discretion accept prerequisite preparatory courses from other CNME approved institutions. This option is generally reserved for students who apply as transfer students. It is preferable for first year applicants to complete their prerequisite courses through a recognized university or college.

SUGGESTIONS

In addition, prospective students would benefit by completing additional courses in some or all of the following areas: Anatomy; Business (300+ level only); Calculus; Cell Biology; Genetics; Human Physiology; Leadership (300+ level only); Management (300+ levels only); Marketing (300+ level only); Microbiology; Nutrition; Physics; Research; Sociology; Statistics.

PROCESS

The Boucher Institute of Naturopathic Medicine evaluates all applicants in accordance with the constitutional guidelines that protect the rights of individuals. The primary objective of the applicant screening process is to assure that applicants accepted into the program have made an informed commitment to naturopathic medicine as a career and that there is a good match between the applicant's goals and expectations and what the Boucher's unique program has to offer. Applicants must be temperamentally and morally suited to the profession, and must have a reasonable probability of successfully completing the program and becoming licensed to practice in a regulated jurisdiction. The successful applicant is expected to: have demonstrated reasonable academic ability in previous educational endeavours; have reasonable knowledge of and realistic attitudes towards health and healing and towards naturopathic medicine in particular, understand the importance of self-care, demonstrate a reasonable understanding of holistic health care, and be able to discuss the role of the healer.

CANADIAN COLLEGE OF NATUROPATHIC MEDICINE

CANADIAN COLLEGE OF NATUROPATHIC MEDICINE

1255 SHEPPARD AVENUE EAST, TORONTO, ON M2K 1E2 • ADMISSION: 416-498-1255 x245 • FAX: 416-498-3197
E-MAIL: INFO@CCNM.EDU • WEBSITE: WWW.CCNM.EDU

STUDENT BODY

Type	Private
Enrollment of parent institution	542
Enrollment of medical school	542
% male/female	20/80
% underrepresented minorities	10
# countries represented	6
Average age of entering class	26

FACULTY

Total faculty	95
Student-faculty ratio	17.0:1

ADMISSIONS

# applied	175
% accepted	73
% enrolled	63

Average GPA and MCAT Scores

Overall GPA	3.4

Application Information

Regular application	8/15
Early application	12/31
Are transfers accepted?	Yes
Admissions may be deferred?	Yes
Admissions need-blind?	No
Application fee	$115

Academics

CCNM's ND program is a post-university professional program requiring a Bachelor's degree for admission. We provide an intensive four-year program that includes more than 1,200 hours of clinical experience and involves more than 3,000 hours of classroom training. Our program covers three major areas of study: biomedical sciences, clinical sciences and naturopathic therepeutics. CCNM is accredited by the Council on Naturopathic Medical Education (CNME), the North American accrediting agency for naturopathic colleges and programs recognized by the US Department of Education.

BASIC SCIENCES: The biomedical sciences segment of the curriculum provides an in-depth study of the human body through lectures and labs. Students take courses in anatomy (including gross anatomy, prosection, neuroanatomy, embryology and histology), physiology, biochemistry, immunology, clinical pathology, environmental and public health (including infectious diseases), pharmacology, and pharmacognosy.

CLINICAL TRAINING
The clinical sciences segment of the curriculum thoroughly prepares students to educate patients and the public in health promotion and disease prevention. It also prepares them to diagnose the causes of a range of primary care conditions and to effectively help patients manage their conditions using a broad range of therapeutics. Laboratory and clinical demonstrations are utilized to foster the development of practical skills. Diagnostics courses include physical and clinical diagnosis, integrated clinical pathology and differential diagnosis and diagnostic imaging. A range of primary care issues are covered in courses ranging from maternal and newborn care to pediatrics. Primary care management is covered in the study of botanical medicine, homeopathy, emergency medicine, nutrition, physical medicine (including naturopathic, osseous and soft tissue manipulative therapy, physiotherapy, sports medicine, therapeutic exercise and hydrotherapy), psychological counseling, nature cure, acupuncture and Asian medicine, and minor surgery.

Students

Campus facilities include: NSA student centre: A spacious area for student use is located on the second floor of the academic wing. The lounge area has a satellite TV, games room, meditation room and piano room. It also houses the student newspaper, extracurricular clubs and the Naturopathic Students' Association offices. Fitness centre: A fully equipped indoor fitness centre with change rooms and saunas is located on the lower level of the College. A tennis/basketball court is located behind the building on the northwest corner. A variety of campus and intra-mural sports teams are organized by students each year, based on interest. Courtyard and herb garden: Students, staff and faculty are encouraged to visit our treed courtyard for group meetings, studying or simply relaxing. Brick barbecues and picnic tables are available for student use. The Paracelsus Herb Garden offers a relaxing oasis for reflection and meditation and is used as a teaching garden for CCNM students and visitors. Lockers: Each student is entitled to a locker and combination lock for the academic year free of charge. Please see Admissions and Student Services for more information. Recycling and composting and re-use: CCNM's Facilities Department oversees a comprehensive waste reduction program. Cans, bottles and paper are collected throughout the campus. Food waste is collected in the student residence kitchens, staff and student lounges, and in the cafeteria. Used household batteries are also collected. Food waste and yard waste are recycled into compost that is used on campus lawns and gardens. Public transit: In accordance with its environmental program, CCNM encourages the use of public transit and has direct access to Toronto's subway system. Students can purchase monthly TTC Metropasses at a discounted rate. Career Resource Centre: CCNM has an on-site Career Resource Centre located in the administration wing near Student Services. Students can also access career resources on Moodle and Integra Practice Management. Hearty Catering offers healthy foods at reasonable prices in a pleasant, welcoming atmosphere. Adjacent to the courtyard. Open Monday to Friday from 7:45 a.m. to 5:30 p.m. during the regular academic year, excluding holidays. Closed during August. Operates on a limited basis during reading weeks. It also offers catering services to the CCNM community. Learning Resources Centre: The Learning Resources Centre houses more than 22,740 resources on naturopathic and complementary health care. Bookstore: Body and Mind is an on-campus textbook and medical supply store. Body and Mind provides students with textbooks, software and medical equipment. Body and Mind also serves the wider community of complementary health-care professionals, carrying a range of clinic supplies. The store sells an assortment of organic foods, textbooks, software and medical equipment. It also serves the wider community of complementary health-care professionals, carrying a complete line of clinic supplies. Stocks a range of organic foods and healthy snacks. Naturopathic Students' Association (NSA): Naturopathic Students' Association includes all students in the ND program. Each year 14 executive members are elected from the student body to represent the interests of the students in all aspects pertaining to their education, clinical experiences and everyday life as a future naturopathic doctor. Parking: A limited number of parking spaces are available at the front of the College by entering from Sheppard Ave. East or Old Leslie Street. The monthly parking rate is $90 and the maximum daily rate is $25 (subject to change). Monthly permits are issued on a first-come, first-served basis and are available at the front desk through an application process.

STUDENT LIFE

CCNM's location in Toronto offers a wealth of entertainment, leisure, and cultural activities for students to enjoy. Whether your tastes lead you to exotic cuisines, multicultural festivals, sports events or the theatre district, there's always something to capture your interest in Toronto.

Admissions

REQUIREMENTS

To be considered for admission to the ND program, applicants must have completed a three- or four-year bachelor's degree in any discipline at an accredited institution. A minimum cumulative grade point average of 2.7 is required. Prerequisites include organic chemistry, biology, physiology, psychology, and humanities.

SUGGESTIONS

In addition to the required courses outlined above, we recommend that applicants complete courses in some or all of the following areas to prepare for the ND program curriculum: anatomy, environmental science, genetics, microbiology, physics, sociology, statistics and/or English composition

PROCESS

CCNM is committed to excellence in naturopathic education and to the success of our graduates. All candidates for admission are evaluated based on their academic history and personal interview, as well as their motivation for becoming a naturopathic doctor, leadership skills, problem solving and critical-thinking skills, and specific personal qualities and characteristics.

Admissions Requirements (Required)

Essays, Science GPA, Extracurricular activities, Non-Science GPA, Recommendation, Interview

Admissions Requirements (Optional)

StandardizedTest, Exposure to medical profession, State Residency

COSTS AND AID

Tuition & Fees

Annual tuition (in-state out-of-state)	$20,100/$21,990
Room & board (on-campus off-campus)	$700/$475
Cost of books	$1,800
Fees	$585/$585

Financial Aid

% students receiving any aid	70
% students receiving grants	15
% students receiving loans	70
% aid that is merit-based	15
Average grant	$1,000
Average loan	$13,000
Average debt	$65,000

NATIONAL COLLEGE OF NATURAL MEDICINE

NATIONAL COLLEGE OF NATURAL MEDICINE

049 SW PORTER STREET, PORTLAND, OR 97201 • ADMISSION: 503-552-1660 • FAX: 503-499-0027
E-MAIL: ADMISSIONS@NCNM.EDU • WEBSITE: WWW.NCNM.EDU

STUDENT BODY

Type	Private
Enrollment of parent institution	517
Enrollment of medical school	422
% male/female	20/80
% underrepresented minorities	2
% international	15
# countries represented	5
Average age of entering class	28

FACULTY

Total faculty	80
% female faculty	56
% minority faculty	12
% part-time faculty	78
Student-faculty ratio	5.0:1

ADMISSIONS

# applied	224
% accepted	82
% enrolled	55

Average GPA and MCAT Scores

Overall GPA	3.4

Application Information

Regular application	2/1
Early application	11/1
Are transfers accepted?	Yes
Admissions may be deferred?	Yes
Admissions need-blind?	No
Application fee	$75

Academics

The National College of Natural Medicine is the oldest naturopathic medical college in North America. Its mission is clear: To educate and train physicians and pre-professionals in the art, science and research of natural medicine. Naturopathic medicine is a patient-centered primary care approach that uses natural means to restore and optimize health. It is a distinct system of health care—an art, science, philosophy and practice of diagnosing, treating and preventing disease. Naturopathic medicine emphasizes the treatment of disease through the stimulation, enhancement, and support of the inherent healing power of the body. Methods of treatment respect this natural healing process and emphasize maintaining wellness over suppressing symptoms. Therapeutic modalities include clinical nutrition, botanical medicine, homeopathy, mind/body medicine, minor surgery, naturopathic midwifery, IV therapy, physical medicine and pharmacotherapy. In addition to its naturopathic medicine program, NCNM also offers masters degree programs in classical Chinese medicine and integrative medicine research. Concurrent with the naturopathic degree program, many students elect to take an additional degree program to expand the scope of their knowledge.

Established in June of 2003 at the National College of Natural Medicine, the Helfgott Research Institute (Helfgott) is a professionally independent, nonprofit institute whose mission is to conduct rigorous, high-quality research on the art and science of healing, specifically working to understand natural forms of medicine. Together, scientists from the fields of naturopathic medicine, Chinese medicine, acupuncture, immunology, and nutrition work with students to apply their expertise to the study of natural medicine.

The NCNM library has one of the best collections of books on natural medicine in North America. It houses over 18,000 volumes and maintains a large collection of rare and historic books. The Rare Book Room began with donations from the estate of Dr. Benedict Lust in 1985. Dr. Lust, regarded as the "Father of Naturopathy," emigrated from Germany to the United States in 1892 after studying with many prominent European Nature Cure doctors, including Sebastian Kneipp.

BASIC SCIENCES: Students are trained as primary care physicians, with the first two years of study focused on basic sciences and clinical diagnosis. Courses include biochemistry; human physiology; histology; anatomy; macro-and microbiology; immunology; human pathology; neuroscience; and pharmacology. The curriculum is structured to provide a solid scientific understanding of the body while maintaining the philosophies inherent to naturopathic medicine. Students of naturopathic medicine use Western medical sciences as a foundation on which to build a thorough knowledge of natural, holistic therapies, such as botanical medicine, nutrition and homeopathy, while they develop skills in diagnosis, disease prevention and wellness optimization.

CLINICAL TRAINING

Naturopathic clinical sciences present both the conventional and naturopathic perspective on diagnosis, prevention and treatment of disease by system. NCNM prides itself on offering the most complete clinical experience available. Students assist doctors in providing comprehensive patient care in all aspects of diagnosis and treatment. Naturopathic students can observe a broad range of acute or chronic medical conditions among a culturally diverse patient base at NCNM Clinic or at one of 12 other Portland-area community clinics, where NCNM offers free and low-cost health care to underserved populations.

Students

A haven for those seeking well-being, community, culture, and an environment steeped in natural beauty, Portland, Oregon, is an ideal place for studying natural medicine. Students enroll from every state in the U.S. and more than a dozen countries worldwide. The city offers an eclectic mix of people and ideas with a common thread of sustainability and social justice. A model of livability, Portland is surrounded by sweeping vistas of natural beauty, and close to an astonishing array of natural environments, including the Columbia Gorge, old-growth forests, coastal ocean towns, majestic mountain peaks, and high desert. Portland is home to a variety of medical schools including naturopathic medicine, classical and traditional Chinese medicine, conventional Western medicine, and chiropractic medicine, making it unique in its perspective on health and healing.

STUDENT LIFE

Portland offers a wide variety of neighborhoods, community gardens, a diversity of pubs, restaurants and food carts, and an avid culture of bicycle enthusiasts. NCNM has a wide variety of clubs and organizations, including clubs to help students develop their professional skills. There are groups for every interest, from Natural Doctors International and the NCNM Business Club, to AWARE, which supports campus diversity on campus, to the Beth Shalom Club or the Herb Society. Students actively advocate for natural medicine through the American Association of Naturopathic Physicians and state affiliates, the Naturopathic Medical Student Association and by organizing events with medical students from other Portland institutions. NCNM has soccer, basketball, ultimate Frisbee and dragon boat teams.

GRADUATES

NCNM graduates leave school with the knowledge and skills required to succeed in their licensing exams. Graduates also receive institutional support through extensive continuing education and a vast network of alumni. The college is alma mater to over 2,200 alumni who practice medicine across the U.S. and several continents. In addition to maintaining private practices, many NCNM graduates have earned international reputations through publications, research, and conferences and symposia.

Admissions

REQUIREMENTS

Applicants must have a bachelor's degree (or its equivalent) from a regionally accredited college or university. There is no advantage to holding a BS rather than a BA, as long as you have completed the program's prerequisites. Credit will only be given for prerequisite coursework earning a C or better. Applicants may apply with coursework still in progress; however, the Office of Admissions must receive all official transcripts showing completed coursework prior to matriculation. For the purpose of prerequisites, the Office of Admissions defines a "course" as either a quarter or semester term. Prerequisites are as follows: Mathematics (1 course), General Chemistry with lab (2 courses), Organic Chemistry (2 courses), General Biology with lab (2 courses), Physics (1 course), Social Science (2 courses, at least one course must be in general psychology), Humanities (2 courses at least one course must be English composition).

SUGGESTIONS

Strongly recommended courses: Biochemistry or Cellular Biology; Anatomy. Other recommended courses: Statistics; Business; and/or Marketing. Other suggested courses: Biomedical; Ethics; Philosophy of Science; Public Speaking; Microbiology; Immunology; Public Health.

PROCESS

Applicants must submit the following items, which are required to complete an application: 1) Submit an admission application online or mail to NCNM. 2) $75 Application fee. 3) Application essays. 4) Transcripts from all attended colleges and universities mailed directly to NCNM. 5) Two letters of recommendation. 6) On campus interview upon invitation.

Admissions Requirements (Required)

Essays, Science GPA, Non-Science GPA, Recommendation, Interview

Admissions Requirements (Optional)

StandardizedTest, Extracurricular activities, Exposure to medical profession, State Residency

COSTS AND AID

Tuition & Fees

Annual tuition	$24,150
Room & board	$20,400
Cost of books	$3,600
Fees (in-state/out-of-state)	$608

SOUTHWEST COLLEGE OF NATUROPATHIC MEDICINE

SOUTHWEST COLLEGE OF NATUROPATHIC MEDICINE

2140 E. BROADWAY ROAD, TEMPE, AZ 85282 • ADMISSION: 888-882-7266 • FAX: 480-858-9116
E-MAIL: ADMISSIONS@SCNM.EDU • WEBSITE: WWW.SCNM.EDU

STUDENT BODY

Type	Private
Enrollment of parent institution	0
Enrollment of medical school	411
% male/female	27/73
% underrepresented minorities	1
% out-of-state	65
% international	34
# countries represented	11
Average age of entering class	29

FACULTY

Total faculty	80
% female faculty	61
% part-time faculty	66
Student-faculty ratio	9.0:1

ADMISSIONS

# applied	212
% accepted	65
% enrolled	70

Average GPA and MCAT Scores

Overall GPA	3.2

Application Information

Regular application	2/1
Regular notification	3/1
Early application	12/15
Early notification	1/15
Are transfers accepted?	Yes
Admissions may be deferred?	Yes
Admissions need-blind?	No
Application fee	$115

Academics

Celebrating its 20th anniversary, Southwest College of Naturopathic Medicine (SCNM) trains world-class physicians focused on treating the patient's root cause of their condition using research-based natural therapies, as well as conventional medicine when necessary. Students in this four-year, accredited doctoral program receive the same rigorous education as an allopathic medical student and learn how to treat patients with natural, effective treatments. Naturopathic doctors (NDs) are general family practitioners trained as specialist in preventative medicine and natural therapies and see patients for everything from pediatrics to geriatrics, diabetes to pain management and everything in between. Students are trained in the use of natural therapies such as nutrition, botanical medicine, acupuncture, oriental medicine, counseling, homeopathy and hydrotherapy to treat disease, and combine these therapies with conventional medical treatments when appropriate. The Principles of naturopathic medicine, the Therapeutic order and patient centered care are at the core of the SCNM didactic and clinical curriculum. SCNM is accredited by the Council on Naturopathic Medical Education (CNME) and The Higher Learning Commission of the North Central Association of Colleges and Schools.

BASIC SCIENCES: Many of the features of the curriculum are delivered in "blocks" where course content is organized in a meaningful way that provides for ease of learning, the necessary progression of medical education, and also supports the principles of adult learning theory. These content locks represent formerly distinct courses by organizing the content as units of instruction within the block rather than separate courses. for example, in the General Medical Diagnosis block, content is organized by body systems. Within each system, the pathology, diagnostic imaging, and clinical, physical, and lab diagnosis associated with that system are addressed.

CLINICAL TRAINING

The clinical training at SCNM is a key part of your medical education and starts on the first day of class. Under the supervision of attending physicians, students apply the scientific knowledge acquired in class to real-life clinical cases and develop the skills and confidences necessary to deliver patient-oriented care. Clinical rotations with NDs, MDs and DOs are available through the college's on-site medical center, SCNM's nine community clinics for the underserved, and off-site private practices, hospitals and treatment centers. On average, SCNM students treat 1,000 patients during the four-year program, significantly more than the minimum required to graduate.

Students

The campus is set on 15 Acres in the college town of Tempe, Arizona, home to Arizona State University. Campus grounds offer students beautiful and tranquil outdoor spaces to study, relax and play, all of course in the generously sunny and warm climate of Arizona.

STUDENT LIFE

The Southwest College campus culture is easy to sense, yet difficult to describe in words. Once you walk onto our campus, you'll feel the energy. This is a place for meaningful discovery, academic challenge, real-life experience, and lasting friendships. Students enroll at Southwest College and quickly realize they share a common bond in their passion for naturopathic medicine and a unified goal in making an impact in medicine and healthcare. More than 15 student clubs and organizations provide unlimited leadership, educational, social and cultural opportunities, as well as terrific resume-building material and networking opportunities for students. SCNM encourages student involvement in professional and community organizations which can range in variation. Here are just a few of the organization that are here on campus. Naturopaths Without Borders (NWB), a non-profit SCNM student-based organization, provides medical services abroad to underprivileged communities. SGA is the official voice of the SCNM student body. SGA representatives work closely with students and College administrators to work on policies and identify ways to best serve the campus and its students. SGA also sponsors several services and events, such as New Student Welcome Dinners, student activities, and student club/organizations. The American Association of Naturopathic Physicians (AANP) is the national professional society representing naturopathic physicians who are licensed or eligible for licensing as primary care providers. The Arizona Naturopathic Medical Association is the state professional society representing naturopathic physicians who are silenced or eligible for licensure in the state of Arizona. The purpose of the Homeopathic Society is to broaden and strengthen knowledge of homeopathy through readings and discussions of the Organon of Medicine, Materia Medica, and guest lectures. Imhotep Circle's Mission is to encourage and develop programs that promote unity and contribute to the education, welfare, and growth of underserved communities and the students of SCNM. This organization's goals are to raise funds for local programs, volunteer our time to benefit the underserved communities, and establish programs within the SCNM community that promote our mission. Naturopathic Public Awareness Campaign is dedicated to furthering and supporting current and future public awareness efforts for naturopathic medicine in the United States and Canada. In coordination with the AANP and the accredited naturopathic medical schools, we strive to expand public awareness of naturopathic medicine as a viable, affordable option for quality healthcare. As a strong naturopathic student organization, NPAC is an extremely effective vehicle for public health education and community outreach. Naturopathic Society International provides educational opportunities and resources concerning Naturopathic Philosophy for physicians and students of naturopathic medicine.

GRADUATES

The SCNM Alumni community is now more than 700 doctors strong, with graduates practicing across the United States and internationally. Alumni have made an important contribution to communities worldwide as well as the naturopathic medical profession.

Admissions

REQUIREMENTS

Application, application fee, professional essay, 3 letters of reference, official transcripts, professional resume and an in-person interview.

SUGGESTIONS

Visit our website www.scnm.edu for more information on our program and admission requirements. Please do not hesitate to contact us by phone 480-858-9100, toll free 1-888-882-SCNM (7266), or by email at admissions@scnm.edu with any questions you may have regarding application, naturopathic medicine, relocation, naturopathic career opportunities, etc.

PROCESS

Two intakes a year (Winter and Fall). Priority Application deadlines: February 1 for the Fall intake; December 1 for the Winter intake. Admissions process is on a rolling basis.

Admissions Requirements (Required)

Essays, Science GPA, Non-Science GPA, Recommendation, Interview

Admissions Requirements (Optional)

StandardizedTest, Extracurricular activities, Exposure to medical profession, State Residency

COSTS AND AID

Tuition & Fees

Annual tuition	$26,505
Room & board	$16,000
Cost of books	$4,000
Fees	$965

Financial Aid

% students receiving any aid	80
% students receiving grants	4
% students receiving loans	80
% aid that is merit-based	0
Average grant	$1,000
Average loan	$54,000
Average total aid package	$54,000
Average debt	$200,000

UNIVERSITY OF BRIDGEPORT
COLLEGE OF NATUROPATHIC MEDICINE

126 PARK AVENUE, BRIDGEPORT, CT 06604 • ADMISSION: 203-576-4532 • FAX: 203-576-4941
E-MAIL: LPROCTOR@BRIDGEPORT.EDU • WEBSITE: HTTP://WWW.BRIDGEPORT.EDU/ACADEMICS/GRADUATE/NATURO

Academics

University of Bridgeport College of Naturopathic Medicine provides an educational program for the training of generalist naturopathic physicians able to competently provide comprehensive natural health care. The College's mission is to provide appropriate educational experiences to prepare candidates to become doctors of naturopathic medicine. UBCNM's mission is to train the next generation of physicians as competent and caring clinicians; as insightful scholars and researchers; and as courageous leaders in the integration of natural medicine into the health care system. We provide comprehensive natural health care through the Integrated Health Science Center and in conjunction with a variety of community agencies. Students are involved with our research department, which conducts basic and clinical research on natural and alternative therapeutics. We offer joint degree programs as ND/MS in Acupuncture and ND/MS in Nutrition. University of Bridgeport library supports student/faculty research with over 272,000 volumes of classified books and bound journals/indexes and over 1,128,000 microforms, subscribes to more than 1,100 periodicals.

BASIC SCIENCES: First two years of the program focus on basic science courses such as anatomy, physiology, biochemistry, histology, microbiology, embryology, pathology, research methods, public health, clinical and laboratory diagnosis, counseling, nutrition, history and philosophy of naturopathic medicine. These basic science courses are the foundation of clinical education and training at UBCNM.

CLINICAL TRAINING

First and second year students are exposed to the clinic including grand rounds and patient care classes. Third and fourth year of ND education at UBCNM focus on clinical education. Focus of the clinical education is diagnosis and therapeutics which includes botanical medicine, homeopathy, clinical nutrition, physical medicine, obstetrics and gynecology, pediatrics, geriatrics, cardiology, gasteroenterology, Eye & ENT, diagnostic imaging, pharmacology, environmental medicine, endocrinology, neurology, urology/proctology, oncology, dermatology and hydrotherapy. Students receive their clinical training at the University's own Health Science Center and at various off-site clinics through supervised internships.

Students

University of Bridgeport was founded in 1927 as the junior College of Connecticut—the first junior college chartered by any legislature in the northeastern states. The Junior College of Connecticut became the University of Bridgeport in 1947. University is located on a 86 acre picturesque Long Island Sound 50 miles north of New York City. The architectural diversity of UB's seventy five buildings, from stately homes as well as newer structures of modern design, reflects the origins and progress of the university and also embodies its twofold commitment to solidity and change. University of Bridgeport offers a wide range of opportunities for students to learn about other cultures and to understand American culture. Students from approximately 80 countries attend the University. College of Naturopathic Medicine was founded in 1997, is an integral part of the University of Bridgeport. It is the only College of Naturopathic Medicine in the eastern United States. The main Magnus Wahlstrom Library occupies 5 floors in the centrally located Wahlstrom Building, supports student/faculty research with over 272,000 volumes of classified books. UB has a large Dining Hall, Café, Recreation Center. University supports a wide range of clubs, organizations (more than 30 clubs or organizations) and special interest groups that expand and cultivate the academic, professional and cultural interests of the students.

STUDENT LIFE

Being a part of the large university, Naturopathic students at the University of Bridgeport are always involved in activities with other programs within UB or within the Division of Health Sciences programs which includes Naturopathic medicine, Chiropractic, Acupuncture Institute, Human Nutrition and Dental Hygiene. Students are involved in the decision making process of the university as well as the college of Naturopathic Medicine through various committees. Naturopathic Student Government Association and college administration work very closely.

GRADUATES

Graduates of University of Bridgeport College of naturopathic Medicine are trained and qualified primary health care professionals who are qualified to pass professional licensure exams and are prepared to set up and maintain private practices. Some of UB's graduates have joined group practices and are part of research teams in various medical universities. Depending on the state laws their scope of practice varies but includes all aspects of family care.

Admissions

REQUIREMENTS

A completed application through NDCAS with fee, personal statement, three letters of recommendation, one must be from a health care provider, official transcripts from all colleges/universities attended. A bachelors degree is required with 6 semester hours of biology with lab (2 courses), 6 semester hours of general chemistry with lab, 6 semester hours of organic chemistry with lab, 3 semester hours of physics with lab, 3 semester hours of psychology, 6 semester hours (2 courses) of communication/language skills, 3 semester hours of social science, 3 semester hours of humanities and 9 semester hours of elective courses. Earned grades of C- or below are not accepted. All the science courses must be completed within last seven years. Applicants meeting all the requirements are invited for interview.

SUGGESTIONS

Although we have rolling admissions, it is better to apply early. Late applications are considered on a space available basis.

PROCESS

Acceptance decision is made by the admission committee and is based on academic achievement, relevant experience, knowledge of naturopathic philosophy, personal standard of ethics, financial planning and demonstrated verbal communication ability and personal attitude.

Admissions Requirements (Required)

Essays, Science GPA, Non-Science GPA, Recommendation, Interview

Admissions Requirements (Optional)

Extracurricular activities, Exposure to medical profession, State Residency

COSTS AND AID

Tuition & Fees

Annual tuition	$24,750
Room & board	$16,300
Cost of books	$1,000

Financial Aid

% students receiving loans	100
Average loan	$90

9 Osteopathic Profiles

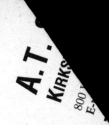

Still University of Health Sciences

...sville College of Osteopathic Medicine

West Jefferson, Kirksville, MO 63501 • **Admission:** 660-626-2237 • **Fax:** 660-626-2969
...ail: ADMISSIONS@ATSU.EDU • **Website:** WWW.ATSU.EDU

STUDENT BODY

Type	Private
Enrollment of parent institution	3,314
Enrollment of medical school	684
% male/female	59/41
% underrepresented minorities	1
% out-of-state	69
% international	14
# countries represented	9
Average age of entering class	25

FACULTY

Total faculty	75
% female faculty	20
% minority faculty	13
% part-time faculty	44
Student-faculty ratio	4.5:1

ADMISSIONS

# applied	4,110
% accepted	10
% enrolled	40

Average GPA and MCAT Scores

Overall GPA	3.6
MCAT Bio	9.4
MCAT Phys	8.5
MCAT Verbal	8.9
MCAT Essay	0

Application Information

Regular application	2/1
Regular notification	
Early application	8/1
Early notification	10/15
Are transfers accepted?	Yes
Admissions may be deferred?	Yes
Admissions need-blind?	No
Application fee	$70

Academics

The Kirksville College of Osteopathic Medicine is the founding school of osteopathic medicine, and is distinguished by offering an education firmly based on holistic care, wellness, and academic excellence. Kirksville has a reputation for training physicians in primary care areas, as well as providing a strong clinical and basic science education for specialization. A clerkship with a primary care physician is included in the first-year curriculum. Traditional tenets of osteopathic medicine are coupled with the use of all modern technology, thus providing a well-rounded, comprehensive education. Problem solving and critical thinking are emphasized in both the basic science courses and clinical training. Clinical rotations currently take place in one of the following areas: Arizona, Illinois, Michigan, Missouri, Ohio, Pennsylvania, Utah, and New Jersey. Kirksville is a community of approximately 20,000 residents. With a 2013 class size of 172, the average age is 25 with a composite MCAT of 27 and an overall GPA of 3.50.

Admissions

REQUIREMENTS

As a private institution, no preference is given to Missouri residents, and almost all states are represented in the student body. Course requirements are Biology (8 semester hours); Chemistry (8 hours); Organic Chemistry (8 hours); Physics (8 hours); and English (6 hours). To be considered for admission, applicants should have a minimum GPA of 2.8 in both the sciences and overall. The MCAT is required and scores must be no more than three years old. About 15 percent of AACOMAS applicants are interviewed, with interviews consisting of two sessions with faculty and/or administrators. Financial aid, both merit- and need-based, is available in the form of grants and loans.

PROCESS

The Kirksville College of Osteopathic Medicine participates with other osteopathic colleges in a centralized application processing service called the American Association of Colleges of Osteopathic Medicine Application Service (AACOMAS) An application may be submitted online at https://aacomas.aacom.org/. Applicants meeting the minimum 2.8 cumulative and science grade point average requirement will receive a KCOM secondary application. A non-refundable application fee of $70 and letters of evaluation from a premed committee/science faculty member and a physician are required at the time the additional information is submitted. Applications should be submitted no later than February 1 of the academic year prior to which admission is sought. Applicants are encouraged to apply far in advance of the February 1 deadline. As "The National College of Osteopathic Medicine," KCOM seeks students from all parts of the United States who are interested in a career in osteopathic medicine. The college also actively seeks and encourages underrepresented minority students to apply.

Admissions Requirements (Required)

MCAT Scores, Essays, Science GPA, Extracurricular activities, Non-Science GPA, Exposure to medical profession, Recommendation, Interview

COSTS AND AID

Tuition & Fees

Annual tuition	$46,950
Cost of books	$3,282
Fees	$787

Financial Aid

% students receiving any aid	97
% students receiving grants	64
% students receiving loans	94
% aid that is merit-based	14
Average grant	$24,371
Average loan	$57,688
Average total aid package	$63,584
Average debt	$211,987

DES MOINES UNIVERSITY
COLLEGE OF OSTEOPATHIC MEDICINE

3200 GRAND AVENUE, DES MOINES, IA 50312-4198 • ADMISSION: 515-271-1451 • FAX: 515-271-7163
E-MAIL: DOADMIT@DMU.EDU • WEBSITE: WWW.DMU.EDU

STUDENT BODY

Type	Private
Enrollment of parent institution	1,783
Enrollment of medical school	872
% male/female	47/53
% underrepresented minorities	2
% out-of-state	71
% international	13
# countries represented	4
Average age of entering class	25

FACULTY

Total faculty	62
% female faculty	32
% minority faculty	1
% part-time faculty	35
Student-faculty ratio	13.0:1

ADMISSIONS

# applied	3,139
% accepted	16
% enrolled	45

Average GPA and MCAT Scores

Overall GPA	3.7
MCAT Bio	9.7
MCAT Phys	8.7
MCAT Verbal	8.8
MCAT Essay	0

Application Information

Regular application	2/1
Are transfers accepted?	Yes
Admissions may be deferred?	Yes
Admissions need-blind?	No
Application fee	$50

Academics

At the Des Moines University College of Osteopathic Medicine, students learn within a supportive environment. This includes a solid basic sciences education, extensive practical experience in the clinical setting, and one-on-one interaction with seasoned educators and clinicians. The curriculum emphasizes state-of-the-art standardized patient assessment laboratories and problem-based learning opportunities which emphasize critical thinking and problem solving. The college is the second-oldest osteopathic school. Located in a safe metropolitan setting, the campus offers proximity to affordable housing. A new 143,000-square-foot Student Education Center provides students with modern facilities and a location to exercise, relax, and learn. Other distinguishing features of DMU include a wireless campus, laptop and hand-held computers for incoming students, and a dual master's degree program in Health Care Administration or Public Health. The College of Osteopathic Medicine provides a flexible program which allows students to explore a range of professional goals. Students learn to consider the overall needs of the patient rather than an isolated medical problem. During the first two years, basic science lectures and laboratory studies are combined with experience in hospitals, clinics, and community service agencies. This pre-clinical phase features a systems approach and the innovative use of simulated patients. The last two years of the four-year program involve clinical training. Third- and fourth-year rotations in hospitals and clinics may be selected from sites across the country.

BASIC SCIENCES: The College of Osteopathic Medicine provides a flexible program which allows students to explore a range of professional goals. Students learn to consider the overall needs of the patient rather than an isolated medical problem. During the first two years, basic science lectures and laboratory studies are combined with experience in hospitals, clinics, and community service agencies. This pre-clinical phase features a systems approach and the innovative use of simulated patients. The last two years of the four-year program involve clinical training. Third- and fourth-year rotations in hospitals and clinics may be selected from sites across the country.

CLINICAL TRAINING
The College of Osteopathic Medicine provides a flexible program which allows students to explore a range of professional goals. Students learn to consider the overall needs of the patient rather than an isolated medical problem. During the first two years, basic science lectures and laboratory studies are combined with experience in hospitals, clinics, and community service agencies. This pre-clinical phase features a systems approach and the innovative use of simulated patients. The last two years of the four-year program involve clinical training. Third- and fourth-year rotations in hospitals and clinics may be selected from sites across the country.

Students

Students enjoy a collaborative environment. Campus facilities include a wellness center, student game room and lounge, on-campus dining, and a library with comfortable study areas.

STUDENT LIFE

Each entering class has about 220 students. A wide variety of undergraduate majors are represented, ranging from biology to the humanities. Though the average age of incoming students is 25, student ages range from the early 20's to the 40's. Beyond classes and labs, students have numerous opportunities to get involved and meet others through community service, clubs, and social events. From the beginning, 1st year students are paired up with 2nd year students as part of Big Sib/Little Sib. DMU also offers peer tutoring. Over 40 professional clubs and organizations invite students to become part of a larger community of students and student concerns. Many students also get involved in community outreach. Through events such as the Senior Health Fair, they provide free medical screening. The Literacy Army tutors reading and other subjects to elementary schools. At various local races and marathons DMU students provide free OMM to the involved athletes.

GRADUATES

Graduates may enter residency programs in any specialty or subspecialty area. Des Moines University has over 9,000 alumni in virtually every state in the nation.

Admissions

REQUIREMENTS

Eight semester hours (with lab) each in biology, chemistry,and physics (or four hours of physics and a statistics course); four hours of organic chemistry; and three semester hours of biochemistry are required. In addition, applicants must have taken six semester hours of English. We accept students without regard to legal state of residence. Usually 70 percent of students are from states other than Iowa. You can apply while working on your undergraduate degree but you should have plans to receive it by the time you register with the College. The MCAT (taken within the last two years) is required.

SUGGESTIONS

Recommended courses include: cell biology, microbiology, immunology, physiology, and anatomy.

PROCESS

AACOMAS application required. Those AACOMAS applicants who meet the minimum requirements for GPA and MCAT are sent secondary applications and about half of those who return secondary applications are invited for an interview. Notification occurs on a rolling basis.

Admissions Requirements (Required)

MCAT Scores, Essays, Science GPA, Extracurricular activities, Non-Science GPA, Exposure to medical profession, Recommendation, Interview

Admissions Requirements (Optional)

State Residency

COSTS AND AID

Tuition & Fees

Annual tuition	$35,840
Cost of books	$3,966
Fees	$0

Financial Aid

% students receiving any aid	95
% students receiving grants	32
% students receiving loans	88
Average grant	$22,287
Average loan	$47,865
Average total aid package	$52,333
Average debt	$171,257

EDWARD VIA COLLEGE OF OSTEOPATHIC MEDICINE

EDWARD VIA COLLEGE OF OSTEOPATHIC MEDICINE-CAROLINAS CAMPUS

VCOM OFFICE OF ADMISSIONS, 350 HOWARD STREET SPARTANBURG, SC 29303 • ADMISSION: 864-327-9800
FAX: 864-804-6986 • E-MAIL: ADMISSIONS-CAROLINAS@CAROLINAS.VCOM.EDU • WEBSITE: WWW.VCOM.VT.EDU

STUDENT BODY

Type	Private
Enrollment of medical school	321
% male/female	47/53
% out-of-state	50
% international	14
Average age of entering class	24

FACULTY

Total faculty	1,013
% female faculty	21
% minority faculty	12
% part-time faculty	98
Student-faculty ratio	1.1:1

ADMISSIONS

# applied	2,305
% accepted	10
% enrolled	68

Average GPA and MCAT Scores

Overall GPA	3.6
MCAT Bio	9.0
MCAT Phys	8.0
MCAT Verbal	8.0
MCAT Essay	0

Application Information

Regular application	2/1
Early application	11/1
Are transfers accepted?	Yes
Admissions may be deferred?	Yes
Admissions need-blind?	Yes
Application fee	$50

Academics

The MISSION of the Edward Via College of Osteopathic Medicine (VCOM) is to prepare globally minded, community-focused physicians for the rural and medically underserved areas of Virginia, North Carolina, South Carolina and the Appalachian Region, and to improve human health especially of those most in need. VCOM's faculty, staff, and students VALUE: Professionalism, integrity, duty, compassion, altruism, knowledge, and critical thinking. VCOM Goals 1) To provide education in the art and science of osteopathic medicine. 2) To recruit and graduate students who will address health care disparities including those related to rural locations, minority populations, or poverty status. Priority 1) Recruit students from, and educate students in, rural and medically underserved areas of Virginia, North Carolina, South Carolina, and the Appalachian Region. Priority 2) Recruit students with a strong desire to care for medically underserved populations. 3) To provide medical students with experiences that promote an understanding of global healthcare and disaster medicine. 4) To provide osteopathic medical education and research focused on evidence-based medicine, patient centered care, the body's innate ability to heal, the relationship of structure to function, and the clinical application of osteopathic manipulation. 5) To generate, promote, and disseminate medical knowledge in disease prevention, chronic disease management, community health, and public health practices. 6) To advance scientific knowledge through biomedical and clinical research. 7) To partner with hospitals, healthcare organizations, and health care providers who value medical education and healthcare for the medically underserved. 8) To serve as an advocate for osteopathic medicine, rural health, and affordable, accessible healthcare for the medically underserved. In 2010, VCOM added a second campus in Spartanburg, South Carolina. VCOM – Carolinas Campus, the sister campus to the VCOM – Virginia Campus, matriculated it's inaugural class in 2011. The addition of the Carolinas Campus allows VCOM to increase the presence and involvement in the Appalachian region as well as the ability to greater meet the mission of the school.

BASIC SCIENCES: All courses in the first two years are available to students on computer through Scholar. The computer based materials are placed on Scholar in order to augment student learning where minimal note taking is required in class. This leaves valuable classroom time for faculty/student interaction. Block 1) begins the curriculum at the cellular level with courses including: Cell Biology and Physiology, Microbiology, Immunology, Genetics and Embryology. In addition students are introduced to Pathology and Pharmacology, as well as a course in Professionalism and Medical Ethics. Blocks 2-8) are comprehensive system based blocks and include courses in Anatomy, Physiology, Pharmacology and Pathology. Principles of Primary Care is extended throughout all blocks and includes Physical Diagnosis, Introduction to Osteopathic Manipulation and Behavioral Medicine topics. Clinical Case Correlations brings the cases with the medical disciplines aligned with the blocks. These include Immunology and Hematology, Dermatology, Cardiopulmonary System, Neurological, Psychiatry, and Musculoskeletal Systems, Gastrointestinal and Endocrine Systems, Nutrition, and Renal and Genitourinary Systems. Students also have Early Clinical Experiences throughout the pre-clinical years which include experiences such as: Geriatrics, Palliative care, Free Clinics, Appalachian Medical Missions, Gynecologic experience, Clinical Skills training, Laboratory Medicine, and Radiology rounds.

Students

Via Wellness – VCOM sponsors social, fitness, spiritual, cultural, and vocational activities throughout the year. "Via Wellness" strives to promote balance in the busy lives of medical students and provides incentives for participation in a spectrum of activities. Information and a schedule of activities sponsored through "Via Wellness" are available from the VCOM Office of Student Services and are listed on the Activities Calendar. VCOM operates with a collaborative agreement with Virginia Tech for research and for student activities. The VCOM Passport provides osteopathic medical students full access to recreational and athletic facilities on the Virginia Tech campus, admittance to social and cultural events, use of the library and bus transportation to the main campus and the bus routes. In instances where Virginia Tech assesses a fee for its students for activities (e.g., rental of equipment, admittance fees to special events, etc.), VCOM students are typically required to pay the same fee as a Virginia Tech student. Following are a partial list of activities and services available to VCOM students through the collaborative agreement with Virginia Tech. Hokie Sports – Tickets for Hokie Varsity Sports are available to VCOM students in the same manner they are available to Virginia Tech students. Recreational Access – Access to swimming pools and fitness centers in McComas and War Memorial Halls, as well as golf and tennis facilities, are available to VCOM students. Venture Out sponsors low risk outdoor adventures and rental of camping gear, canoes, and stoves for outdoor activities. The Venture Out Resource Center located at 117C Squires Student Center on the Virginia Tech campus. Intramural sports at Virginia Tech are available to VCOM students. Visit www.recsports.vt.edu for a listing of programs and registration deadlines. BreakZone provides billiard tables, bowling, table tennis, and pottery and is located in 117 Squires Student Center on the Virginia Tech campus.

Admissions

PROCESS

Step 1: AACOMAS Application. Submit an application to the centralized application service, American Association of Colleges of Osteopathic Medicine Application Service (AACCOMAS), and designate VCOM. Applications may not be submitted directly to VCOM. In order to process your application, AACOMAS will require official copies of your transcripts from all colleges/universities you attended. Please also submit your official MCAT scores from AAMC to AACOMAS. Remember to send transcripts directly to AACOMAS. Request your MCAT scores to be sent from AAMC to AACOMAS. AACOMAS Application Deadline: February 1. Step 2: Secondary Application. Once VCOM receives your AACOMAS application, your file will undergo initial screening. VCOM will invite competitive applicants to submit a Secondary Application. Please be advised, VCOM screens applications before sending the invitation to submit the Secondary Application and not all applicants will receive the invitation. The Secondary Application deadline in March 15. Step 3: Letters of Recommendation. VCOM requires two letters of recommendation – one from an osteopathic physician and one from a premedical committee or science faculty member. All letters must be written on professional letterhead, signed, and submitted directly to VCOM. VCOM is willing to accept letters through VirtualEvals, Interfolio, and college/university service. Candidates are welcome to submit additional letters of recommendation including a letter of recommendation from an allopathic physician (MD). However, the letter of recommendation from a MD cannot be substituted for the required letter of recommendation from a DO. VCOM provides evaluation forms for the osteopathic physician and premedical advisor or science faculty member as a resource. The evaluation forms are not required.

Admissions Requirements (Required)

MCAT Scores, Essays, Science GPA, Extracurricular activities, Non-Science GPA, Exposure to medical profession, Recommendation, Interview, State Residency

COSTS AND AID

Tuition & Fees

Annual tuition	$39,740
Cost of books	$2,137
Fees	$250

Financial Aid

% students receiving any aid	95
% students receiving grants	11
% students receiving loans	94
Average grant	$22,899
Average loan	$57,634
Average total aid package	$57,875

Kansas City University of Medicine and Biosciences
College of Osteopathic Medicine

Office of Admissions, 1750 Independence Ave, Kansas City, MO • **Admission:** 800-234-4847
Fax: 816-460-0566 • **E-mail:** admissions@kcumb.edu • **Website:** www.kcumb.edu

STUDENT BODY

Type	Private
Enrollment of parent institution	100
Enrollment of medical school	887
% male/female	50/50
% underrepresented minorities	2
% out-of-state	75
% international	18
# countries represented	9
Average age of entering class	24

FACULTY

Total faculty	54
% female faculty	54
% minority faculty	6
% part-time faculty	100
Student-faculty ratio	8.0:1

ADMISSIONS

# applied	2,400
% accepted	20
% enrolled	51

Average GPA and MCAT Scores

Overall GPA	3.5
MCAT Bio	8.6
MCAT Phys	8.1
MCAT Verbal	8.1
MCAT Essay	Q

Application Information

Regular application	2/6
Are transfers accepted?	No
Admissions may be deferred?	Yes
Admissions need-blind?	No
Application fee	$50

Academics

Kansas City University of Medicine and Biosciences is both the largest medical school in the state of Missouri and the oldest in Kansas City, Missouri. Affordable and friendly, Kansas City's metropolitan area encompasses counties in both Kansas and Missouri. The University's core values, leadership, humility, faith and positivity, integrity, compassion and service. These core values, coupled with exemplary basic sciences and clinical training, are at the heart of the KCUMB educational process from a student's first day on campus to the end of postdoctoral training and beyond. In 2006, 51 percent of the entering class was female, and the average age was 24. The age range of the class was 20–48 with a class size of 250. During their years at KCUMB, the University helps its students build on that foundation by offering a progressive and innovative 21st-century curriculum that emphasizes early clinical experience and an integrated, patient-centered approach to medicine. An outstanding faculty who keep students' interests uppermost and state-of-the-art facilities provide unparalleled educational opportunities. High standards and educational excellence make KCUMB an award-winning academic institution, but it is the human dimension that makes KCUMB such a meaningful and special place.

CLINICAL TRAINING

KCUMB puts the patient at the center of the learning process with an innovative new curriculum launched in 2000. This curriculum eliminates the artificial separation of the basic and clinical sciences, integrating all essential concepts and information into a seamless continuum of clinical presentations. The foundations of anatomy, biochemistry, epidemiology, genetics, immunology, pathology, pharmacology, physiology, and the clinical disciplines of internal medicine, pediatrics, family medicine, surgery, Ob/Gyn and psychiatry are incorporated into clinical presentations. Topics such as health-care policy, medical informatics, and health and wellness are integrated into the curricular structure. The case-based, patient-centered curriculum prepares students to begin analyzing and integrating medical information in a format used by medical practitioners. This approach integrates the basic and clinical sciences from the first day of medical school rather than the traditional postponing of meaningful clinical interaction and decision-making until the third year of medical school. A variety of teaching and learning methods are used in the first two years. These methods include classroom lectures, laboratory exercises, small-group discussions, computer-assisted instruction, specialized workshops, the use of standardized patients and other simulated clinical activities.

Students

While the Kansas City area might be best known for its smooth jazz, beautiful fountains and superior barbecue, the area has so much to offer—from upscale shopping districts and world-class entertainment to ample recreational activities and thrilling professional sporting events, to name a few. Located at the junction of the Missouri and Kansas rivers, Kansas City sits in the middle of the United States, about 1,900 miles from each coast. Approximately 1.8 million people live in the Kansas City metro area, which includes more than 135 cities in 11 counties on both sides of the state line. In the historic northeast area of Kansas City, the KCUMB campus is just minutes from the Country Club Plaza, Arrowhead and Kauffman stadiums, the Nelson-Atkins Museum of Art, the Negro Leagues Baseball Museum, Worlds of Fun, Oceans of Fun, Union Station and the River Market. The city and its surrounding communities offer a combination of urban sophistication and small-town friendliness that is distinctly Kansas City.

Admissions

REQUIREMENTS

The minimum academic requirements for admission to the first year class are: 1. The Medical College Admissions Test (MCAT). The MCAT is administered in April and August of every year. 2. A baccalaureate degree, or commendable completion of at least three-fourths (90 semester hours or 135 term credit hours) of the required credits for a baccalaureate degree, from a regionally accredited college or university. The baccalaureate degree is preferred and preference is given to those candidates who will have earned the degree prior to matriculation in the medical school program. 3. Satisfactory completion, with a grade of C or higher, of the following college courses, including laboratory work: Biological Sciences (12 Semester Hours); Chemistry (13 Semester Hours); Bio Chemistry (in addition to Chemistry hours—3 Semester Hours); Genetics (in addition to Biological Sciences—3 Semester Hours); Physics (8 Semester Hours); English Composition/Literature (6 Semester Hours); Total 45 Semester Hours.

SUGGESTIONS

Applicants are encouraged to begin the application process a year prior to matriculation. The following represents a monthly guide for application preparation. May Contact all colleges and universities attended and have official transcripts forwarded directly from the educational institution to AACOMAS. May Submit AACOMAS application. Supplemental application or materials are mailed to qualified applicants immediately upon receipt of the AACOMAS application in the admissions office. Sept. Personal interviews begin. Feb. 1 Application deadline (AACOMAS). Supplemental applications are accepted and processed until all interview positions have been filled. Feb. 15 Transcript deadline to AACOMAS.

PROCESS

All application materials, including detailed instructions, can be accessed through the AACOM website, http://www.aacom.org. AACOMAS gathers all the necessary material about each applicant and transmits the information in a standardized format to the college(s) of osteopathic medicine selected by the applicant. AACOMAS has no participation in the selection process. The applicant will receive from AACOMAS a computer-generated applicant profile with a calculation of GPA and MCAT averages. KCUMB also will receive the applicant profile, accompanied by a photocopy of the AACOMAS application and personal statement. KCUMB conducts an initial review of the transmitted AACOMAS application, MCAT scores, and academic record to determine which applications will be further processed. Applicants meeting the initial review criteria will receive a KCUMB supplemental application. A supplemental application may be forwarded to an applicant under some circumstances when specific information is not available or will be submitted later. These circumstances generally relate to applicants who have not taken the MCAT and/or are registered to take the next scheduled MCAT exam. Applicants are encouraged to include the scheduled MCAT test dates on the AACOMAS application to indicate the intent of taking or retaking the exam.

Admissions Requirements (Required)

MCAT Scores, Essays, Science GPA, Extracurricular activities, Non-Science GPA, Exposure to medical profession, Recommendation, Interview

Admissions Requirements (Optional)

State Residency

COSTS AND AID

Tuition & Fees

Annual tuition	$41,013
Room & board	$16,500
Cost of books	$1,400
Fees	$175

Financial Aid

% students receiving any aid	96
% students receiving grants	7
% students receiving loans	93
% aid that is merit-based	0
Average grant	$1,500
Average loan	$40,000
Average total aid package	$46,000
Average debt	$154,000

LAKE ERIE COLLEGE OF OSTEOPATHIC MEDICINE

LAKE ERIE COLLEGE OF OSTEOPATHIC MEDICINE

OFFICE OF ADMISSIONS, 1858 WEST GRANDVIEW BOULEVARD, ERIE, PA 16509 • ADMISSION: 814-866-6641
FAX: 814-866-8123 • E-MAIL: ADMISSIONS@LECOM.EDU • WEBSITE: WWW.LECOM.EDU

STUDENT BODY

Type	Private
Enrollment of parent institution	0
Enrollment of medical school	1,091
% male/female	54/46
% out-of-state	67
# countries represented	0
Average age of entering class	25

ADMISSIONS

# applied	4,398

Average GPA and MCAT Scores

Overall GPA	3.4
MCAT Bio	9.0
MCAT Phys	8.0
MCAT Verbal	9.0
MCAT Essay	0

Application Information

Regular application	4/1
Early application	7/1
Early notification	9/1
Are transfers accepted?	No
Admissions may be deferred?	No
Admissions need-blind?	Yes
Application fee	$50

Academics

The Lake Erie College of Osteopathic Medicine main campus is located in Erie, Pennsylvania with an additional location in Greensburg, Pennsylvania. The College has a branch campus in Bradenton, Florida, is the nation's largest medical college. Its mission is to train physicians to meet the country's growing demand for health care professionals. The majority of LECOM graduates become primary care physicians. LECOM has introduced a new Primary Care Scholars Pathway that condenses four years of medical education into three years by concentrating on specific courses and clinical training required to become a family physician. LECOM recognizes student-centered learning styles by offering three additional curriculum pathways. The traditional, lecture-discussion curriculum begins with core basic science and preclinical courses and progresses with a systems-based curriculum in year two. Problem-based learning offers small group training following patient cases and Independent Study allows qualified students to use educational modules based on the core and systems curricula.

BASIC SCIENCES: All students are required to complete 12 weeks of Gross Anatomy in the first semester. Microbiology, immunology, physiology, pharmacology, biochemistry, pathology, health care management, and spirituality, medicine and ethics are the core of the Lecture-Discussion and Independent Study Pathways and integrated into the cases of the Problem-Based Learning Pathway.

CLINICAL TRAINING

Clinical education and training at LECOM begins in the first year through the History and Physical (H&P) Examination courses. Having documented competency in obtaining histories and physical examinations, all students are prepared to participate in clinical preceptor encounters during the second year. These encounters occur at the clinical preceptor's offices where students will have the opportunity to actively participate in actual patient encounters, obtaining histories and performing examinations. This begins the clinical experience that intensifies in years three and four as LECOM prepares students to become an osteopathic physician possessing the highest competencies in the profession. The program will educate students to become competent physicians who clearly recognize their roles as providers of comprehensive healthcare to the individual, to the family as a unit, and to communities. Osteopathic physicians must be able to function in the role of leader of the healthcare team to bring about needed change from the level of the individual to the level of the community. The ultimate intent of the program is to prepare physicians who will impact positively on the equality of healthcare and healthcare delivery systems and will improve access for individuals and their families.

Students

LECOM's main campus is located in Pennsylvania's fourth largest city and overlooks Lake Erie. The city is a resort community with a large number of tourist, entertainment and recreational facilities. Erie County has five colleges and supports several professional minor league teams in baseball, football and hockey. LECOM Bradenton is located in a master-planned community in one of the fastest growing regions of Florida. LECOM Bradenton is just a few miles east of the Florida Gulf Coast and located in Lakewood Ranch, a master-planned community between Sarasota and Bradenton. Tampa is less than an hour north of the campus. LECOM at Seton Hill is located on the campus of

Seton Hill University. This additional location of LECOM Erie is located among 200 beautiful acres of tree-lined hills in Greensburg, Pennsylvania. The campus is just 30 miles southeast of Pittsburgh.

STUDENT LIFE

LECOM encourages students to participate in community service and extra-curricular activities. LECOM clubs offer social activities and opportunities to become involved in local events. LECOM students have organized mentoring programs for under-served children, Boy Scout and Girl Scout Troops, and provided health care screening and other related services to local citizens.

GRADUATES

While the majority of LECOM graduates become primary care physicians, many alumni have completed residencies and fellowships in other medical specialties. LECOM has developed post-graduate training at 32 hospitals. Graduates have matched for residencies at major hospitals around the country.

Admissions

REQUIREMENTS

LECOM seeks applicants who not only have shown success in their science courses, but also have proven themselves as well-rounded individuals who have done well overall in their academic careers. Applicants must meet the following minimum admissions requirements: Applicants must complete a baccalaureate degree from an accredited college or university by the time of enrollment. Applicants participating in special affiliated programs with LECOM and other exceptions to this policy will be considered on an individual basis. Applicants must have a minimum 2.7 science grade point average. Successful candidates typically have both science and overall grade point averages of 3.2 or above. Applicants must meet the following specific course requirements: Biology: A minimum of eight semester hours, including two semester hours of laboratory work. These eight hours may consist of general biology or zoology, or a combination of biology, zoology, and botany. Inorganic Chemistry: A minimum of eight semester hours, including two semester hours of laboratory work. Organic Chemistry: A minimum of eight semester hours, including two semester hours of laboratory work. Physics: A minimum of eight semester hours, including two hours of laboratory work. English: A minimum of six semester hours of composition and literature. Behavioral Sciences: A minimum of six semester hours of courses in the behavioral sciences; i.e., psychology, sociology, anthropology, medical ethics, or philosophy. LECOM recommends that prospective students consider taking advanced coursework, such as biochemistry, physiology, microbiology, and/or anatomy, if at all possible. Each candidate must submit his or her most recent Medical College Admission Test (MCAT) scores. MCAT scores taken within the past three years are acceptable.osteopathic physician. Science course requirements are: 8 semester hours of Biology, Chemistry, Organic Chemistry, and Physics. In addition, 6 semester hours of English and Behavioral Science are required.

SUGGESTIONS

LECOM encourages applicants to learn more about the profession by getting to know an osteopathic physician to enhance awareness of the osteopathic medical philosophy and prepare for the admissions interview. The College looks for students who exemplify the osteopathic philosophy of compassionate, total person health care.

PROCESS

LECOM makes it easy to apply for the osteopathic medicine and pharmacy degrees. You begin with the centralized application services—AACOMAS for osteopathic medicine. When LECOM receives the AACOMAS application, the admissions office will contact the applicant with details on completing process. Candidates for the Post Baccalaureate and Master of Science in Medical Education programs apply directly to LECOM.

Admissions Requirements (Required)

MCAT Scores, Essays, Science GPA, Non-Science GPA, Exposure to medical profession, Recommendation, Interview

Admissions Requirements (Optional)

Extracurricular activities, State Residency

COSTS AND AID

Tuition & Fees

Annual tuition (in-state out-of-state)	$26,700/$28,100
Room & board	$11,500
Cost of books	$1,000
Fees	$800

Financial Aid

% students receiving any aid	92
% students receiving grants	31
% students receiving loans	90
% aid that is merit-based	0
Average grant	$16,500
Average loan	$35,000
Average total aid package	$45,000
Average debt	$158,000

MICHIGAN STATE UNIVERSITY
COLLEGE OF OSTEOPATHIC MEDICINE

965 FEE ROAD, A136 EAST FEE HALL EAST LANSING, MI • **ADMISSION:** 517-353-7740 • **FAX:** 517-355-3296
E-MAIL: COM.ADMISSIONS@HC.MSU.EDU • **WEBSITE:** COM.MSU.EDU

STUDENT BODY

Type	Public
Enrollment of parent institution	49,300
Enrollment of medical school	1,252
% male/female	57/43
% out-of-state	12
Average age of entering class	23

ADMISSIONS

# applied	4,588

Average GPA and MCAT Scores

Overall GPA	3.6

Application Information

Regular application	12/2
Are transfers accepted?	Yes
Admissions may be deferred?	Yes
Admissions need-blind?	No

Academics

The Michigan State University College of Osteopathic Medicine (MSUCOM), originally a private school established in 1969, was created by the Michigan legislature in 1971 to provide osteopathic physicians to meet the health care needs of the state's population. The college now has preclinical programs in three sites: at the MSU campus in East Lansing, at the Detroit Medical Center downtown, and at the Macomb University Center in Clinton Township. Educating primary care and specialty care osteopathic physicians occurs in a spectrum that includes premedical programs, osteopathic medical college, internships, residencies and fellowships. The college has been recognized as being in the top 11% of all medical schools—M.D. and D.O.—for primary care education. The college has partnerships for clinical education with 47 hospitals and 31 Federally Qualified Health Centers in Michigan in its Statewide Campus System, and it also occurs in private clinics and other environments. Medical research is a high priority of the college, and MSUCOM provides educational opportunities for physician/scientists, especially in its joint D.O./Ph.D. curriculum. The curriculum, based on a study of the body's organ systems, emphasizes osteopathic principles and practices, early patient care, behavioral and diversity aspects of medicine, lifelong learning, professionalism and use of technology. MSUCOM is a close-knit community known for compassionate care and its volunteer work in the communities.

BASIC SCIENCES: Basic science courses are generally taught in the first year, and then reinforced in body systems courses in the second year.

CLINICAL TRAINING
Clinical training occurs in 20 "base hospitals" affiliated with the college, and in the office of preceptors and other clinical faculty.

Admissions

REQUIREMENTS

Requirements are eight semester hours each of biology/zoology, inorganic chemistry, organic chemistry, and physics, three hours of biochemistry, and six hours each of English and behavioral science. The MCAT is required, and scores can be no more than three years old. Supplemental application requirements: Cumulative and science GPA of 2.7, MCAT total 20 and minimum subject scores: 6 verbal, 6 physical sciences, 8 biology. Supplemental application includes essagy, nonacademic information and two completed evaluation forms.

SUGGESTIONS

Recommend completed AACOMAS application no later than mid-July; supplemental completed by mid-August

PROCESS

Primary application service: AACOMAS

Admissions Requirements (Required)

MCAT Scores, Essays, Science GPA, Extracurricular activities, Non-Science GPA, Exposure to medical profession, Recommendation

Admissions Requirements (Optional)

Interview, State Residency

COSTS AND AID

Tuition & Fees

Annual tuition (in-state out-of-state)	$38,634/$80,526
Room & board	$14,616
Fees	$85

Financial Aid

% students receiving any aid	85
Average debt	$195,079

MIDWESTERN UNIVERSITY
ARIZONA COLLEGE OF OSTEOPATHIC MEDICINE

OFFICE OF ADMISSIONS, 19555 NORTH 59TH AVENUE, GLENDALE, AZ 85308 • **ADMISSION:** 623-572-3275
FAX: 623-572-3229 • **E-MAIL:** ADMISSAZ@MIDWESTERN.EDU • **WEBSITE:** WWW.MIDWESTERN.EDU

STUDENT BODY

Type	Private
Enrollment of parent institution	1,301
% male/female	54/46
% out-of-state	70
% international	54
Average age of entering class	25

FACULTY

Total faculty	345
% female faculty	24
% minority faculty	12
% part-time faculty	22
Student-faculty ratio	2.0:1

ADMISSIONS

# applied	3,746
% accepted	15
% enrolled	47

Average GPA and MCAT Scores

Overall GPA	3.5
MCAT Bio	10.0
MCAT Phys	9.0
MCAT Verbal	9.0
MCAT Essay	O

Application Information

Regular application	1/2
Regular notification	3/1
Are transfers accepted?	Yes
Admissions may be deferred?	Yes
Admissions need-blind?	Yes
Application fee	$50

Academics

The Arizona College of Osteopathic Medicine (AZCOM) was founded in 1995. The College, along with its sister college, the Chicago College of Osteopathic Medicine (CCOM), is part of Midwestern University. In addition to the Colleges of Osteopathic Medicine, Midwestern University also includes a college of pharmacy and a college of health sciences. The school is located on a 124-acre site in scenic Glendale, Arizona, a suburb of Phoenix. Facilities include three main academic centers housing lecture halls, conference rooms, a student services facility, numerous lecture and laboratory classrooms boasting the finest in educational equipment, cadavers for anatomy laboratories rather than plastic models, on-campus housing which features one- and two-bedroom student apartments and a heated pool, a comprehensive library with computer resources and study rooms, a researcy facility, a clinic, and a student clubhouse. The mission of Arizona College of Osteopathic Medicine of Midewestern University responds to the contemporary societal need for physicians by emphasizing primary care and education experiences needed to serve in rural and underserved urban communities.

Admissions

REQUIREMENTS

As a private institution, the college attracts a national applicant pool, and out-of-state residents account for over 80 percent of the group. Only 125 positions are available in each class, and in recent years there have been over 3,000 applicants. The average GPA of successful applicants is about 3.4 in both Sciences and overall. Minimum course work includes six semester hours in English and eight semester hours in each of the following: biology, inorganic chemistry, organic chemistry, and physics. The MCAT is required and must be no more than three years old. In addition to the AACOMAS application, applicants must submit a supplemental application (provided by the College after the AACOMAS application has been received).

Admissions Requirements (Required)

MCAT Scores, Essays, Science GPA, Extracurricular activities, Non-Science GPA, Exposure to medical profession, Recommendation, Interview

Admissions Requirements (Optional)

State Residency

COSTS AND AID

Tuition & Fees

Annual tuition	$50,129
Room & board (on-campus off-campus)	$16,490/$13,090
Cost of books	$3,398
Fees	$512

Financial Aid

Average grant	$1,910
Average loan	$23,500

MIDWESTERN UNIVERSITY
CHICAGO COLLEGE OF OSTEOPATHIC MEDICINE

MIDWESTERN UNIVERSITY, 555 31ST STREET DOWNERS GROVE, IL 60515 • ADMISSION: 800-458-6253
FAX: 630-971-6086 • E-MAIL: ADMISSIL@MIDWESTERN.EDU • WEBSITE: WWW.MIDWESTERN.EDU

STUDENT BODY

Type	Private
Enrollment of parent institution	1,978
Enrollment of medical school	690
% male/female	42/58
% underrepresented minorities	1
% out-of-state	56
% international	29
# countries represented	0
Average age of entering class	24

FACULTY

Total faculty	345
% female faculty	24
% minority faculty	12
% part-time faculty	22
Student-faculty ratio	2.0:1

ADMISSIONS

# applied	2,934
% accepted	15
% enrolled	39

Average GPA and MCAT Scores

Overall GPA	3.6
MCAT Bio	9.1
MCAT Phys	8.5
MCAT Verbal	8.6
MCAT Essay	O

Application Information

Regular application	1/1
Are transfers accepted?	Yes
Admissions may be deferred?	Yes
Admissions need-blind?	Yes
Application fee	$50

Academics

Midwestern University administers the Chicago College of Osteopathic Medicine (CCOM), the Chicago College of Pharmacy, and the College of Health Sciences, in addition to related programs in Glendale, Arizona. The MWU campus is located in a western suburb of Chicago, Illinois. Clinical training takes place at various sites around the city and throughout the Midwest region. Students enjoy early clinical exposure through volunteering, preceptor programs, and formal patient contact in the second semester of year one. Research is also important at CCOM, which offers a combined D.O./Ph.D program and has summer research awards for medical students. The Downers Grove campus offers modern academic and recreational facilities, in addition to on-campus housing. The male/female ratio is 40/60, and average age of incoming students is about 27. In Fall 2002, the Downers Grove campus enrolled 1,590 students while the Glendale, AZ campus enrolled 1,154 students.

Admissions

REQUIREMENTS

Residents of Illinois account for 65 percent of the student body on the Downers Grove campus. Residents of Arizona account for 42 percent of the student body on the Glendale, AZ campus. See www.midwestern.edu for specific admissions requirements.

Admissions Requirements (Required)

MCAT Scores, Essays, Science GPA, Extracurricular activities, Non-Science GPA, Exposure to medical profession, Recommendation, Interview

COSTS AND AID

Tuition & Fees

Annual tuition	$51,680
Room & board (on-campus off-campus)	$16,250/$13,543
Cost of books	$2,212
Fees	$550

Financial Aid

% students receiving any aid	90
% aid that is merit-based	0
Average loan	$50,000
Average total aid package	$50,000
Average debt	$151,270

NEW YORK INSTITUTE OF TECHNOLOGY
NEW YORK COLLEGE OF OSTEOPATHIC MEDICINE

DIRECTOR OF ADMISSIONS, NYCOM/NYIT, OLD WESTBURY, NY 11568 • **ADMISSION:** 516-626-6947
FAX: 516-626-6946 • **E-MAIL:** • **WEBSITE:** WWW.NYIT/NYCOM/NYCOM

Academics

The New York College of Osteopathic Medicine is part of the New York Institute of Technology, an independent institution that encompasses numerous academic and professional programs at the undergraduate and graduate level. In conjunction with some of these programs, medical students may pursue joint degrees, such as a D.O./M.B.A. or D.O./M.S. The College of Medicine is located 22 miles east of New York City and uses more than 20 clinical facilities in and around Manhattan, on Long Island, in upstate New York, and in northern New Jersey. With such a diverse patient population, students learn to be excellent clinicians in both primary and specialty fields. The medical student population itself is diverse, largely as a result of special efforts at recruiting women, minorities, and immigrants who were trained as physicians in other countries. Women account for 48 percent of the student body, and underrepresented minorities account for about 13 percent.

Admissions

REQUIREMENTS

Course requirements are 8 semester hours of Biology, Chemistry, Organic Chemistry, and Physics in addition to 6 semester hours of English. A minimum grade of 2.75/4.0 is expected in all of the required courses, and applicants' combined Science and overall GPAs must be higher than 2.75 for serious consideration. The MCAT is required as well as a baccalaureate degree. About 20 percent of AACOMAS applicants are interviewed, with interviews taking place between November and May. The supplementary application is given to candidates at the time of interview. Interviews are conducted with basic science faculty and/or osteopathic physicians from the community. About two-third of those interviewed are accepted. Preference is given to New York residents and to residents of states in the northeastern United States.

Admissions Requirements (Required)

Science GPA, Extracurricular activities, Non-Science GPA, Exposure to medical profession, Recommendation, Interview, State Residency

Admissions Requirements (Optional)

Standardized Test, Essays

COSTS AND AID

Tuition & Fees

Annual tuition	$34,984

NOVA SOUTHEASTERN UNIVERSITY
COLLEGE OF OSTEOPATHIC MEDICINE

3200 SOUTH UNIVERSITY DRIVE, FORT LAUDERDALE, FL 33328 • ADMISSION: 954-262-1101 • FAX: 954-262-2282
E-MAIL: COM@NOVA.EDU • WEBSITE: WWW.MEDICINE.NOVA.EDU

STUDENT BODY

Type	Private
Enrollment of parent institution	18,000
Enrollment of medical school	822
% male/female	50/50
% underrepresented minorities	1
% out-of-state	26
% international	24
# countries represented	15
Average age of entering class	25

FACULTY

Total faculty	604
% female faculty	88
% minority faculty	20
% part-time faculty	2

ADMISSIONS

# applied	2,800
% accepted	15
% enrolled	55

Average GPA and MCAT Scores

Overall GPA	3.4
MCAT Bio	8.6
MCAT Phys	8.0
MCAT Verbal	8.5
MCAT Essay	O

Application Information

Regular application	1/15
Are transfers accepted?	Yes
Admissions may be deferred?	Yes
Admissions need-blind?	Yes
Application fee	$50

Academics

The Colleges of Osteopathic Medicine, Optometry, Allied Health, Pharmacy, and Biomedical Science are among the many schools featured at Nova Southeastern University, which is situated on a 232-acre campus in Fort Lauderdale. The curriculum includes two years of basic science instruction, followed by two years of clinical training. One of the required clinical rotations is a three month clerkship in a rural, underserved area. Some students are admitted to a special seven year primary medicine track that ensures residency placement, and others jointly pursue an M.P.H. along with the D.O. Seventy percent of graduates enter primary care fields. The male/female ratio is 70/30, and the average age of incoming students is approximately 26.

Admissions

REQUIREMENTS

Nova Southeastern University receives over 3,000 application each year to fill a class of 180 students. All AACOMAS applicants receive a secondary application, but not everyone that applies is granted an interview. Interviews begin in October and consist of a session with a panel of health professionals including a DO. Science pre-requisites must include 8 hours of each (with labs) in Biology, Chemistry, Organic Chemistry and Physics. In addition, three semester hours of English Literature and three hours of English Composition are required. The MCAT is required and should be no more than three years old. The best set of scores will be used.

SUGGESTIONS

Because of the time it takes for AACOMAS to provide all of the student information, and the fact that NSU is on rolling admissions, making application early is advisable.

Admissions Requirements (Required)

MCAT Scores, Essays, Science GPA, Extracurricular activities, Non-Science GPA, Exposure to medical profession, Recommendation, Interview, State Residency

COSTS AND AID

Tuition & Fees

Annual tuition	$25,785
Room & board	$12,040
Cost of books	$2,000
Fees	$925

Financial Aid

% students receiving any aid	96
% students receiving grants	19
% students receiving loans	98
Average loan	$42,944
Average total aid package	$43,599
Average debt	$225,000

OHIO UNIVERSITY

OHIO UNIVERSITY COLLEGE OF OSTEOPATHIC MEDICINE

102 GROSVENOR HALL, ATHENS, OH 45701 • ADMISSION: 800-345-1560 • FAX: 740-593-2256
E-MAIL: ADMISSIONS@EXCHANGE.OUCOM.OHIOU.EDU • WEBSITE: WWW.OUCOM.OHIOU.EDU

STUDENT BODY

Type	Public
Enrollment of parent institution	20,000
Enrollment of medical school	433
% male/female	42/58
% underrepresented minorities	0
% out-of-state	16
% international	26
# countries represented	0
Average age of entering class	24

FACULTY

Total faculty	115
% female faculty	30
% minority faculty	15
% part-time faculty	33
Student-faculty ratio	4.0:1

ADMISSIONS

# applied	3,651
% accepted	5
% enrolled	72

Average GPA and MCAT Scores

Overall GPA	3.7
MCAT Bio	9.1
MCAT Phys	8.2
MCAT Verbal	8.4
MCAT Essay	P

Application Information

Regular application	2/1
Are transfers accepted?	Yes
Admissions may be deferred?	Yes
Admissions need-blind?	No
Application fee	$50

Academics

The Ohio University College of Osteopathic Medicine (OU-COM) is dedicated to preparing well-rounded primary care and specialty physicians for service to the state of Ohio as well as the nation. Students begin their first two years of training in Athens while the final two years taking place at one of twenty-six hospitals in our Centers for Osteopathic Research and Education (CORE). The learning environment at OU-COM and the CORE is constructed based on the principles of adult learning which include student empowerment and clinical relevance. Students will enroll in one of two tracks , the Patient-Centered Continuum (PCC) curriculum or the Clinical Presentation Continuum (CPC) curriculum. Both curricula view medical education as an organized building process that extends from the first day of medical school through residency training and beyond. Students in both curricula begin interacting with real patients in the first weeks of their medical education. The PCC curriculum is a student-directed approach that uses a problem-based learning environment and places emphasis on small group discussions, case analysis, collaborative learning, and problem solving as its primary educational tools. The CPC curriculum provides students with opportunities to learn the biomedical science fundamentals of medicine in an integrated, clinically relevant environment. This faculty-directed curriculum uses the most common and/or important symptoms that patients present to primary care providers as its organizing focus.

CLINICAL TRAINING

In order to become a patient-centered osteopathic physician, we feel that it is extremely important to have patient contact from the very beginning of your undergraduate medical education. As part of the OU-COM curricula, you will receive patient contact within the first week of your first year through our Clinical and Community Experience (CCE) program. Students are able to see first-hand the roles of other health-care professionals and become aware of cultural, economic and social issues that can affect health status and health-care delivery. Through OU-COM's pioneering Simulated Patient Program, students begin to hone their history taking, psychosocial and physical examination skills. One of the first in the country, this program, in place for over 25 years, features "patient actors" who role play a variety of conditions. Whenever possible, patients with actual symptoms or illnesses such as diabetes or rheumatoid arthritis are used as part of the simulated patient experience. Students are also able to get involved in health-care initiatives and community health service programs related to rural Southeastern Ohio. The Childhood Immunization Program and the Breast and Cervical Cancer Screening Clinic are both delivered through one of the college's two Mobile Health Units. Opportunities for clinical service also abound at University Medical Associates, an ambulatory health-care facility in Athens, and in OU-COM's satellite clinics in the outlying rural areas. Clinical rotations at one of our twenty-six CORE hospitals will take place in the third and fourth years of study.

Students

Being part of a major university has its advantages! From cultural and athletic events to phenomenal student recreation opportunities, OU-COM students enjoy it all. Located within minutes of Strouds Run State Park students can relax by hiking, swimming or fishing or they can blade, walk, bike, or jog our nineteen-mile, paved fitness path that extends from Athens to Nelsonville. Even more outdoor adventure is available in nearby Wayne National Forest. Ohio University also provides a nine-hole golf course, a natatorium, ice arena as well as indoor and outdoor tennis courts all within walking distance of the OU-COM campus. Intramural sports are also very popular. OU-COM has produced championship teams in both basketball and broomball over the past two years.

STUDENT LIFE

While it is no surprise that most of a med student's day is spent studying, there is still time for fun. Students can enjoy the many amenities offered by the university or get involved in OU-COM student government or other medically related student organizations. The environment at OU-COM is one of collegiality and cooperativeness. Students are often seen studying together, having a meal together or even living in close proximity to one another. The quality of life for an OU-COM student is high. Support from caring and dedicated faculty and staff alongside the beauty and history of Ohio University make OU-COM an extraordinary place to obtain a medical education. The environment at OU-COM is one of collegiality and cooperativeness. Students are often seen studying together, having a meal together or even living in close proximity to one another. The quality of life for an OU-COM student is high. Support from caring and dedicated faculty and staff alongside the beauty and history of Ohio University make OU-COM an extraordinary place to obtain a medical education.

GRADUATES

OU-COM was founded for the express purpose of providing outstanding primary care physicians for the state of Ohio. Since our first graduating class in 1980 we have accomplished that and more. Sixty percent of our graduates do go on to specialize in family medicine, internal medicine or pediatrics, with 50 percent going specifically into family medicine. The remaining 40 percent are pursuing specialties such as orthopedic surgery, neurology, nephrology, psychiatry, anesthesiology, and ophthalmology just to name a few.

Admissions

REQUIREMENTS

Eight semester hours each in Biology, Chemistry, Organic Chemistry, and Physics are required. In addition, applicants must have taken 6 semester hours of English and Behavioral Science. As a state-affiliated institution, the college gives preference to Ohio residents, who make up about 80 percent of the student body. About 80 percent of AACOMAS applicants are sent supplemental applications. About 16 percent of those who submit supplemental applications are invited to interview. Interviews take place from September through April, and consist of three 30-minute sessions with members of the faculty and administration. Approximately half of interviewees are accepted, with notification occurring on a rolling basis. In the past, successful candidates have had a mean GPA of 3.7 and an average of at least 8 on each section of the MCAT.

SUGGESTIONS

Additional coursework in biochemistry, histology, gross anatomy, and immunology is recommended but not required.

PROCESS

Students may begin the application process through AACOMAS on May 1. Primary applications will be reviewed to determine the eligibility of a secondary application. If a secondary application is granted, students will need to supply letters of recommendation, a supplemental essay and, if from outside Ohio, a signed contract of admission. A letter from a DO is strongly encouraged. Application status notices are sent electronically so it is imperative that students provide AACOMAS with a valid email address. Only complete files will go before the selection committee for review. Students are responsible for making sure their file is complete. Interviews begin in September and end in April. Admission decisions are made on a rolling basis with accepted candidates being notified via email the next business day after the interview.

Admissions Requirements (Required)

MCAT Scores, Essays, Science GPA, Extracurricular activities, Non-Science GPA, Exposure to medical profession, Recommendation, Interview

Admissions Requirements (Optional)

State Residency

COSTS AND AID

Tuition & Fees

Annual tuition (in-state out-of-state)	$26,580/$38,619
Room & board	$12,992
Cost of books	$7,548
Fees	$2,523

Financial Aid

% students receiving any aid	100
% students receiving grants	23
% students receiving loans	96
% aid that is merit-based	0
Average grant	$3,940
Average loan	$35,297
Average total aid package	$40,720
Average debt	$132,927

OKLAHOMA STATE UNIVERSITY

OKLAHOMA STATE UNIV. COLLEGE OF OSTEO. MEDICINE

1111 WEST 17TH STREET, OFFICE OF STUDENT AFFAIRS TULSA, OK 74107 • **ADMISSION:** 918-561-8421
FAX: 918-561-8243 • **E-MAIL:** AMANDA.GUTIERREZ@OKSTATE.EDU • **WEBSITE:** WWW.HEALTHSCIENCES.OKSTATE.EDU

STUDENT BODY

Type	Public
Enrollment of parent institution	23,307
Enrollment of medical school	351
% male/female	52/48
% underrepresented minorities	0
% out-of-state	9
% international	19
# countries represented	0
Average age of entering class	24

FACULTY

Total faculty	536
% female faculty	20
% minority faculty	10
% part-time faculty	84
Student-faculty ratio	2.0:1

ADMISSIONS

# applied	486
% accepted	30
% enrolled	61

Average GPA and MCAT Scores

Overall GPA	3.6
MCAT Bio	9.0
MCAT Phys	8.0
MCAT Verbal	9.0
MCAT Essay	0

Application Information

Regular application	2/1
Are transfers accepted?	Yes
Admissions may be deferred?	No
Admissions need-blind?	Yes
Application fee	$40

Academics

The curriculum at OSU College of Osteopathic Medicine includes hands-on clinical experiences, student-centered, and problem-based methods of instruction, as well as frequent consultation with faculty and community-based physicians. The first year focuses on biomedical sciences, and the second year emphasizes case-based learning and problem solving as it relates to conditions seen in primary care environments. The third and fourth years are composed of clinical rotations, most of which take place at OSU Medical Center, the country's largest osteopathic hospital (521 beds). Students also rotate to adjacent rural areas, and they may fulfill requirements at various medical institutions across the country. Although 64 percent of graduates enter primary care, they are prepared to enter residencies in all medical specialty fields. The medical school, a college of Oklahoma State University, is located in Tulsa, a very livable city of of 386,000.

Admissions

REQUIREMENTS

Of the 88 positions in a class, 68 are reserved for Oklahoma residents. Prerequisites for application are 8–10 semester hours of Biology, Physics, Chemistry, and Organic Chemistry with labs, in addition to 6–8 hours of English, and at least 1 upper division science course. The minimum overall undergraduate GPA is 3.0, with a minimum Science GPA of 2.75. An average score of 7.0 (21 total) on the MCAT is required. Approximately 10 percent of all qualified applicants are interviewed. Interviews begin in October and continue through April. Applicants are interviewed simultaneously by 2 faculty members (1 D.O. and 1 Ph.d.) for 35–40 minutes. Notification of admission occurs on a rolling basis, and about 35 to 40 percent of interviewees are accepted.

Admissions Requirements (Required)

MCAT Scores, Essays, Science GPA, Extracurricular activities, Non-Science GPA, Exposure to medical profession, Recommendation, Interview

Admissions Requirements (Optional)

State Residency

COSTS AND AID

Tuition & Fees

Annual tuition (in-state out-of-state)	$16,045/$31,265
Room & board (on-campus off-campus)	
Cost of books	$3,500
Fees (in-state out-of-state)	$893/$893

Financial Aid

% students receiving any aid	96
% students receiving grants	36
% students receiving loans	92
% aid that is merit-based	6
Average grant	$2,500
Average loan	$30,000
Average total aid package	$34,000
Average debt	$150,000

PHILADELPHIA COLLEGE OF OSTEOPATHIC MEDICINE

PHILADELPHIA COLLEGE OF OSTEOPATHIC MEDICINE

OFFICE OF ADMISSIONS, 4170 CITY AVENUE PHILADELPHIA, PA 19131 • **ADMISSION:** 800-999-6998
FAX: 215-871-6719 • **E-MAIL:** ADMISSIONS@PCOM.EDU • **WEBSITE:** WWW.PCOM.EDU

STUDENT BODY

Type	Private
Enrollment of parent institution	1,762
Enrollment of medical school	1,086
% male/female	50/50
% underrepresented minorities	1
% out-of-state	41
% international	25
# countries represented	9
Average age of entering class	25

FACULTY

Total faculty	1,370
% female faculty	22
% minority faculty	5
% part-time faculty	94
Student-faculty ratio	1.0:1

ADMISSIONS

# applied	4,880
% accepted	9
% enrolled	64

Average GPA and MCAT Scores

Overall GPA	3.5
MCAT Bio	9.6
MCAT Phys	8.5
MCAT Verbal	8.8

Application Information

Regular application	2/1
Are transfers accepted?	No
Admissions may be deferred?	Yes
Admissions need-blind?	No
Application fee	$50

Academics

Established in 1899, Philadelphia College of Osteopathic Medicine (PCOM) is one of the nation's oldest osteopathic medical institutions and a multidisciplinary, multistate health science educational institution. The college encompasses a main campus in Philadelphia and a branch campus, Georgia Campus—Philadelphia College of Osteopathic Medicine (GA-PCOM), established in 2004, located in the suburbs of Atlanta, Georgia (Suwannee, Gwinnett County). The College offers the doctor of osteopathic medicine (DO) degree and joint DO/MBA, DO/MPH, DO/PhD, DO/MS, and DO/MA degrees, as well as graduate programs in biomedical sciences; clinical, counseling and clinical health and school psychology; organizational development and leadership; physician assistant studies; forensic medicine and pharmacy—enrolling nearly 1750 medical and graduate students in Pennsylvania and 565 students in Georgia. Integral to the medical program is the strong osteopathic tradition upon which the college was founded—an approach that treats the patient's body, lifestyle and behavior as a whole. As an osteopathic medical school, PCOM graduates physicians who are in all respects equal to graduates of non-osteopathic medical schools, but who have additional training in the osteopathic tradition. The college has nearly 11,750 living alumni. Although the College is solidly focused on teaching, research is also an important component of the institution's mission; in fact, the college houses a Center for the Chronic Disorders of Aging for collaborative research. Integral, too, is the institution's commitment to community service. This commitment is exemplified in the college's establishment of five affiliated Healthcare Centers that serve the medical needs of urban and rural Pennsylvania communities.

BASIC SCIENCES: PCOM and GA-PCOM students begin preparation for the world of clinical medicine from their first day as medical students. The curriculum combines basic science and clinical course content with integrated courses, as well as integrated approaches to the pharmacology, pathology, medicine and surgery related to respiratory, genitourinary, cardiovascular and gastrointestinal systems. The first two years lay the foundation with intense concentration on the basic sciences, anatomy, biochemistry, molecular biology, neuroscience, physiology, microbiology, pathology, and pharmacology, taught in integrated course units that emphasize clinical applications. The College also recognizes that medical practice is more than science. Coursework in ethics and patient communication helps the student relate well to patients, while content in evidence-based medicine and public health prepares the student for the complex world of private practice. The basic sciences are complemented by instruction in clinical subjects such as internal medicine, surgery, neurology, psychiatry, pediatrics, epidemiology, OB/GYN, family medicine, rehabilitation medicine, geriatrics, radiology, oncology and physical diagnosis. The principles and practice of osteopathic medicine are taught throughout the medical curriculum. All students attend small group sessions during the first and second year to develop communication and diagnostic skills. These special instructional activities include patient observation, case conferences and basic clinical skills workshops. In addition, a state-of-the-art standardized patient and robotic simulation program introduces students to patient care through examinations of patient actors in a simulated practice setting, augmented by clinical exercises on high-fidelity manikins and laparoscopic and arthroscopic surgical and cardiac simulators and other various trainers. This competency-based assessment offers an outstanding tool for acquiring diagnostic skills and practicing medical procedures

CLINICAL TRAINING

The last two years of the DO program emphasize clinical training experiences. There are a total of twenty-three clerkship periods of four weeks each (clinical training) for DO students. Fifteen are assigned in a manner prescribed by the curriculum to ensure that each student obtains the core experience needed to become a well-trained osteopathic generalist physician. Assigned clerkship sites are predominately in Pennsylvania (for PCOM students) and in Georgia and the Southeast (for GA-PCOM students). The sites comprise affiliated hospitals, the college's five Healthcare Centers (urban and rural), numerous outpatient units and scores of physicians' offices. In addition, flexibility is provided by six months of elective time and three months of selective time to give the student ample opportunity to pursue his/her special interests. The program is designed to afford progressive student responsibility for all phases of patient care under the direction of experienced physicians. Because of admissions increases at many medical schools, graduate medical training opportunities (internships and residencies) are often disjointed. Countering this trend, PCOM and GA-PCOM retain students in Pennsylvania and Georgia (respectively) by exposing them to and matching them into internships and residencies in a Consortium of affiliated hospitals known as the PCOM MEDnet. This extensive network of thirty-three hospitals ensures the highest standard of education in the clinical education of PCOM and GA-PCOM students who wish to continue their graduate medical education under the auspices of the college and its osteopathic affiliates.

STUDENT LIFE

PCOM and GA-PCOM campuses are noted for their spirit of collegiality and camaraderie, rather than competitiveness. There is a warm, family atmosphere that inspires friendly interaction and advances academic and personal growth as well as professional and career development. Students are encouraged to participate in community service and co-curricular activities. More than fifty chapter and national organizations, academic interest groups, athletic teams and charitable groups and clubs offer social activities and leadership opportunities. Those who embrace the College's osteopathic philosophy are often drawn to service; PCOM and GA-PCOM students actively participate in blood drives, fundraising events, medical mission trips and free health screenings in community locations and PCOM Healthcare Centers.

Admissions

REQUIREMENTS

Prior to matriculation each applicant must meet the following admissions requirements: 1. A bachelor's degree from a regionally accredited college or university. Applications from students with at least 3 years of exceptional undergraduate work will be considered. 2. Eight semester hours each, including 2 semester hours of laboratory: general chemistry, organic chemistry, biology and physics. 3. Six semester hours of English composition and literature. 4. Each applicant must sit for the Medical College Admissions Test (MCAT), which is given multiple times each year. Prospective students are urged to take the test as early as possible and certainly not later than August of the year prior to matriculation. The MCAT must be taken within 3 years of desired matriculation. Application to the DO program is comprehensive and competitive. The Faculty Committee on Admissions recommends applicants to the program have at least an 8 or higher in each section of the MCAT.

SUGGESTIONS

Admission to PCOM is competitive and selective. We seek well-rounded, achievement-oriented persons whose character, maturity and sense of dedication point to a successful and productive life as an osteopathic physician. We are an institution that has historically sought diversity in our student population. We actively recruit under-represented minority students and non-traditional students who often offer exceptional potential for becoming outstanding physicians.

Admissions Requirements (Required)

MCAT Scores, Essays, Science GPA, Non-Science GPA, Recommendation, Interview

Admissions Requirements (Optional)

Extracurricular activities, Exposure to medical profession, State Residency

COSTS AND AID

Tuition & Fees

Annual tuition	$45,036
Room & board	$13,230
Cost of books	$2,802
Fees	$725

Financial Aid

% students receiving any aid	89
% students receiving grants	64
% students receiving loans	80
% aid that is merit-based	10
Average grant	$7,765
Average loan	$56,446
Average total aid package	$58,493
Average debt	$182,446

TOURO UNIVERSITY CALIFORNIA
TOURO UNIVERSITY COLLEGE OF OSTEOPATHIC MEDICINE

OFFICE OF ADMISSIONS, 1310 CLUB DRIVE VALLEJO, CA 94592 • ADMISSION: 707-638-5270 • FAX: 707-638-5250
E-MAIL: ADMIT@TU.EDU • WEBSITE: WWW.TU.EDU

STUDENT BODY

Type	Private
Enrollment of parent institution	1,357
Enrollment of medical school	540
% male/female	55/45
% underrepresented minorities	0
% out-of-state	28
% international	7
Average age of entering class	25

FACULTY

Student-faculty ratio	15.0:1

ADMISSIONS

# applied	4,689
% accepted	7
% enrolled	44

Average GPA and MCAT Scores

Overall GPA	3.5
MCAT Bio	10.3
MCAT Phys	9.9
MCAT Verbal	9.9

Application Information

Regular application	3/15
Are transfers accepted?	Yes
Admissions may be deferred?	Yes
Admissions need-blind?	Yes
Application fee	$100

Academics

The Touro University California College of Osteopathic Medicine is located in the northeast part if San Francisco Bay, on Mare Island. Touro University California is an international institution based in New York, with branches in Irael and the Russian Federation. The mission of TUCOM California is to train Osteopathic, family practice physicians to help meet the need for primary care practitioners in California and throughout the country. Though preventative medicine and primary care are emphasized, graduates are also prepared to enter residency programs that train osteopathic specialists. Patient contact begins in the first year, and clinical training takes place at sites throughout the greater Bay Area including hospitals, clinics, and physicians' offices. Students have the opportunity to experience both urban and rural patient populations.

Admissions

REQUIREMENTS

TUCOM requires eight semester units each of Biology/Zoology, Inorganic Chemistry, Organic Chemistry and Physics. Six semester units each of English, Humanities and Behavioral Science courses are also required. Computers are an integral part of the educational process and candidates are strongly encouraged to be computer literate. TUOCOM participates in AACOMAS. The MCAT is required and scores must be no more than three years old. Successful candidates typically have minimum Science and Cumulative GPA's of 3.0, with a minimum cumulative MCAT score of 23 or higher.

Admissions Requirements (Required)

MCAT Scores, Essays, Science GPA, Non-Science GPA, Exposure to medical profession, Recommendation, Interview

Admissions Requirements (Optional)

Extracurricular activities, State Residency

COSTS AND AID

Tuition & Fees

Annual tuition	$47,100
Cost of books	$8,000

Financial Aid

% students receiving any aid	89
Average grant	$0
Average loan	$0

University of Medicine and Dentistry of New Jersey
UMDNJ - School of Osteopathic Medicine

One Medical Center Drive, Suite 210, Stratford, NJ 8084 • Admission: 856-566-7050 • Fax: 856-566-6895
E-mail: SOMADM@UMDNJ.EDU • Website: SOM.UMDNJ.EDU

STUDENT BODY

Type	Public
Enrollment of parent institution	0
Enrollment of medical school	382
% male/female	43/57
% underrepresented minorities	1
% out-of-state	1
% international	53
# countries represented	1
Average age of entering class	24

FACULTY

Total faculty	187
% female faculty	39
% minority faculty	18
% part-time faculty	19

ADMISSIONS

# applied	2,401
% accepted	12
% enrolled	34

Average GPA and MCAT Scores

Overall GPA	3.5
MCAT Bio	9.2
MCAT Phys	9.0
MCAT Verbal	8.5
MCAT Essay	Q

Application Information

Regular application	2/1
Are transfers accepted?	Yes
Admissions may be deferred?	Yes
Admissions need-blind?	No
Application fee	$90

Academics

All applicants are processed and reviewed without regard to state of residence. The minimum course requirements are eight semester hours of Biology, Physics, Chemistry, and Organic Chemistry, all with associated labs and six semester hours each of English, Math and Social Sciences. Applicants should have at least a 3.0 GPA in both sciences and overall, as the average GPA of successful applicants is 3.4. The MCAT is required and must be no more than three years old. The average MCAT of successful applicants is in the 89 range. Just over 15 percent of approximately 2000 applicants are interviewed, with interviews taking place between August and April. About one half (1/2) of interviewees are accepted. Wait list candidates may send supplementary information to update their files.

Admissions

REQUIREMENTS

All applicants are processed and reviewed without regard to state of residence. The minimum course requirements are eight semester hours of Biology, Physics, Chemistry, and Organic Chemistry, all with associated labs, and six semester hours each of English, Math, and Social Sciences. Applicants should have at least a 3.0 GPA in both sciences and overall, as the average GPA of successful applicants is about 3.4. The MCAT is required, and must be no more than three years old. The average MCAT of successful applicants is in the 8–9 range. Just under 10 percent of approximately 3,200 applicants are interviewed, with interviews taking place between August and April. About one-third of interviewees are accepted. Wait-listed candidates may send supplementary information to update their files.

Admissions Requirements (Required)

MCAT Scores, Essays, Science GPA, Extracurricular activities, Non-Science GPA, Exposure to medical profession, Recommendation, Interview

Admissions Requirements (Optional)

State Residency

COSTS AND AID

Tuition & Fees

Annual tuition (in-state out-of-state)	$21,390/$33,472
Room & board	$10,000
Cost of books	$8,536
Fees	$2,587

Financial Aid

% students receiving any aid	92
% students receiving grants	45
% students receiving loans	98
Average grant	$2,690
Average loan	$32,759
Average total aid package	$35,652
Average debt	$104,005

University of New England
College of Osteopathic Medicine

Office of Constituent Services, 11 Hills Beach Road Biddeford, ME 04005 • **Admission:** 207-602-2329
Fax: 207-602-5967 • **E-mail:** UNECOMADMISSIONS@UNE.EDU • **Website:** WWW.UNE.EDU/COM

STUDENT BODY

Type	Private
Enrollment of parent institution	5,666
Enrollment of medical school	500
% male/female	45/55
% underrepresented minorities	1
% out-of-state	80
% international	11
# countries represented	4
Average age of entering class	25

FACULTY

% part-time faculty	97
Student-faculty ratio	10.0:1

ADMISSIONS

# applied	3,868
% accepted	6
% enrolled	55

Average GPA and MCAT Scores

Overall GPA	3.5
MCAT Bio	9.8
MCAT Phys	9.1
MCAT Verbal	9.5
MCAT Essay	Q

Application Information

Regular application	2/1
Are transfers accepted?	Yes
Admissions may be deferred?	No
Admissions need-blind?	No
Application fee	$55

Academics

The University of New England College of Osteopathic Medicine (UNECOM) transforms students into health care leaders who advance patient-centered, high quality osteopathic primary care, community health, and research for the people of Maine, New England and the nation. UNECOM's core values include professionalism, compassion, excellence, collaboration, innovation, and critical thinking. The academic environment is one of collaboration and support among the student body and with faculty members. The typical class size is 115-124 students, who come from a wide variety of educational and professional backgrounds. We will be increasing our class size in 2013 to 165–175.[MD1] While approximately 60-70 percent of the class is from New England, there are students from around the country. Some come directly from undergraduate studies, while others have completed master's and professional degrees. The male/female ratio is about 50/50 and the average age of entering students is 25 years old. UNECOM offers academic excellence, a supportive learning environment and a beautiful ocean-side campus.

BASIC SCIENCES: UNECOM's curriculum is based upon the belief that medical students are adult learners who assume responsibility for their own learning. Our curriculum is designed to guide and support students as they become life-long, self-directed learners and prepare for graduate medical training. Case-driven curricula, which allows for learning in context, is delivered in active, collaborative learning activities designed to engage the student in the learning process. During the first year students take Osteopathic Medical Knowledge and Osteopathic Clinical Skills. Osteopathic Medical Knowledge is a multidisciplinary course designed to introduce medical science knowledge that undergirds the practice of osteopathic medicine. Osteopathic Clinical Skills is a course designed to transform learners into student physicians who demonstrate superior clinical skills and medical professionalism, and embody empathetic, patient centered medical care in preparation for clinical clerkship training. Year two curriculum focuses on the various body systems and builds on the foundation established in the first year.

CLINICAL TRAINING
The third year is devoted to clerkships in core disciplines of internal medicine, family medicine, obstetrics, pediatrics, surgery, psychiatry, and community health at partner clinical campuses around the Northeast. Students are involved in patient care and didactic sessions in ambulatory, hospital and rural settings. The third year concludes with a student colloquium for the assessment of acquired skills in the simulated patient program. Year four requires clerkships in internal medicine and surgery sub-specialties, emergency medicine and osteopathic manipulative medicine, while providing an opportunity for electives throughout the United States and overseas as the student completes their preparation for residency.

Students

The UNE College of Osteopathic Medicine is one of six colleges of the University of New England. The College of Osteopathic Medicine and the College of Arts and Sciences are located on the waterfront campus in Biddeford, Maine; the Portland Campus is home to the Westbrook College of Health Professions, the College of Pharmacy, the College of Dental Medicine, and the College of Graduate Studies. Osteopathic medical students have access to a full-range of student services on both campuses. Most students live less than six miles from campus in the cities of Biddeford (22,000) and Saco (17,000).

STUDENT LIFE

With an active COM Student Government Association, class officers, and nearly 40 clubs and organizations, there are many opportunities for first- and second-year osteopathic medical students to be involved on campus and assume leadership positions. First- and second-year students also serve the Biddeford and Southern Maine communities through various programs including the Biddeford Free Clinic, local soup kitchen, mentoring program with one of the elementary schools, and volunteering at hospitals and nursing homes. Students maintain a healthy balance in their lives by utilizing the Campus Center (including the fitness room, racquetball court, gym, indoor track, pool and hydro-spa, and saunas) and participating in the University's intramural leagues and tournaments. The campus sits at the mouth of the Saco River where it meets the Atlantic Ocean, and the southern coastal Maine area is ideal for jogging and running, cycling, mountain biking, kayaking and canoeing, and cross-country skiing. Hiking, backpacking, camping, climbing, downhill skiing and snowboarding opportunities are less than two hours away in the White Mountains. Portland, Maine's largest city, is only a half-hour to the north, and Boston is just over an hour and a half to the south.

GRADUATES

UNECOM has more than 2,600 graduates working in primary care and specialty fields around the country. Approximately sixty-five percent of each class pursues residency programs in family practice, general internal medicine, pediatrics and obstetrics. Others choose to bring a patient-centered approach to a wide variety of specialties including emergency medicine, anesthesiology, psychiatry, general and orthopedic surgery, sports medicine, and physical medicine and rehabilitation, to name a few. Others will specialize in neuromuscular medicine (NMM). Graduates continue to serve the osteopathic community by serving in leadership positions in state societies and specialty colleges.

Admissions

REQUIREMENTS

Specific academic requirements include eight semester hours of biology, eight semester hours of physics, and six hours of English composition or literature or comparable courses. Four semesters of chemistry are also required, one of which must be biochemistry. Appropriate labs are required for all science courses with the exception of biochemistry. The catalog-posted minimum GPA is 2.7 in both the sciences and overall, while the class average is in the 3.3-3.5 range. The MCAT is required and should be no more than two years old at time of application. The class average MCAT was 28 for the classes entering in 2012. The following non-academic achievements are important in the evaluation process as well: leadership experience and organizational involvement; hands-on, patient-centered healthcare experience, whether volunteer or paid employment; and community service and volunteer experience. Passion and commitment to working with and serving others is important to the Committee on Admissions. There is some preference for candidates from the six New England states, but approximately forty (40) percent of the class is from the rest of the country.

PROCESS

The primary application to the University of New England College of Osteopathic Medicine (UNECOM) is through the American Association of Colleges of Osteopathic Medicine Application Service (AACOMAS). UNECOM received 3,800 AACOMAS applications during the 2011–12 application cycle. Applicants who meet all prerequisites are invited to complete a UNECOM specific online supplemental application and submit letters of recommendation. A letter from an osteopathic physician is not required, but strongly encouraged. Once all materials have been received, applicant's files are reviewed for possible interview. On campus interviews are generally conducted September through April. Qualified candidates are offered acceptance on a modified rolling admissions basis.

Admissions Requirements (Required)

MCAT Scores, Essays, Science GPA, Extracurricular activities, Non-Science GPA, Exposure to medical profession, Recommendation, Interview

Admissions Requirements (Optional)

State Residency

COSTS AND AID

Tuition & Fees

Annual tuition	$48,800
Room & board	$12,000
Cost of books	$2,400
Fees	$715

Financial Aid

% students receiving any aid	88
% students receiving grants	28
% students receiving loans	92
% aid that is merit-based	6
Average grant	$30,327
Average loan	$62,717
Average total aid package	$66,148
Average debt	$231,664

UNIVERSITY OF NORTH TEXAS HEALTH SCIENCE CENTER

TEXAS COLLEGE OF OSTEOPATHIC MEDICINE

OFFICE OF ADMISSIONS AND OUTREACH, EAD-248, 3500 CAMP BOWIE BOULEVARD FORT WORTH, TX
ADMISSION: 817-735-2204 • FAX: 817-735-2225 • E-MAIL: TCOMADMISSIONS@HSC.UNT.EDU
WEBSITE: WWW.HSC.UNT.EDU / EDUCATION / TCOM / ADMISSIONS.CFM

STUDENT BODY

Type	Public
Enrollment of parent institution	0
Enrollment of medical school	492
% male/female	48/52
% underrepresented minorities	0
% out-of-state	6
% international	9
# countries represented	0
Average age of entering class	25

FACULTY

Total faculty	198
% female faculty	22
% minority faculty	8

ADMISSIONS

# applied	1,350
% accepted	11
% enrolled	82

Average GPA and MCAT Scores

Overall GPA	3.6
MCAT Bio	9.2
MCAT Phys	8.7
MCAT Verbal	8.5
MCAT Essay	0

Application Information

Regular application	11/1
Regular notification	2/1
Early application	8/1
Early notification	10/1
Are transfers accepted?	Yes
Admissions may be deferred?	Yes
Admissions need-blind?	No
Application fee	$0

Academics

The University of North Texas Health Science Center at Fort Worth trains osteopathic physicians, physician assistants, biomedical scientists, and public health professionals. Its academic components are the Texas College of Osteopathic Medicine, the Graduate School of Biomedical Sciences, and the School of Public Health. Dual-degree programs combine medical training with research and public health. U.S. News & World Report and the Texas Academy of Family Physicians have both recognized TCOM's commitment to primary care.

BASIC SCIENCES: The first portion of the curriculum is designed to help students integrate the basic and clinical sciences, further develop their ability to diagnose illness, and increase their understanding of the context within which medicine is practiced. The integrated systems approach is built on the same strong foundation of scientific and clinical knowledge that has long characterized TCOM's outstanding academic program.

CLINICAL TRAINING

During the third and fourth years of study, students pursue a number of clinical training programs throughout the state at university sites, clinics, and affiliated teaching hospitals. A rural medicine track provides extensive preparation for those who wish to practice in small communities.

Students

UNT Health Science Center is located on a 17-acre, $107 million medical care complex in Fort Worth, Texas, in the city's beautiful Cultural District. Downtown Fort Worth, major thoroughfares, parks, museums, theaters, restaurants, shops, and affordable housing are all within minutes of campus.

STUDENT LIFE

The campus is located in the midst of a world-renowned cultural district, near parks and a variety of arts and entertainment facilities. The DFW Metroplex is home to several major and minor league sports teams, including the Dallas Cowboys, Texas Rangers, and Dallas Stars. A variety of student organizations bring a sense of community and camaraderie to campus. The health science center does not provide on-campus student housing, but a variety of affordable housing options are available in the area. Every student is responsible for making his or her own housing arrangements.

GRADUATES

Named as one of the nation's top 50 medical schools for primary care medicine by U.S. News & World Report, TCOM is a leader in training physicians skilled in comprehensive primary care. Approximately 65 percent of TCOM's graduates practice primary care medicine (family practice, general internal medicine, pediatrics, obstetrics and gynecology). One of the distinct advantages of an osteopathic medical education is that it prepares students to enter all three of the nation's residency programs: allopathic, military and osteopathic. Our graduates have been placed in residency and internship positions throughout the United States. UNT Health Science Center offers residency programs through the Texas Osteopathic Postdoctoral Training Institutions (OPTI) in the following areas: Family Medicine, Internal Medicine, Obstetrics & Gynecology, Orthopedics,

Radiology, Surgery and Manipulative Medicine. The Health Science Center also offers fellowship programs in Osteopathic Manipulative Therapy, Geriatric Medicine, Sports Medicine and Vascular Surgery.

Admissions

REQUIREMENTS

At least 90 percent of the positions in each class of 150 are reserved for Texas residents. Traditional pre-medical science training at an accredited undergraduate institution is necessary to prepare for matriculation. In addition applicants are required to submit MCAT scores, test results must be from within the past three years. Applications are accepted through the Texas Medical and Dental Schools Application Service (TMDSAS). Selected applicants are invited to interview between August and December. Initial offers of acceptance are sent on February 1 and continue until the incoming class is full. Applications are accepted through the Texas Medical and Dental Schools Application Service (TMDSAS). Selected applicants are invited to interview between August and December. Initial offers of acceptance are sent on February 1 and continue until the incoming class is full.

SUGGESTIONS

In addition to the required science course work, it is recommended that students take advanced course work in Bio-chemistry and Genetics in order to prepare for the rigors of medical education.

Admissions Requirements (Required)

MCAT Scores, Essays, Science GPA, Non-Science GPA, Exposure to medical profession, Recommendation, Interview

Admissions Requirements (Optional)

Extracurricular activities, State Residency

COSTS AND AID

Tuition & Fees

Annual tuition (in-state out-of-state)	$6,550/$19,650
Room & board	$10,098
Cost of books	$2,426
Fees	$2,480

Financial Aid

% students receiving any aid	91
% students receiving grants	49
% students receiving loans	91
Average grant	$5,000
Average loan	$24,418
Average total aid package	$26,878
Average debt	$86,000

UNIVERSITY OF PIKEVILLE
KENTUCKY COLLEGE OF OSTEOPATHIC MEDICINE

147 SYCAMORE STREET, PIKEVILLE, KY 41501 • ADMISSION: 606-218-5409 OR 606-218-5406 • FAX: 606-218-5405
E-MAIL: KYCOMADMISSIONS@UPIKE.EDU • WEBSITE: WWW.UPIKE.EDU

STUDENT BODY

Type	Private
Enrollment of parent institution	2,205
Enrollment of medical school	432
% male/female	52/48
% underrepresented minorities	0
% out-of-state	48
% international	16
# countries represented	0
Average age of entering class	24

FACULTY

Total faculty	25
% female faculty	32
% minority faculty	12
% part-time faculty	0
Student-faculty ratio	11.0:1

ADMISSIONS

# applied	3,187
% accepted	4
% enrolled	100

Average GPA and MCAT Scores

Overall GPA	3.5
MCAT Bio	8.4
MCAT Phys	7.5
MCAT Verbal	8.0
MCAT Essay	0

Application Information

Regular application	2/1
Are transfers accepted?	Yes
Admissions may be deferred?	Yes
Admissions need-blind?	No
Application fee	$75

Academics

The KYCOM Advantage KYCOM's tuition is very competitive compared to other osteopathic medical schools. Further, KYCOM provides its students with benefits of significant value that include the following: 1. A new laptop computer and iPad. 2. All required texts and workbooks (to be provided each year). 3. All necessary anatomy dissection equipment. 4. A new portable osteopathic treatment table. 5. Stethoscope. 6. Ophthalmoscope. 7. Otoscope. 8. Lab Coats. 9. Scrub suits. 10. Level 1 Board preparation sessions. 11. The cost of taking Level 1 and Level 2CE of NBOME once.

CLINICAL TRAINING

Given KYCOM's commitment to primary care, about 30 percent of required clinical rotations take place in ambulatory primary care settings such as physician's offices and rural clinics. At least 90 percent of this training occurs at sites in the Appalachian region.

Students

As a smaller medical school, KYCOM students, faculty, staff, and administrators interact in a family atmosphere. Students readily have access to faculty and administrators who maintain an open-door policy for students.

STUDENT LIFE

KYCOM students are encouraged to balance their studies with extracurricular activities. KYCOM sponsors nearly twenty student professional and special interest groups in various specialty areas of osteopathic medicine. Further, students frequently contribute to the wellness of the local community through programs that offer residents free health screening and osteopathic manipulative medical services.

GRADUATES

Approximately 60 percent of KYCOM alumni practice in the Appalachian region. Many serve as clinical preceptors to KYCOM students during their clinical education program.

Admissions

PROCESS

KYCOM participates in the AACOMAS application process. Requirements for admission include twelve hours of Biology, four hours of Chemistry, eight hours of Physics, and eight hours of Organic Chemistry. The MCAT exam is required.

Admissions Requirements (Required)

MCAT Scores, Essays, Science GPA, Extracurricular activities, Non-Science GPA, Exposure to medical profession, Recommendation, Interview

Admissions Requirements (Optional)

State Residency

COSTS AND AID

Tuition & Fees

Annual tuition	$38,950
Cost of books	$0
Fees	$0

Financial Aid

% students receiving any aid	96
% students receiving grants	31
% students receiving loans	94
% aid that is merit-based	0
Average grant	$7,346
Average loan	$53,438
Average total aid package	$54,378
Average debt	$165,086

VIRGINIA POLYTECHNIC INSTITUTE AND STATE UNIVERSITY

EDWARD VIA COLLEGE OF OSTEOPATHIC MEDICINE—VIRGINIA CAMPUS

OFFICE OF ADMISSIONS, VCOM, 2265 KRAFT DRIVE BLACKSBURG, VA 24060 • ADMISSION: 540-231-6138
FAX: 540-231-5252 • E-MAIL: ADMISSIONS@VCOM.VT.EDU • WEBSITE: WWW.VCOM.VT.EDU

STUDENT BODY

Type	Private
Enrollment of medical school	756
% male/female	51/49
% underrepresented minorities	0
% out-of-state	60
% international	10
# countries represented	1
Average age of entering class	24

FACULTY

Total faculty	1,013
% female faculty	22
% minority faculty	12
% part-time faculty	99
Student-faculty ratio	1.1:1

ADMISSIONS

# applied	3,504
% accepted	8
% enrolled	65

Average GPA and MCAT Scores

Overall GPA	3.6
MCAT Bio	9.0
MCAT Phys	8.0
MCAT Verbal	8.0
MCAT Essay	0

Application Information

Regular application	2/1
Early application	11/1
Are transfers accepted?	Yes
Admissions may be deferred?	Yes
Admissions need-blind?	Yes
Application fee	$50

Academics

The MISSION of the Edward Via College of Osteopathic Medicine (VCOM) is best described through both the primary mission and the goals of the institution. The MISSION of the Edward Via College of Osteopathic Medicine (VCOM) is to prepare globally-minded, community-focused physicians to meet the needs of rural and medically underserved populations and promote research to improve human health.

BASIC SCIENCES: All courses in the first two years are available to students on computer through Scholar. The computer based materials are placed on Scholar to give students an opportunity preview and review the material outside of class and minimize in-class note-taking, to augment student learning and preserve valuable classroom time for faculty/student interaction. Block 1 provides a foundational introduction to curriculum that focuses learning at the cellular level with courses including: Cell Biology and Physiology, Microbiology, Immunology, Pathology, Genetics, and Embryology. In addition students are introduced to the Principles of Primary Care and Osteopathic Manipulative Medicine, as well as a course in Professionalism and Medical Ethics. Blocks 2–7 are comprehensive system based blocks and include courses in Anatomy, Physiology, Pharmacology and Pathology. Principles of Primary Care is extended throughout all blocks and includes Physical Diagnosis, Introduction to Osteopathic Manipulation and Behavioral Medicine topics. Clinical Medicine brings the cases with the medical disciplines aligned with the blocks. These include Immunology and Hematology, Dermatology, Cardiopulmonary System, Neurological, Psychiatry, and Musculoskeletal Systems, Gastrointestinal and Endocrine Systems, Nutrition, and Renal and Genitourinary Systems. Block 8 is a comprehensive review block that brings together all of the material learned in blocks 1–7, to prepare the students for step 1 board exams and clinical rotations. Students also have Early Clinical Experiences throughout the pre-clinical years which include experiences such as: Geriatrics, Free Clinics, mini med school, resident shadowing, athletic trainer shadowing, EMS ride along, ICU nurse shadowing, hospital pharmacist shadowing, gynecologic experience, Obstetrics and Pediatric simulations, clinical Skills training, Laboratory Medicine and Radiology rounds. Please see our college catalog for more information: http://www.vcom.vt.edu/catalog

CLINICAL TRAINING

VCOM Clinical faculty provide the Clinical Medicine Course and the Principles of Primary Care Course during the first two years of osteopathic medical school. The clinical curriculum is integrated throughout the eight blocks to augment the learning of the biomedical curriculum in a meaningful way and to build each block upon medical knowledge. The Clinical Curriculum is planned by the Clinical Chairs. VCOM begins early clinical experiences in the second year through various clinical experiences with preceptors and clinical simulations in the VCOM Simulation and Technology laboratories. In the third year students complete a variety of clinical experiences including family medicine, internal medicine (1 and 2), pediatrics, obstetrics, geriatrics, surgery, psychiatry, and primary care in an underserved setting to complete a broad understanding of those conditions most likely to be seen in the primary care setting. In the fourth year students complete Emergency Medicine, two medical subspecialties, and two surgical subspecialties of their choice to complete a solid medical knowledge base required to begin their Internship. In addition students have four electives in the fourth year where they may visit various residency programs to choose and be seen by the program. VCOM partners with community based hospitals in the target region of Virginia, North Carolina, South Carolina, and bordering West Virginia for the third year Core rotations. VCOM appoints and employs a dedicated clinical faculty within each region in ambulatory settings and affiliated community based hospitals. The clinical faculty who are located in each core site are hired by VCOM as faculty members in clinical departments and fully engage in curriculum development, student teaching in the clinical setting, curriculum development and feedback, and many provide on-campus classroom teaching as well. This partnership with the community-based hospitals and clinical faculty allow a structured academic health center model in a community based setting. VCOM delivers a core medical curriculum in each region that includes a monthly lecture series, on-line clinical presentations, videos, and cases. Students have access to the electronic library, VCOM TV, and web-based videoconferencing. Additional Core Academic Conferences are held three to four times yearly. In addition to the Associate Dean for Clinical Affairs, each core regional site is administered by a Director of Student Medical Education who oversees the development of the academic program in that site and who assists with continued faculty recruitment and development. A Student Coordinator is employed in each region to assist students and regional preceptors with the coordination and scheduling of the academic program. VCOM students also have unique educational opportunities. In the third and fourth year, the opportunity exists to do a Global Medicine Outreach month in the Dominican Republic, Honduras, or El Salvador. Please see our college catalog for more information: http://www.vcom.vt.edu/catalog

Students

STUDENT LIFE

VCOM promotes an environment where students balance curricular, extra-curricular, and personal experiences. Introductory meetings for student organizations occur during the first three months of the first year. Students are encouraged to learn about all organizations and participate in those that will advance career and personal interests. Examples of student organizations formally recognized by VCOM include: American College of Osteopathic Emergency Physicians (ACOEP); American College of Osteopathic Family Practitioners (ACOFP); American College of Osteopathic Pediatricians (ACOP); American College of Osteopathic Internist (ACOI); American College of Osteopathic Obstetricians and Gynecologists (ACOOG); American Osteopathic Academy of Sports Medicine (AOASM); American Medical Women's Association/ National Osteopathic Women Association (AMWA/NOWPA); American Osteopathic Academy of Sports Medicine (AOASM); Student Association of Military Osteopathic Physicians and Surgeons (SAMOPS); Christian Medical and Dental Association (CMDA); Student Associate Auxiliary (SAA); Student Government Association (SGA); Student National Medical Association (SNMA); Student Osteopathic Medical Association (SOMA); Student Osteopathic Surgical Association (SOSA); Undergraduate American Academy of Osteopathy (UAAO); Via Wellness Program—Via Wellness promotes balance for VCOM students by offering social, spiritual, exercise fitness, vocational and intellectual programs. Virginia Rural Health Association/Appalachian Medical Volunteers VCOM also currently has interest groups in: Anesthesia; Neurology/Mental Health and Addiction Medicine; Complementary and Integrative Medicine; Radiology; and the Hispanic Community Medical Outreach Organization (HCMO).

Admissions Requirements (Required)

MCAT Scores, Essays, Science GPA, Extracurricular activities, Non-Science GPA, Exposure to medical profession, Recommendation, Interview, State Residency

COSTS AND AID

Tuition & Fees

Annual tuition	$39,740
Cost of books	$2,137
Fees	$250

Financial Aid

% students receiving any aid	93
% students receiving grants	46
% students receiving loans	90
Average grant	$11,867
Average loan	$54,089
Average total aid package	$55,884

WEST VIRGINIA SCHOOL OF OSTEOPATHIC MEDICINE

WEST VIRGINIA SCHOOL OF OSTEOPATHIC MEDICINE

WEST VIRGINIA SCHOOL OF OSTEOPATHIC MEDICINE

DEPT OF ADMISSIONS AND STUDENT RECRUITMENT, 400 NORTH LEE STREET LEWISBURG, WV 24901
ADMISSION: 800-356-7836 • FAX: 304-645-4859 • E-MAIL: ADMISSIONS@OSTEO.WVSOM.EDU
WEBSITE: WWW.WVSOM.EDU

STUDENT BODY

Type	Public
Enrollment of parent institution	0
Enrollment of medical school	817
% male/female	53/47
% underrepresented minorities	0
% out-of-state	68
% international	23
# countries represented	0
Average age of entering class	22

FACULTY

Total faculty	65
% female faculty	48
% minority faculty	3
% part-time faculty	2
Student-faculty ratio	8.0:1

ADMISSIONS

# applied	4,330
% accepted	11
% enrolled	42

Average GPA and MCAT Scores

Overall GPA	3.5
MCAT Bio	8.7
MCAT Phys	7.7
MCAT Verbal	8.2
MCAT Essay	0

Application Information

Regular application	2/15
Are transfers accepted?	Yes
Admissions may be deferred?	Yes
Admissions need-blind?	No
Application fee	$40

Academics

West Virginia School of Osteopathic Medicine is part of the West Virginia State System of Higher Education. As a state school located in rural Appalachia, it is geared towards meeting the primary care needs of West Virginia's significantly rural population. Nine other states have loose affiliations with the School and are also served by its programs. This curriculum includes clinical training at community sites. Among all students the average age is 25, and the male/female ratio is 54/46.

BASIC SCIENCES: Students are exposed to a broad array of medical topics ranging from biochemistry and gross anatomy to pharmacology and immunology.

CLINICAL TRAINING

Our Clinical Evaluation Center is equipped with 19 state-of-the-art robotic patient simulators that train students in a variety of medical procedures. Additionally, the CEC employs numerous Standardized Patients to present students with real-life patient care scenarios. During their third and fourth years, students participate in clinical rotations. Many of them do rotations at any of our Statewide Campus Locations.

Students

WVSOM's campus is located in Lewisburg, WV and nestled in the heart of beautiful Greenbrier River Valley. WVSOM has spent more than $38 million on construction and renovation projects while increasing from one building in 1972 to 12 campus facilities across its more than 50-acre campus.

STUDENT LIFE

The Roland P. Sharp Alumni Center is home to a cafeteria. We are also planning to build a new student center.

GRADUATES

WVSOM has 2,716 total graduates (1978–2013). WVSOM grads practice medicine in 47 states and the District of Columbia. WVSOM ranks #1 in the nation for physicians practicing in rural settings and a leader in primary care. There are approximately 750 licensed osteopathic physicians practicing medicine in West Virginia; 657 of those are WVSOM alumni. WVSOM graduates practice medicine in 46 of West Virginia's 55 counties.

Admissions

REQUIREMENTS

Historically, residents of West Virginia account for 50 percent of the student body and are given priority in admissions. However, that number has shifted and is now approximately 40%. The minimum course requirements are eight semesters of Biology, Physics, General Chemistry, and Organic Chemistry, all with associated labs, and six semester hours of English. The MCAT is required and the test must be taken no later than the fall prior to the entering class year. Average MCAT of successful applicants is in the 7-8 range. About 17 percent of approximately 3,500 applicants are interviewed, with interviews taking place between September and April.

PROCESS

The admission process at WVSOM is initiated by completing the American Association of Colleges of Osteopathic Medicine Application Service (AACOMAS) On-Line Application. The web-based application allows a prospective student to apply to WVSOM through a secure web server. In order to apply on-line, applicants only need access to a computer with an internet connection. Access to AACOMAS On-Line, which includes all application materials and instructions, is available through the American Association of Colleges of Osteopathic Medicine (AACOM) web site. WVSOM uses the American Association of Colleges of Osteopathic Medicine Application Service (AACOMAS) to process its applications. The following information must be submitted before applications are reviewed by the WVSOM Admissions Committee.

WESTERN UNIVERSITY OF HEALTH SCIENCES
COLLEGE OF OSTEOPATHIC MEDICINE OF THE PACIFIC

OFFICE OF ADMISSIONS, POMONA, CA • **ADMISSION:** 909-469-5335 • **FAX:** 909-469-5570
E-MAIL: ADMISSIONS@WESTERNU.EDU • **WEBSITE:** WWW.WESTERNU.EDU

STUDENT BODY

Type	Private
Enrollment of parent institution	2,130
Enrollment of medical school	762
% male/female	49/51
% underrepresented minorities	2
% out-of-state	38
% international	45
# countries represented	0
Average age of entering class	23

FACULTY

Total faculty	35
% female faculty	26
% minority faculty	29
% part-time faculty	17
Student-faculty ratio	22.0:1

ADMISSIONS

# applied	2,631
% accepted	20
% enrolled	42

Average GPA and MCAT Scores

Overall GPA	3.5
MCAT Bio	9.6
MCAT Phys	9.2
MCAT Verbal	9.6
MCAT Essay	0

Application Information

Regular application	4/15
Are transfers accepted?	Yes
Admissions may be deferred?	Yes
Admissions need-blind?	No
Application fee	$60

Academics

Founded in 1977, Western University of Health Sciences is a nonprofit, graduate university for the health professions located next to Southern California's historic downtown Pomona. With 5 colleges and 1,885 students studying toward advanced degrees in osteopathic medicine, pharmacy, graduate nursing, physical therapy, physician assistant studies, health professions education, and veterinary medicine, Western University is one of the largest graduate schools for the health professions in California.

BASIC SCIENCES: The educational program is centered on the basic concepts of osteopathic medicine. The College of Osteopathic Medicine of the Pacific identifies and develops the knowledge, cognitive and psychomotor skills, and the personal and professional behaviors required of an osteopathic physician to provide competent and comprehensive health care to all members of a family, on a continuing basis. The first semester of the first year is designed to introduce the students to the basic concepts of anatomy (gross, embryology, and histology), biochemistry, microbiology, pathology, pharmacology, and physiology. Interwoven throughout the curriculum are osteopathic principles and practice.

The second phase begins in the second semester of the first year and continues throughout the year 2. The basic and clinical sciences concerned with one particular organ system of the body are integrated in classroom instruction. This approach emphasizes the relevance of basic sciences to clinical practice. The osteopathic approach is continually emphasized by lecture and laboratory demonstration, including manipulative techniques.

CLINICAL TRAINING

Clinical training via rotation through each of the major medical disciplines (Family Practice, Internal Medicine, Surgery, Pediatrics, Obstetrics/Gynecology, Pathology, Psychiatry, Emergency Medicine, and Radiology) is accomplished in the third and fourth years of training. Twenty-two rotations of 4 weeks each provide an opportunity for clinical skill development in primary care medicine. Several elective options are also offered during this two-year period. The goal of the clinical curriculum is to prepare each and every student with the knowledge, attitudes, and skills to excel in his or her chosen postdoctoral-training program.

Campus Life

The main campus of Western University is in Pomona, a city of approximately 150,000, located about 35 miles east of Los Angeles near the foothills of the San Gabriel Mountains.

STUDENT LIFE

Western University provides YMCA or designated fitness club individual memberships for students at a minimal cost. The YMCA is within walking distance of the Pomona campus and offers coeducational facilities for swimming, racquetball, basketball, exercise programs, and so on.

GRADUATES

The College of Osteopathic Medicine of the Pacific supports Western University of Health Sciences (WesternU) in its mission to increase the availability of physicians to serve the needs of the people living in the western region of the United States. The College of Osteopathic Medicine provides the educational basis for internship and residencies in all medical specialties.

Admissions

REQUIREMENTS

Applicants applying for admission to the DO program must meet the following minimum academic requirements at the time of application: a minimum of 90 semester hours at a regionally accredited college or university; a completed application, which can be submitted prior to taking the MCAT; scores from the MCAT, which must be taken prior to January of the entering year; 8 semester units each of biology, inorganic chemistry (with a lab), organic chemistry (with a lab), physics; and 6 semester units of English and behavioral science.

PROCESS

Prospective applicants must submit a primary application through AACOMAS. Applications can be submitted electronically by accessing http://AACOMAS.AACOM.org, or a request for application material can be made by mail at the following address: AACOMAS, 550 Friendship Boulevard, Suite 310, Chevy Chase, MD 20815-7231, 301-968-4190. The AACOMAS deadline is April 15.

Once the AACOMAS application is received, selected applicants are contacted by postcard or e-mail with instructions on how to submit the supplementary application. At this time, applicants are instructed to complete the supplementary application online. The supplementary application and all supporting documents should be received by the Admissions Office within 30 days of the date we contact you regarding the supplementary application. The AACOMAS application, together with the supplemental application, letters of recommendation, and official MCAT score constitutes an application ready for evaluation. Once the interview process begins, students are admitted to the program on a rolling basis; therefore, students are encouraged to apply early.

As part of the application process, you are required to submit letters of recommendation from a pre-health professions committee (or the committee on your campus responsible for writing recommendations) and one physician. If such a committee does not exist at your college, you are required to submit two evaluations from science professors (i.e., biology, chemistry, or physics), one evaluation from a non-science professor, and one evaluation from a physician, DO, or MD who you have worked with or observed in a clinical setting. A recommendation letter from a DO is preferred. The science/non-science letters must be from professors who have instructed you, and the recommender should specify the course(s). All recommendations must be on the Western University form provided or on college or professional letterhead. Applicants who wish to use course work completed outside the United States must submit the transcripts for evaluation to one of the following services: World Education Services, PO Box 745, Old Chelsea Station, New York, New York, 10113-0745, 212-966-6311, WES.org; Josef Silny & Associates, 7101 SW 102 Avenue, Miami, Florida, 33173, 305-273-1616, JSilny.com; Educational Credential Evaluators, Inc., PO Box 514070, Milwaukee, Wisconsin, 53203-3470, 414-289-3400, ECE.org; International Educational Research Foundation, Inc., PO Box 3665, Culver City, California, 90231-3665, IERF.org.

A course-by-course evaluation is required, and all course work must be designated as undergraduate, graduate, or professional. Western University will only honor evaluations from one of these services. The evaluation must be included with the application.

Admissions Requirements (Required)

MCAT Scores, Essays, Science GPA, Extracurricular activities, Non-Science GPA, Exposure to medical profession, Recommendation, Interview

Admissions Requirements (Optional)

State Residency

COSTS AND AID

Tuition & Fees

Annual tuition	$37,190
Room & board	$10,380
Cost of books	$2,320
Fees	$60

Financial Aid

% students receiving any aid	94
% students receiving grants	21
% students receiving loans	91
% aid that is merit-based	5
Average grant	$23,663
Average loan	$45,651
Average total aid package	$49,415
Average debt	$159,768

10 Post-baccalaureate Premedical Schools

Colleges and universities offer organized post-baccalaureate premedical programs. Although this list is quite comprehensive, it may be incomplete because many schools have just recently adopted post-bacc programs. In addition, many undergraduate institutions that do not offer formal programs have flexible enrollment policies that facilitate post-bacc studies.

For further listings of post-bacc programs, Syracuse University Health Professions Advisory Program (315-443-2321) has an online compilation at: http://services.aamc.org/postbac/.

ADELPHI UNIVERSITY
Certificate in Basic Sciences for Health
Professions
Robert Schwartz
Director, Office of Pre-Professional
Advising and Fellowships
One South Avenue
P.O. Box 701
Garden City, NY 11530
516-877-3410
E-mail: rschwartz@adelphi.edu

AGNES SCOTT COLLEGE
Post-baccalaureate Premedical Program
Andrea L. Clark, MBA
Health Professions Coordinator
141 East College Avenue
Decatur, GA 30030-3797
404-471-5395
Fax: 404-471-5838
E-mail: post-bacc@agnesscott.edu

AMERICAN UNIVERSITY
Post-baccalaureate Premedical Certificate
Program
Dr. Lynne Arneson
Programs Coordinator
Hurst 101
American University
4400 Massachusetts Avenue Northwest
Washington, DC 20016-8014
202-885-2186
Fax: 202-885-1752
E-mail: premed@american.edu

ASSUMPTION COLLEGE
Steven Theroux, Ph.D.
Biology Department, Assumption College
Program Director
500 Salisbury Street
Worcester, MA 01609-0005
508-767-7545
E-mail: stheroux@assumption.edu

AVILA UNIVERSITY
Post-baccalaureate Premedical Program
Dr. C. Larry Garrison Sullivan,
Prehealth Professional Advisor
11901 Wornall Road
Kansas City, MO 64145
816-501-3655
Fax: 816-501-2457
E-mail: Larry.Sullivan@avila.edu

BARRY UNIVERSITY
Biomedical Sciences
Dr. Jonathan Coffman, Program Director
College of Health Sciences
11300 Northeast Second Avenue
Miami Shores, FL 33161-6695
305-899-3279 or 800-756-6000, ext. 3379
Fax: 305-899-3232
Program Contact: Mrs. Denise Deen
E-mail: healthsciences@mail.barry.edu

BENNINGTON COLLEGE
Post-baccalaureate Premedical Program
Dr. Janet Foley, Program Director
Office of Admissions
Bennington College
One College Drive
Bennington, VT 05201
802-440-4485
Program Contact: Ferrilyn Sourdiffe
E-mail: fsourdiffe@bennington.edu

BOSTON UNIVERSITY
Post-baccalaureate Certificate in
Premedical Studies
PMC Program Coordinator
755 Commonwealth Avenue, Room 102
Boston, MA 02215
617-353-2980
Fax: 617-353-4190
E-mail: metuss@bu.edu

BOSTON UNIVERSITY
Master of Arts in Medical Sciences
Program
Dr. Gwynneth Offner, Program Director
GMS, Boston Univ. School of Medicine
72 East Concord Street, Room L-315
Boston, MA 02118
617-638-8221 or 617-638-5255
Fax: 617-638-5740
Program Contact: Gwynneth Offner
E-mail: goffner@bu.edu

BRANDEIS UNIVERSITY
Post-baccalaureate Certificate Program
Nicole Labrecque
Post-Baccalaureate Premedical Program
Coordinator
Usdan/Mailstop 001
415 South St.
Waltham, MA 02453-2728
781-736-3461
Fax: 781-736-2003
E-mail: nicolab@brandeis.edu

BRYN MAWR COLLEGE
Post-baccalaureate Premedical Program
Jodi Domsky, Program Director
Bryn Mawr College Canwyll House
101 North Merion Ave.
Bryn Mawr, PA 19010-2899
610-526-7350
Fax: 610-526-7353
E-mail: postbac@brynmawr.edu

CALIFORNIA STATE UNIVERSITY— LOS ANGELES
Post-Baccalaureate Certificate Program
for Pre-Health Professionals
Department of Biological Sciences
5151 State University Drive
Los Angeles, CA 90032
323-343-2050
Fax 323-343-6451
Biomicr@calstatela.edu

CALIFORNIA STATE UNIVERSITY— FULLERTON
Certificate in Pre-Health Professions
Studies
Brandy Schaal
2600 Nutwood Ave. Suite 100
Fullerton, CA 92831
657-278-7269
bschaal@fullerton.edu

CALIFORNIA STATE UNIVERSITY, EAST BAY
Pre-Health Sciences Professional
Certificate Program
Dr. Oscar Wambuguh
California State University, East Bay
25800 Carlos Bee Blvd - North Science,
Room 231
Hayward, CA 94542
510-885-2366
Fax: 510-885-2035
Program Contact: Linda Steele
E-mail: linda.steele@csueastbay.edu

CARSON-NEWMAN COLLEGE
Steve Karr, Postbaccalaureate Program
Program Director
Carson-Newman College
2130 Branner Ave.
Jefferson City, TN 37760
865-471-3252
Fax: 865-471-3578
E-mail: stkarr@cn.edu

CASE WESTERN RESERVE UNIVERSITY
Master of Science in Medical Physiology
Dr. Thomas Nosek, Program Director
10900 Euclid Avenue
Department of Physiology and
Biophysics
Cleveland, OH 44106-4970
216-368-2084
Fax: 216-368-5529
Program Contact: Ms. Jean Davis
E-mail: Jean.Davis@Case.edu

CHAPMAN UNIVERSITY

Post Baccalaureate Program
Kenneth Sumida, PhD
One University Drive
Orange, CA 92866
Fax: 714-997-6995
E-mail: sumida@chapman.edu

CHARLES R. DREW UNIVERSITY

Post Baccalaureate Certificate in Pre
Medicine
Program Director
Suzanne Porszasz-Reisz
1731 East 120th Street
Los Angeles, CA 90059
Office of Admissions
323-563-4838
Fax: 323-563-4837
E-mail: admissionsinfo@cdrewu.edu

THE CITY COLLEGE OF NEW YORK

Belinda Smith
Program in Premedical Studies
Convent Avenue & 138th Street
Marshak Science Building, Room J529
New York, NY 10031
212-650-6622
Fax: 212-650-7816
Program Contact: Belinda Smith
E-mail: premedical@sci.ccny.cuny.edu

CLEVELAND STATE UNIVERSITY

Post-Baccalaureate Program
Cheryl Laubacher, Program Director
Cleveland State University
Post-Baccalaureate Program Cleveland
State University
COSHP Advising 2121 Euclid, MC 218B
Cleveland, OH 44115-2214
(216) 687-9321
E-mail: postbacPP@csuohio.edu

COLORADO STATE UNIVERSITY

Professional Master's Program (MS- B) in
Biomedical Sciences
Merk Frasier, Program Director
Program Contact: Erin Bisenius
970-491-6188
Email: Bmsgradinformation@colostate.edu

COLUMBIA UNIVERSITY MEDICAL CENTER

Institute of Human Nutrition
Dr. Sharon Akabas, Program Director
630 W. 168th Street
PH15E-1512
New York, NY 10032
212-305-4808
Fax: 212-305-3079
Program Contact: Erin Paxson
E-mail: nutrition@columbia.edu

COLUMBIA UNIVERSITY

Post-baccalaureate Premedical Program
404 Lewisohn Hall, MC 4101
2970 Broadway
New York, NY 10027
212-854-7961
Fax: 212-854-6316
Email: postbac@columbia.edu

THE COMMONWEALTH MEDICAL COLLEGE

Master's of Biomedical Science
Dr. Jennifer Smith, Program Director
The Commonwealth Medical College
525 Pine Street
Scranton, PA 18509
570-504-9638
Fax: 570-504-9663
Program Contact: Jennifer Smith
E-mail: jsmith@tcmedc.org

CORNELL UNIVERSITY
The Cornell/Division of Nutritional Sciences Post-baccalaureate Program in Health Studies
Joy Swanson
B20 Day Hall
Ithaca, NY 14853
607-255-7259
E-mail: cusp@cornell.edu

CREIGHTON UNIVERSITY
Premedical Post-baccalaureate
Dr. Sade Kosoko-Lasaki
Program Director
2500 California Plaza
Omaha, NE 68178
402-280-3029
Fax: 402-280-4030
Program Contact: Channing Bunch
E-mail: cbunch@creighton.edu

DARTMOUTH MEDICAL SCHOOL
The Dartmouth Institute for Health Policy and Clinical Practice
Mr. Adam Keller, Program Director
Hinman Box 7252
30 Lafayette St., 1st Floor
Lebanon, NH 03766
603-653-3234
Fax: 603-653-3266
Program Contact: Courtney Theroux
Recruitment & Admissions
E-mail: Courtney.L.Theroux@dartmouth.edu

DOMINICAN UNIVERSITY
Post-baccalaureate Premedical Program
Drs. Louis Scannichio and Hughes, Program Directors
7900 West Division Street
River Forest, IL 60305
708-355-2490
Fax: 708-524-6032
E-mail: postbacc@dom.edu

DREXEL UNIVERSITY
Master of Biological Science (MBS) Program
Drexel University College of Medicine
245 North Fifteenth Street, MS 344,
New College Building Room 4-104
Philadelphia, PA 19102
215-762-4692
Fax: 215-762-8651
Program Contact: Joy Henderson
E-mail: joy.henderson@drexelmed.edu

DREXEL UNIVERSITY
Medical Science Preparatory Program (MSP)
Drexel University College of Medicine
245 North Fifteenth Street, MS 344,
New College Building Room 4-104
Philadelphia, PA 19102
215-762-4692
Fax: 215-762-8651
Program Contact: Joy Henderson
E-mail: joy.henderson@drexelmed.edu

DREXEL UNIVERSITY
College of Medicine
Office of Professional Studies in the Health Sciences: Interdisciplinary Health Sciences (IHS) program
Dr. Nancy Minugh-Purvis, Program Director
245 North 15th Street Mail Stop #344
New College Building Room 4-104
Philadelphia PA 19102
215-762-3948
Fax: 215-762-8803
Program Contact: Tara Sarica
E-mail: Tara.Sarica@drexelmed.edu

DREXEL UNIVERSITY

College of Medicine
Office of Professional Studies in the
Health Sciences: Master of
Interdisciplinary Health
Sciences (MIHS) program
Dr. Nancy Minugh-Purvis, Program
Director
245 North 15th Street Mail Stop #344
New College Building Room 4-104
Philadelphia PA 19102
215-762-3948
Fax: 215-762-8803
Program Contact: Tara Sarica
E-mail: Tara.Sarica@drexelmed.edu

DREXEL UNIVERSITY

Drexel Pathway to Medical School (DPMS)
Drexel University College of Medicine
Dr. Loretta Walker, Program Director
245 North 15th Street,
MS 344, New College Building
Room 4-104
Philadelphia, PA 19102
215-762-7125
Fax: 215-762-8651
E-mail: loretta.walker@drexelmed.edu

DREXEL UNIVERSITY

Evening Post-baccalaureate Premedical
Program (PMED)
Drexel University College of Medicine
Dr. Laura Mangano, Program Director
245 North 15th Street, MS 344
North College Building Room 4-104
Philadelphia, PA 19102
215-762-4692
Fax: 215-762-8651
Program Contact: Joy Henderson
E-mail: Joy.Henderson@drexelmed.edu

DREXEL UNIVERSITY

Interdepartmental Medical Science
Program (IMS)
Drexel University College of Medicine
245 North 15th Street,
MS 344
New College Building Room 4-104
Philadelphia, PA 19102
Program Contact: Joy Henderson
215-762-4692
Fax: 215-762-8651
E-mail: Joy.Henderson@drexelmed.edu

DREW UNIVERSITY

Pre-Medical Preparation Program
36 Madison Avenue
Madison, NJ 07940
Program Contact: Patricia Laprey
973-408-3400
Fax: 973-408-3004
Email: plaprey@drew.edu

DUQUESNE UNIVERSITY

Post-Baccalaureate Pre-Medical Program
Kyle Selcer, Program Director
600 Forbes Avenue
700 Fisher Hall
Pittsburgh, PA 15282
412-396-6335
Fax: 412-396-5587
Program Contact: Amy Whittington
Email: postbacpremed@duq.edu

EASTERN MENNONITE UNIVERSITY

MA in Biomedicine
1200 Park Rd.
Harrisonburg, VA 22802
540-432-4400
Fax: 540-432-4488
Program Contact: Cheryl Doss
Email: ma-biomed@emu.edu

EASTERN VIRGINIA MEDICAL SCHOOL

Medical Master's Program
Program Contact: Rose Mwayungu
700 West Olney Road
Norfolk, VA 23507
757-446-7153
Fax: 757-446-8915
E-mail: mwayunra@evms.edu

EDWARD VIA COLLEGE OF OSTEOPATHIC MEDICINE, VIRGINIA CAMPUS

Post-Baccalaureate Pre-Med Program
Dr. Brian Hill, Program Director
VCOM Post-Baccalaureate Pre-Med
Program
309 N. Knollwood Drive
Blacksburg, VA 24060
540-231-5090
Fax: 540-231-2001
Program Contact: Jean Herndon
E-mail: jherndon@vcom.vt.edu

ELMS COLLEGE

Post-baccalaureate Premedical Program
Dr. Janet Williams
291 Springfield Street
Chicopee, MA 01013
413-265-2381
Fax: 413-592-4871
E-Mail: williamsj@elms.edu

FARMINGDALE STATE COLLEGE

Certificate in Sciences for Health
Professions
Charles Adair, Program Director
2350 Broadhollow Rd.
Farmingdale, NY 11735
631-420-2175
Program Contact: Matthew Bahamonde
Ph.D.
Email: bahamonde@farmingdale.edu

FLORIDA STATE UNIVERSITY

Bridge to Clinical Medicine Program
College of Medicine
Helen Livingston, Program Director
West Call Street
P.O. Box 3064300
Tallahassee, FL
850-645-2826
Program Contact: Ms. Kit Clayton
Email: kit.clayton@med.fsu.edu

GEORGETOWN UNIVERSITY

Special Master's Program, Department of
Physiology
Dr. Susan Mulroney, Program Director
3900 Reservoir Rd. NW,
Washington, DC 20057
Program Contact: Amy Richards
202-687-1179
Fax: 202-687-8825
E-mail: physio@georgetown

GEORGETOWN UNIVERSITY

Post-baccalaureate Pre-medical Certificate
Program
Dr. Edward Meyertholen, Program
Director
180 White Gravenor
Washington, DC 20057
202-687-4853
E-mail: premed@georgetown.edu

GEORGETOWN UNIVERSITY
MS Physiology & Biophysics -
Complementary & Alternative Medicine
(CAM) Program
Dr. Hakima Amri, Program Director
3900 Reservoir Rd NW
237 Basic Science
Washington, DC 20057
202-687-7979
Fax: 202-687-8919
Program Contact: Aureller Cabiness
E-mail: camprogram@georgetown.edu

**GEORGETOWN UNIVERSITY/
GEORGE MASON UNIVERSITY**
Advanced Biomedical Sciences Graduate
Certificate Program
Dr. Donna Fox, Program Director
10900 University Blvd.
MSN 6E3, Bull Run Hall 308
Manassas, VA 20110
703-993-7136
Fax: 703-993-7139
Program Contact: Ms. Tanneh Kamara
E-mail: gsquared@gmu.edu

**GEORGETOWN UNIVERSITY/
GEORGE MASON UNIVERSITY**
MS Biomedical Sciences with emphasis in
Systems Biology
Dr. Donna Fox, Program Director
10900 University Blvd.
MSN 6E3, Bull Run Hall 308
Manassas, VA 20110
703-993-7136
Fax: 703-993-7139
Program Contact: Ms. Tanneh Kamara
E-mail: gsquared@gmu.edu

GOUCHER COLLEGE
Post-baccalaureate Premedical Program
Betsy Merideth, Program Director
1021 Dulaney Valley Road
Baltimore, MD 21204-2794
800-414-3437
Fax: 410-337-6461
E-mail: pbpm@goucher.edu

HAMPTON UNIVERSITY
Medical Science Masters Program
Michael Druitt, Program Director
School of Science
110 Turner Hall
Hampton, VA 23668
757-728-6757
Fax: 757-727-5832
E-mail: Michael.druitt@hamptonu.edu

HARVARD UNIVERSITY
Health Careers Program
Dr. William Fixsen, Program Director
51 Brattle Street
Cambridge, MA 02138
617-495-2926
Program Contact: Owen Peterson
E-mail: peterson@hudce.harvard.edu

HOFSTRA UNIVERSITY
Post-baccalaureate Premedical Program
Ellen Miller, Program Director
Hofstra University
Memorial Hall Room 101
Hempstead, NY 11549
516-463-4900
Fax: 516-463-6674
E-mail: premedpostbach@hofstra.edu

JOHN CARROLL UNIVERSITY

Pre-Medical Post-Baccalaureate Program
Dr. Kathy Lee, Program
Director
John Carroll University
20700 N. Park Blvd.
University Heights, OH 44118
216-397-4902
Program Contact: Vivienne Porter
E-mail: vporter@jcu.edu

JOHNS HOPKINS UNIVERSITY

Post-baccalaureate Premedical Program
Liza Thompson, Program Director
3400 N. Charles Street
28 Shriver Hall
Baltimore, MD 21218
410-516-7748
Fax: 410-516-5233
E-mail: postbac@jhu.edu

KECK GRADUATE INSTITUTE

Postbaccalaureate Premedical Certificate
Program
Dr. Joon Kim
535 Watson Drive
Claremont, CA 91711
909-607-8590
Fax: 909-607-8086
Program Contact: Sofia Toro, MBA
E-mail: admissions@kgi.edu

LAKE ERIE COLLEGE OF OSTEOPATHIC MEDICINE

Health Science Post Baccalaureate
Program
1858 W. Grandview Blvd.
Erie, PA 16509
814-866-6641
Email: postbac@lecom.edu

LASALLE UNIVERSITY

Postbaccalaureate Premedical Certificate
Program
Dr. Geri Seitchik, Program Director
1900 W. Olney Ave
Philadelphia PA 19141
215-951-1248
E-mail: seitchik@lasalle.edu

LINCOLN MEMORIAL UNIVERSITY

Post-Baccalaureate Medical Science
Certificate
Amiel Jarstfer, Program Director
6965 Cumberland Gap Parkway
Harrogate, TN 37752
423-869-6328
Fax: 423-869-7093
Program Contact: F. Ryan Stump, M.D.
Email: frank.stump@lmunet.edu

LOYOLA MARYMOUNT UNIVERSITY

Post-baccalaureate Premedical Program
Dr. Rebecca Pazdral, Program Director
1 LMU Drive, North Hall 213
Los Angeles, CA 90045-2659
310-338-7704
E-mail: prehealth@lmu.edu

LOYOLA UNIVERSITY OF CHICAGO

Master of Arts in Medical Sciences
Dr. F. Bryan Pickett, Graduate
Program Director
Department of Biology
1032 W. Sheridan Road
Chicago, IL 60660
773-508-3285
E-mail: mams@luc.edu

MANHATTANVILLE COLLEGE

Post-baccalaureate Pre-health Professions
Program
Daniel Gerger, Program Director
Academic Advising Office
2900 Purchase Street
Purchase, NY 10577
914-323-5446
Fax: 914-323-5338
E-mail: Daniel.gerger@mville.edu

MEREDITH COLLEGE

Pre-Health Post Baccalaureate Certificate
Dr. Francie Cuffney
3800 Hillsborough Street
Raleigh, NC 27607
919-760-8058
Fax: 919-760-2898
Program Contact: Sylvia Horton
Email: hortons@meredith.edu

MIDWESTERN UNIVERSITY

Master of Arts in Biomedical Services
Leonard Bell, Program Director
19555 N. 59th Ave.
Glendale, AZ 85308
623-572-3620
Fax: 623-572-3647
E-mail: lbellx@midwestern.edu

MILLS COLLEGE

Post-baccalaureate Program
5000 MacArthur Boulevard
Oakland, CA 94613
510-430-2317
Fax: 510-430-3314
Program Contact: Jo Scullion
E-mail: jscullio@mills.edu

MISSISSIPPI COLLEGE

Masters of Medical Sciences
Dr. Stan Baldwin
Box 445
Mississippi College
Clinton, MS 39058
601-925-3321
Email: sbaldwin@mc.edu

MONTANA STATE UNIVERSITY

Post-baccalaureate Premedical Certificate
Program
Dr. Sheila Nielsen-Preiss, Program
Director
MSU Division of Health Sciences
317 Leon Johnson Hall
Bozeman, MT 59717
406-994-1670
Program Contact: Sarah Karlsgodt
E-mail:hpa@montana.edu

MONTANA STATE UNIVERSITY

Master of Science in Health Science
Dr. Sheila Nielsen-Preiss, Program
Director
315 Leon Johnson Hall
Bozeman, MT 59717
406-994-1670
Fax: 406-994-4398
Program Contact: Sarah Karlsgodt
E-mail:hpa@montana.edu

MOUNT HOLYOKE

Post-baccalaureate Prehealth Program
Studies Program
Dr. David Gardner, Program Director
50 College Street
South Hadley, MA 01075
413-538-3389
Fax: 413-538-3398
E-mail: posttbac@mtholyoke.edu

NEW YORK CHIROPRACTIC COLLEGE

Masters of Applied Clinical Nutrition
Dr. Anna R. Kelles, Program Director
2360 State Route 89
Seneca Falls, NY 13148
315-568-3312
Fax: 315-568-3017
Program Contact: Maria Golonski
E-mail: mgolonski@nycc.edu

NEW YORK MEDICAL COLLEGE

Basic Medical Science Interdisciplinary
Program Traditional Track
Dr. Ken Lerea, Program Director
Basic Sciences Building, Room A41
Valhalla, NY 10595
Program Contact: Carolyn J. Chiarieri,
M.S.
914-594-3464
Fax: 914-594-4944
E-mail: carolyn_chiareri@nymc.edu

NEW YORK MEDICAL COLLEGE

Basic Medical Science Interdisciplinary
Program Accelerated Track
Dr. Norman Levine, Program Director
Graduate School of Basic Medical
Sciences
Basic Sciences Building, Room
Valhalla, NY 10595
Program Contact: Carolyn J. Chiarieri,
M.S.
914-594-3464
Fax: 914-594-4944
E-mail: carolyn_chiareri@nymc.edu

NEW YORK UNIVERSITY

Post-baccalaureate Pre-health Studies
Program
100 Washington Square East
Silver Center, Room 901
New York, NY 10003
212-998-8160
Fax: 212-995-4549
NYU Preprofessional Center
E-mail: postbacc@nyu.edu

NORTHEASTERN STATE UNIVERSITY

Postbaccalaureate Prehealth Certificate
Program
Dr. Craig Clifford, Program Director
College of Science & Health Professions
611 N. Grand Ave
Tahlequah, OK 74464
918-449-6474
Fax: 918-458-2325
E-mail: prehealth@nsuok.edu

NORTHWESTERN UNIVERSITY SCHOOL OF CONTINUING STUDIES

Premedical Professional Health Careers
Program
Admissions Coordinator
339 E. Chicago Ave.
Wieboldt Hall, 6th Floor
Chicago, IL 60611
312-503-0875
Fax: 312-503-4942
E-mail: scsadmissions@northwestern.edu

NORTHWESTERN UNIVERSITY

Program in Public Health
680 N Lake Shore Dr., Suite 1400
Chicago, IL 60611
312-503-0500
Fax: 312-908-9588
Program Contact: Maureen Moran, MPH
E-mail: m-moran@northwestern.edu

THE OHIO STATE UNIVERSITY

MEDPATH
Leon McDougle, Program Director
370 West 9th Avenue
061Meiling Hall
Columbus, OH 43210
614-292-3161
Program Contact: Nikki Radcliffe
E-mail: nikki.radcliffe@osumc.edu

OREGON STATE UNIVERSITY

OSU Postbac Premed Program
Chere Pereira, Program Director
Corvallis, OR 97331
541-737-4811
Fax: 541-737-1009
E-mail: chere.pereira@oregonstate.edu

PENN STATE BRANDYWINE

Accelerated Postbaccalaureate Medical
Sciences Certificate
Margaret Bacheler, Program Director
25 Yearsley Mill Road
Media, PA 19063-5596
610-892-1306
Fax: 610-892-1320
E-mail: mbw10@psu.edu

THE PENNSYLVANIA STATE UNIVERSITY

Post-Baccalaureate Premedical Certificate
Program
Dr. Mildred Rodriguez, Program Director
213 Whitmore Lab
University Park, PA 168802
814-865-7620
Fax: 814-865-7214
Email: mxr22@psu.edu

PHILADELPHIA COLLEGE OF OSTEOPATHIC MEDICINE

Biomedical Sciences Program
Office of Admissions
4170 City Avenue
Philadelphia, PA 19131
800-999-6998
Fax: 215-871-6719
E-mail: gradadmissions@pcom.edu

REGIS UNIVERSITY

Master of Science in Biomedical Sciences
Dr. Joan Betz, Program Director
Dept. Biology D-8
3333 Regis Blvd
Denver, CO 80221-1099
303-458-6114
E-mail: BiomedMS@regis.edu

RICHARD STOCKTON COLLEGE OF NEW JERSEY

Post-baccalaureate Certificate Program in
Health Professions
Dr. Ralph Werner, Program Director
101 Vera King Farris Drive
Galloway, NJ 08205
609-652-4462
E-mail: ralph.werner@stockton.edu

RIDER UNIVERSITY

Premedical Studies Program
Dr. Bryan Spiegelberg, Program Director
2083 Lawrenceville Road
Lawrenceville, NJ 08648
609-896-7729
E-mail: bspiegelber@rider.edu

ROCKHURST UNIVERSITY

Post-baccalaureate Premedical Program
Dr. James Wheeler, Program Director
1100 Rockhurst Road
Kansas City, MO 64110
816-501-4068
Fax: 816-501-4802
E-mail: james.wheeler@rockhurst.edu

ROSALIND FRANKLIN UNIVERSITY OF MEDICINE & SCIENCE

Master of Science in Biomedical Sciences
Catherine Gierman-Riblon, Program Director
3333 Green Bay Rd.
North Chicago, IL 60064
847-578-8789
E-mail:Catherine.giermanriblon@rosalindfranklin.edu

RUTGERS UNIVERSITY—NEW BRUNSWICK

Post-baccalaureate Pre-health Program
Dr. Elizabeth Vogel, Program Director
604 Allison Rd.
Nelson Biological Laboratories, Room A-207
Piscataway, NJ 08854
732-445-5667
Fax: 732-445-6341
Program Contact: Bonnie Katz
E-mail: bkatz@biology.rutgers.edu

SAN DIEGO STATE UNIVERSITY

Pre-professional Health Advising Office
Barbara Huntington
5500 Campanile Drive
MC-1017
San Diego, CA 92182-1017
619-594-6638
Fax: 619-594-0244
E-mail: healthpr@sciences.sdsu.edu

SAN FRANCISCO STATE UNIVERSITY

Pre-Health Professions Certificate Program
Dr. Barry S. Rothman, Program Director
Department of Biology,
1600 Holloway Avenue
San Francisco, CA 94132
415-405-4239
Fax: 415-338-2295
E-mail: PBAdmit@sfsu.edu

SCRIPPS COLLEGE

Post-baccalaureate Premedical Program
DeEttra Mulay, Program Director
1030 Columbia Ave
Claremont, CA 91711
909-621-8764
Fax: 909-621-8588
E-mail: dmulay@scrippscollege.edu

SEATTLE UNIVERSITY

Post-baccalaureate Premedical Program
Ms. Rebecca Bregel, Program Director
901 Twelfth Avenue, PO Box 222000
300 ENGR: Science and Engineering Advising Center
Seattle, WA 98122-1090
206-296-2500
Fax: 206-296-2179
E-mail: bregelr@seattleu.edu

SOUTHERN ILLINOIS UNIVERSITY

SCHOOL OF MEDICINE
Medical/Dental Education Preparatory Program (MEDPREP)
Dr. Harold Bardo, Program Director
975 S. Normal Ave., MC 4323
Carbondale, IL 62901-4323
618-453-1554
Fax: 618-453-1919
Program Contact: Layla Murphy
E-mail: MedPrepAdmissions@siumed.edu

STONY BROOK UNIVERSITY

Post-baccalaureate Pre-Health Program
E2360 Melville Library
Stony Brook University
Stony Brook, NY 11794-3353
631-632-7082
Program Contact: Joanie Maniaci
Email: prehealth@notes.cc.sunysb.edu

TEMPLE UNIVERSITY SCHOOL OF MEDICINE

Advanced Core in Medical Science Post Baccalaureate PreMedical Program
Grace Hershman, Program Director
3500 North Broad Street
Suite 124
Philadelphia, PA 19140
215-707-3342
Fax: 215-707-6932
E-mail: postbac@temple.edu

TEMPLE UNIVERSITY SCHOOL OF MEDICINE

Basic Core In Medical Science (BCMS) Post Baccalaureate PreMedical Program
Grace Hershman, Program Director
3500 North Broad Street
Suite 124
Philadelphia PA 19140
215-707-3342
Fax: 215-707-6932
E-mail: postbac@temple.edu

TEXAS TECH UNIVERSITY

Health Sciences Center
Pre-Medical Sciences, M.S. in Biomedical Sciences
Dr. Brandt Schneider, Program Director
3601 4th St., STOP 6540
Lubbock, TX 79430
806-743-2701
Fax: 806-743-2990
Program Contact: Terri Lloyd
E-mail: terri.lloyd@ttuhsc.edu

THOMAS JEFFERSON UNIVERSITY

Postbaccalaureate Pre-Professional Program
Dr. Adrienne Dolberry, Program Director
1020 Locust Street
M-46
Philadelphia, PA 19107
215-503-6905
Fax: 215-503-3433
Email:postbac@jefferson.edu

TOURO COLLEGE/TOURO COLLEGE OF OSTEOPATHIC MEDICINE

Interdisciplinary Studies in Biological and Physical Sciences
230 W. 125th Street
Suite 425
New York, NY 10027
646-981-4602
Fax: 212-678-1782
Program Contact: Lissette Mercado
E-mail: Lissette.Mercado@touro.edu

TUFTS UNIVERSITY

Post-baccalaureate Premedical Program
Carol Baffi-Dugan, Program Director
419 Boston Avenue
Dowling Hall
Medford, MA 02155
Program Contact: Liz Regan
617-627-2321
Fax: 617-627-3907
E-mail: liz.regan@tufts.edu

TULANE UNIVERSITY

Cell and Molecular Biology One Year Masters
Dr. Fiona Inglis, Program Director
2000 Percival Stern Hall
Tulane University
New Orleans, LA 70118
504-865-5618
Fax: 504-865-6785
Program Contact: Marnie Mercado
E-mail: mmercado@tulane.edu

TULANE UNIVERSITY

Master's Degree in Human Genetics
-Hayward Genetics Center
1430 Tulane Avenue
Hayward Genetics Center SL-31
New Orleans, LA 70112
504-988-6242
Fax: 504-988-1763
Program Contact: Dr. Karen Weisbecker
E-mail: kremer@tulane.edu

TULANE UNIVERSITY SCHOOL OF MEDICINE

One Year Masters in Pharmacology
Program
Dr. Craig Clarkson, Program Director
Dept of Pharmacology SL83, School of
Medicine
1430 Tulane Avenue
New Orleans, LA 70112
504-988-5444
Fax: 504-988-6761
E-mail: cclarks@tulane.edu

TULANE UNIVERSITY SCHOOL OF MEDICINE

One Year Masters Program in
Biochemistry & Molecular Biology
David Franklin, Program Director
Dept. of Biochemistry and Molecular
Biology
1430 Tulane Avenue
New Orleans, LA 70112
504-988-8868
Fax: 504-988-2739
E-mail: franklin@tulane.edu

UMDNJ-GSBS-ROBERT WOOD JOHNSON MEDICAL SCHOOL

Master of Biomedical Sciences
674 Hoes Lane
Piscataway, NJ 08854
732-235-5016
E-mail: rwjmsmasters@umdnj.edu

UMDNJ—GRADUATE SCHOOL OF BIOMEDIAL SCIENCES AT NJ MEDICAL SCHOOL

Master of Biomedical Sciences
Dr. BJ Wagner, Program Director
Medical Science Building C696
185 South Orange Avenue
Newark, NJ 07101
973-972-5335/973-972-4511
Fax: 973-972-7148
E-mail: wagner@umdnj.edu

UNIVERSITY OF CALIFORNIA—BERKELEY

Post-Baccalaureate Health Professions
Certificate Program
Dr. Alexandra Tan, Program Director
1995 University Avenue, Suite 110
Berkeley, CA 94704-7000
510-643-0598
Fax: 510-643-0599
E-mail: atan@unex.berkeley.edu

UNIVERSITY OF CINCINNATI

Special Master's Program in Physiology
(12 Month Premedical Program)
Dr. Robert Banks, Program Director
231 Albert B. Sabin Way
Cincinnati, OH 45267-0576
513-558-3102
Fax: 513-558-5738
Program Contact: Jeannie Cummins
E-mail: Jeannie.cummins@uc.edu

UNIVERSITY OF COLORADO AT BOULDER

Postbaccalaureate PreMedical Certificate
Program- Career Changer
Dr. Anne Bekoff, Program Director
303-492-3963
Fax: 303-492-3962
Program Contact: Carol Drake
E-mail: pstbacmd@colorado.edu

UNIVERSITY OF LOUISVILLE

Post-Bac Pre-med Certificate Program
Mrs. Tonia Thomas
University of Louisville
College of A & S Advising Gardiner Hall,
Louisville, KY 40292
502-852-2712
Fax: 502-852-7230
E-mail: pbpmed@louisville.edu

UNIVERSITY OF MASSACHUSETTS, DARTMOUTH

Pre-Health Certificate
Eileen Carreiro-Lewandowski
285 Old Westport Rd
N Dartmouth, MA 02747-2300
508-999-8213
E-mail: ecarreiro@umassd.edu

UNIVERSITY OF MIAMI

Pre-medical Post-baccalaureate Program
Eva Alonso, Program Director
205 Ashe Building PO Box 248004
Coral Gables, FL 33124-4622
Program Contact: Alixsa Rodriguez
305-284-5176
Fax: 305-284-4686
E-mail: postbaccum@miami.edu

UNIVERSITY OF MICHIGAN MEDICAL SCHOOL

M.S. Program in Physiology
Elizabeth Rust, Program Director
1301 E. Catherine Street
7744 Med Sci II
Ann Arbor, MI 48109-5622
734-936-2921
Fax: 734-936-8813
Program Contact: Elizabeth Rust or
Michael Ferrari
E-mail: msphysiology@umich.edu

UNIVERSITY OF NORTH CAROLINA— GREENSBORO

Premedical Program
Robert E. Cannon, PhD
Post-Baccalaureate Premed Program,
UNC—Greensboro
Department of Biology, PO Box 26170
Greensboro, NC 27402-6170
336-256-0071
Fax: 336-334-5839
E-mail: Robert_Cannon@uncg.edu

UNIVERSITY OF NORTHERN COLORADO

Master's in Biomedical Science
Dr. Ginger Fisher, Program Director
501 20th Street
Greeley, CO 80639
970-351-2921
E-mail: Ginger.Fisher@unco.edu

UNIVERSITY OF OREGON

Post-baccalaureate Premedical Program
Ms. Jenni VanWyk, Program Director
Office of Academic Advising
University of Oregon
Eugene, OR 97403
541-346-3211
Fax: 541-346-6048
E-mail: jvanwyck@uoregon.edu

UNIVERSITY OF PENNSYLVANIA

Post-baccalaureate Pre-health Specialized
Studies
Ms. Valerie Dorn, Program Director
3440 Market Street, Suite 100
College of Liberal Arts and Professional
Studies
Philadelphia, PA 19104
Program Contact: Sally Cardy
215-898-1684
Fax: 215-573-2053
E-mail: cardy@sas.upenn.edu

UNIVERSITY OF PENNSYLVANIA, LPS

Pre-Health Programs
Ms. Valerie Dorn, Program Director
3440 Market Street, Suite 100
Philadelphia, PA 19104
Program Contact: Sally Cardy
215-898-7326
Fax: 215-573-2053
E-mail: cardy@sas.upenn.edu

UNIVERSITY OF ROCHESTER

Post-baccalaureate Pre-medical Program
Ms. Suzanne O'Brien, Program Director
312 Lattimore Hall
RC Box 270402
Rochester, NY 14627
585-275-4559
Fax: 585-461-5901
Program Contact: Juliet Sullivan
E-mail: postbac@mail.rochester.edu

UNIVERSITY OF SOUTH FLORIDA

One Year master of Science in Medical
Sciences
Dr. Michael Barber, Program Director
Biomedical Sciences
12901 Bruce B. Downs Blvd., MDC40
Tampa, FL 33612
813-974-2256
Program Contact: Katie Carson
E-mail: KCarson1@health.usf.edu

UNIVERSITY OF SOUTHERN CALIFORNIA

Post-baccalaureate Premedical Program
Admissions Coordinator
Department of Chemistry
University of Southern California
Los Angeles, CA 90089-00744
213-821-2354
E-mail: postbacc@usc.edu

UNIVERSITY OF SOUTH CAROLINA, SCHOOL OF MEDICINE

Graduate Certificate in Biomedical
Sciences
Dr. Chandrashekhar Patel, Program
Director
USC School of Medicine, Bldg 1 Rm B34
6439 Garners Ferry Rd
Columbia, SC 20209
803-216-3818
Email: chandrashekhar.patel@uscmed.sc.edu

UNIVERSITY OF SOUTHERN MAINE

Department of Biology
Dr. Patricia O'Mahoney-Damon, Program
Director
96 Falmouth St.
University of Southern Maine
Portland, ME 04103
207-780-4263
Fax: 207-228-8116
E-mail: pato@usm.maine.edu

UNIVERSITY OF TOLEDO— HEALTH SCIENCE CAMPUS

MSBS in Medical Sciences
Dr. Carol Bennett-Clarke, Program
Director
300 Arlington Avenue
Mail Stop #1050
Toledo,OH 43614-5805
419-383-4903
E-mail: Carol.Bennett-Clarke@utoledo.edu

UNIVERSITY OF VERMONT

Post-baccalaureate Premedical Program
Polly Allen
Continuing Education
322 South Prospect Street
Burlington, VT 05401
802-639-3210
Fax: 802-656-3891
Program Contact: Weston Sherherd
E-mail: weston.shepherd@uvm.edu

UNIVERSITY OF VIRGINIA

U.Va. Post-Baccalaureate Pre-Medical Program
Dr. Beth Bailey, Program Director
Zehmer Hall
104 Midmont Lane
Charlottesville, VA 22903
434-982-5288
E-mail: bab7g@virginia.edu

UNIVERSITY OF WISCONSIN-MILWAUKE

Certificate of Premedical Studies
Patricia Cobb, Program Director
UW-Milwauke
2442 E. Hartford Ave. Holton Hall 131
Milwaukee, WI 53211
414-229-4654
Fax: 414-229-4628
Email: pacobb@uwm.edu

VIRGINIA COMMONWEALTH UNIVERSITY

Premedical Graduate Certificate Program
Dr. Louis De Felice, Program Director
Office of Graduate Education
VCU School of Medicine
1101 East Marshall Street, PO
 Box 980565
Richmond, VA 23298-0565
804-828-0641
Program Contact: Mr. Harold Greenwald
E-mail: haroldg@vcu.edu

WASHINGTON UNIVERSITY IN ST. LOUIS

Post-baccalaureate Premedical Program
Elizabeth Fogt, Program Director
One Brookings Drive, Campus Box 1085
St. Louis, MO 63130-4899
314-935-6778
Fax: 314-935-4847
E-mail: efogt@wustl.edu

WAKE FOREST UNIVERSITY SCHOOL OF MEDICINE

Post-baccalaureate Premedical Program
Brenda Latham-Sadler, Program Director
Medical Center Boulevard
Diversity Development Initiatives
Winston-Salem, NC 27157
Program Contact: Shirley Dockery
336-716-3884
Fax: 336-716-0613
E-mail: pbprogram@wfubmc.edu

WEST CHESTER UNIVERSITY

Premedical Program
Dr. Stephen Zimniski, Program Director
117 Schmucker Science Center South
West Chester, PA 19383
610-436-2978
Fax: 610-436-3277
E-mail: pmed@wcupa.edu

WESTERN UNIVERSITY OF HEALTH SCIENCES

Master of Science in Medical Science
Ms. Jodi Olson, Program Director
309 E. Second Street
Pomona, CA 91766-1854
909-706-3842
E-mail: olsonj@westernu.edu

WILLIAM CAREY UNIVERSITY COLLEGE OF OSTEOPATHIC MEDICINE

Master of Biomedical Science
Dr. Robert Bateman, Program Director
William Carey University, Box 207
498 Tuscan Avenue
Hattiesburg, MS 39401
601-318-6316
Fax: 601-318-6410
Program Contact: Ms. Donna Day, MBS Secretary
Email: dday@wmcarey.edu

WILLIAM PATERSON UNIVERSITY OF NJ

Postbaccalaureate Premedical Program
Dr. Carey Waldburger, Program Director
300 Pompton Rd.
Wayne, NJ 07470
973-720-2486
E-mail: waldburgerc@wpunj.edu

WORCESTER STATE COLLEGE

Post-baccalaureate Premedical Program
Dr. Margaret Kerr. Program Director
486 Chandler Street
Worcester, MA 01602
E-mail: mkerr@worcester.edu

SCHOOL SAYS . . .

In this section you'll find schools with extended listings describing admissions, curriculum, internships, and much more. This is your chance to get in-depth information on programs that interest you. The Princeton Review charges each school a small fee to be listed, and the editorial responsibility is solely that of the university.

ST. GEORGE'S UNIVERSITY
School of Medicine

St. George's University is an international institution of higher education that was founded in Grenada, West Indies, in 1976 as an independent School of Medicine. In the years since, the University broadened its mission to offer undergraduate and graduate degrees in veterinary medicine, public health, science, business, and liberal studies, and now draws students and faculty from over 140 countries to its 53 academic programs. These programs are marked by a strong network of affiliations with educational institutions worldwide, including in the United States, the United Kingdom, Canada, Australia, and Ireland. St. George's has been honored with numerous accreditations and approvals from international institutions and governing bodies.

Over 12,000 St. George's MD graduates have practiced in all 50 US states and over 50 countries in every medical specialty and subspecialty around the globe. "One Health, One Medicine," the concept of collaboration between scientists, physicians, and veterinarians, is integral to St. George's and a key driver of the University's mission.

MEDICAL SCHOOL CURRICULUM

St. George's University provides a wide range of entry options and an extensive foundation for students with varied academic qualifications in the 4-, 5-, 6-, or 7-year MD program that lead to the Doctor of Medicine degree. Students may enter St. George's 7-year Bachelor of Science/Doctor of Medicine program after high school through programs such as those offered through affiliations with the New Jersey Institute of Technology and Caldwell College. However, most students from North America who hold a bachelor's degree with the appropriate premedical courses enter directly into the 4-year medical program.

Most medical students will begin their study on Grenada's True Blue campus. However, the Keith B. Taylor Global Scholars Program provides students with an opportunity to spend the first year of the 4-year medical program in Newcastle, United Kingdom, on the Northumbria University campus. Immersed in the UK culture, students follow a program identical to the first-year program offered in Grenada, further encouraging their international experience.

The clinical sciences take place in the final two years. Students are placed at one of over 70 clinical centers and affiliated hospitals in the United States, the United Kingdom, Canada, and Grenada, all of which are done on services with approved postgraduate training programs.

DUAL-DEGREE OPTIONS

Students may choose to advance their knowledge in specific areas of medical study with dual degree programs offered within the School of Medicine.

The 15-year-old St. George's Master of Public Health program is accredited by the US Council on Education for Public Health, one of only a few outside the US to receive this distinction, and is delivered in the School of Medicine. Students may pursue independent MPH degrees or the dual MD/MPH degree.

The Masters in Business Administration degrees in Multi-Sector Health Management and in International Business offered at St. George's combine online learning with ongoing collegial collaboration developed from the initial one-week, professor-directed residence on campus that kicks off each program. A second, one-week residency takes place towards the end of the program. Students may pursue independent MBA degrees or a dual degree MD/MBA in Multi-Sector Health Management.

GRENADA CAMPUS

The stunning True Blue campus is the heart of the University. This $250+ million state-of-the-art University community is located on the southwestern corner of Grenada, on a peninsula overlooking the Caribbean Sea. The wireless-enhanced campus has more than 65 buildings, including a library, anatomy labs, dormitories, lecture halls, and a research institute. The campus houses over 1,800 students. Free bus transportation is available from 7 am to 2 am to accommodate those students living off campus in various areas of the island.

Students enjoy a rich campus life, with over 50 diverse student organizations and a wide variety of organized athletic programs. In addition, all students have access to the 17,000-square-foot Student Center, which houses a cafeteria, food court, offices for student organizations, a fitness center, lockers, showers, and many more amenities.

A DEDICATION TO STUDENT SUCCESS

Student support services are deeply ingrained into the culture of the St. George's University community. In fact, St. George's has more faculty members and staff devoted to student support services than some regional schools have on their entire faculty.

The University's dedicated Department of Educational Services teaches students how to learn and teachers how to teach more effectively. The Department of Educational Services faculty is the largest on campus, and is an important component of our students' and graduates' successes. Almost all of the University's students and many of the professors in all schools avail themselves of the support offered through a variety of innovative programs, including time management, note-taking skills, and utilizing technology effectively in teaching and learning.

SCHOLARSHIPS AND LOANS

St. George's University's MD and DVM programs qualify for US Department of Education federally sponsored loans. Additionally, the University funds a wide range of academic and need-based scholarships. High academic achievers may be eligible for scholarships such as the Chancellor's Circle of the Legacy of Excellence Scholarship which is automatically awarded to qualified students and provides a one-third tuition discount.

SUCCESSFUL STUDENT AND GRADUATE PERFORMANCE

St. George's students excel in all qualifying examinations. In 2013, the first-time pass rate for St. George's students on United States Medical Licensing Examination (USMLE) Step 1 Exam was 98%, exceeding the overall pass rate of 97 % for all US and Canadian medical schools.1

St. George's graduates have obtained prestigious and diverse US residencies every year and many are matched in the positions of their choice, including sought-after residencies such as surgery, radiology, orthopedics, neurology, and emergency medicine. Within one year of graduation, 96% of 2013's eligible US graduates obtained US residencies.2 In the past three years combined, SGU graduates have obtained more first-year US residency positions than any other medical school, with over 770 residency placements in the US and Canada in 2014.2

FACULTY

St. George's University has more than 2,300 faculty members, with over 400 campus-based in the Basic Sciences part of the curriculum. Each year, more than 400 visiting scholars lecture in the School of Medicine; they come from institutions such as Cambridge University, Georgetown University, and Emory University.

CONTACT

To learn more about St. George's University, visit www.sgu.edu or call 1 (800) 899-6337, extension 1280. Information on the University is also available through YouTube, Facebook and Twitter at StGeorgesU.

ALPHABETICAL INDEX

INDEX BY LOCATION

INTERNATIONAL

INDEX BY COST

MORE THAN $50,000

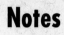

Notes

Notes

Notes